A Practical Guide to Breast Cancer Treatment

Eun Sook Lee
Editor

A Practical Guide to Breast Cancer Treatment

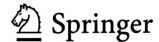

Editor
Eun Sook Lee
Center for Breast Cancer
National Cancer Center
Goyang, Kyonggi-do, Korea (Republic of)

ISBN 978-981-19-9043-4   ISBN 978-981-19-9044-1   (eBook)
https://doi.org/10.1007/978-981-19-9044-1

© The Editor(s) (if applicable) and The Author(s), under exclusive license to Springer Nature Singapore Pte Ltd. 2023
This work is subject to copyright. All rights are solely and exclusively licensed by the Publisher, whether the whole or part of the material is concerned, specifically the rights of reprinting, reuse of illustrations, recitation, broadcasting, reproduction on microfilms or in any other physical way, and transmission or information storage and retrieval, electronic adaptation, computer software, or by similar or dissimilar methodology now known or hereafter developed.
The use of general descriptive names, registered names, trademarks, service marks, etc. in this publication does not imply, even in the absence of a specific statement, that such names are exempt from the relevant protective laws and regulations and therefore free for general use.
The publisher, the authors, and the editors are safe to assume that the advice and information in this book are believed to be true and accurate at the date of publication. Neither the publisher nor the authors or the editors give a warranty, expressed or implied, with respect to the material contained herein or for any errors or omissions that may have been made. The publisher remains neutral with regard to jurisdictional claims in published maps and institutional affiliations.

This Springer imprint is published by the registered company Springer Nature Singapore Pte Ltd. The registered company address is: 152 Beach Road, #21-01/04 Gateway East, Singapore 189721, Singapore

Contents

Detection and Diagnosis of Breast Cancer 1
Ji Young You, Soojin Park, Eun-Gyeong Lee, and Eun Sook Lee

Benign and Proliferative Case Series 19
Chan Wha Lee, Youngmi Kwon, Yunju Kim, and Bo Hwa Choi

Carcinoma In Situ 51
Eun Sook Lee, Chan Wha Lee, Youngmi Kwon, Yunju Kim,
and Bo Hwa Choi

Brief Overview of Breast Cancer Treatment 147
Ji Young You, Soojin Park, and Eun Sook Lee

HR(+) HER2(−) Breast Cancer 173
Yunju Kim, Bo Hwa Choi, Eun-Gyeong Lee, Ji Young You,
and Youngmi Kwon

HR(+) HER2(+) Breast Cancer 299
Soojin Park, Ran Song, Yunju Kim, Bo Hwa Choi, Eun Sook Lee,
Chan Wha Lee, and Eun-Gyeong Lee

HR(−) HER2(+) Breast Cancer 427
Youngmi Kwon, Yunju Kim, Bo Hwa Choi, Ji Young You,
Ran Song, Jeayeon Woo, and Soojin Park

HR(−) HER2(−) Breast Cancer 575
Eun Sook Lee, Chan Wha Lee, Youngmi Kwon, Jeayeon Woo,
and Yunju Kim

Local Recurrence 717
Yunju Kim, Eun-Gyeong Lee, Ran Song, and Eun Sook Lee

Metastatic Breast Cancer 861
Youngmi Kwon, Yunju Kim, Bo Hwa Choi, Eun-Gyeong Lee,
Ji Young You, and Eun Sook Lee

Treatment Roadmap and Summaries 941
Eun Sook Lee

Contributors

Bo Hwa Choi Department of Radiology, National Cancer Center, Goyang, Gyeonggi, Republic of Korea

Yunju Kim Department of Pathology, National Cancer Center, Goyang, Gyeonggi, Republic of Korea

Youngmi Kwon Department of Radiology, Center for Breast Cancer, National Cancer Center, Goyang, Gyeonggi, Republic of Korea

Chan Wha Lee Department of Radiology, National Cancer Center, Goyang, Republic of Korea

Eun Sook Lee Center for Breast Cancer, National Cancer Center, Goyang, Kyonggi-do, Republic of Korea

Eun-Gyeong Lee Division of Surgery, Center for Breast Cancer, National Cancer Center, Goyang, Republic of Korea

Soojin Park Department of Surgery, Wonkwang University Sanbon Hospital, Gunpo, Gyeonggi-do, Republic of Korea

Ran Song Division of Surgery, Center for Breast Cancer, National Cancer Center, Goyang, Republic of Korea

Jeayeon Woo Division of Surgery, Center for Breast Cancer, National Cancer Center, Goyang, Republic of Korea

Ji Young You Division of Breast and Endocrine, Department of General Surgery, Korea University Medical Center, Seoul, Republic of Korea

Detection and Diagnosis of Breast Cancer

Ji Young You, Soojin Park, Eun-Gyeong Lee, and Eun Sook Lee

1 Epidemiology of Breast Cancer

Breast cancer is the most common female cancer worldwide. It accounts for a major proportion of cancer deaths in women in their 20s and 50s. Over two million new breast cancer cases occur worldwide each year, and more than 680,000 patients die of breast cancer (2018 base). Recently, the global trend in breast cancer incidence continues to increase by about 0.5% each year. The circumstances are a little different depending on the country. This increasing trend in the incidence of breast cancer is considered to be due to the following reasons. First, changes in reproductive factors associated with breast cancer risk factors such as decreased menarche age, increased age at first birth, low birth, and decreased breastfeeding. Second is the increase in early detection through regular mammography.

The incidence of breast cancer in South Korea has also steadily increased, rising from 24.5 per 100,000 women in 1999 to 39.9 in 2007. In 2018, approximately 60 people from Asian countries belong to the highest breast cancer incidence group (Fig. 1) [1].

Approximately 22,000 new cases occur annually, according to the Central Cancer Registration Report of the Ministry of Health and Welfare of South Korea. In 2019, breast cancer ranked fifth among all cancers in South Korea at 9.6% and first among all cancers in women at 20.6%. The proportion of patients with breast cancer risk factors is also increasing, in particular, the proportion of patients with early or late births, non-breastfeeding patients, obese patients, and patients with a family history of breast cancer. Along with these factors, the rate of early detection of breast cancer through regular examinations such as mammography is increasing, and the number of patients is expected to continue to increase. A characteristic phenomenon of breast cancer patients in South Korea is that the proportion of premenopausal young women is higher than in Western Europe (Fig. 2).

J. Y. You (✉)
Division of Breast and Endocrine, Department of General Surgery, Korea University Medical Center, Seoul, Republic of Korea
e-mail: joliejean@korea.ac.kr

S. Park
Department of Surgery, Wonkwang University Sanbon Hospital, Gunpo, Gyeonggi-do, Republic of Korea

E.-G. Lee
Division of Surgery, Center for Breast Cancer, National Cancer Center, Goyang, Republic of Korea
e-mail: bnf333@ncc.re.kr

E. S. Lee
Center for Breast Cancer, National Cancer Center, Goyang, Kyonggi-do, Republic of Korea
e-mail: eslee@ncc.re.kr

© The Author(s), under exclusive license to Springer Nature Singapore Pte Ltd. 2023
E. S. Lee (ed.), *A Practical Guide to Breast Cancer Treatment*,
https://doi.org/10.1007/978-981-19-9044-1_1

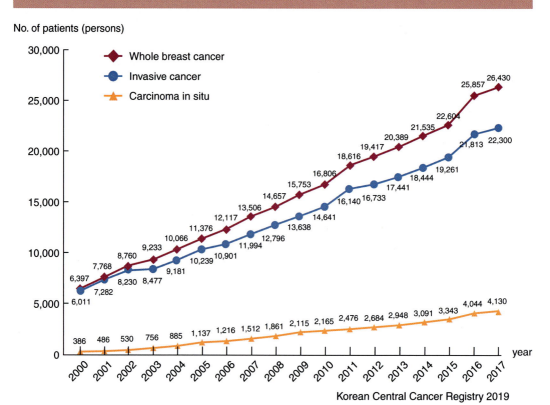

Fig. 1 Annual incidence of breast cancer in South Korean women

In Western countries such as the United States, more than 70% of all breast cancer patients are menopausal women, whereas, in South Korea, the median age at diagnosis in 2017 was 51.9 years, with a minimum age of 15 years and a maximum age of 99 years. Of these, 8867 were in their 40s, the age group with the highest incidence of breast cancer, followed by 7944 in their 50s, 4491 in their 60s, and 2413 in their 30s.

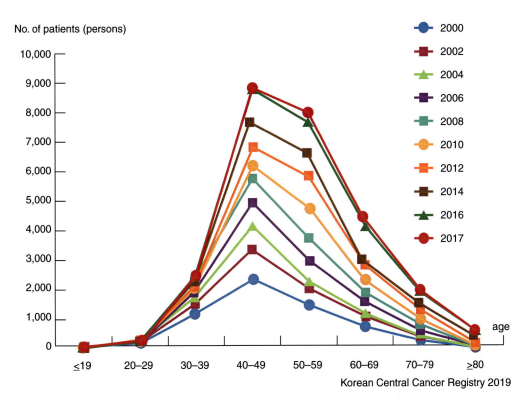

Fig. 2 Annual age-specific breast cancer occurrence in South Korea

2 Anatomy of the Breast

The breast is located between the second or third rib and the sixth or seventh rib on the vertical axis and between the sternal edge and the midaxillary line on the horizontal axis. The structure of the breast is composed of parenchymal tissue and the substrate tissue that supports it [2, 3]. Parenchymal tissue includes lobules and intralobular body tissue, substrate tissues include adipose tissue and the body tissue between them. The parenchymal tissue extends between the substrate tissues. The breast consists of an average of 15–20 leaves, and the average size of the breast is about 10–12 cm in diameter and about 5–7 cm in thickness (Fig 3).

The nipple–areolar complex looks like a plate with increased pigmentation when viewed from the outside. There are 15–20 openings at the tip of the nipple, where collecting ducts gather and breast milk is secreted. During pregnancy, the areola grows and pigmentation increases further. The areola contains abundant sebaceous glands and Montgomery nodules.

The system of branching tubes is arranged in segments and is radial. Therefore, the other areas of the breast are just below the nipple and consist of structures that extend outward from the nipple, breast milk is secreted through a collecting duct that is open to the nipple. The collecting duct just below the nipple is relatively wide, this part is called the lactiferous sinus [4].

The tip of the flow tube is the area of the blocked glandular part. The glandular part is the unit that produces breast milk. The last part of the transport system in the breast is called the disap-

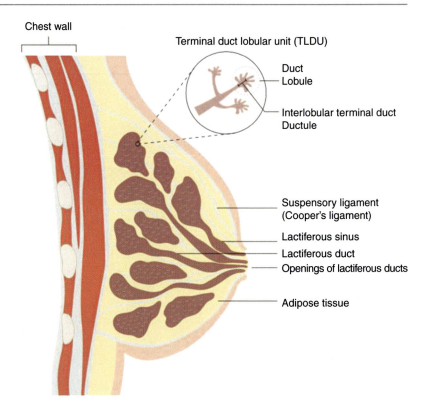

Fig. 3 Anatomy of the breast

pearing or terminal breast duct, this terminal breast duct is also designed to secrete and has both transport and secretory functions.

The main sources of blood in the breast are the perforating branches of the internal mammary artery, the pectoral branch of the thoracoacromial artery or the lateral thoracic artery.

(external mammary artery), a branch of the intercostal artery. A significant amount of lateral circulation of the arteries exists in the breast, even after mastectomy, a part of the artery supplies blood, and it is responsible for supplying blood and nutrition to the remaining breast.

The second anterolateral intercostal nerve among the sensory nerves involved in the breast is known as the intercostobrachial nerve, responsible for the inner sensation of the upper arm through the axillary part. Care should be taken during surgery as this may cause numbness or dysesthesia if it is cut during axillary lymph node dissection.

The lymphatic embryonic pathway of the breast is very important and has four parts: cutaneous, axillary, internal thoracic, and posterior intercostal [5, 6]. The axillary reaches about 75% (as seen by self-radiography) to 97% (as seen by the radioactive colloidal gold uptake study during radical mastectomy) where most of the lymph vessels in the breast collect [7]. The axillary lymph nodes can be divided into three stages relative to pathological anatomy and tumor metastasis [8]. The first group (level I) is the lymph node outside the outer edge of the pectoralis minor muscle, the second group (level II) is below the pectoralis minor muscle, and the third group (level III) is the lymph node inside the pectoralis minor muscle internal organs. The lymph nodes between the pectoralis major and pectoralis minor are sometimes called Rotter's lymph nodes and are classified separately. Most breast cancer lymph node metastases are found in the axillary. The clavicle lymph node is the innermost and is located on the non-lateral, ventral side of the axillary veins. In the past, it was not considered to be in the area of local lymph nodes, but recently it has been included in local metastases [9].

The main muscles around the breast are the pectoralis major, pectoralis minor, serratus anterior, latissimus dorsi, and the rectus abdominis and aponeurosis of the external oblique.

3 Patient History Taking

When treating a patient with suspected breast disease, checking the medical history and symptoms is the most basic matter. The medical history can provide clues to possible underlying causes of abnormal symptoms, abnormal physical examination, and laboratory findings. If breast cancer is confirmed, it is also essential to determine future treatment options. Common items of medical history include the age of the patient, fertility, first menstrual age, regular menstrual cycle, menopausal age, past surgical ability, and confirmation of a family history of breast and ovarian cancer. Especially when a past breast tissue examination has been performed, the pathological examination result must be confirmed, and whether an ovarian or hysterectomy has occurred must also be confirmed. When a hysterectomy has been performed, it is difficult to confirm the presence or absence of menopause, so it is useful to determine whether or not there are menopausal-related symptoms. For women in their childbearing years, matters related to pregnancy, childbirth, and breastfeeding should be checked. Regarding drugs, it is important to confirm the presence or absence of postmenopausal hormone replacement therapy and the history of contraceptives. Relative to the breast, whether there is breast pain (mastalgia), nipple discharge, nipple changes, changes in the skin or symmetry of the left and right breasts, or in the breast axillary part. Check if any new lumps can be detected by touch. Breast pain is the most common symptom of female patients referred to a breast clinic, most appear as part of the normal menstrual phenomenon. Initially, it is necessary to confirm whether the pain is periodic or aperiodic, or whether the cause may be outside the breast. When breast cancer is found, the most common early symptom is a painless mass. Whether there are changes after it was discovered and whether it is related to the menstrual cycle

must be checked. Nipple discharge should be distinguished from hyperlactation. Pathological nipple discharge should be suspected when the discharge is naturally secreted without compression, shows continuous bloody secretions in a single duct, the patient is over 40 years old, or the symptoms are accompanied by a detectable mass. If breast cancer is suspected, systemic symptoms such as weight loss, fatigue, cough, dyspnea, or bone pain should be confirmed.

4 Symptom and Physical Examination

Breast pain and discomfort are common symptoms that can occur at any age, from young women to postmenopausal women, and usually improves spontaneously. Patients who complain of breast pain should undergo a physical examination, mastectomy, and breast ultrasonography to confirm that there is no suspicion of breast cancer. It is important to reassure the patient that most breast pain is not a peculiar symptom suggestive of latent breast cancer. The causes of nipple discharge are diverse and include physiological factors, intraductal papilloma, breast cancer, pregnancy, drugs, hyperprolactinemia, hypothyroidism, fibrocystic disease, and ductal dilatation. In the case of breast mass, a physical examination, as well as mastectomy and breast ultrasound, is performed. The results of the imaging test are reported by the Breast Imaging Reporting and Data System (BI-RADS), which is the breast imaging reporting system of the American College of Radiology. If the final category is C4a or higher, a histological examination should be performed.

Breast examinations should be performed in a comfortable and quiet environment with plenty of time allowed, and with consideration so that the patient does not feel shame [10]. Beginning with an inspection of the breast, with the patient sitting upright, assess bilateral breast symmetry, skin changes such as edema and skin retraction, erythema, dents, excoriation, etc., and observe changes in the papilla. It is a misconception that skin dimpling usually appears when breast cancer progresses, often this is due to small scirrhous tumors. In the presence of skin edema, redness, tenderness, and fever, the possibility of inflammatory breast cancer should always be differentiated along with acute mastitis and abscesses. Skin changes in the papilla and areola can manifest as simple dermatitis such as eczema and Paget's disease, a type of carcinoma in situ. Eczema generally begins in the areola, while Paget's disease begins in the nipple and shows a difference that secondarily invades the areola.

Breast palpation should be performed gently with clean hands and both hands together, it should include both the bilateral breast and axillary and the upper and lower clavicle where the lymph nodes that drain from the breast are located. If there is a breast mass, the size, shape, hardness, position, presence or absence of movement, etc. should be described. When displaying a mass, the patient is usually viewed from the front and in a clockwise position, the distance from the nipple and the depth at the surface are noted. It is important to check for lymphadenopathy, especially if breast cancer is suspected. Generally, the presence or absence of mass in the axillary lymph node is confirmed while the patient is sitting and the shoulder joint is relaxed. Check for lymphadenopathy in the axillary, upper and lower clavicle, around the sternum, and neck, if there is a vertical stand, the size, hardness, shape, presence or absence of movement, etc. must be confirmed in the same way as a breast mass.

5 Breast Imaging Study

5.1 Mammography

Mammography is a simple but basic X-ray test to detect and diagnose all breast disorders. The purpose is to obtain detailed images of intramammary structures to diagnose breast cancer at an early stage. The mammography should include as much breast tissue as possible, which requires the proper compression and correct posture of the breast. Internal and external slave photography (mediolateral oblique view, MLO) and vertical photography (craniocaudal view, CC) are the basics of mammography. Auxiliary imaging is added to confirm the presence or absence of a lesion after basic imaging, to evaluate the lesion, and to grasp the position. There are spot compression view, magnification view, 90° lateral view, exaggerated CC view, valley view, cleavage view, tangential view, implant displacement view, axillary view, etc. In addition, mammography is performed after injecting a contrast medium containing iodine, which is used for tomosynthesis and computed tomography (CT). This obtains a single three-dimensional breast image by obtaining multiple sections from various angles. New tests, such as contrast-enhanced digital mammography, are being used to make a more accurate diagnosis of breast cancer. Normal breast tissue appears white in mammography, normal adipose tissue generally surrounds the mammary gland tissue and is also mixed between the mammary gland tissues and appears black on mammography. The Cooper's ligament appears as a white linear structure, clearly visible from the fat breast of older women. Normal breasts exhibit various aspects depending on the distribution and composition of fat, fibrous, and mammary gland tissue. Normal breasts vary by age and individual, but maintain symmetry, so fine lesions can be found by observing bilateral breast photographs together. American College of Radiology (ACR) Breast Imaging Reporting and Data System (BI-RADS) is used for lesion analysis, reporting, and evaluation, and the report will record major findings such as breast parenchymal aspect, seed mass and calcification, and final evaluation results. BI-RADS evaluations are divided into categories 0–6, where category 0 is incomplete and requires additional testing, category 1 is negative, category 2 is clearly benign, category 3 is probably benign, category 4 is suspicious abnormality, and category 5 is highly suggestive of malignancy, category 6 is when breast cancer is diagnosed (known malignancy). Of these, categories 4 and 5 are subject to histological examination, and with category 3 a 6-month follow-up is recommended to reassess the group with a malignancy probability of 1–2% or less. Category 4 is a group with a malignant probability of 2–94%, which is subdivided into a, b, and c.

Group 4a has a malignant probability of 2–10%, 4b has an 11–50% probability, and 4c has a malignant probability of 50–94%. In the case of group 4a, when the tissue test result is positive, it is considered that the image and the tissue test result match, and a 6-month follow-up test is recommended. In the case of 4b or 4c, when the histological examination result is benign, it is considered that the image and the histological examination result do not match, and rehabilitation examination or surgery is recommended.

Breast cancer mammography findings vary, but microcalcifications and mass are the main findings [11, 12]. Other findings include new or changing calcifications or shadows, structural distortions, asymmetric shadows, etc [13–15]. Advanced breast cancer may have findings such as skin thickening and contraction, nipple depression, and axillary lymphadenopathy. Breast cancer is multiple and has many multiple viscosities, and there are bilateral breast cancers in about 1–5%. Therefore, a thorough examination is required before surgery, and enlarged radiography must be performed on all lesions for analysis of microcalcified lesions, range grasping, and postoperative follow-up. If microcalcification is observed, it is likely to be malignant. Malignant calcification is usually small in size and multimorphic, with irregular shapes, sizes, and concentrations. Malignancy must be suspected if there are at least 5 calcifications within 1 cm^3 that are dense and have a strange and irregular shape in various vortices of various sizes or shapes or have a bizarre branching irregular or linear form and are smaller than 0.5 mm. Ductal Carcinoma in situ may also be observed around invasive breast cancer.

A mass is a space-occupying lesion that is visible on breast imaging in at least two directions and has a convex outer surface. When analyzing mass, size, shape, edge, position, density, etc., the shape and edge observations are the most important in the differential diagnosis. A mass showing needle-like protrusions or a mass with an unclear boundary is likely to be a malignant mass. The breast imaging density of mass is also an important finding in differentiating malignancy. Most malignant masses are denser than normal tissue or benign masses of the same volume. In rare cases, there may be a benign pattern of calcification in the malignant mass, so if malignancy is suspected in the form of the mass, tissue examination must be performed even if the calcification is benign.

5.2 Breast Ultrasound

The great advantage of breast ultrasonography is that there is no risk of radiation and no discomfort during the examination. One of the important roles of ultrasound is to distinguish between well-bound solid mass and cysts without the calcification seen in mammography. Breast ultrasound can be used as a primary examination in young women under the age of 30 and pregnant or lactating women requiring a breast examination [16, 17]. Breast ultrasound is in direct contact with the patient and can be examined in real-time, and unlike mammography, which is a planar image, ultrasound can distinguish between normal and abnormal structures with different echoes without overlap as in tomographic images. Physiological information can also be provided through elastic ultrasound (elastography), Doppler test, and the like. It is also useful for assessing lesions located in the margins, axillae, and deep areas that are difficult to include in mammography and for guiding histological examination [18, 19]. Currently, confirmation and evaluation of tactile abnormalities, evaluation of clinical symptoms other than mass (nipple discharge, pain, discomfort, dents in the skin and nipple, etc.), evaluation of abnormal findings of mammography, the guidance of intervention surgery, surgery pre-scope and postoperative follow-up, breast insert assessment, and high-risk group screening are standard indications, and breast ultrasound is widely used [20]. Malignancy can be suspected if findings on breast ultrasound indicate spiculated, angular, microlobulated margin, echogenic halo, not parallel, posterior acoustic shadowing, etc. There is no provision that any of the findings fit into some categories of the final verdicts when describing lesions using the terms presented in ultrasound BI-RADS. Therefore, the experience of the physician performing ultrasound is very important in the final decision. The ultrasound report has a simple clinical history and the reason why the examination was decided, the presence or absence of the previous ultrasonic examination and comparison, the examination range and the technique used, the size and position of the lesion in the analysis for the lesion (includes directions expressed in terms of distance and direction from the nipple), physical findings, mammography, comparison with other imaging findings such as magnetic resonance imaging, and recommendations for final determination and subsequent treatment. The final judgment is divided into categories 1–6 according to its clinical significance. Category 1 is negative, category 2 is benign, category 3 is probably benign, category 4 is suspicious abnormality, category 5 is highly suggestive of malignancy, category 6 is breast cancer that has already been confirmed by histological examination. Category 4 is subdivided into a, b, and c according to the possibility of malignancy, The experience of the reading physician is important and is still a process that needs research, as no provisions have been established for each finding. Category 5 is a lesion in which breast cancer is almost definite, and category 6 is a state in which malignancy has already been confirmed and no histological examination is required. The reason we created category 6 is to exclude it from subsequent follow-up and medical monitoring.

What is important is that the judgment by only one breast ultrasonography is incomplete and should always be interpreted relative to the mammography that is the basis of the breast imaging [21, 22]. It can be used conveniently to determine whether breast cancer is malignant such as in elastic ultrasound (elastography), which is a technique that visualizes the hard characteristics of the tissue that is firmer than a benign mass, and the Doppler test, which grasps the state of blood vessel distribution.

5.3 Breast Magnetic Resonance Imaging, MRI

Magnetic resonance images have no risk of radiation exposure, have excellent image contrast, are easy to evaluate objectively, and are used as an auxiliary examination method for mammography [13]. In particular, dynamic contrast examinations using contrast media have been introduced. Breast magnetic resonance imaging has reduced the number of unnecessary histological examinations. Non-invasive methods that help detect and determine multiple breast cancers are of great interest. In addition, lesions are found on magnetic resonance imaging but are not seen on mammography or ultrasonography, magnetic resonance imaging-guided histology (MR-guided biopsy), and immersion value determination (MR-guided wire localization). Therefore, it is expected that the role of magnetic resonance images will be further expanded because of their ability to perform [23].

The most suitable time for breast magnetic resonance imaging is on the 7th–14th day of the menstrual cycle. A breast surface coil is a device designed to transmit and accept radio frequency signals from breast tissue to provide a sufficient signal-to-noise ratio. A special breast coil designed for tissue biopsy with the breast compressed and fixed has also been developed. The patient should be in a lying position, with the extended breast firmly positioned in the center of the breast coil, and then with both arms raised sufficiently to include the axillary in the maximum breast coil. Therefore, the breast shape taken by MRI is different from the breast shape of the photographs of the breast taken by pressing in the erect position, and it is different from breast ultrasound in a supine position and during surgery.

Breast MRI scans aim to obtain high-resolution images of the thinnest possible sections before and after the injection of a contrast agent. The most important image is the dynamic enhanced image, it is basically based on obtaining T2-weighted images before the injection of contrast medium and T1-weighted images and comparing them with the images after contrast enhancement. T2-weighted images are important for finding cystic lesions and may help predict the histological features of the axillary. When combined with the fat suppression technique, it is possible to suppress the high signal intensity of fat and enhance the lesion. The images of both breasts can be viewed simultaneously in an axial plane or a sagittal plane with excellent resolution. When the size of the malignant mass grows to 2 mm or more, nutrition is supplied through microneovascularization. Unlike in normal tissue, these vessels have thin vessel walls, form irregular spaces and arteriovenous shunts at the ends, lack vasomotor, increased fragility, and increased permeability to the surroundings. Because of these characteristics such as leakage to stromal cells (leaking), a dynamic contrast enhancement image using a contrast medium is obtained by using the characteristics of such a malignant mass.

Breast MRI analysis divides the lesions that are contrast-enhanced primarily according to the ACR BI-RADS Lexicon First Edition into foci, mass, and non-mass enhancement relative to morphological features. The foci show a very small contrast enhancement site where no lesions appear in the pre-enhancement image and clearly do not occupy space. The mass analyzes the shape, edge, and internal contrast surface. Non-mass enhancement uses common terms that are categorized as linear, ductal, segmental, regional, and diffuse. In addition, nipple retraction, nipple inversion, T1-weighted image before injection of contrast agent, high signal intensity in the flow tube, skin dimpling, skin thickening, skin infiltration, edema, lymphadenopathy, pectoralis major muscle invasion, hematoma, abnormal signal disappearance, cysts, etc. are classified by findings. A method for visually evaluating the aspect of the dynamic contrast enhancement graph was studied. Classified by the shape of the graph, type I is rapidly increasing in signal strength consistently, type II is rapidly increasing in the early stage and maintained at the apex, and type III is rapidly increasing in the early stage. This is the case when contrast enhancement is shown but the signal strength is rather decreased. Kuhl et al. [24, 25] found that 83% of positives showed type I, 11.5% showed type II, 5.5% showed type III, in benign disease. But it was reported in malignancy, 57.4% showed type III, 33.6% showed type II, and 8.9% showed type I. In conclusion, he argued that the type III contrast enhancement

aspect was a strong suggestion of malignancy. However, because there are common findings in both benign and malignant lesions in morphological features and dynamic contrast enhancement graphs, it is possible to improve the sensitivity and specificity by analyzing both, rather than performing only the morphological analysis or analyzing only the dynamic contrast enhancement graph.

Breast magnetic resonance images provide a more accurate picture of the extent of breast cancer infiltration before surgery (especially the relationship between the chest wall and the nipple) and confirm the presence or absence of multiple breast cancers on the same or opposite side of the breast, which helps to determine the exact stage and plan the surgery. It is also useful for assessing the effects of anticancer chemotherapy in breast cancer and for distinguishing recurrent breast cancer from normal changes such as breast preservation, fibrotic scars after irradiation, and granulation tissue. Breast cancer that is not found by mastectomy or breast ultrasound can be identified with positive hormone receptors, especially in metastatic cancer and for multiple lesions where it is difficult to characterize the lesion with both tests alone; additional information can be obtained when deciding whether to perform a follow-up or tissue biopsy. Breast MRI also helps diagnose intra- and extra-capsular rupture of breast-molded inserts, and it is not only the best but the only inspection method when a foreign substance such as paraffin or silicone is injected into the breast parenchyma. It can be used for breast cancer screening in young women with dense breasts in the high-risk group. Breast cancer is reported to be detected by MRI screening with a probability of 3–7.6% and a false positive rate of 6–9% [26].

Breast MRI is a very sensitive and useful test for the detection of breast cancer, but it has low specificity, is difficult to diagnose by breast MRI alone, and cannot be used in place of mastectomy. Nonetheless, it is an effective, valuable, sensitive, and useful screening test as a method that is complementary to other diagnostic methods for patients in the high-risk group.

5.4 Other Diagnostic Imaging Methods

If nipple discharge is found, galactography can be used, and CT can be used for patients who have a pacemaker or metallic implant inserted, or who have claustrophobia and are unsuitable for MRI examination. Various nuclear medicine tests using various radiopharmaceuticals are also used to diagnose and stage breast cancer, for instance, breast scintimammography, lymphoscintigraphy to detect monitored lymph nodes, positron emission tomography (PET), and PET-CT with 18F-fluorodeoxyglucose (FDG).

6 Pathologic Reports

6.1 Malignant Tumor

Lesions that occur in the breast vary, but some types are predominantly observable in breast tissue. Lesions can be classified into different types based on the anatomy and histological structure of the breast. To facilitate the pathological approach to breast lesions, various breast disorders can be organized by type and divided into benign and malignant. Cancer development is a multi-step process that occurs over time. It consists of a series of genetic changes, each of which potentially gives cells high growth potential and induces them to convert from normal cells to cancer cells. Invasive breast cancer is distinguished by clinical, imaging, pathological, and biological characteristics, and its classification generally follows the World Health Organization health classification. This classification system is determined by the growth morphology and cytological shape of invasive tumor cells and is not based on the origin of their development but is broadly classified into tube carcinoma and lobular carcinoma. When the epithelial cells of the breast are "malignant" but still limited to the normal ducts or lobules, it is called carcinoma in situ.

6.1.1 Ductal Carcinoma In Situ (DCIS)

In DCIS, cancer cell proliferation is localized in the breast duct and does not invade the epithelium. It is not well distinguished from normal breast tissue by the naked eye, but when it grows in size, it forms a mass on the cross-section, and when there is a calcified substance, it is distinguished by a crunching feeling [27]. It is classified into comedo, cribriform, papillary, micropapillary, and solid according to the growth form. This classification is independent of prognosis. Local recurrence after surgery is predicted, grading is presented, and it is generally classified into nuclear grade, low grade, intermediate grade, and high grade. Findings that must be included in the pathology report are nuclear grade, presence or absence of necrosis, and growth morphology. Microinvasive carcinoma refers to the case where some DCIS shows epithelial infiltration and the infiltrated site is 1 mm or less, and even if microinfiltration is observed in some places, it is not added up. The prognosis is similar to that of DCIS [28].

6.1.2 Lobular Carcinoma In Situ (LCIS)

LCIS occurs in the terminal duct lobular unit, and biochemical findings are similar to those of low-grade DCIS. It shows typical lobular lesion findings [29].

6.1.3 Invasive Ductal Carcinoma

Invasive ductal carcinoma accounts for 70% of breast cancers and is mostly the pure type. In the case of the complex type, the prognosis is classified as invasive coronary carcinoma along with invasive ductal carcinoma. The longest diameter is chosen as the size because it is macroscopically hard, shows nodules with unclear boundaries, and has an irregular morphology. The prognosis is better than that of a well-defined carcinoma. The microscopic findings of invasive duct carcinoma are very diverse. Therefore, establish an objective classification system that influences clinical prognosis and classify using nuclear and histological grades. Histological grades are divided into 1–3 grades according to the total scored, and based on the tubular formation, nuclear atypia, and mitosis. The higher the histological grade of invasive cancer, the higher the rate of axillary lymph node metastasis, the more frequent recurrence, and the higher the mortality rate from metastasis. This is an important factor for determining prognosis in stage I carcinoma. In stage II carcinoma, the effect of histologi-

Detection and Diagnosis of Breast Cancer

cal grade on prognosis is uncertain, but it has been reported to be a major determinant of response to adjuvant anticancer therapy. Vascular and lymphatic infiltration are among the poor prognostic factors. According to the 2009 St. Gallen guideline, factors that influence treatment decisions for breast cancer patients include hormone receptor status, histological grade, degree of proliferative capacity, lymph node metastasis, vascular lymphatic vessel infiltration, and the size of the tumor.

6.1.4 Other Invasive Cancer Type Characteristics

Invasive lobular carcinoma accounts for 10–15% of all breast cancers, with more than 95% showing hormone receptor positivity. It has a better prognosis than invasive ductal carcinoma. However, pleomorphic lobular carcinoma is often HER2-positive and, similar to invasive ductal carcinoma, has a poor prognosis. Histologically, tubular carcinoma is a carcinoma with a coronary structure of 90% or more, rare in 2% or less overall, and is usually characterized by being positive for hormone receptors and having a good prognosis. Invasive cribriform carcinoma has a good prognosis with histological findings similar to the cribriform type of DCIS. Medullary carcinoma accounts for 5% of breast cancer tumors and 60% of patients develop it at a relatively young age, under 50. The frequency of triple-negative is high, whereas the prognosis is better when compared to the same subtype of relatively invasive ductal carcinoma. Mucinous carcinoma (and carcinoma with signet ring cell differentiation) is a carcinoma that produces large amounts of mucus in most cells. In those with a late onset age, 90% or more are hormone receptor-positive, HER2 negative, and have a good prognosis [23]. Invasive papillary carcinoma is characterized by papillary proliferation, which accounts for about 2%, but is mostly postmenopausal [30]. Micropapillary carcinoma accounts for about 2% of the recently described types and has a poor prognosis, unlike invasive papillary carcinoma [31]. Metaplastic carcinoma is a carcinoma that exhibits squamous epithelial or substrate differentiation despite being an adenocarcinoma. Mostly hormone-negative, the prognosis resembles invasive ductal carcinoma. Carcinoma with apocrine differentiation

also has a low hormone-positive rate and shows a prognosis similar to that of invasive ductal carcinoma [32]. Carcinoma with neuroendocrine features in the breast may have metastasized from other organs and need to be differentiated. Although it is benign, it is distinguished from small cell carcinoma of the lung by its characteristics such as the observation of coronary intracutaneous cancer components. Inflammatory carcinoma is not a histological type, but a clinical form of invasive breast cancer that presents with redness of the entire breast, a burning sensation, and edema [33]. It is a grade 3 poorly differentiated invasive carcinoma, and embolization of subcutaneous cancer cells is observed in the lymphatic vessels dilated in the dermis. There are many triple-negative subtypes, and the prognosis is very poor. Twenty-five percent of other breast metastatic cancers occur in occult carcinomas where the primary lesion is unknown. Malignant tumors of other organs that often invade the breast include lymphoma, leukemia, malignant melanoma, and lung cancer, and rarely kidney cancer, ovarian cancer, gastric cancer, and uterine cancer.

6.2 Classification of Tumor, Lymph Node, and Metastasis (TNM Staging)

Breast cancer staging is used when classifying patients with similar degrees of illness into the same population, finding appropriate treatments for individual patients, predicting prognosis, and comparing the results of treatments that are applied separately [34]. In the 1940s, breast cancer was classified into four categories that began to be used in the United Kingdom based on clinical findings. Since then, several classifications have been used, in early stage breast cancer, the effect of tumor size on prognosis is not considered, it is difficult to determine objectively axillary lymph node metastasis, and the drawback of not considering non-invasive breast cancer is highlighted [35]. In 1954, the International Union against Cancer (UICC) developed a cancer classification system that could be shared worldwide and introduced the current TNM classification system. In 1962, it started to be used by the American Joint Committee on Cancer (AJCC) [36].

As breast cancer treatments evolved, there were changes in treatment targets and treatments. The TNM staging system for breast cancer has also undergone several revisions, with the eighth revised edition released in 2018. Since the breast cancer disease classification system is the same worldwide, it is a great help for multinational and multi-institutional research. Modern molecular biological techniques have been mobilized to subdivide the stage, and patients receiving prior anticancer chemotherapy are staged twice, before and after treatment. Recently, consideration for tumor display has been reflected, and the prognosis can be evaluated more accurately.

In the initial TNM classification, the patient status was judged only by the presence or absence of each TNM element, and it was only classified into 8 patient groups by the combination of T0, T1, N0, N1, M0, and M1. Now, the clinical characteristics of breast cancer are known in detail and the system has changed to the current classification. The T stage is divided into 6 stages (T0, Tis, T1, T2, T3, T4), the N stage is divided into 4 stages (N0, N1, N2, N3), and the M classification is divided into 2 stages (M0, M1). As such, it has become possible to classify small groups. A prerequisite is to identify the cancer cells and the histological type of cancer from the breast tissue under a microscope. After confirmation of pathological cancer, breast cancer staging is possible before surgery based on clinical findings, and clear staging is performed after surgery based on pathological findings. In addition, the skin on the same side of the breast where the breast cancer is located, the breast tissue and lower muscles, the surrounding lymph nodes, and the distant lymph nodes should be investigated in detail. In addition, various molecular biological techniques and various imaging tests excluding lymphatic scintigraphy are also required. The breast cancer stage can be classified pathologically after surgery to remove the primary breast tumor and surrounding lymph nodes. At this time, the surgical resection margin must be able to confirm pathologically that no tumor remains, and at least one level of axillary lymph nodes (usually 6 or more) must be removed. Pure coronary carcinoma, mucinous carcinoma, and microinvasive cancers smaller than 1 cm may not require axillary lymph node dissection because few axillary lymph nodes are involved in metastases. If prior chemotherapy was received before surgery, the prefix "y" is added and it is expressed as ypTNM. For bilateral breast cancer, different stages are given (Fig 4).

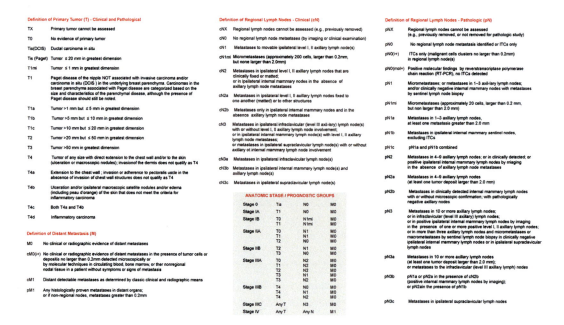

Fig. 4 AJCC eighth TNM staging system

6.3 Important Markers for the Diagnosis and Treatment of Breast Cancer (Basic Biomarkers and Special Studies)

Whether breast cancer patients should receive additional hormone therapy or anticancer chemotherapy after receiving surgical treatment depends on the individual. It depends on the extent of tumor spillover such as stage and prognosis and predictors. Prognostic factors are those that affect patient survival without additional treatment other than surgery. Predictive factors are those related to the response to a particular treatment. Breast cancer prognostic factors are also predictors. There are hormone receptors (estrogen receptor, ER; progesterone receptor, PR), human epidermal growth factor receptor 2 (HER2), and Ki-67, which indicate proliferative ability.

6.3.1 Hormone Receptors

ER and PR are typical hormone receptors for breast cancer. As a transcription factor present in the nucleus, ER is involved in breast development, growth, differentiation, and cancer development and regulates gene expression such as pS2, PR, and bcl-2. Therefore, the presence of PR indicates that ER-related pathways are active and, at the same time, the presence of ER. Hormone receptor-positive breast cancer means ER-positive or PR-positive breast cancer, which has a better prognosis and a better response to hormone treatment than hormone receptor-negative breast cancer. Breast cancer recurrence or death Is significantly reduced after hormone treatment with estrogen antagonist tamoxifen or aromatase inhibitor in patients with hormone receptor-positive intraepithelial carcinoma, invasive breast cancer, and metastatic breast cancer [37, 38]. Hormone receptor tests should always be done at the time of initial diagnosis and initial recurrence of breast cancer in patients. Accurate test results are essential for treatment policy decisions, as the test results determine the presence or absence of hormone therapy. The hormone receptor test method that is commonly used in breast cancer tissue is immunohistochemistry. This method is difficult but not complicated; however, many factors affect the results such as rectification of tissue fixative, fixation time, antigen exposure method, primary antibody type, staining method, and reading standard, among others. In addition, strict quality control is required. In 2010, the American Society for Clinical Cancer (ASCO) and the American-Canada Pathology Society (CAP) jointly published a draft recommendation for ER/PR testing for breast cancer, which is being assessed worldwide [39–41]. Most hormone receptor-positive breast cancers are positive for ER and PR at the same time. However, it is known that about 10% of all breast cancers are positive only for ER and less than 5% of breast cancers are positive only for PR. Regardless of the staining intensity, if at least 1% of tumor cells are stained in the nucleus (corresponding to an Allred score of 3 or higher), the reading criteria will be positive and will be the target of hormone therapy. It is known that even if the hormone receptor is positive, the therapeutic effect differs depending on the degree of staining [42]. Therefore, for pathological results, it is helpful to describe the amount and staining intensity of positively stained cells together with positive or negative results in the treatment of the patient. The ER-positive rate for Korean breast cancer was reported to be about 59–69%, and the PR-positive rate was about 52% [43, 44] (Fig 5).

6.3.2 Human Epidermal Growth Factor Receptor 2 (HER2)

HER2 encodes epidermal growth factor receptor 2, which is a proto-tumor gene and has tyrosine kinase activity. HER2 gene amplification is the major mechanism of HER2 protein overexpression, and this finding appears in about 15–20% of all breast cancers, which are known as HER2-positive breast cancer. This is exactly what was reported in a national multicenter study, HER2 overexpression was observed in 17.3% of all invasive breast cancers and gene amplification was observed in 21% [43, 44]. HER2-positive breast cancer has a worse prognosis than HER2-negative breast cancer without anticancer chemotherapy. Administration of trastuzumab, a therapeutic agent targeting overexpressed HER2,

Allred Score for Estrogen and Progesterone Receptor Evaluation			
Proportion Score (PS)	% Positive Cells	Intensity Score (IS)	Intensity of Positivity
0	0	0	None
1	<1%	1	Weak
2	1% to 10%	2	Intermediated
3	11% to 33%	3	Strong
4	34% to 66%		
5	>67%		
The proportion score and intensity score are added together for a total score			
Total score		Interpretation	
0,2		Negative	
3,4,5,6,7,8		Positive	

Fig. 5 Allred scoring system

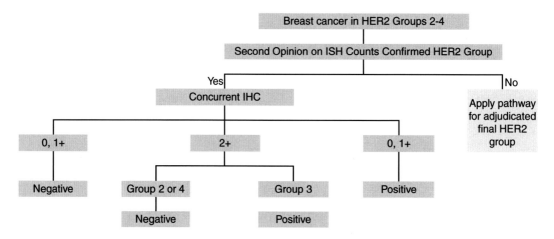

Fig. 6 HER2 test flowchart

to patients with HER2-positive breast cancer can be expected to have a favorable therapeutic effect. HER2 status is an essential factor in determining treatment strategies for breast cancer patients, and all invasive breast cancer patients must be tested for HER2 at diagnosis or at the time of recurrence [45]. There are methods of testing for the HER2 protein and expression using immunohistochemical staining and a method of testing for HER2 gene amplification using in situ hybridization (ISH). In Korea, immunohistochemical staining is performed as a primary test, whereas ISH is performed restrictedly according to the results. If the immunohistochemical staining is 0 or 1+, it is read as HER2-negative breast cancer, and if it is 3+, it is read as HER2-positive breast cancer. For 2+ staining, gene amplification is checked by fluorescence in situ hybridization (FISH) or silver in situ hybridization (SISH) and read as HER2-positive or negative breast cancer depending on the results (Fig 6).

6.3.3 Ki-67

Proliferative activity is closely associated with tumor malignancy. Although high proliferative potential in breast cancer is associated with poor prognosis, it may also show good therapeutic effects on common anticancer drugs that target proliferative cells. To measure the proliferative potential of tumor cells, the mitotic count can be determined directly from the tissue slide, or the S phase cell fraction can be measured by flow cytometry. However, a widely used method in practice is immunohistochemical staining for the Ki-67 protein. The Ki-67 protein is located in the nucleus and is expressed in all cell cycles except

G_0. It is an international recommendation to count 500–1000 tumor cells in 3 or more high-power fields at the margin of invasive breast cancer and to display the number of cells showing Ki-67 positive as a percentage. If the cells stained positive in the tumor have more "hot spots" than the surroundings, this part is included in the measurement, and it is recommended to report an average with peripheral measurements. Studies have shown that Ki-67 can remain useful as a prognostic factor when cutoffs are set within the Ki-67 labeling index of 4–15% [46]. However, it is not advisable to have a cutoff and report it as high or low, or as a grade.

6.3.4 Markers Useful for Other Diagnostic and Differential Diagnosis

Staining for E-cadherin and β-catenin may be useful for differentiation from ductal carcinoma in the diagnosis of LCIS or invasive lobular carcinoma. Cancer cells have the property of penetrating the myocutaneous cell layer and basement membrane and infiltrating the substrate, and when markers are used to stain calponin, smooth muscle myosin-heavy chain, and p63 the disappearance of the myosin cell layer can be confirmed. This makes it possible to distinguish between invasive carcinoma and carcinoma in situ. CK 5/6 staining is used as an adjunct to the diagnosis to distinguish between usual ductal hyperplasia, atypical ductal hyperplasia, and low-grade DCIS. There is also a study that has reported a sensitivity of 75% and specificity of 100% by using CK 5/6 and EGFR together for confirmation of basal-like breast cancer [47, 48]. In addition, vimentin, P-cadherin, CK14, etc., are used as markers.

References

1. National Central Cancer Registry Statistics Report 2019. Republic of Korea.
2. Parks AG. The micro-anatomy of the breast. Ann R Coll Surg Engl. 1959;25:235–51.
3. Spratt JS. Anatomy of the breast. Major Probl Clin Surg. 1979;5:1–13.
4. Moffat DF, Going JJ. Three dimensional anatomy of complete duct systems in human breast: pathological and developmental implications. J Clin Pathol. 1996;49(1):48–52. https://doi.org/10.1136/jcp.49.1.48.
5. Nathanson SD, Wachna DL, Gilman D, Karvelis K, Havstad S, Ferrara J. Pathways of lymphatic drainage from the breast. Ann Surg Oncol. 2001;8(10):837–43. https://doi.org/10.1007/s10434-001-0837-3.
6. Turner-Warwick RT. The lymphatics of the breast. Br J Surg. 1959;46:574–82. https://doi.org/10.1002/bjs.18004620004.
7. Egan RL, McSweeney MB. Intramammary lymph nodes. Cancer. 1983;51(10):1838–42. https://doi.org/10.1002/1097-0142(19830515)51:10<1838::aid-cncr2820511014>3.0.co;2-8.
8. Berg JW. The significance of axillary node levels in the study of breast carcinoma. Cancer. 1955;8(4):776–8. https://doi.org/10.1002/1097-0142(1955)8:4<776::aid-cncr2820080421>3.0.co;2-b.
9. Paganelli G, Galimberti V, Trifiro G, Travaini L, De Cicco C, Mazzarol G, et al. Internal mammary node lymphoscintigraphy and biopsy in breast cancer. Q J Nucl Med. 2002;46(2):138–44.
10. O'Malley MS, Fletcher SW. US preventive services task force. Screening for breast cancer with breast self-examination. A critical review. JAMA. 1987;257(16):2196–203.
11. Holland R, Hendriks JH. Microcalcifications associated with ductal carcinoma in situ: mammographic-pathologic correlation. Semin Diagn Pathol. 1994;11(3):181–92.
12. Feig SA. Ductal carcinoma in situ. Implications for screening mammography. Radiol Clin N Am. 2000;38(4):653–68, vii. https://doi.org/10.1016/s0033-8389(05)70192-5.
13. Ikeda DM, Andersson I. Ductal carcinoma in situ: atypical mammographic appearances. Radiology. 1989;172(3):661–6. https://doi.org/10.1148/radiology.172.3.2549563.
14. Stomper PC, Connolly JL, Meyer JE, Harris JR. Clinically occult ductal carcinoma in situ detected with mammography: analysis of 100 cases with radiologic-pathologic correlation. Radiology. 1989;172(1):235–41. https://doi.org/10.1148/radiology.172.1.2544922.
15. Dershaw DD, Abramson A, Kinne DW. Ductal carcinoma in situ: mammographic findings and clinical implications. Radiology. 1989;170(2):411–5. https://doi.org/10.1148/radiology.170.2.2536185.
16. Moon WK, Im JG, Noh DY, Han MC. Nonpalpable breast lesions: evaluation with power Doppler US and a microbubble contrast agent-initial experience. Radiology. 2000;217(1):240–6. https://doi.org/10.1148/radiology.217.1.r00oc03240.
17. Buchberger W, DeKoekkoek-Doll P, Springer P, Obrist P, Dunser M. Incidental findings on sonography of the breast: clinical significance and diagnostic workup. AJR Am J Roentgenol. 1999;173(4):921–7. https://doi.org/10.2214/ajr.173.4.10511149.
18. Moon WK, Myung JS, Lee YJ, Park IA, Noh DY, Im JG. US of ductal carcinoma in situ. Radiographics.

18. 2002;22(2):269–80; discussion 80–1. https://doi.org/10.1148/radiographics.22.2.g02mr16269.

19. Cho N, Moon WK, Cha JH, Kim SM, Kim SJ, Lee SH, et al. Sonographically guided core biopsy of the breast: comparison of 14-gauge automated gun and 11-gauge directional vacuum-assisted biopsy methods. Korean J Radiol. 2005;6(2):102–9. https://doi.org/10.3348/kjr.2005.6.2.102.

20. Berg WA, Gutierrez L, NessAiver MS, Carter WB, Bhargavan M, Lewis RS, et al. Diagnostic accuracy of mammography, clinical examination, US, and MR imaging in preoperative assessment of breast cancer. Radiology. 2004;233(3):830–49. https://doi.org/10.1148/radiol.2333031484.

21. Dronkers DJ. Stereotaxic core biopsy of breast lesions. Radiology. 1992;183(3):631–4. https://doi.org/10.1148/radiology.183.3.1584909.

22. Leconte I, Feger C, Galant C, Berliere M, Berg BV, D'Hoore W, et al. Mammography and subsequent whole-breast sonography of nonpalpable breast cancers: the importance of radiologic breast density. AJR Am J Roentgenol. 2003;180(6):1675–9. https://doi.org/10.2214/ajr.180.6.1801675.

23. Monzawa S, Yokokawa M, Sakuma T, Takao S, Hirokaga K, Hanioka K, et al. Mucinous carcinoma of the breast: MRI features of pure and mixed forms with histopathologic correlation. AJR Am J Roentgenol. 2009;192(3):W125–31. https://doi.org/10.2214/AJR.07.4021.

24. Kuhl CK, Mielcareck P, Klaschik S, Leutner C, Wardelmann E, Gieseke J, et al. Dynamic breast MR imaging: are signal intensity time course data useful for differential diagnosis of enhancing lesions? Radiology. 1999;211(1):101–10. https://doi.org/10.1148/radiology.211.1.r99ap38101.

25. Kuhl CK, Klaschik S, Mielcarek P, Gieseke J, Wardelmann E, Schild HH. Do T2-weighted pulse sequences help with the differential diagnosis of enhancing lesions in dynamic breast MRI? J Magn Reson Imaging. 1999;9(2):187–96. https://doi.org/10.1002/(sici)1522-2586(199902)9:2<187::aid-jmri6>3.0.co;2-2.

26. Orel SG, Schnall MD. MR imaging of the breast for the detection, diagnosis, and staging of breast cancer. Radiology. 2001;220(1):13–30. https://doi.org/10.1148/radiology.220.1.r01jl3113.

27. Silverstein MJ, Parker R, Grotting JC, Cote RJ, Russell CA. Ductal carcinoma in situ (DCIS) of the breast: diagnostic and therapeutic controversies. J Am Coll Surg. 2001;192(2):196–214. https://doi.org/10.1016/s1072-7515(00)00791-2.

28. Silverstein MJ, Poller DN, Waisman JR, Colburn WJ, Barth A, Gierson ED, et al. Prognostic classification of breast ductal carcinoma-in-situ. Lancet. 1995;345(8958):1154–7. https://doi.org/10.1016/s0140-6736(95)90982-6.

29. Fisher ER, Fisher B. Lobular carcinoma of the breast: an overview. Ann Surg. 1977;185(4):377–85. https://doi.org/10.1097/00000658-197704000-00001.

30. Pal SK, Lau SK, Kruper L, Nwoye U, Garberoglio C, Gupta RK, et al. Papillary carcinoma of the breast: an overview. Breast Cancer Res Treat. 2010;122(3):637–45. https://doi.org/10.1007/s10549-010-0961-5.

31. Adrada B, Arribas E, Gilcrease M, Yang WT. Invasive micropapillary carcinoma of the breast: mammographic, sonographic, and MRI features. AJR Am J Roentgenol. 2009;193(1):W58–63. https://doi.org/10.2214/AJR.08.1537.

32. Gunhan-Bilgen I, Memis A, Ustun EE, Zekioglu O, Ozdemir N. Metaplastic carcinoma of the breast: clinical, mammographic, and sonographic findings with histopathologic correlation. AJR Am J Roentgenol. 2002;178(6):1421–5. https://doi.org/10.2214/ajr.178.6.1781421.

33. Robertson FM, Bondy M, Yang W, Yamauchi H, Wiggins S, Kamrudin S, et al. Inflammatory breast cancer: the disease, the biology, the treatment. CA Cancer J Clin. 2010;60(6):351–75. https://doi.org/10.3322/caac.20082.

34. Elston CW, Ellis IO. Pathological prognostic factors in breast cancer. I. the value of histological grade in breast cancer: experience from a large study with long-term follow-up. Histopathology. 1991;19(5):403–10. https://doi.org/10.1111/j.1365-2559.1991.tb00229.x.

35. Rosen PP. The pathological classification of human mammary carcinoma: past, present and future. Ann Clin Lab Sci. 1979;9(2):144–56.

36. American Joint Committee on Cancer (AJCC) 8th TNM staging system.

37. Allred DC, Carlson RW, Berry DA, Burstein HJ, Edge SB, Goldstein LJ, et al. NCCN task force report: estrogen receptor and progesterone receptor testing in breast cancer by immunohistochemistry. J Natl Compr Cancer Netw. 2009;7(Suppl 6):S1–21; quiz S2–3. https://doi.org/10.6004/jnccn.2009.0079.

38. Allred DC, Anderson SJ, Paik S, Wickerham DL, Nagtegaal ID, Swain SM, et al. Adjuvant tamoxifen reduces subsequent breast cancer in women with estrogen receptor-positive ductal carcinoma in situ: a study based on NSABP protocol B-24. J Clin Oncol. 2012;30(12):1268–73. https://doi.org/10.1200/JCO.2010.34.0141.

39. Hammond ME, Hayes DF, Wolff AC, Mangu PB, Temin S. American Society of Clinical Oncology/College of American pathologists guideline recommendations for immunohistochemical testing of estrogen and progesterone receptors in breast cancer. J Oncol Pract. 2010;6(4):195–7. https://doi.org/10.1200/JOP.777003.

40. Hammond ME, Hayes DF, Dowsett M, Allred DC, Hagerty KL, Badve S, et al. American Society of Clinical Oncology/College of American pathologists guideline recommendations for immunohistochemical testing of estrogen and progesterone receptors in breast cancer. J Clin Oncol. 2010;28(16):2784–95. https://doi.org/10.1200/JCO.2009.25.6529.

41. Hammond ME, Hayes DF, Dowsett M, Allred DC, Hagerty KL, Badve S, et al. American Society of

Clinical Oncology/College of American pathologists guideline recommendations for immunohistochemical testing of estrogen and progesterone receptors in breast cancer. Arch Pathol Lab Med. 2010;134(6):907–22. https://doi.org/10.1043/1543-2165-134.6.907.

42. Harvey JM, Clark GM, Osborne CK, Allred DC. Estrogen receptor status by immunohistochemistry is superior to the ligand-binding assay for predicting response to adjuvant endocrine therapy in breast cancer. J Clin Oncol. 1999;17(5):1474–81. https://doi.org/10.1200/JCO.1999.17.5.1474.

43. Bae YK, Gong G, Kang J, Lee A, Cho EY, Lee JS, et al. HER2 status by standardized immunohistochemistry and silver-enhanced in situ hybridization in Korean breast cancer. J Breast Cancer. 2012;15(4):381–7. https://doi.org/10.4048/jbc.2012.15.4.381.

44. Bae YK, Gong G, Kang J, Lee A, Cho EY, Lee JS, et al. Hormone receptor expression in invasive breast cancer among Korean women and comparison of 3 antiestrogen receptor antibodies: a multi-institutional retrospective study using tissue microarrays. Am J Surg Pathol. 2012;36(12):1817–25. https://doi.org/10.1097/PAS.0b013e318267b012.

45. Wolff AC, Hammond ME, Hicks DG, Dowsett M, McShane LM, Allison KH, et al. Recommendations for human epidermal growth factor receptor 2 testing in breast cancer: American Society of Clinical Oncology/College of American Pathologists clinical practice guideline update. J Clin Oncol. 2013;31(31):3997–4013. https://doi.org/10.1200/JCO.2013.50.9984.

46. Gudlaugsson E, Skaland I, Janssen EA, Smaaland R, Shao Z, Malpica A, et al. Comparison of the effect of different techniques for measurement of Ki67 proliferation on reproducibility and prognosis prediction accuracy in breast cancer. Histopathology. 2012;61(6):1134–44. https://doi.org/10.1111/j.1365-2559.2012.04329.x.

47. Nielsen TO, Andrews HN, Cheang M, Kucab JE, Hsu FD, Ragaz J, et al. Expression of the insulin-like growth factor I receptor and urokinase plasminogen activator in breast cancer is associated with poor survival: potential for intervention with 17-allylamino geldanamycin. Cancer Res. 2004;64(1):286–91. https://doi.org/10.1158/0008-5472.can-03-1242.

48. Nielsen TO, Hsu FD, Jensen K, Cheang M, Karaca G, Hu Z, et al. Immunohistochemical and clinical characterization of the basal-like subtype of invasive breast carcinoma. Clin Cancer Res. 2004;10(16):5367–74. https://doi.org/10.1158/1078-0432.CCR-04-0220.

Benign and Proliferative Case Series

Chan Wha Lee, Youngmi Kwon, Yunju Kim, and Bo Hwa Choi

1 Case 1

1.1 Patient History and Progress

Female/37 years old, pre-menopause.

Screen detected mass lesion on left breast 8 o'clock and 5 o'clock direction.

Outside result of biopsy: Papillary neoplasm.
No family history.
No comorbidities.

1.2 Important Radiologic Findings

See Figs. 1 and 2.

1.3 Courses of Treatment

→ 2022-02-11 Excision, Lt. (8H and 5H).

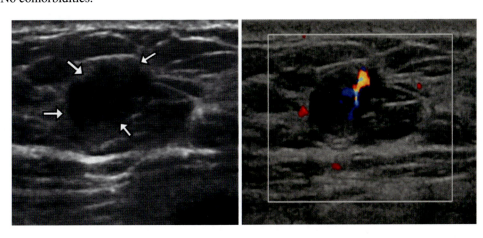

Fig. 1 A 1 cm sized complex cystic and solid mass with increased vascularity (IDP with UDH)

C. W. Lee · B. H. Choi (✉)
Department of Radiology, National Cancer Center, Goyang, Republic of Korea
e-mail: cwlee@ncc.re.kr; iawy82@ncc.re.kr

Y. Kwon
Department of Radiology, Center for Breast Cancer, National Cancer Center, Goyang, Gyeonggi, Republic of Korea
e-mail: ymk@ncc.re.kr

Y. Kim
Department of Pathology, National Cancer Center, Goyang, Gyeonggi, Republic of Korea
e-mail: radkyj@ncc.re.kr

© The Author(s), under exclusive license to Springer Nature Singapore Pte Ltd. 2023
E. S. Lee (ed.), *A Practical Guide to Breast Cancer Treatment*,
https://doi.org/10.1007/978-981-19-9044-1_2

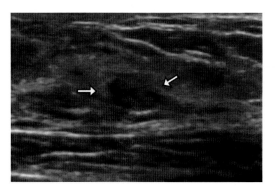

Fig. 2 A 0.6 cm oval circumscribed isoechoic mass (sclerosing adenosis)

1.3.1 Pathology Report

- Breast, left 8 o'clock, excision:
  - Intraductal papilloma with usual ductal hyperplasia.
- Breast, left 5 o'clock, excision:
  - Sclerosing adenosis.

2 Case 2

2.1 Patient History and Progress

Female/47 years old, pre-menopause.
Screen detected mass lesion on left breast 2 o'clock direction.
Outside result of biopsy: Intraductal papilloma.
No family history.
No comorbidities.

2.2 Important Radiologic Findings

See Fig. 3.

2.3 Courses of Treatment

→ 2022-02-14 Excision, Lt.

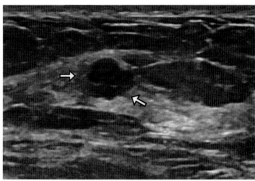

Fig. 3 Ultrasonography shows a 0.6 cm lobulated hypoechoic mass in the left breast

2.3.1 Pathology Report

- Breast, left, excision:
  - Atypical ductal hyperplasia with microcalcification.
  - Intraductal papilloma with usual ductal hyperplasia.

3 Case 3

3.1 Patient History and Progress

Female/72 years old, post-menopause.
Screen detected nodular lesion on right breast 9 o'clock direction.
No family history.
Hypertension.

3.2 Important Radiologic Findings

See Figs. 4 and 5.

3.3 Courses of Treatment

→ 2021-12-10 Excision, Rt.

Benign and Proliferative Case Series

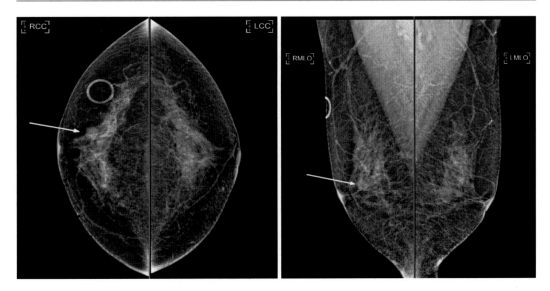

Fig. 4 Mammogram shows a round circumscribed iso-dense mass (white arrow) in the right subareolar area. The ring-shaped marker represents the skin wart

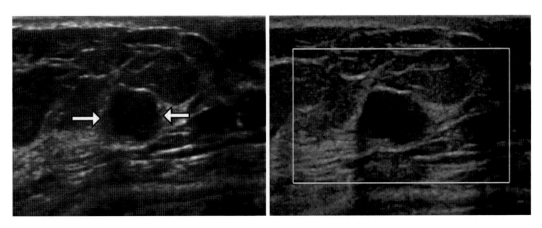

Fig. 5 Ultrasonogram shows a 0.8 cm round, parallel, lobulated, complex cystic and solid mass with internal vascularity in the right breast

3.3.1 Pathology Report

Diagnosis
- Breast, right, excision:
  – Intraductal papilloma.

4 Case 4

4.1 Patient History and Progress

Female/60 years old, post-menopause.
Screen detected mass lesion on left breast 12 o'clock direction.

Family history of pancreatic cancer, mother. Hypertension, dyslipidemia (taking medication).

4.2 Important Radiologic Findings

See Fig. 6.

4.3 Courses of Treatment

→ 2021-12-14 Excision, Lt.

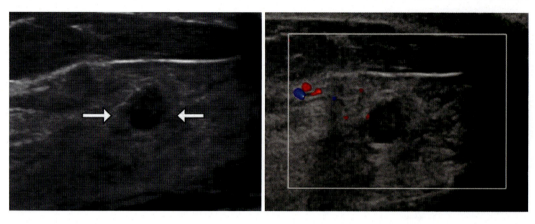

Fig. 6 Ultrasonogram shows a 0.6 cm round, parallel, microlobulated hypoechoic mass without vascularity in the left breast

4.3.1 Pathology Report

Diagnosis
- Breast, left, excision:
  - Intraductal papilloma.

5 Case 5

5.1 Patient History and Progress

Female/48 years old, pre-menopause.

Screen detected microcalcification on upper outer portion of left breast.

Family history of breast cancer, mother and sister.

No comorbidities.

BRCA 1 and 2 mutation: Not detected.

5.2 Important Radiologic Findings

See Figs. 7 and 8.

5.3 Courses of Treatment

→2021-12-17 Excision, Lt. (11H, 1H).

5.3.1 Pathology Report
- Breast, left, excision:
  - Atypical ductal hyperplasia (#1. 1 o'clock & #2. 11 o'clock) involving intraductal papilloma with microcalcification.

Benign and Proliferative Case Series

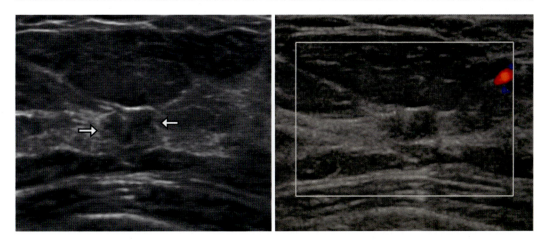

Fig. 7 Ultrasonogram shows a 0.8 cm irregular shaped, microlobulated hypoechoic mass without vascularity in the left upper inner breast

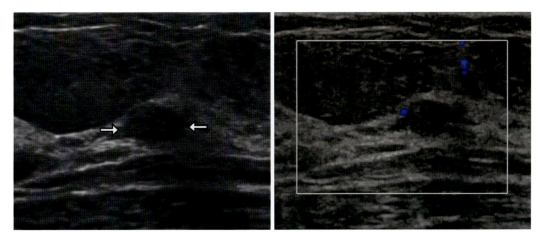

Fig. 8 Ultrasonogram shows a 0.7 cm oval shaped, circumscribed hypoechoic mass without vascularity in the left upper outer breast

6 Case 6

6.1 Patient History and Progress

Female/48 years old, pre-menopause.
Bloody discharge from right nipple.
No family history.
Hypertension.

6.2 Important Radiologic Findings

See Figs. 9 and 10.

6.3 Courses of Treatment

→ 2021-12-31 excision, both.

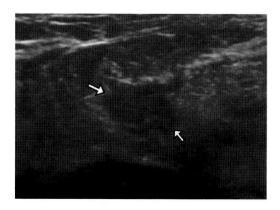

Fig. 9 Ultrasonogram shows an oval shaped, angular margin, hypoechoic mass

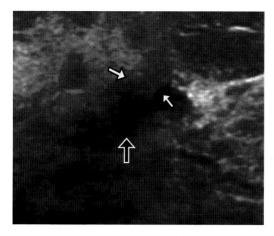

Fig. 10 Ultrasonogram shows irregular ductal dilatation (black arrow) with irregular shaped isoechoic intraductal lesion (white arrow)

6.3.1 Pathology Report
- Breast, right, excision:
  - Intraductal papilloma with (1) usual ductal hyperplasia, (2) microcalcification.
- Breast, left, excision:
  - Intraductal papilloma with (1) usual ductal hyperplasia, (2) microcalcification.

7 Case 7

7.1 Patient History and Progress

Female/58 years old, post-menopause.
    Screen detected microcalcification on upper portion of right breast.
    No family history.
    No comorbidities.

7.2 Important Radiologic Findings

See Fig. 11.

7.3 Courses of Treatment

→2021-10-29 Rt upper, stereotactic biopsy.

7.3.1 Pathology Report

Diagnosis
- Breast, right upper, stereotactic biopsy:
  - Atypical ductal hyperplasia (#1. Ca++) with microcalcification.
  - Flat epithelial atypia (#2. no Ca++) with microcalcification.

→2021-11-26 excision, Rt.

Diagnosis
- Breast, right, excision:
  - Atypical ductal hyperplasia with microcalcification.
        Post-stereotactic biopsy status.

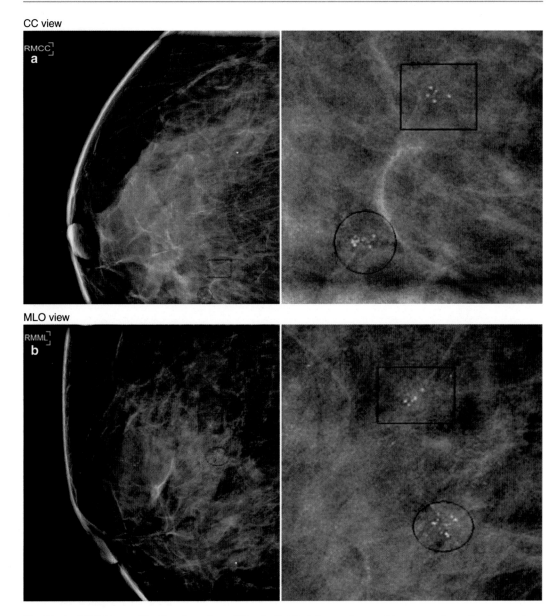

Fig. 11 (**a, b**) Right magnification views show diffusely distributed amorphous and two grouped round and amorphous microcalcifications. The right image is zoomed in

8 Case 8

8.1 Patient History and Progress

Female/54 years old, pre-menopause.

Screen detected microcalcification on upper outer portion of left breast.

No family history.
No comorbidities.

8.2 Important Radiologic Findings

See Fig. 12.

8.3 Courses of Treatment

→2021-11-12 excision, Lt.

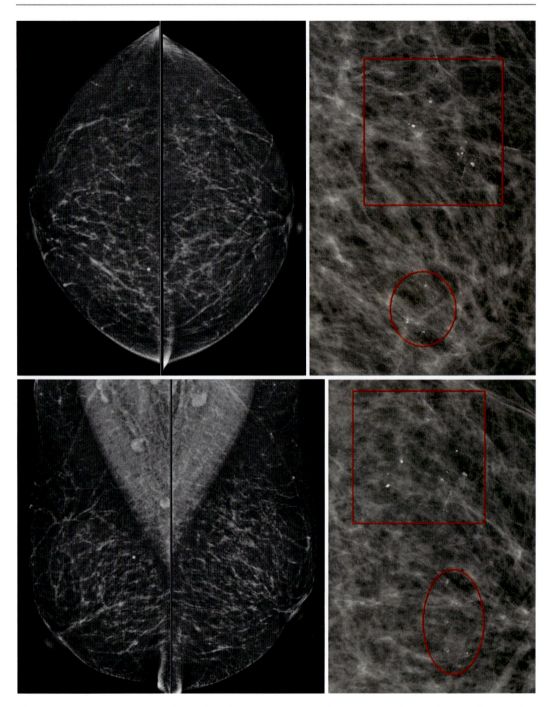

Fig. 12 Both mammogram and left magnification view show regional and some linear distribution of amorphous and round microcalcifications in left upper outer (red rectangle), and grouped amorphous and round microcalcifications in left upper central (red circle)

8.3.1 Pathology Report

Diagnosis
- Breast, left, excision:
  - Atypical ductal hyperplasia with microcalcification.

9 Case 9

9.1 Patient History and Progress

Female/32 years old, pre-menopause.

Screen detected mass lesion on right breast 8 o'clock direction.

Family history of breast cancer, mother and maternal aunt.

No comorbidities.

9.2 Important Radiologic Findings

See Figs. 13, 14 and 15.

9.3 Courses of Treatment

→ 2021-11-12 Excision, Rt.

9.3.1 Pathology Report

Diagnosis
- Breast, right, excision:
  - Atypical ductal hyperplasia, focal.

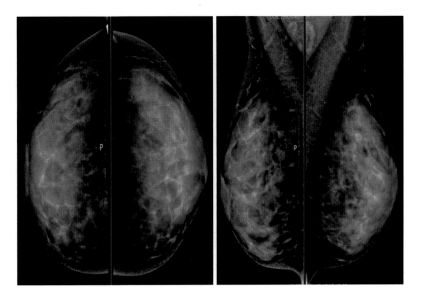

Fig. 13 Mammography shows no discernable abnormality

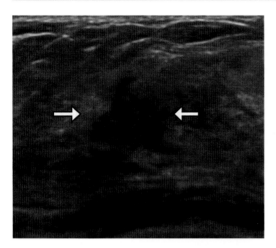

Fig. 14 Ultrasonography shows a 1 cm irregular shaped hypoechoic mass in right lower outer breast

10 Case 10

10.1 Patient History and Progress

Female/33 years old, pre-menopause.
  Bloody discharge from left nipple.
  No family history.
  No comorbidities.

10.2 Important Radiologic Findings

See Figs. 16 and 17.

10.3 Courses of Treatment

→2021-11-09 excision (Lt. 3H SA, Lt. nipple mass).

10.3.1 Pathology Report
- Breast, "left subareolar 3 o'clock", excision:
  - Atypical ductal hyperplasia.
- Breast, "left nipple mass," excision:
  - Nipple adenoma (florid papillomatosis).

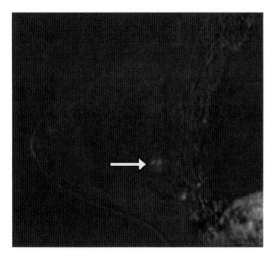

Fig. 15 MR image shows a 1 cm focal heterogeneous non-mass enhancement in the right lower outer breast

Benign and Proliferative Case Series

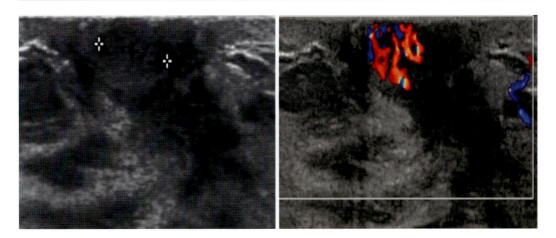

Fig. 16 US shows 0.8 cm oval hyper-vascular isoechoic nodule in the nipple

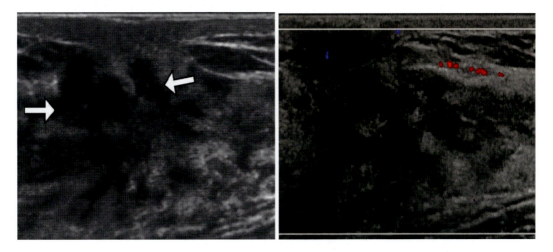

Fig. 17 The US shows 1.3 cm hypoechoic non-mass lesions without vascularity in the left subareolar area

11 Case 11

11.1 Patient History and Progress

Female/39 years old, pre-menopause.
　Serous discharge from right nipple.
　No family history.
　Asthma, hyperthyroidism.

11.2 Important Radiologic Findings

See Fig. 18.

11.3 Courses of Treatment

→2021-10-29 excision, Rt.

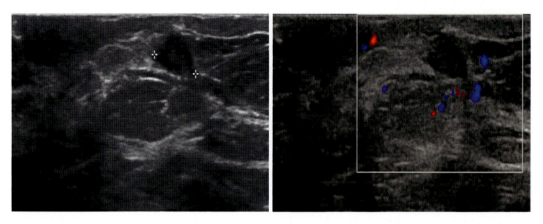

Fig. 18 US shows a 0.7 cm oval, angular margin, hypoechoic mass without vascularity

11.3.1 Pathology Report

Diagnosis
- Breast, right, excision:
  - Intraductal papilloma.

12 Case 12

12.1 Patient History and Progress

Female/70 years old, post-menopause.

Screen detected mass lesion on left breast 2 o'clock and 5 o'clock and 9 o'clock direction.

No family history.

s/p Right breast conserving surgery (right breast cancer), hypertension, diabetes mellitus.

12.2 Important Radiologic Findings

See Figs. 19 and 20.

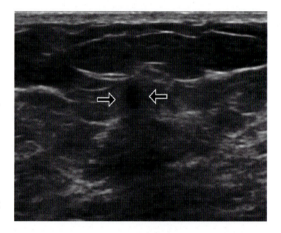

Fig. 19 The US shows a round shaped, not parallel oriented hypoechoic mass in left upper outer breast

12.3 Courses of Treatment

→2021-10-29 excision, Lt.

12.3.1 Pathology Report

Diagnosis
- Breast, left, excision:
  - Intraductal papilloma (#1. 2 o'clock, #2. 5 o'clock & #3. 9 o'clock) with (1) usual ductal hyperplasia, (2) apocrine metaplasia.

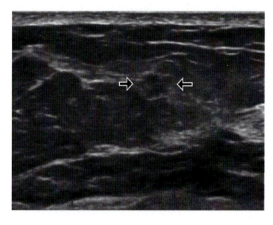

Fig. 20 The US shows an irregular shaped hypoechoic mass in the left inner central breast

13 Case 13

13.1 Patient History and Progress

Female/45 years old, pre-menopause.
Screen detected microcalcification on upper center of right breast.
No family history.
No comorbidities.

13.2 Important Radiologic Findings

See Figs. 21 and 22.

13.3 Courses of Treatment

→2021-10-26 excision, Rt.

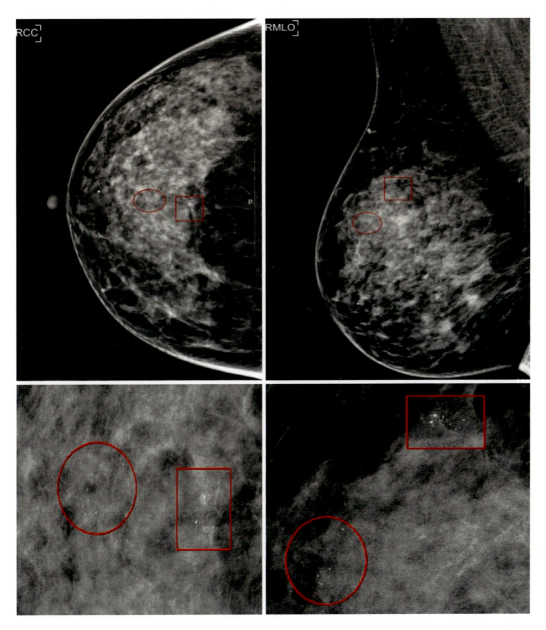

Fig. 21 Right mammogram with magnification view (lower column) shows two groups of round and amorphous microcalcifications in the right upper central area

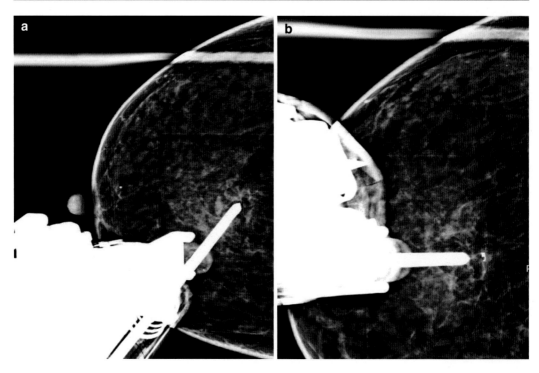

Fig. 22 Stereotactic vacuum assisted biopsy was performed at the site of microcalcifications (**a**). After the successful biopsy, the marker was inserted at the site of biopsy (**b**)

13.3.1 Pathology Report
- Breast, right 12 o'clock, excision:
  - Flat epithelial atypia with microcalcification
- Breast, right 2 o'clock, excision:
  - Atypical ductal hyperplasia with microcalcification.

14 Case 14

14.1 Patient History and Progress

Female/60 years old, post-menopause.

Screen detected mass lesion on right breast 9 o'clock direction.

Family history of breast cancer, mother.

s/p Total hysterectomy (leiomyoma) and Left salpingo-oophorectomy.

14.2 Important Radiologic Findings

See Figs. 23 and 24.

14.3 Courses of Treatment

→2021-10-15 excision, Rt.

14.3.1 Pathology Report
- Breast, right, excision:
  - Atypical ductal hyperplasia involving intraductal papilloma with marked cautery artifact.

Benign and Proliferative Case Series

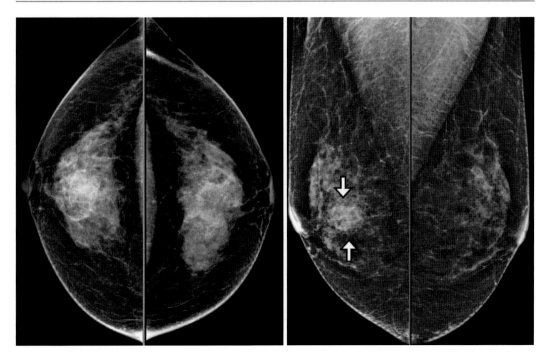

Fig. 23 Right MLO view of the mammogram shows asymmetry of right central portion (white arrow)

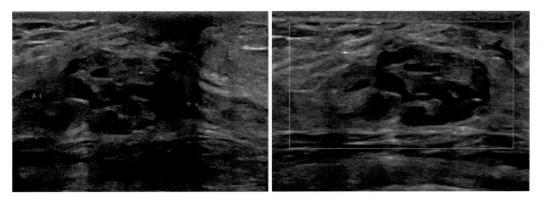

Fig. 24 Ultrasonogram shows about 2 cm extent, aggregations of dilated ducts without vascularity

15 Case 15

15.1 Patient History and Progress

Female/33 years old, pre-menopause.

Screen detected mass lesion on left breast 3 o'clock direction.

Family history of pancreatic cancer, maternal grandmother.

No comorbidities.

BRCA 1 and 2 mutation: Not detected.

15.2 Important Radiologic Findings

See Figs. 25 and 26.

15.3 Courses of Treatment

→2021-10-12 excision, Lt.

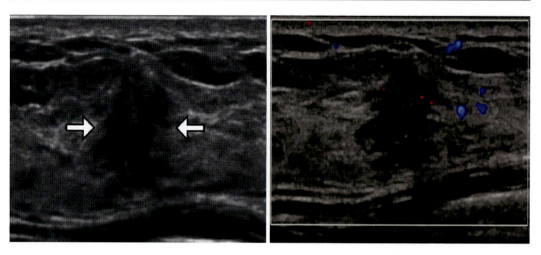

Fig. 25 Ultrasonogram shows 1.2 cm irregular hypoechoic mass (white arrow) without significant vascularity in left outer central breast

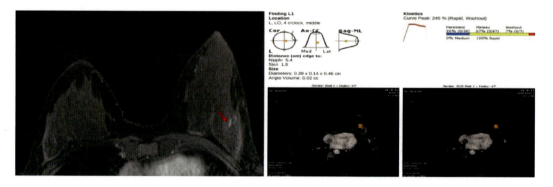

Fig. 26 MR image shows an enhancing focus with washout kinetics in left outer central breast

15.3.1 Pathology Report
- Breast, left, excision:
  - Atypical ductal hyperplasia, focal
  - Fibroadenomatous change.

16 Case 16

16.1 Patient History and Progress

Female/59 years old, post-menopause.
Screen detected mass lesion on right breast 7 o'clock direction.
No family history.
s/p Total hysterectomy, s/p left nephrectomy (donor), s/o cholecystectomy.

16.2 Important Radiologic Findings

See Figs. 27, 28 and 29.

16.3 Courses of Treatment

→2021-09-13 needle biopsy.

16.3.1 Pathology Report

Diagnosis
- Breast, right, needle biopsy:
  - Ductal carcinoma in situ.
    Nuclear grade: low.
    Necrosis: present.

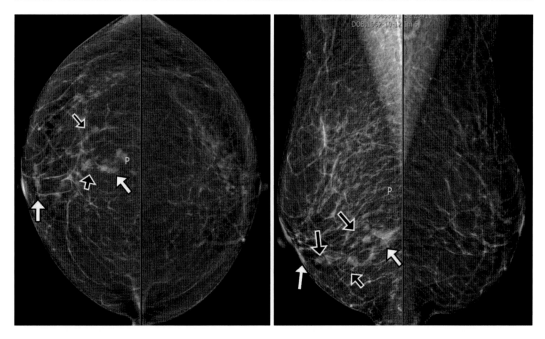

Fig. 27 Mammogram shows multiple oval and round circumscribed iso-dense masses (black arrows) and focal asymmetry (white arrows) with round microcalcifications in the right lower outer breast, extending to subareolar area

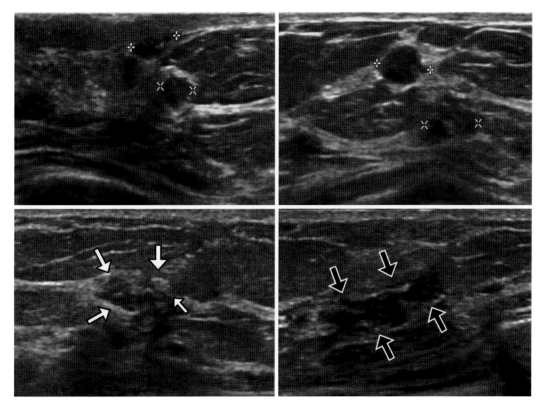

Fig. 28 Ultrasonogram shows multifocal circumscribed round and irregular indistinct hypoechoic masses in the right breast from subareolar to right lower outer breast

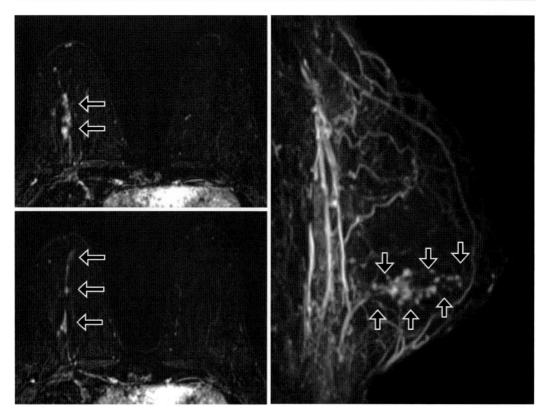

Fig. 29 MRI shows about 8 cm extent heterogeneous segmental non-mass enhancement at right subareolar to the right 7 o'clock direction

Architectural pattern: micropapillary/cribriform/comedo.
Microcalcification: present, tumoral.

→2021-10-08 Rt. BCS + Lt. mastopexy.

16.3.2 Pathology Report

Diagnosis
1. Breast, right, lumpectomy: Microinvasive Ductal Carcinoma.
   (a) Size of tumor: <0.1 cm (pT1mi).
   (b) Size of in situ component: 4.0 cm.
   (c) Histologic grade: not applicable.
   (d) Intraductal component: present, intratumoral/extratumoral (>95%) (nuclear grade: high, necrosis: present, architectural pattern: micropapillary/cribriform/solid/comedo, extensive intraductal component: present).
   (e) Skin: no involvement of tumor.
   (f) Surgical margins:
      • Nipple margin: positive for ductal carcinoma in situ (Fro 10) (see Note 1).
      • Superior margin: (see Note 2).
      • Inferior margin: 20 mm.
      • Medial margin: (see Note 3).
      • Lateral margin: 5 mm.
      • Deep margin: <1 mm from ductal carcinoma in situ (slides 1 & 2).
      • Superficial margin: 10 mm
   (g) Lymph nodes: no metastasis in three axillary lymph nodes (pN0(sn)) (sentinel LN: 0/3).
   (h) Arteriovenous invasion: absent.
   (i) Lymphovascular invasion: absent.

(j) Tumor border: infiltrative.
(k) Microcalcification: present, tumoral.
(l) Pathological TN category (AJCC 2017): pT1miN0(sn).
   Note: 1. Ductal carcinoma in situ is present only in the permanent section of Fro 10.
2. The superior margin of the lumpectomy specimen (slide 3) is positive for ductal carcinoma in situ but this margin submitted for frozen diagnosis (Fro 2) is free of tumor.
3. The medial margin of the lumpectomy specimen (slide 6) is close to ductal carcinoma in situ (2 mm) but this margin submitted for frozen diagnosis (Fro 4) is free of tumor.
4. Histologic mapping has been done.

	Result	Intensity	Positive%
Estrogen receptor	Strong (2/8)	1	<1%
Progesterone receptor	Strong (0/8)	0	0
C-erbB2	Negative (3+)		
Ki-67	Positive in 20% of tumor cells		

Diagnosis
- Breast, left, excision:
  - Usual ductal hyperplasia, focal.
    Postoperative radiotherapy for right breast.

17 Case 17

17.1 Patient History and Progress

Female/39 years old, pre-menopause.
Screen detected mass lesion on right breast 9 o'clock direction.
No family history.
s/p appendectomy (cecal cancer), s/p hysterectomy, and bilateral salpingo-oophorectomy.
s/p partial hepatectomy.

17.2 Important Radiologic Findings

See Figs. 30 and 31.

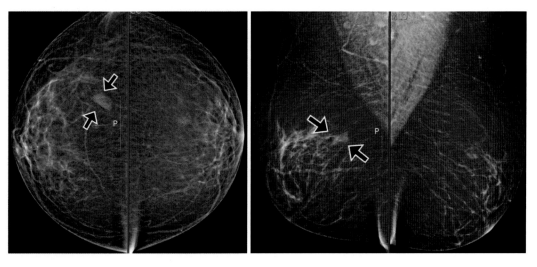

Fig. 30 Mammogram shows an oval circumscribed iso-dense mass in the right upper outer breast

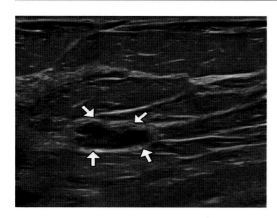

Fig. 31 Ultrasonogram shows an oval lobulated hypoechoic mass in the right 9 o'clock direction

17.3 Courses of Treatment

→2021-09-17 excision, Rt.

17.3.1 Pathology Report

Diagnosis
- Breast, right, excision:
  - Atypical ductal hyperplasia involving mammary cyst.
  - Usual ductal hyperplasia, focal with microcalcification.

18 Case 18

18.1 Patient History and Progress

Female/57 years old, pre-menopause.
  Screen detected mass lesion on right breast 9 ~ 10 o'clock direction.
  No family history.
  No comorbidities.
  s/p Right breast excision.

18.2 Important Radiologic Findings

See Figs. 32 and 33.

18.3 Courses of Treatment

→2021-08-27 excision, Rt.

18.3.1 Pathology Report

Diagnosis
- Breast, right, excision:
  - Atypical ductal hyperplasia with microcalcification.
    Post-excision status.
  - Intraductal papilloma.

Benign and Proliferative Case Series

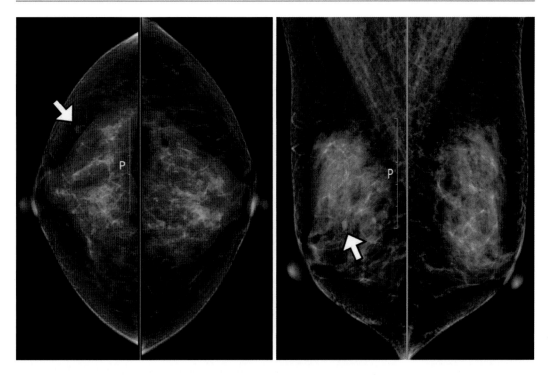

Fig. 32 Mammogram shows an oval circumscribed iso-dense mass in the right outer central breast

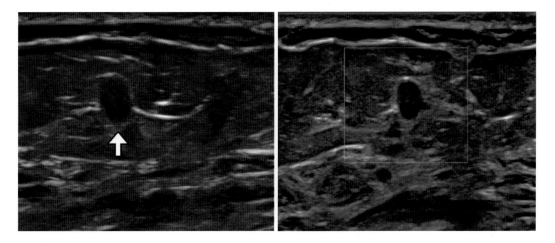

Fig. 33 The US shows an oval, not parallel, circumscribed hypoechoic mass without vascularity in the right 9 o'clock direction

19 Case 19

19.1 Patient History and Progress

Female/42 years old, pre-menopause.
　Screen detected mass lesion on left breast 8 o'clock direction.
　Outside result of biopsy: papillary neoplasm.
No family history.
No comorbidities.

19.2 Important Radiologic Findings

See Figs. 34, 35 and 36.

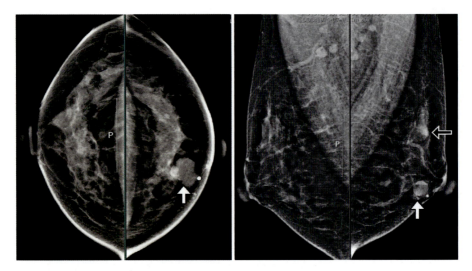

Fig. 34 Mammogram shows 2 cm oval circumscribed lobulated mass in left subareolar with BB marker (white arrow) and questionable iso-dense mass in left upper breast (black arrow)

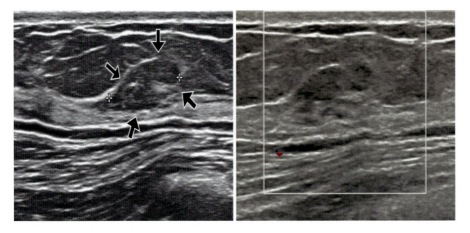

Fig. 35 Ultrasonogram shows an oval shaped, angular margin, isoechoic mass without vascularity in the left 1 o'clock direction

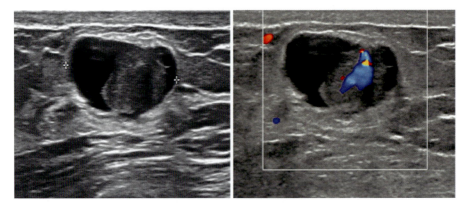

Fig. 36 Ultrasonogram shows oval shaped, circumscribed, complex cystic and solid mass with increased vascularity of solid portion in left subareolar area

19.3 Courses of Treatment

→2021-08-03 excision, Lt.

19.3.1 Pathology Report

Diagnosis
- Breast, left 1 o'clock, excision:
  - Fibroadenoma.
  - Intraductal papilloma with usual ductal hyperplasia.
- Breast, left 8 o'clock, excision:
  - Intraductal papilloma with (1) usual ductal hyperplasia, (2) microcalcification.

20 Case 20

20.1 Patient History and Progress

Female/44 years old, pre-menopause.
Screen detected microcalcification on upper outer portion of left breast.
Family history of breast cancer, sister.
No comorbidities.

20.2 Important Radiologic Findings

See Figs. 37 and 38.

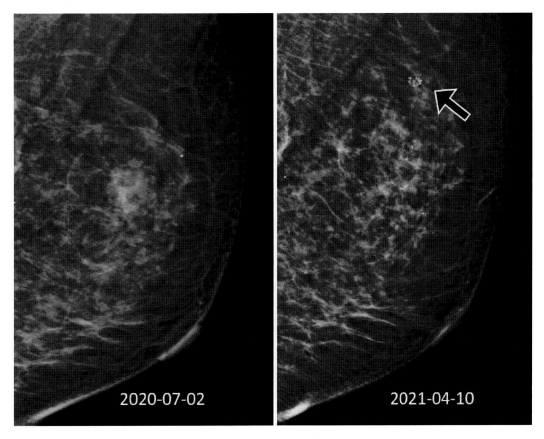

Fig. 37 Serial mammograms revealed newly developed microcalcifications in the left upper breast

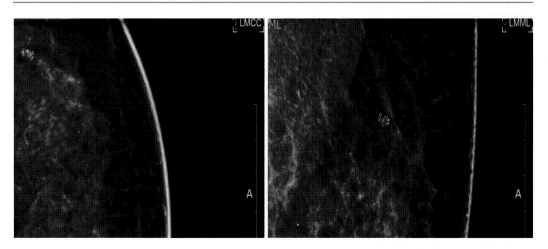

Fig. 38 Left magnification view shows grouped coarse heterogeneous microcalcifications in the upper breast

20.3　Courses of Treatment

→2021-05-10 excision, Lt.

20.3.1　Pathology Report

Diagnosis
- Breast, left, excision:
  - Atypical ductal hyperplasia.
  - Fibrocystic change with microcalcification.

21　Case 21

21.1　Patient History and Progress

Female/42 years old, pre-menopause.

Screen detected mass lesion on right breast 7 o'clock direction and left 1 o'clock direction.

Outside result of biopsy: both papillary neoplasm.

No family history.

s/p Right breast mammotome biopsy (result: fibroadenoma).

21.2　Important Radiologic Findings

See Figs. 39, 40 and 41.

21.3　Courses of Treatment

→2021-07-07 excision, both.

21.3.1　Pathology Report

Diagnosis
- Breast, left, excision:
  - Intraductal papilloma.
  - Sclerosing adenosis with microcalcification.

Diagnosis
- Breast, right, excision:
  - Intraductal papilloma.
  - Sclerosing adenosis with microcalcification.

Benign and Proliferative Case Series

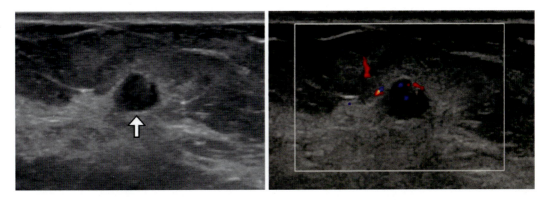

Fig. 39 Ultrasonogram shows a round circumscribed hypoechoic mass with internal vascularity in the left 1 o'clock direction

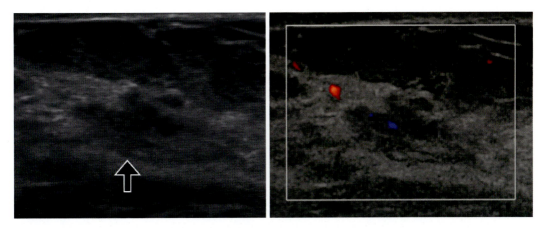

Fig. 40 Ultrasonogram shows an irregular hypoechoic mass with minimal vascularity in left 2 o'clock direction

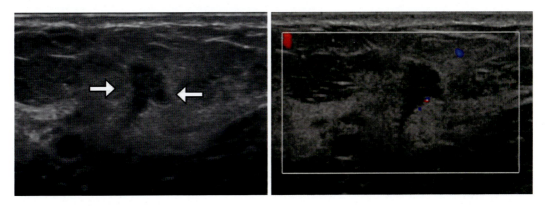

Fig. 41 Ultrasonography shows an irregular microlobulated mass without vascularity in the right 7 o'clock direction

22 Case 22

22.1 Patient History and Progress

Female/50 years old, peri-menopause.

Screen detected microcalcification on upper outer portion of right breast.

No family history.

Hypertension (taking medication), carotid atherosclerosis.

22.2 Important Radiologic Findings

See Fig. 42.

22.3 Courses of Treatment

→2021-07-07 excision, Rt.

22.3.1 Diagnosis

- Breast, right, excision:
  - Atypical ductal hyperplasia with microcalcification.

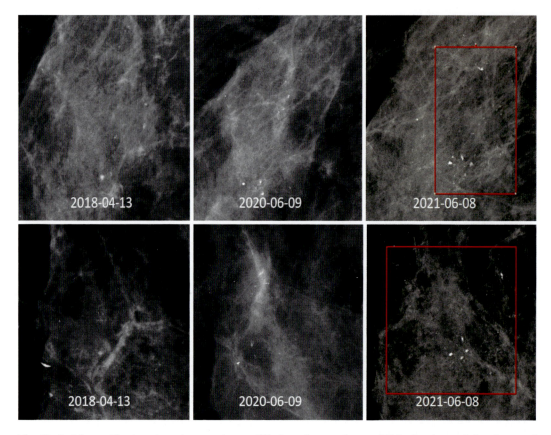

Fig. 42 Serial magnification views (upper column—CC views, lower column—MLO views) revealed an increased number of regional coarse heterogeneous microcalcifications and newly developed amorphous microcalcifications

23 Case 23

23.1 Patient History and Progress

Female/47 years old, pre-menopause.
Screen detected mass lesion on left breast 1 o'clock direction.
Outside result of biopsy: atypical papilloma.
No family history.
No comorbidities.

23.2 Important Radiologic Findings

See Figs. 43, 44 and 45.

23.3 Courses of Treatment

→2021-07-13 Excision, Lt.

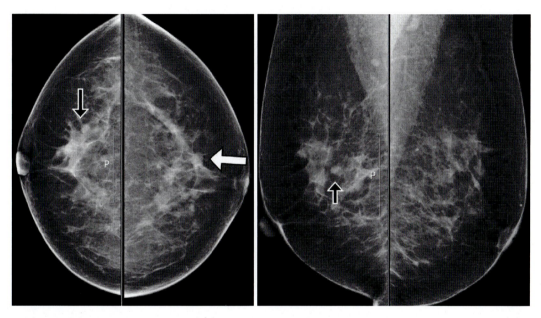

Fig. 43 Mammogram shows a round circumscribed iso-dense mass (black arrow) in the right upper outer and questionable asymmetry in left outer breast (white arrow)

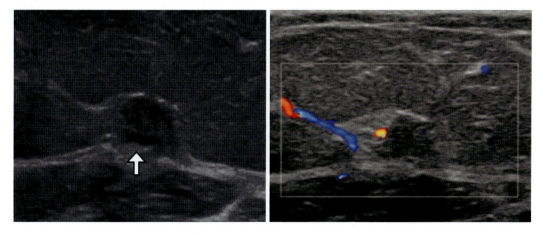

Fig. 44 Ultrasonogram shows an oval shaped, angular margin hypoechoic mass without vascularity in the left 1 o'clock direction

23.3.1 Pathology Report

Diagnosis
- Breast, left, excision:
  - Atypical ductal hyperplasia involving intraductal papilloma with microcalcification.

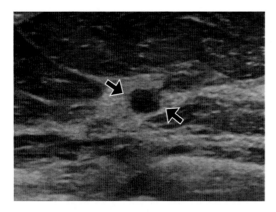

Fig. 45 Ultrasonogram shows a round circumscribed isoechoic mass in the right upper outer breast, which seems to be corresponding to the lesion detected in mammogram

24 Case 24

24.1 Patient History and Progress

Female/44 years old, pre-menopause.
Screen detected mass lesion in both breasts.
No family history.
s/p total thyroidectomy (thyroid cancer), s/p right breast excision (intraductal papilloma).

24.2 Important Radiologic Findings

See Figs. 46, 47 and 48.

24.3 Courses of Treatment

→2021-07-14 excision, both.

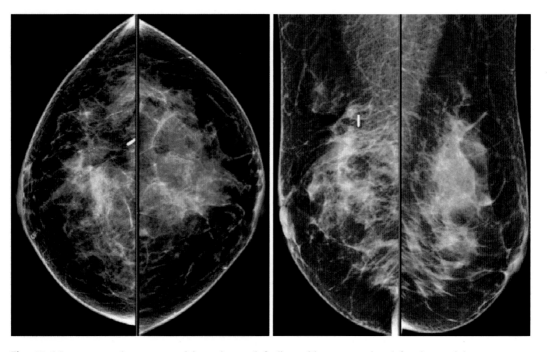

Fig. 46 Mammogram shows no suspicious abnormal finding with postoperative deformity at right upper outer portion

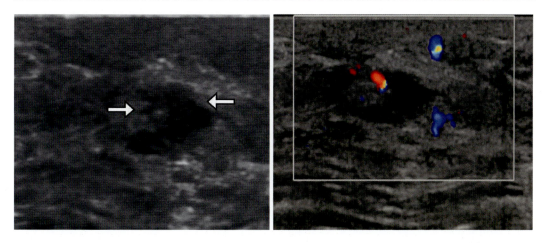

Fig. 47 US shows a 0.5 cm angular margin hypoechoic mass with adjacent increased vascularity in the left subareolar area

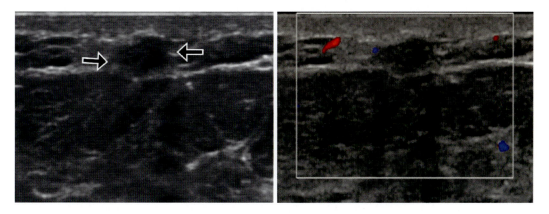

Fig. 48 US shows a 0.7 cm angular margin hypoechoic mass in the right subareolar area

24.3.1 Pathology Report

Diagnosis
- Breast, right, excision:
  – Intraductal papilloma.
    Post-excision status.
    Usual ductal hyperplasia.
    Apocrine metaplasia.
  – Sclerosing adenosis with microcalcification.

Diagnosis
- Breast, left, excision:
  – Atypical ductal hyperplasia, focal.
  – Intraductal papilloma.

25 Case 25

25.1 Patient History and Progress

Female/46 years old, pre-menopause.
Screen detected mass lesion on left breast 3 o'clock direction.
Outside result of biopsy: Intraductal papilloma.
No family history.
No comorbidities.

25.2 Important Radiologic Findings

See Figs. 49 and 50.

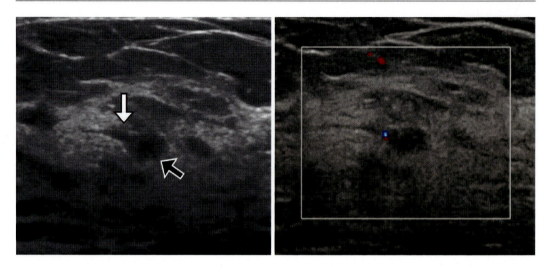

Fig. 49 US shows a 0.5 cm sized oval circumscribed hypoechoic mass (black arrow) with ductal dilatation (white arrow) and minimal vascularity

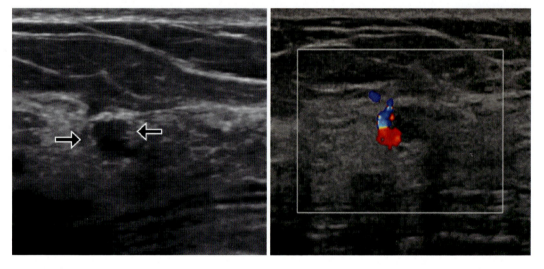

Fig. 50 US shows a 0.5 cm sized, not parallel oriented, lobulated hypoechoic mass with minimal vascularity

25.3 Courses of Treatment

→2021-07-27 excision, Lt.

25.3.1 Diagnosis
- Breast, left, excision:
  - Atypical ductal hyperplasia involving intraductal papilloma.
  - Tubular adenoma.

26 Case 26

26.1 Patient History and Progress

Female/72 years old, post-menopause.

Screen detected nodular asymmetry on outer central portion of right breast.

No family history.

s/p Total thyroidectomy (thyroid cancer).

26.2 Important Radiologic Findings

See Figs. 51 and 52.

26.3 Courses of Treatment

→2021-06-16 excision, Rt.

26.3.1 Pathology Report

Diagnosis
- Breast, right, excision:
  - Intraductal papilloma with usual ductal hyperplasia.

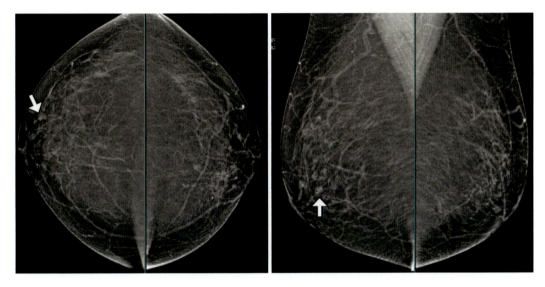

Fig. 51 Mammogram shows an oval circumscribed iso-dense mass in the right outer central breast

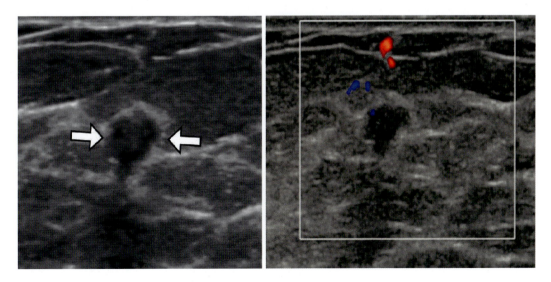

Fig. 52 Ultrasonography shows a round microlobulated hypoechoic mass without vascularity in the right 9 o'clock direction

27 Case 27

27.1 Patient History and Progress

Female/41 years old, pre-menopause.

Screen detected mass lesion on right breast 4 o'clock direction.

Outside result of biopsy: Papillary neoplasm.
No family history.
No comorbidities.

27.2 Important Radiologic Findings

See Fig. 53.

27.3 Courses of Treatment

→2021-06-07 excision, Rt.

27.3.1 Pathology Report

Diagnosis
- Breast, right, excision:
  - Intraductal papilloma with usual ductal hyperplasia.

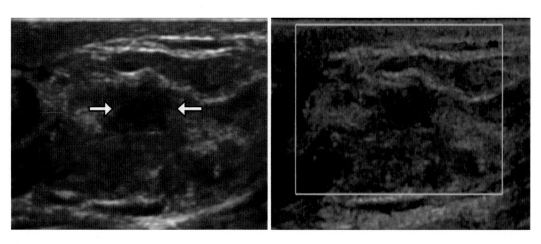

Fig. 53 The US shows a 0.7 cm irregular microlobulated hypoechoic mass with internal vascularity in the right breast

Carcinoma In Situ

Eun Sook Lee, Chan Wha Lee, Youngmi Kwon, Yunju Kim, and Bo Hwa Choi

1 Case 1

1.1 Patient History and Progress

Female/47 years old, pre-menopause.

Screen detected a mass lesion on left breast in 10 o'clock direction.

No family history of breast cancer or other cancers.

S/P Uterine myomectomy.

1.2 Important Radiologic Findings

See Figs. 1, 2, 3 and 4.

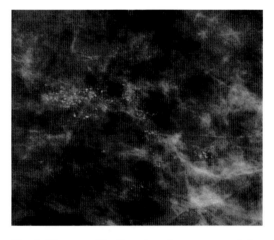

Fig. 1 The magnification view shows segmental fine pleomorphic microcalcifications

E. S. Lee
Center for Breast Cancer, National Cancer Center, Goyang, Kyonggi-do, Republic of Korea
e-mail: eslee@ncc.re.kr

C. W. Lee (✉) · B. H. Choi
Division of Diagnostic Radiology, Center for Breast Cancer, National Cancer Center, Goyang, Republic of Korea
e-mail: cwlee@ncc.re.kr; iawy82@ncc.re.kr

Y. Kwon
Department of Radiology, Center for Breast Cancer, National Cancer Center, Goyang, Gyeonggi, Republic of Korea
e-mail: ymk@ncc.re.kr

Y. Kim
Department of Pathology, National Cancer Center, Goyang, Gyeonggi, Republic of Korea
e-mail: radkyj@ncc.re.kr

© The Author(s), under exclusive license to Springer Nature Singapore Pte Ltd. 2023
E. S. Lee (ed.), *A Practical Guide to Breast Cancer Treatment*,
https://doi.org/10.1007/978-981-19-9044-1_3

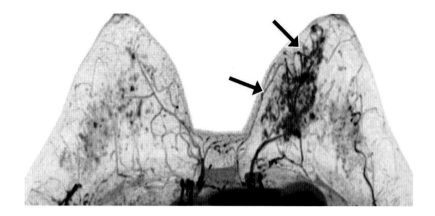

Fig. 2 MRI revealed regional heterogeneous non-mass enhancement in the left upper inner breast

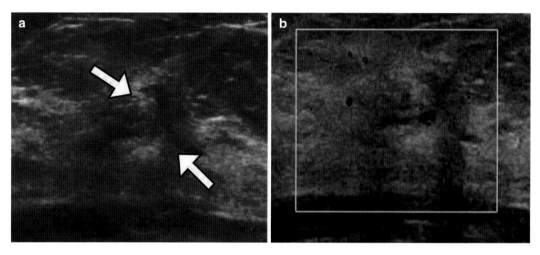

Fig. 3 US shows (**a**) a 1.5 cm irregular hypoechoic mass (white arrow) with (**b**) increased vascularity in color Doppler image

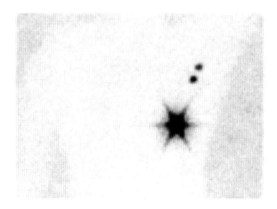

Fig. 4 Lymphoscintigraphy shows visualized sentinel lymph nodes in the left axilla

1.3 Courses of Treatment

Operation + Postoperative radiation therapy + Tamoxifen 20 mg/day for 5 years.

1.3.1 Operation

Nipple–areolar complex sparing mastectomy with immediate implant reconstruction, sentinel lymph node biopsy (Figs. 5 and 6).

1.3.2 Pathology Report

Ductal carcinoma in situ, pathological TN category (AJCC 2017): pTisN0(sn)
1. Size of tumor: 5.2 cm (pTis).
2. Nuclear grade: high.

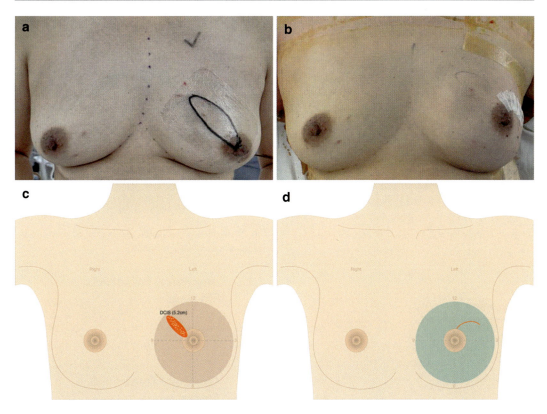

Fig. 5 (**a**, **c**) Preoperative and (**b**, **d**) immediate postoperative appearance

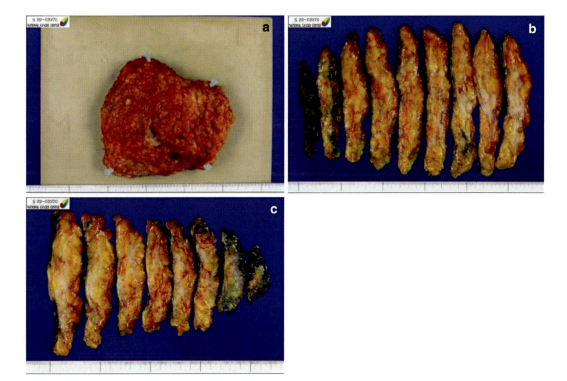

Fig. 6 (**a**) Gross pathology of mastectomy specimen. (**b**, **c**) The margins marked with color and sliced sagittally

3. Necrosis: present.
4. Architectural pattern: papillary/cribriform/solid/comedo.
5. Surgical margins:
   (a) deep margin: 6 mm,
   (b) superficial margin: subareolar margin: (see Note 1).
6. Lymph nodes: no metastasis in one axillary lymph node (pN0(sn)) (sentinel LN: 0/1).
7. Microcalcification: present, tumoral.

   Note: 1. The subareolar margin of the mastectomy specimen (slide 11) is close to ductal carcinoma in situ (<1 mm), but this margin submitted for frozen diagnosis (Fro 2) is free of tumor.

	Result	Intensity	Positive %
Estrogen receptor	Strong (8/8)	3	>2/3
Progesterone receptor	Strong (8/8)	3	>2/3
C-erbB2	Equivocal (2+)		
Ki-67	Positive in 16% of tumor cells		

2 Case 2

2.1 Patient History and Progress

Female/47 years old, pre-menopause.
Nipple discharge on left breast.
Family history of breast cancer, mother and sister, aunt, cousin sister.
Thrombocytopenia (Follow-up at outside hospital).
BRCA 2 VUS (variant of uncertain).

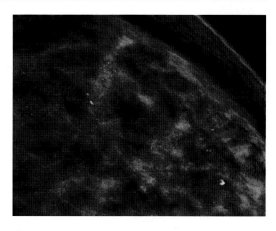

Fig. 7 Mammogram shows regional amorphous microcalcifications in the left breast

2.2 Important Radiologic Findings

See Figs. 7 and 8.

2.3 Course of Treatment: Operation

2.3.1 Operation
Excision (Figs. 9 and 10).

2.3.2 Pathology Report

Lobular carcinoma in situ
1. Size of tumor: 0.2 cm^2.
2. Nuclear grade: low.
3. Necrosis: absent.
4. Architectural pattern: solid.
5. Surgical margin: 2 mm from nearest margin.

Carcinoma In Situ

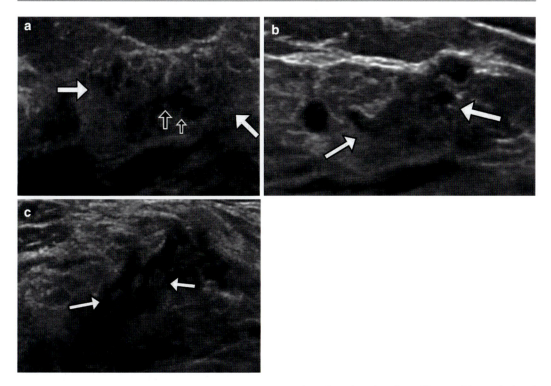

Fig. 8 US demonstrates (**a**) non-mass heterogeneous lesion (white arrow) with echogenic dots (black arrow) suggesting microcalcifications, (**b**, **c**) dilated duct with intraductal mass (white arrow). (**a**, **b**) were pathologically confirmed as intraductal papilloma with usual ductal hyperplasia and (**c**) was confirmed as lobular carcinoma in situ

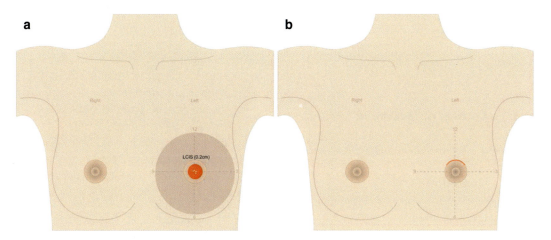

Fig. 9 (**a**) Preoperative, (**b**) immediate postoperative appearance

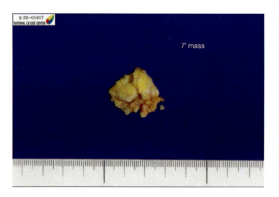

Fig. 10 Gross pathology of breast excision specimen

3 Case 3

3.1 Patient History and Progress

Female/41 years old, pre-menopause.

Screen detected microcalcifications on right breast upper outer.

Outside result of biopsy: Right 10 o'clock. 1. Usual ductal hyperplasia, 2. duct ectasia.

No family history.

S/P Hallux valgus operation.

3.2 Important Radiologic Findings

See Figs. 11 and 12.

3.3 Courses of Treatment

Operation + Tamoxifen 20 mg/day for 5 years.

3.3.1 Operation

First operation: Excision, second operation: Wide excision (Figs. 13 and 14).

3.3.2 Pathology Report
<First operation>

Lobular carcinoma in situ
1. Size of tumor: 0.3 cm.
2. Nuclear grade: low.
3. Necrosis: absent.
4. Architectural pattern: solid.

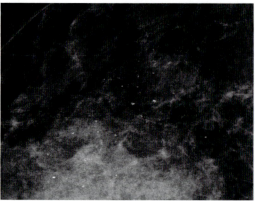

Fig. 11 Magnification view shows regional punctate and amorphous microcalcifications in the right breast

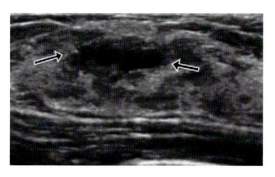

Fig. 12 US demonstrates ill-defined hypoechoic lesion with cystic area, which corresponds to the location of microcalcification

5. Surgical margins:
   (a) superior margin: <1 mm (slide 3),
   (b) inferior margin: 5 mm,
   (c) medial margin: positive (slide 4),
   (d) lateral margin: 5 mm,
   (e) deep margin: 2 mm,
   (f) superficial margin: 2 mm.
6. Microcalcification: present, tumoral/non-tumoral.

	Result	Intensity	Positive %
Estrogen receptor	Strong (7/8)	3	1/3–2/3
Progesterone receptor	Strong (8/8)	3	>2/3
C-erbB2	Negative (1+)		
Ki-67	Positive in 5% of tumor cells		

<Second operation>

Carcinoma In Situ

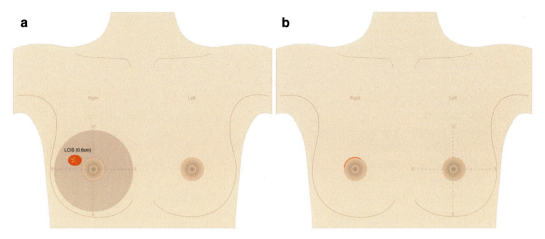

Fig. 13 (**a**) Preoperative, (**b**) immediate postoperative appearance

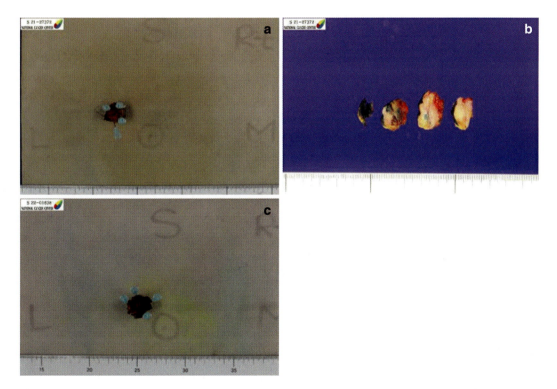

Fig. 14 (**a**, **b**) Gross pathology of breast excision specimen (first operation) and (**c**) gross pathology of wide excision specimen (second operation)

Lobular carcinoma in situ
1. Post-excision status.
2. Size of tumor: 0.3 cm, residual.
3. Nuclear grade: low.
4. Necrosis: absent.
5. Architectural pattern: solid.
6. Surgical margins:
    (a) Superior margin: 5 mm.
    (b) Inferior margin: 5 mm.
    (c) Medial margin: 5 mm.
    (d) Lateral margin: 5 mm.
    (e) Deep margin: 2 mm.
    (f) Superficial margin: 2 mm.
7. Microcalcification: present, non-tumoral.

4 Case 4

4.1 Patient History and Progress

Female/46 years old, pre-menopause.

Self-detected palpable mass on right breast 8 and 9 o'clock direction.

No family history.

No comorbidities.

BRCA 1 and 2: No detected mutation, RAD51C VUS (variant of uncertain).

4.2 Important Radiologic Findings

See Figs. 15, 16, 17 and 18.

4.3 Courses of Treatment

Operation + Postoperative radiation therapy (left side) + Tamoxifen 20 mg/day for 5 years.

4.3.1 Operation

First operation: Excision, second operation: Wide excision (Figs. 19 and 20).

4.3.2 Pathology Report

Right.
<First operation>

Lobular carcinoma in situ
1. Size of tumor: 0.2 cm.
2. Nuclear grade: low.
3. Necrosis: absent.
4. Architectural pattern: solid.
5. Surgical margins:
    (a) superior margin: 5 mm,
    (b) inferior margin: 5 mm,
    (c) medical margin: 10 mm,

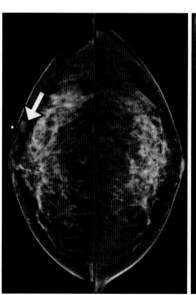
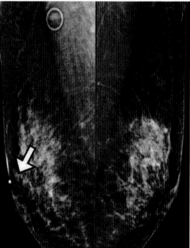

Fig. 15 Mammogram shows no suspicious mass in both breasts, except 1 cm sized circumscribed iso-dense nodule in right upper outer breast, pre-mammary fat layer (white arrow)

(d) lateral margin: 10 mm,
(e) deep margin: 2 mm,
(f) superficial margin: 2 mm.
6. Microcalcification: present, tumoral/non-tumoral.
<Second operation>

Lobular carcinoma in situ
1. Post-excision status.
2. Size of tumor: 0.2 cm, residual.
3. Nuclear grade: low.
4. Necrosis: absent.
5. Architectural pattern: solid.
6. Surgical margins:
   (a) superior margin: 5 mm,
   (b) inferior margin: 5 mm,

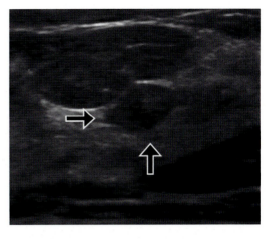

Fig. 17 US shows an oval hypoechoic mass with angular margin in the right 10 o'clock direction (black arrow), confirmed LCIS and fibroadenoma

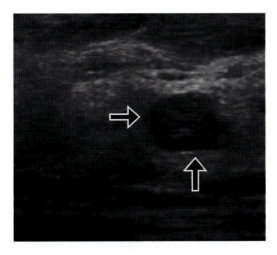

Fig. 16 US shows a round hypoechoic mass with microlobulated margin in left 12 o'clock direction (black arrow), confirmed DCIS and fibroadenoma

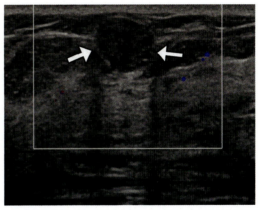

Fig. 18 Color Doppler US shows an oval isoechoic mass without vascularity in the right 10 o'clock direction, premammary fat layer (white arrow), which corresponds to MG detected lesion

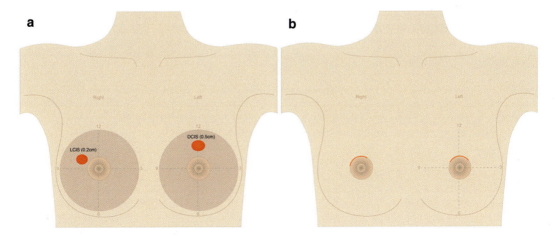

Fig. 19 (**a**) Preoperative and (**b**) immediate postoperative appearance

(c) medial margin: 10 mm,
(d) lateral margin: 30 mm (see Note 1),
(e) deep margin: 10 mm,
(f) superficial margin: 5 mm.
7. Microcalcification: present, non-tumoral.

Note: 1. Atypical ductal hyperplasia is present only in the permanent section of Frozen 10.

Left.
<First operation>

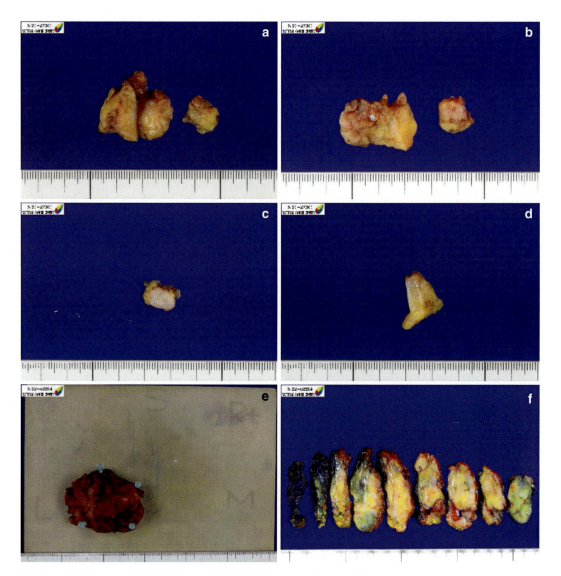

Fig. 20 (a–d) Gross pathology of right breast excision specimen (first operation). (e, f) Gross pathology of right breast wide excision specimen (second operation). (g, h) Gross pathology of left breast excision specimen (first operation). (i, j) Gross pathology of left breast wide excision specimen (second operation)

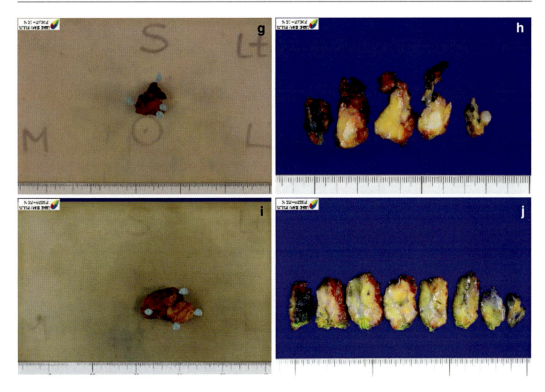

Fig. 20 (continued)

Ductal carcinoma in situ, pathological TN category (AJCC 2017): pTis
1. Size of tumor: 0.5 cm (pTis).
2. Nuclear grade: low.
3. Necrosis: absent.
4. Architectural pattern: micropapillary/cribriform.
5. Surgical margins:
   (a) superior margin: 5 mm,
   (b) inferior margin: 5 mm,
   (c) medial margin: 5 mm,
   (d) lateral margin: 5 mm,
   (e) deep margin: 2 mm,
   (f) superficial margin: 2 mm.
6. Microcalcification: present, tumoral/non-tumoral.

	Result	Intensity	Positive %
Estrogen receptor	Strong (7/8)	2	>2/3
Progesterone receptor	Strong (8/8)	3	>2/3
C-erbB2	Negative (1+)		
Ki-67	Positive in 8% of tumor cells		

<Second operation>

Ductal carcinoma in situ
1. Post-excision status.
2. Size of tumor: 0.4 cm, residual.
3. Nuclear grade: low.
4. Necrosis: absent.
5. Architectural pattern: micropapillary/cribriform.
6. Surgical margins:
   (a) superior margin: 5 mm (see Note 1),
   (b) inferior margin: 5 mm,
   (c) medial margin: (see Note 2),
   (d) lateral margin: 30 mm,
   (e) deep margin: 2 mm,
   (f) superficial margin: 2 mm.
7. Microcalcification: present, tumoral.

Note: 1. Atypical ductal hyperplasia is present only in the permanent section of Fro 1

2. The medial margin of the lumpectomy specimen (slide 4) is close to ductal carcinoma in situ (2 mm) but this margin submitted for frozen diagnosis (Fro 3) is free of tumor

5 Case 5

5.1 Patient History and Progress

Female/52 years old, pre-menopause.

Screen detected mass lesion on left breast 11, 3 and 2 o'clock direction.

Outside result of biopsy:

Left breast 11 o' clock: Intraductal proliferative lesion.

Left breast 3 o' clock: Adenosis and fibrocystic change.

Left breast 2 o'clock: Fibrocystic change.

No family history.

No comorbidities.

5.2 Important Radiologic Findings

See Figs. 21, 22, 23 and 24.

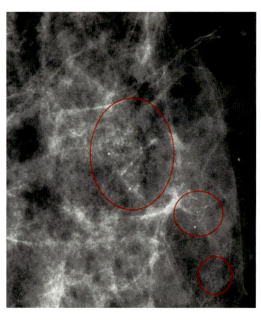

Fig. 21 Magnification view shows three groups of amorphous microcalcifications in left upper breast

5.3 Courses of Treatment

Operation + Postoperative radiation therapy.

5.3.1 Operation

Excision (Figs. 25 and 26).

5.3.2 Pathology Report

Ductal carcinoma in situ, pathological TN category (AJCC 2017): pTis
1. Size of tumor: 0.3 cm (pTis).
2. Nuclear grade: low.
3. Necrosis: absent.
4. Architectural pattern: cribriform.
5. Surgical margins:
    (a) superior margin: 5 mm,
    (b) inferior margin: 5 mm,
    (c) medial margin: <1 mm from ductal carcinoma in situ (slide 12),
    (d) lateral margin: 10 mm,
    (e) deep margin: 2 mm,
    (f) superficial margin: 2 mm.
6. Microcalcification: present, tumoral/non-tumoral.

	Result	Intensity	Positive %
Estrogen receptor	Strong (7/8)	3	1/3–2/3
Progesterone receptor	Weak (4/8)	1	10%–1/3
C-erbB2	Negative (0)		
Ki-67	Positive in <1% of tumor cells		

Carcinoma In Situ

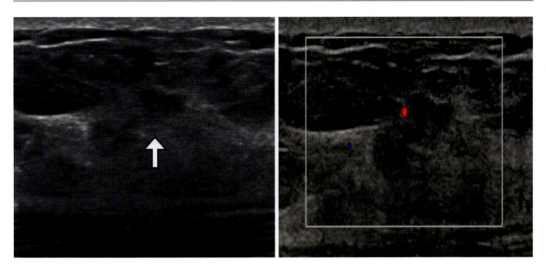

Fig. 22 US shows ill-defined hypoechoic lesion with spotty vascular signal in left 11 o'clock direction, confirmed sclerosing adenosis with microcalcification

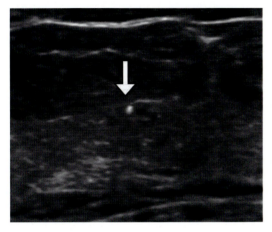

Fig. 23 US shows a few echogenic dots, suggesting microcalcifications

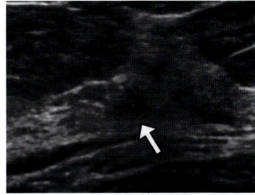

Fig. 24 US shows ill-defined triangular shaped mass in left 2 o'clock direction, confirmed DCIS

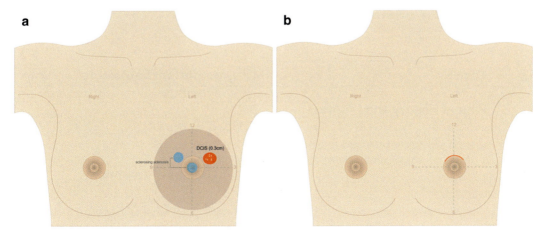

Fig. 25 (**a**) Preoperative and (**b**) immediate postoperative appearance

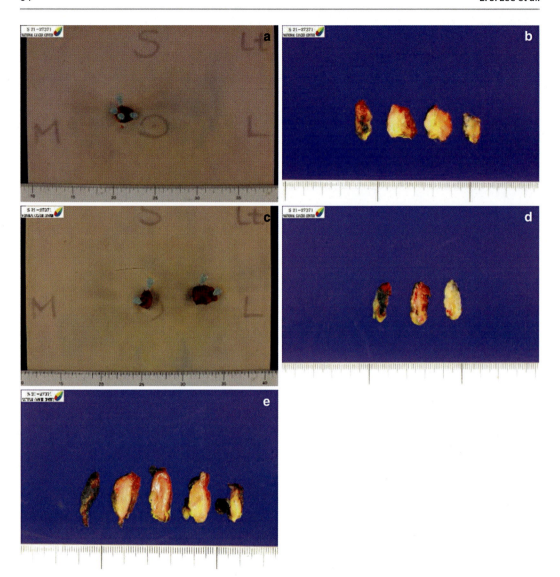

Fig. 26 (**a**, **b**) Mass in 11 o'clock direction was identified as sclerosing adenosis. (**c**, **d**) mass in 12 o'clock direction was identified as sclerosing adenosis. (**c**, **e**) mass in 2 o'clock direction (black arrow) was identified as ductal carcinoma in situ

6 Case 6

6.1 Patient History and Progress

Female/42 years old, pre-menopause.

Screen detected microcalcification on left breast upper outer.

No family history.

s/p Lt mammotome biopsy in 2018 (result: benign).

6.2 Important Radiologic Findings

See Fig. 27.

6.3 Courses of Treatment

Operation + Tamoxifen 20 mg/day for 5 years.

6.3.1 Operation

First operation: Excision, second operation: Wide excision (Figs. 28 and 29).

6.3.2 Pathology Report

<First operation>

Fig. 27 Left magnification view shows grouped amorphous microcalcifications

Ductal carcinoma in situ, pathological TN category (AJCC 2017): pTis

1. Size of tumor: 0.3 cm (pTis).
2. Nuclear grade: low.
3. Necrosis: absent.
4. Architectural pattern: micropapillary/cribriform.
5. Skin: no involvement of tumor.
6. Surgical margins: positive.
7. Microcalcification: present, tumoral/non-tumoral.

	Result	Intensity	Positive %
Estrogen receptor	Strong (7/8)	3	1/3–2/3
Progesterone receptor	Strong (8/8)	3	>2/3
C-erbB2	Equivocal (2+)		
Ki-67	Positive in 2% of tumor cells		

<Second operation>
No residual tumor with foreign body reaction.
1. Post-excision status.

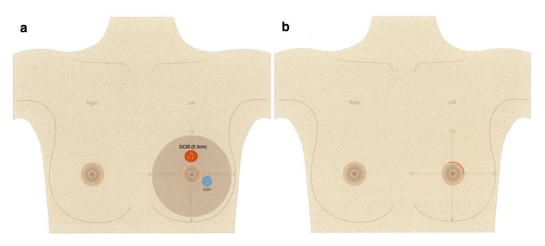

Fig. 28 (**a**) Preoperative and (**b**) immediate postoperative appearance

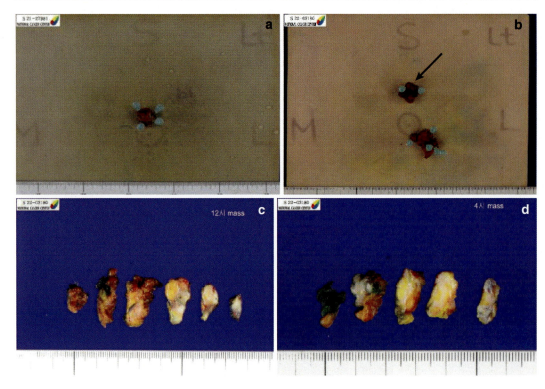

Fig. 29 (**a**) Gross pathology of left breast excision specimen (first operation). (**b–d**) Gross pathology of breast wide excision specimen (black arrow) (second operation). (**b**) Mass in 4 o'clock direction was excised and identified as atypical ductal hyperplasia

7 Case 7

7.1 Patient History and Progress

Female/48 years old, pre-menopause.

Screen detected mass lesion on right breast 1 and 9 o'clock direction.

Outside result of mammotome excision:

Right breast 1 o'clock, DCIS.

Right breast 9 o'clock, intraductal papilloma with atypical ductal hyperplasia.

No family history.

No comorbidities.

7.2 Important Radiologic Findings

See Figs. 30 and 31.

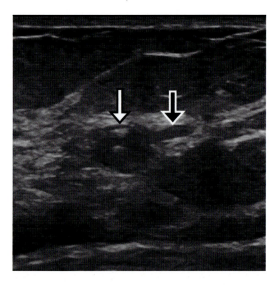

Fig. 30 Round hypoechoic mass (white arrow) with microlobulated margin and macrocalcifications within the mass. Note associated ductal dilatation (black arrow)

Carcinoma In Situ

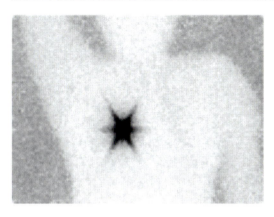

Fig. 31 Lymphoscintigraphy shows visualized sentinel lymph node in right axilla

7.3 Courses of Treatment

Operation + Postoperative radiation therapy + Tamoxifen 20 mg/day for 5 years.

7.3.1 Operation

Breast conserving surgery, sentinel lymph node biopsy (Fig. 32 and 33).

7.3.2 Pathology Report

Ductal carcinoma in situ
1. Post-mammotome excision status.
2. Size of tumor: 0.3 cm, residual.

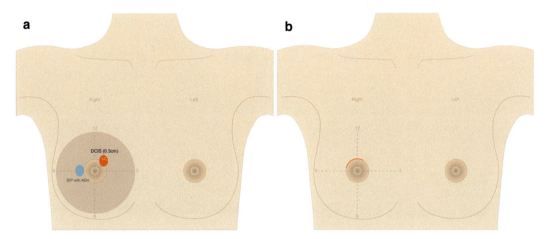

Fig. 32 (**a**) Preoperative and (**b**) immediate postoperative appearance

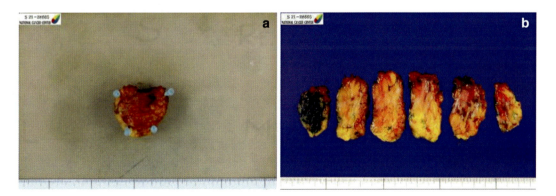

Fig. 33 Gross pathology of right breast (**a**) total (**b**) sliced lumpectomy specimen

3. Nuclear grade: low.
4. Necrosis: absent.
5. Architectural pattern: papillary/cribriform.
6. Skin: no involvement of tumor.
7. Surgical margins:
   (a) superior margin: 10 mm,
   (b) inferior margin: 10 mm,
   (c) medial margin: 5 mm,
   (d) lateral margin: 15 mm,
   (e) deep margin: 2 mm,
   (f) superficial margin: 2 mm.
8. Lymph nodes: no metastasis in one axillary lymph node (pN0(sn)) (sentinel LN: 0/1).
9. Microcalcification: present, tumoral/non-tumoral.

	Result	Intensity	Positive %
Estrogen receptor	Strong (8/8)	3	>2/3
Progesterone receptor	Strong (8/8)	3	>2/3
C-erbB2	Negative (1+)		
Ki-67	Positive in <1% of tumor cells		

8 Case 8

8.1 Patient History and Progress

Female/41 years old, pre-menopause.
   Detected bloody discharge in left nipple.
   No family history.
   No comorbidities.
   ATM VUS (variant of uncertain).

8.2 Important Radiologic Findings

See Figs. 34 and 35.

8.3 Courses of Treatment

Operation + Postoperative radiation therapy (right side) + Tamoxifen 20 mg/day for 5 years.

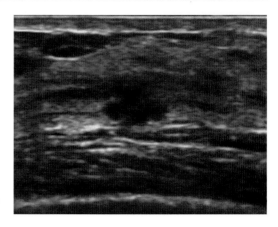

Fig. 34 US shows irregular hypoechoic mass with microlobulated margin in right breast

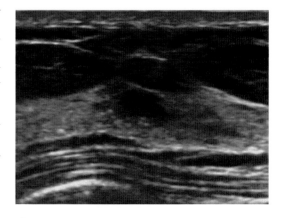

Fig. 35 US shows oval hypoechoic mass with angular margin in left breast

8.3.1 Operation
First operation: Both excision, second operation: Wide excision (right side) (Figs. 36 and 37).

8.3.2 Pathology Report
Right.
   <First operation>

Ductal carcinoma in situ, pathological TN category (AJCC 2017): pTis
1. Size of tumor: 0.3 cm (pTis).
2. Nuclear grade: low.
3. Necrosis: absent.
4. Architectural pattern: papillary.
5. Surgical margins: positive (slide 2).
6. Microcalcification: present, non-tumoral.

Carcinoma In Situ

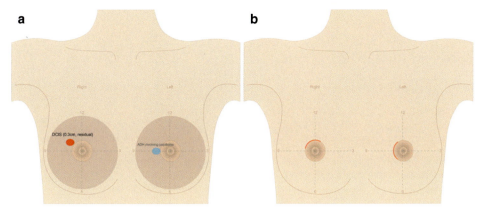

Fig. 36 (**a**) Preoperative and (**b**) immediate postoperative appearance

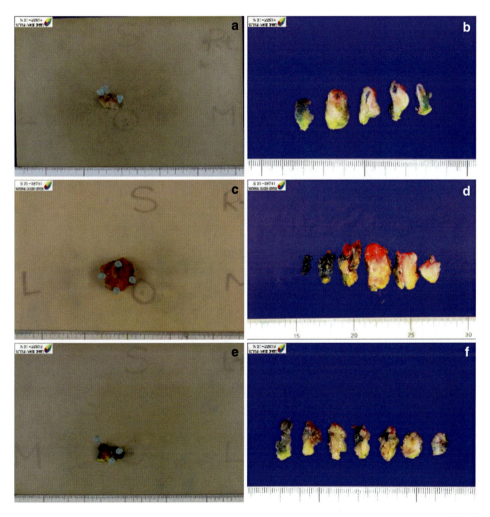

Fig. 37 (**a, b**) Gross pathology of right breast excision specimen (first operation). (**c, d**) Gross pathology of right breast wide excision specimen (second operation). (**e, f**) Gross pathology of left breast excision specimen

	Result	Intensity	Positive %
Estrogen receptor	Weak (4/8)	2	1%–10%
Progesterone receptor	Strong (8/8)	3	>2/3
C-erbB2	Equivocal (2+)		
Ki-67	Positive in 2% of tumor cells		

<Second operation>
Atypical ductal hyperplasia involving intraductal papilloma.
1. Post-excision status.

Left.
Intraductal papilloma.

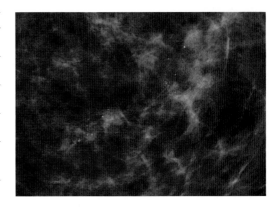

Fig. 38 Left mammography shows regional punctate or amorphous microcalcifications

9 Case 9

9.1 Patient History and Progress

Female/50 years old, pre-menopause.
 Screen detected microcalcification on inner portion of left.
 Outside result of biopsy: Ductal carcinoma in situ, left.
 Family history of breast cancer, maternal aunt.
 No comorbidities.
 BRCA 1 and 2 mutation: Not examination.

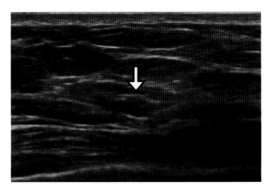

Fig. 39 US shows an irregular hypoechoic mass with angular margin

9.2 Important Radiologic Findings

See Figs. 38, 39 and 40.

9.3 Courses of Treatment

Operation + Tamoxifen 20 mg/day for 5 years.

9.3.1 Operation
Nipple–areolar complex sparing mastectomy with immediate implant reconstruction, sentinel lymph node biopsy (Figs. 41 and 42).

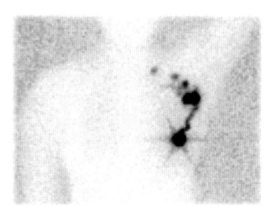

Fig. 40 Lymphoscintigraphy shows visualized sentinel lymph nodes in the left axilla

Carcinoma In Situ

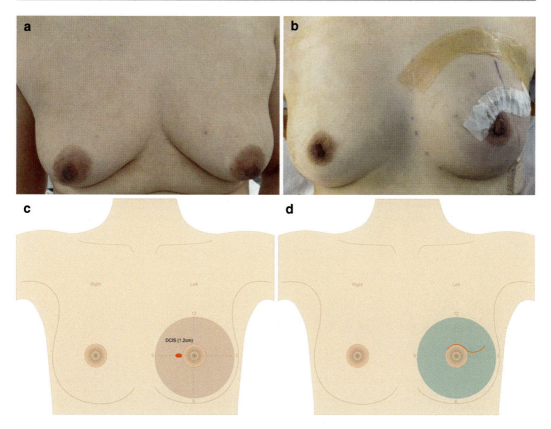

Fig. 41 (**a**, **c**) Preoperative and (**b**, **d**) immediate postoperative appearance

9.3.2 Pathology Report

Ductal carcinoma in situ, pathological TN category (AJCC 2017): pTisN0(sn)

1. Size of tumor: 1.2 cm (pTis).
2. Nuclear grade: high.
3. Necrosis: present.
4. Architectural pattern: solid/comedo.
5. Skin: no involvement of tumor.
6. Surgical margins:
    (a) deep margin: 2 mm,
    (b) superficial margin: 2 mm.
7. Lymph nodes: no metastasis in one axillary lymph node (pN0(sn)) (sentinel LN: 0/1)).
8. Microcalcification: present, tumoral/non-tumoral.

	Result	Intensity	Positive %
Estrogen receptor	Strong (8/8)	3	>2/3
Progesterone receptor	Strong (8/8)	3	>2/3
C-erbB2	Equivocal (2+)		
Ki-67	Positive in 9% of tumor cells		

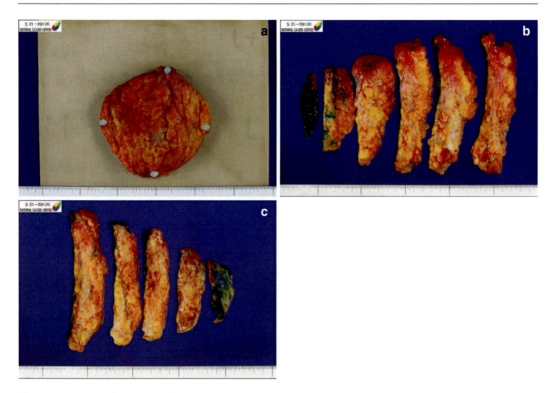

Fig. 42 (a) Gross pathology of left breast mastectomy specimen. (b, c) The margins get marked and sliced with different colors on each direction

10 Case 10

10.1 Patient History and Progress

Female/52 years old, pre-menopause.

Screen detected microcalcification on mid inner portion left breast.

Outside result of biopsy:

Left 9:30 o'clock, ductal carcinoma in situ.

Right 11 o'clock, flat epithelial atypia with microcalcification.

No family history.

BRCA 1 and 2 mutation: Not detected.

10.2 Important Radiologic Findings

See Figs. 43, 44, 45 and 46.

10.3 Courses of Treatment

Operation + Tamoxifen 20 mg/day for 5 years.

10.3.1 Operation

Nipple–areolar complex sparing mastectomy with immediate implant reconstruction, sentinel lymph node biopsy (Figs. 47 and 48).

10.3.2 Pathology Report

Ductal carcinoma in situ, pathological TN category (AJCC 2017): pTisN0(sn)
1. Size of tumor: 2.0 cm (pTis).
2. Nuclear grade: low.
3. Necrosis: absent.
4. Architectural pattern: solid.
5. Skin: no involvement of tumor.
6. Surgical margins:
    (a) deep margin: 2 mm,
    (b) superficial margin: 2 mm.

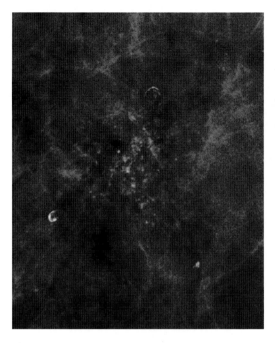

Fig. 43 Left magnification view shows grouped amorphous or fine pleomorphic microcalcifications

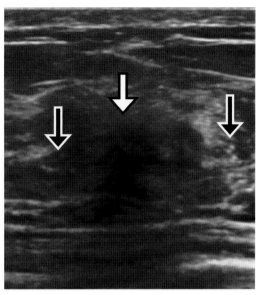

Fig. 44 US shows an irregular hypoechoic mass with indistinct margin (white arrow) and microcalcifications (black arrows) outside of the mass

Fig. 45 MRI shows focal heterogeneous non-mass enhancement

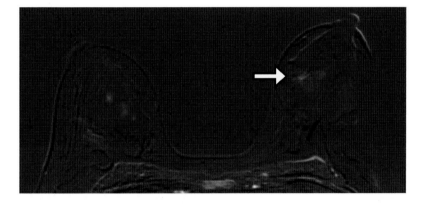

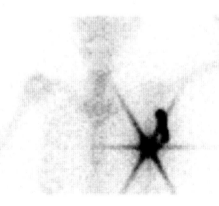

Fig. 46 Lymphoscintigraphy shows visualized sentinel lymph nodes in left axilla

7. Lymph nodes: no metastasis in one axillary lymph node (pN0(sn)) (sentinel LN: 0/1).
8. Microcalcification: present, tumoral/non-tumoral.

	Result	Intensity	Positive %
Estrogen receptor	Strong (8/8)	3	>2/3
Progesterone receptor	Intermediate (6/8)	3	10%-1/3
C-erbB2	Negative (1+)		
Ki-67	Positive in 1% of tumor cells		

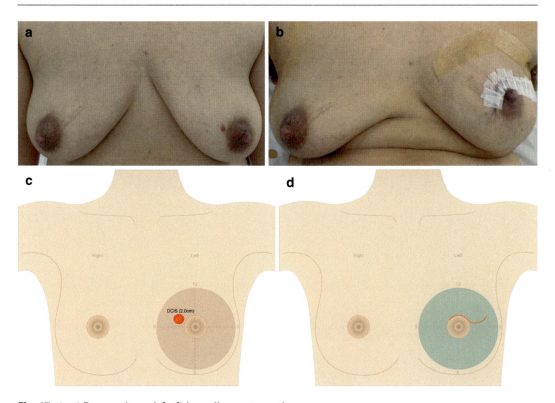

Fig. 47 (**a**, **c**) Preoperative and (**b**, **d**) immediate postoperative appearance

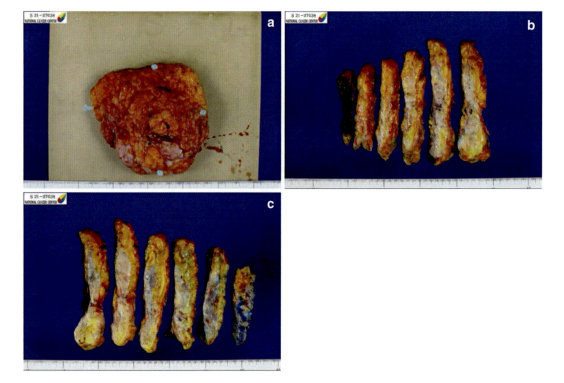

Fig. 48 (**a**) Gross pathology of left breast mastectomy specimen. (**b**, **c**) The margins get marked and sliced with different colors on each direction

11 Case 11

11.1 Patient History and Progress

Female/44 years old, pre-menopause.

Screen detected mass lesion on right breast 8 o'clock direction.

Outside result of biopsy:

Right breast, 8 o'clock, (1) adenosis, (2) fibrocystic change, (3) flat epithelial atypia.

Family history, Father: Prostate cancer.

S/P Percutaneous closure of congenital ventricular septal detected.

11.2 Important Radiologic Findings

See Fig. 49.

11.3 Courses of Treatment: Operation

11.3.1 Operation

First operation: Excision, second operation: Nipple–areolar complex sparing mastectomy with immediate implant reconstruction (Figs. 50 and 51).

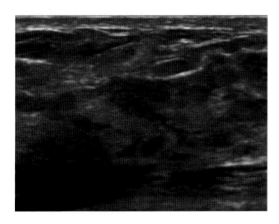

Fig. 49 US shows an irregular hypoechoic mass with microlobulated margin

11.3.2 Pathology Report

<First operation>

1. Ductal Carcinoma In Situ, Pathological TN Category (AJCC 2017): pTis
   (a) Size of tumor: 0.3 cm (pTis).
   (b) Nuclear grade: low.
   (c) Necrosis: absent.
   (d) Architectural pattern: micropapillary/cribriform.
   (e) Skin: no involvement of tumor.
   (f) Surgical margins:
       - superior margin: 10 mm,
       - inferior margin: 2 mm from ductal carcinoma in situ (slide 3),
       - medial margin: 10 mm,
       - lateral margin: <1 mm from lobular carcinoma in situ (slide 5),
       - deep margin: 2 mm,
       - superficial margin: 2 mm.
   (g) Microcalcification: present, tumoral/non-tumoral.
2. Lobular Carcinoma In Situ
   (a) Size of tumor: 0.2 cm.
   (b) Nuclear grade: low.
   (c) Necrosis: absent.
   (d) Architectural pattern: solid.

	Result	Intensity	Positive %
Estrogen receptor	Strong (8/8)	3	>2/3
Progesterone receptor	Strong (8/8)	3	>2/3
C-erbB2	Equivocal (2+)		
Ki-67	Positive in 3% of tumor cells		

<Second operation>

No residual tumor with foreign body reaction.

1. Post-excision status.

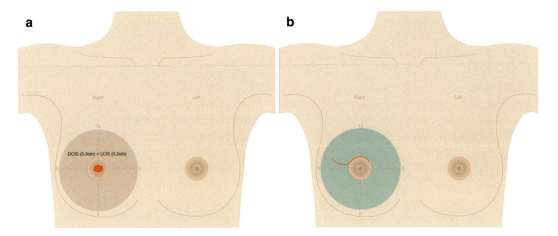

Fig. 50 (**a**) Preoperative and (**b**) immediate postoperative appearance

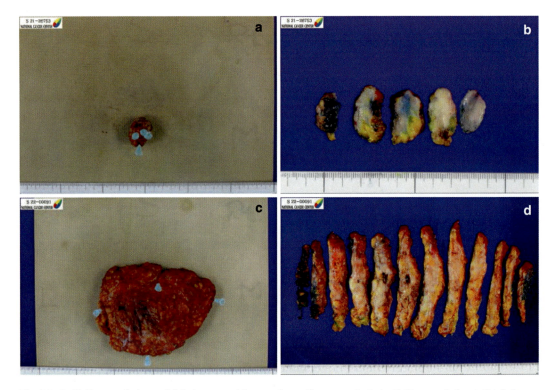

Fig. 51 (**a**, **b**) Gross pathology of right breast excision specimen (first operation). (**c**, **d**) Gross pathology of right breast mastectomy specimen

12 Case 12

12.1 Patient History and Progress

Female/49 years old, pre-menopause.

Screen detected mass lesion on right breast 4:30 and 9 o'clock direction.

Outside result of biopsy:

Left breast 4: 30 o'clock, ductal carcinoma in situ.

Left breast 9 o'clock, intraductal papilloma.

Family history of breast cancer, sister at her 48 years old.

No comorbidities.
BRCA 1 and 2 mutation: Not detected.

12.2 Important Radiologic Findings

See Figs. 52, 53 and 54.

12.3 Courses of Treatment

Operation + Tamoxifen 20 mg/day for 5 years.

12.3.1 Operation

(Robot-assisted) Nipple–areolar complex sparing mastectomy with immediate implant reconstruction, sentinel lymph node biopsy (Figs 55 and 56).

12.3.2 Pathology Report

Ductal carcinoma in situ, pathological TN category (AJCC 2017): pTisN0(sn)

1. Size of tumor: 1.0 cm (pTis).
2. Nuclear grade: high.
3. Necrosis: present.
4. Architectural pattern: cribriform/solid/comedo.
5. Surgical margins:
   (a) deep margin: 10 mm,
   (b) superficial margin: 12 mm.
6. Lymph nodes: no metastasis in two axillary lymph nodes (pN0(sn)) (sentinel LN: 0/1, left intramammary LN: 0/1).
7. Microcalcification: present, non-tumoral.

	Result	Intensity	Positive %
Estrogen receptor	Strong (8/8)	3	>2/3
Progesterone receptor	Strong (8/8)	3	>2/3
C-erbB2	Negative (1+)		
Ki-67	Positive in 16% of tumor cells		

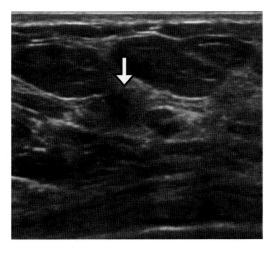

Fig. 52 US shows an irregular hypoechoic mass with angular margin

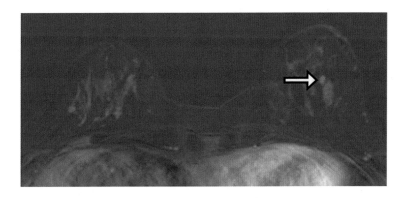

Fig. 53 MRI shows round homogeneous enhancing nodule at the corresponding area of the mass on US

Fig. 54 Lymphoscintigraphy shows visualized sentinel lymph node in left axilla

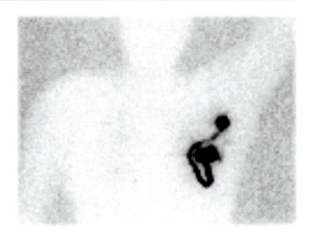

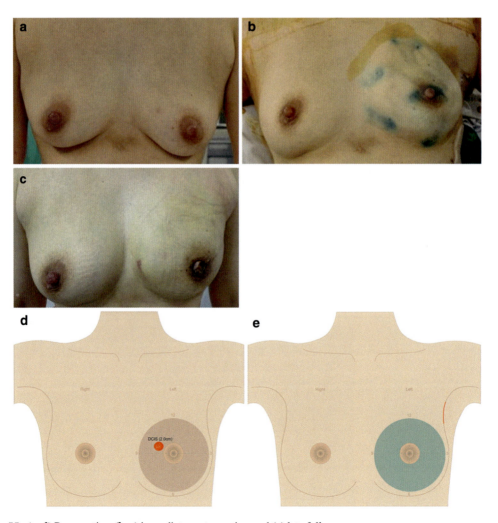

Fig. 55 (**a**, **d**) Preoperative, (**b**, **e**) immediate postoperative, and (**c**) late follow-up appearance

Carcinoma In Situ

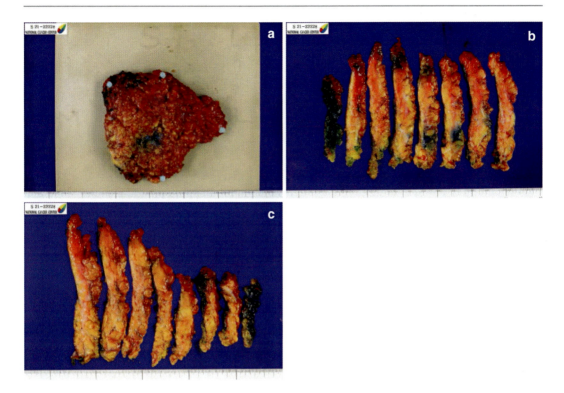

Fig. 56 (**a**) Gross pathology of left breast mastectomy specimen. (**b**, **c**) The margins get marked and sliced with different colors on each direction

13 Case 13

13.1 Patient History and Progress

Female/61 years old, post-menopause.

Screen detected mass lesion on left breast 10 o'clock direction.

Outside result of biopsy: Left breast 10 o'clock, papillary neoplasm.

Family history of breast cancer, sister.

No comorbidities.

BRCA 1 and 2: Not check.

13.2 Important Radiologic Findings

See Fig. 57.

13.3 Courses of Treatment

Operation + Tamoxifen 20 mg/day for 5 years.

13.3.1 Operation

First operation: Excision, second operation: Wide excision (Figs. 58 and 59).

13.3.2 Pathology Report

<First operation>

Ductal carcinoma in situ, pathological TN category (AJCC 2017): pTis

1. Size of tumor: 0.5 cm (pTis).
2. Nuclear grade: low.
3. Necrosis: absent.
4. Architectural pattern: papillary/cribriform.
5. Surgical margins: positive for ductal carcinoma in situ.
6. Microcalcification: present, tumoral/nontumoral.

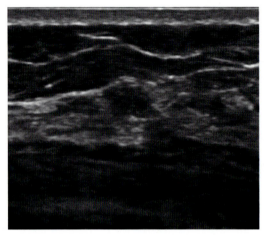

	Result	Intensity	Positive %
Estrogen receptor	Strong (8/8)	3	>2/3
Progesterone receptor	Strong (7/8)	2	>2/3
C-erbB2	Negative (0)		
Ki-67	Positive in 1% of tumor cells		

<Second operation>
No residual tumor with foreign body reaction.

1. Post-excision status.

Fig. 57 US shows an oval isoechoic mass with angular margin

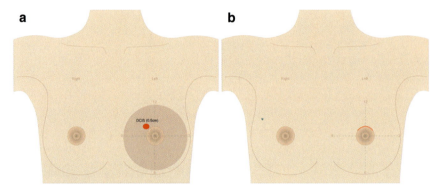

Fig. 58 (**a**) Preoperative, (**b**) immediate postoperative appearance

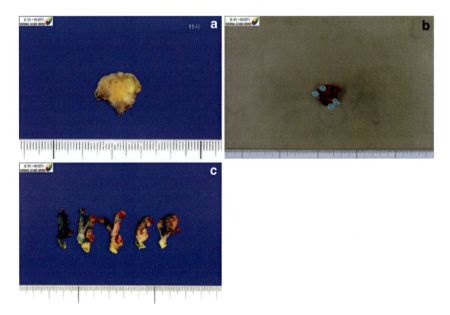

Fig. 59 (**a**) Gross pathology of left breast excision specimen (first operation). (**b**, **c**) Gross pathology of breast wide excision specimen (second operation)

14 Case 14

14.1 Patient History and Progress

Female/54 years old, pre-menopause.
Screen detected microcalcification on upper inner portion of left.
No family history.
Taking medication for bladder dysfunction.

14.2 Important Radiologic Findings

See Fig. 60.

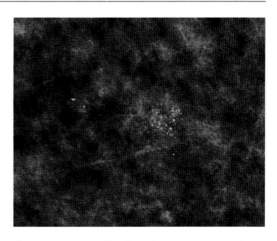

Fig. 60 Left magnification view shows grouped fine pleomorphic microcalcifications

14.3 Courses of Treatment: Operation

14.3.1 Operation
First operation: Excision, second operation: Wide excision (Figs.61 and 62).

14.3.2 Pathology Report
<First operation>

Ductal carcinoma in situ, pathological TN category (AJCC 2017): pTis
1. Size of tumor: 0.3 cm (pTis).
2. Nuclear grade: low.
3. Necrosis: absent.
4. Architectural pattern: papillary.
5. Surgical margins:
   (a) superior margin: 5 mm,
   (b) inferior margin: 7 mm,
   (c) medial margin: 20 mm,
   (d) lateral margin: positive for ductal carcinoma in situ (slide 5),
   (e) deep margin: positive for ductal carcinoma in situ (slide 5),
   (f) superficial margin: 5 mm.
6. Microcalcification: present, tumoral.

	Result	Intensity	Positive %
Estrogen receptor	Weak (4/8)	2	1%–10%
Progesterone receptor	Negative (0/8)	0	0
C-erbB2	Negative (1+)		
Ki-67	Positive in 1% of tumor cells		

<Second operation>
No residual tumor with foreign body reaction.

1. Post-excision status.
   Note: Atypical ductal hyperplasia is present only in the frozen section of Fro 1

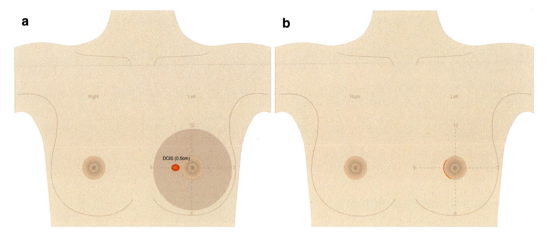

Fig. 61 (**a**) Preoperative, (**b**) immediate postoperative appearance

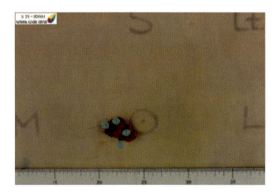

Fig. 62 Gross pathology of left breast excision specimen (first operation)

15 Case 15

15.1 Patient History and Progress

Female/52 years old, pre-menopause.
 Screen detected mass lesion on right breast 1 o'clock direction.
 No family history.
 No comorbidities.

15.2 Important Radiologic Findings

See Figs. 63, 64, 65 and 66.

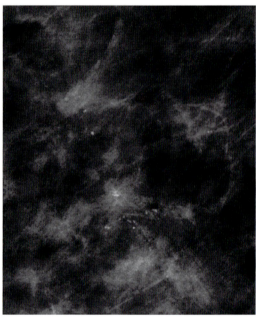

Fig. 63 Right magnification view shows grouped fine linear microcalcifications

15.3 Courses of Treatment

Operation + Postoperative radiation therapy + Tamoxifen 20 mg/day for 5 years.

15.3.1 Operation
Breast conserving surgery, sentinel lymph node biopsy (Figs. 67 and 68).

Carcinoma In Situ

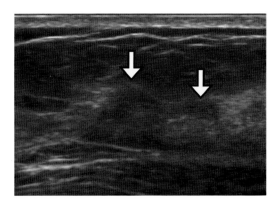

Fig. 64 US shows indistinct irregular isoechoic mass at the corresponding area of the microcalcifications on mammography

15.3.2 Pathology Report

Ductal carcinoma in situ, pathological TN category (AJCC 2017): pTisN0(sn)

1. Size of tumor: 4.0 cm (pTis).
2. Nuclear grade: high.
3. Necrosis: present.
4. Architectural pattern: micropapillary/cribriform/solid/comedo.
5. Skin: no involvement of tumor.
6. Surgical margins:
   (a) superior margin: 5 mm,
   (b) inferior margin: 15 mm,
   (c) medial margin: 10 mm,
   (d) lateral margin: 20 mm,

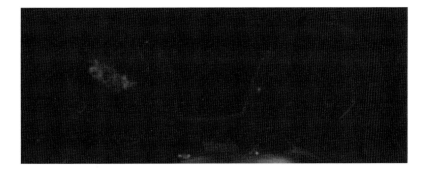

Fig. 65 MRI shows focal clumped non-mass enhancement at the corresponding area of the microcalcifications on mammography

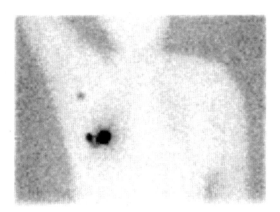

Fig. 66 Lymphoscintigraphy shows visualized sentinel lymph nodes in right axilla

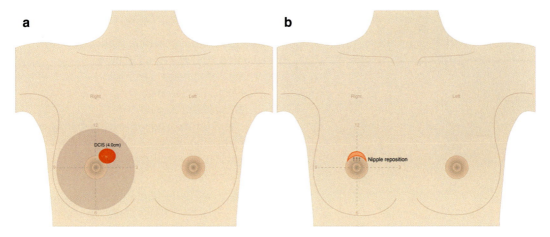

Fig. 67 (**a**) Preoperative, (**b**) immediate postoperative appearance

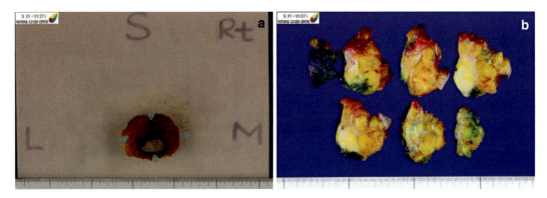

Fig. 68 (**a**) Gross pathology of right breast lumpectomy specimen. (**b**) The margins get marked and sliced with different colors on each direction

    (e) deep margin: 1 mm from ductal carcinoma in situ (slide 1),
    (f) superficial margin: 15 mm.
7. Lymph nodes: no metastasis in two axillary lymph nodes (pN0(sn)) (sentinel LN: 0/2).
8. Arteriovenous invasion: absent.
9. Lymphovascular invasion: absent.
10. Tumor border: infiltrative.
11. Microcalcification: present, tumoral/non-tumoral.

	Result	Intensity	Positive %
Estrogen receptor	Strong (7/8)	3	1/3–2/3
Progesterone receptor	Negative (0/8)	0	0
C-erbB2	Positive (3+)		
Ki-67	Positive in 11% of tumor cells		

16 Case 16

16.1 Patient History and Progress

Female/75 years old, post-menopause.

Screen detected microcalcification on left breast 12 o'clock direction.

Outside result of biopsy: Left breast 12 o'clock, fibrosis.

Family history of breast cancer, mother.

Hypertension.

BRCA 1 and 2: Not examination.

16.2 Important Radiologic Findings

See Figs. 69, 70, 71 and 72.

Carcinoma In Situ

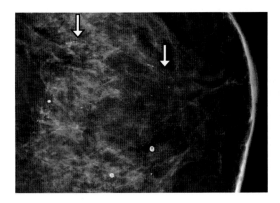

Fig. 69 Left magnification view shows regional fine pleomorphic or fine linear microcalcifications in left breast and some microcalcifications in the nipple–areolar complex

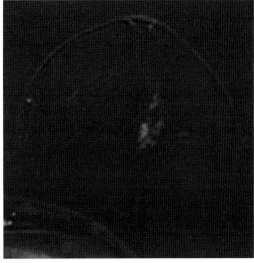

Fig. 71 MRI shows segmental heterogeneous non-mass enhancement at the corresponding area of the microcalcifications on mammography

16.3 Courses of Treatment: Operation

16.3.1 Operation

Skin sparing mastectomy with immediate implant reconstruction, sentinel lymph node biopsy (Fig. 73 and 74).

16.3.2 Pathology Report

Ductal carcinoma in situ, pathological TN category (AJCC 2017): pTis(Paget)N0 (sn)
1. Size of tumor: 1.5 cm (pTis(Paget)).
2. Nuclear grade: high.
3. Necrosis: present.

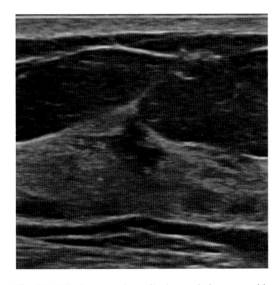

Fig. 70 US shows an irregular hypoechoic mass with associated microcalcifications

Fig. 72 Asymmetric enhancement and thickening were shown in left nipple–areolar complex

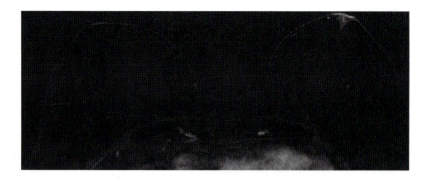

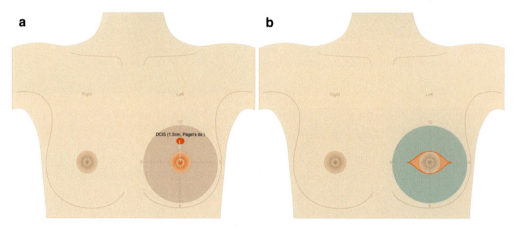

Fig. 73 (**a**) Preoperative, (**b**) immediate postoperative appearance

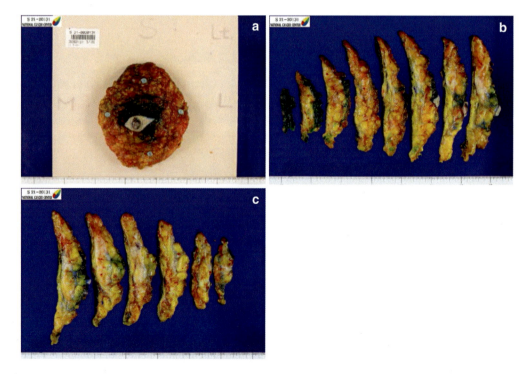

Fig. 74 (**a**) Gross pathology of left breast mastectomy specimen. (**b, c**) The margins get marked and sliced with different colors on each direction

4. Architectural pattern: cribriform/solid/comedo.
5. Nipple: Paget disease with involvement of lactiferous duct.
6. Surgical margins:
   (a) deep margin: 10 mm,
   (b) superficial margin: 10 mm.
7. Lymph nodes: no metastasis in one axillary lymph node (pN0(sn)) (sentinel LN: 0/1).
8. Microcalcification: present, tumoral/non-tumoral.

	Result	Intensity	Positive %
Estrogen receptor	Negative (2/8)	1	<1%
Progesterone receptor	Negative (0/8)	0	0
C-erbB2	Positive (3+)		
Ki-67	Positive in 30% of tumor cells		

17 Case 17

17.1 Patient History and Progress

Female/40 years old, pre-menopause.
Screen detected nodule and microcalcification on upper outer portion of right breast.
No family history.
No comorbidities.

17.2 Important Radiologic Findings

See Figs. 75, 76, 77 and 78.

17.3 Courses of Treatment

Operation + Tamoxifen 20 mg/day for 5 years.

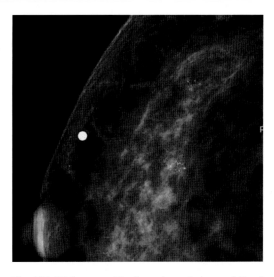

Fig. 75 Right magnification view shows multifocal grouped fine pleomorphic microcalcifications in right upper outer quadrant

17.3.1 Operation

Nipple–areolar complex sparing mastectomy with immediate implant reconstruction, sentinel lymph node biopsy (Figs 79 and 80).

17.3.2 Pathology Report

Ductal carcinoma in situ, pathological TN category (AJCC 2017): pTis(Paget)N0(sn)
1. Size of tumor: 1.5 cm (pTis(Paget)).
2. Nuclear grade: high.
3. Necrosis: present.
4. Architectural pattern: cribriform/solid/comedo.
5. Nipple: Paget disease with involvement of lactiferous duct.
6. Surgical margins:
   (a) deep margin: 10 mm,
   (b) superficial margin: 10 mm.
7. Lymph nodes: no metastasis in one axillary lymph node (pN0(sn)) (sentinel LN: 0/1).
8. Microcalcification: present, tumoral/non-tumoral.

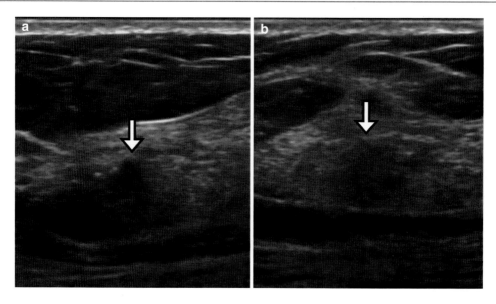

Fig. 76 US shows (**a**) an indistinct irregular hypoechoic mass with associated microcalcifications at the 11 o'clock location and (**b**) an indistinct irregular isoechoic mass at the 10 o'clock location of right breast

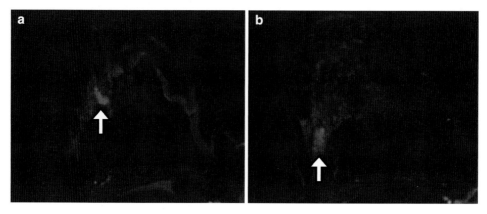

Fig. 77 MRI shows (**a**) an irregular enhancing mass with irregular margin at the 11 o'clock location and (**b**) focal homogeneous non-mass enhancement at the 10 o'clock location of right breast

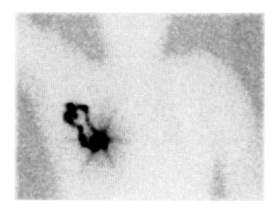

	Result	Intensity	Positive %
Estrogen receptor	Weak (3/8)	1	1%–10%
Progesterone receptor	Weak (4/8)	3	<1%
C-erbB2	Positive (3+)		
Ki-67	Positive in 11% of tumor cells		

Fig. 78 Lymphoscintigraphy shows visualized sentinel lymph nodes in right axilla

Carcinoma In Situ

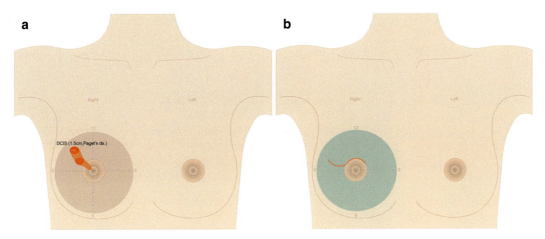

Fig. 79 (**a**) Preoperative, (**b**) immediate postoperative appearance

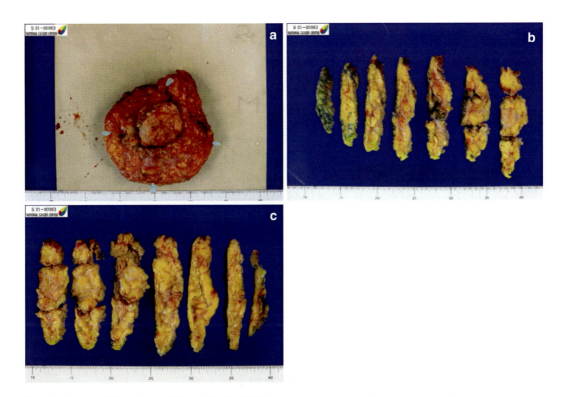

Fig. 80 Gross pathology (**a**: total, **b**, **c**: sliced) of right breast mastectomy specimen

18 Case 18

18.1 Patient History and Progress

Female/64 years old, post-menopause.

Screen detected mass lesion on right breast 8 o'clock direction.

Outside result of biopsy:

Right breast 8 o'clock, atypical intraductal papillary neoplasm, favor ductal carcinoma in situ.

No family history.

Hypertension, diabetes mellitus.

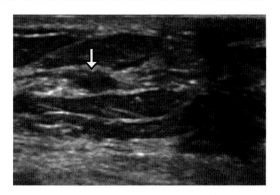

Fig. 81 US shows a microlobulated oval hypoechoic mass

18.2 Important Radiologic Findings

See Figs. 81 and 82.

18.3 Courses of Treatment

Operation + Postoperative radiation therapy.

18.3.1 Operation

Breast conserving surgery (Figs. 83 and 84).

18.3.2 Pathology Report

Ductal carcinoma in situ, pathological TN category (AJCC 2017): pTis
1. Size of tumor: 1.1 cm (pTis).
2. Nuclear grade: low.
3. Necrosis: present.
4. Architectural pattern: micropapillary/cribriform/solid.
5. Surgical margins:
    (a) superior margin: 20 mm,
    (b) inferior margin: (see Note 1),
    (c) medial margin: 5 mm,
    (d) lateral margin: (see Note 2),
    (e) deep margin: 2 mm,
    (f) superficial margin: 5 mm.
6. Microcalcification: present, non-tumoral.

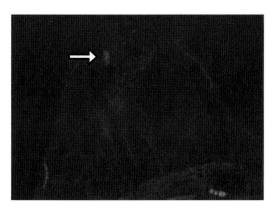

Fig. 82 MRI shows an irregular enhancing mass with irregular margin at the corresponding area of the mass on US

Note: 1. The inferior margin of the lumpectomy specimen (slide 5) is close to ductal carcinoma in situ (2 mm) but this margin submitted for frozen diagnosis (Fro 3) is free of tumor.

2. The lateral margin of the lumpectomy specimen (slide 6) is close to ductal carcinoma in situ (2 mm) but this margin submitted for frozen diagnosis (Fro 7) is free of tumor.

	Result	Intensity	Positive %
Estrogen receptor	Strong (8/8)	3	>2/3
Progesterone receptor	Strong (8/8)	3	>2/3
C-erbB2	Negative (1+)		
Ki-67	Positive in 5% of tumor cells		

Carcinoma In Situ

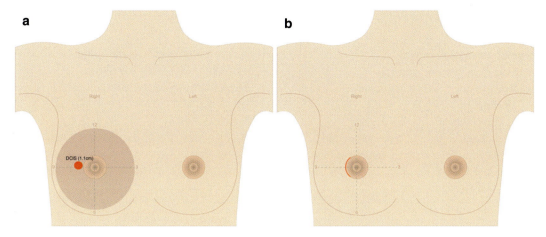

Fig. 83 (**a**) Preoperative, (**b**) immediate postoperative appearance

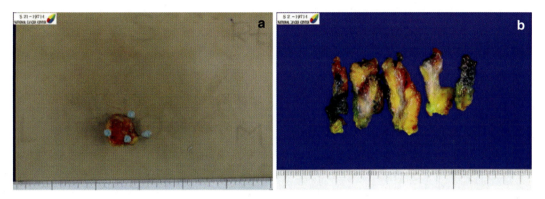

Fig. 84 (**a**, **b**) Gross pathology of right breast lumpectomy specimen. (**b**) The margins get marked and sliced with different colors on each direction

19 Case 19

19.1 Patient History and Progress

Female/48 years old, pre-menopause.

Screen detected diffuse non-mass lesions on upper, central, and lower portion of left breast.

Screen detected microcalcification on inner subareolar of right breast.

Outside result of excisional biopsy: bilateral ductal carcinoma in situ.

No family history.

S/P L-spine operation.

BRCA 1 and 2 mutation: Not detected.

19.2 Important Radiologic Findings

See Figs. 85, 86, 87, and 88.

19.3 Courses of Treatment: Operation

19.3.1 Operation

Both nipple–areolar complex sparing mastectomy with immediate implant reconstruction, sentinel lymph node biopsy (Figs. 89 and 90).

19.3.2 Pathology Report

Right.

Ductal carcinoma in situ

1. Post-mammotome status.
2. Size of tumor: 0.3 cm, residual.
3. Nuclear grade: high.
4. Necrosis: absent.
5. Architectural pattern: cribriform/solid.
6. Skin and nipple: no involvement of tumor.
7. Surgical margins:
   (a) deep margin: 5 mm,
   (b) superficial margin: <1 mm from ductal carcinoma in situ (slide 11).
8. Lymph nodes: no metastasis in two axillary lymph nodes (pN0(sn)) (sentinel LN: 0/2).

9. Microcalcification: present, tumoral.

Left.

Ductal carcinoma in situ, pathological TN category (AJCC 2017): pTisN0(sn)

1. Size of tumor: 6.0 cm (pTis).
2. Nuclear grade: low.
3. Necrosis: absent.
4. Architectural pattern: micropapillary/cribriform/solid.
5. Skin and nipple: no involvement of tumor.
6. Surgical margins: (see note).
   (a) deep margin: 1 mm from ductal carcinoma in situ (slide 4),
   (b) superficial margin: <1 mm from ductal carcinoma in situ (slide 8).
7. Lymph nodes: no metastasis in three axillary lymph nodes (pN0(sn)) (sentinel LN: 0/3).
8. Microcalcification: present, tumoral.

   Note: 1. Atypical ductal hyperplasia is present only in the permanent section of Fro 3.

	Result	Intensity	Positive %
Estrogen receptor	Strong (8/8)	3	>2/3
Progesterone receptor	Strong (8/8)	3	>2/3
C-erbB2	Negative (1+)		
Ki-67	Positive in 14% of tumor cells		

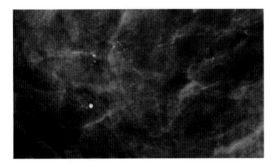

Fig. 85 Right magnification view shows regional amorphous or fine pleomorphic microcalcifications in right inner breast

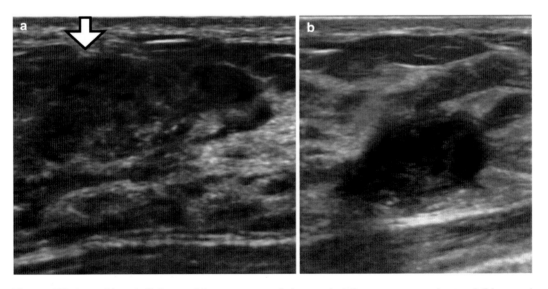

Fig. 86 US shows (**a**) an indistinct oval heterogeneous echoic mass in left upper outer quadrant and (**b**) an oval hypoechoic mass, suggesting stereotactic biopsy-related hematoma at the 1 o'clock direction of the right breast

Carcinoma In Situ

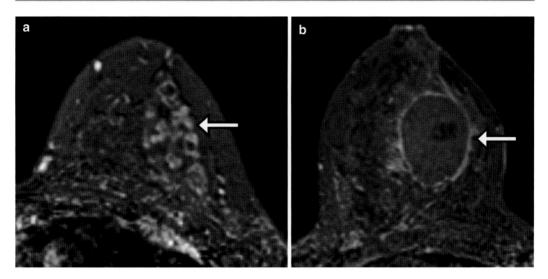

Fig. 87 MRI shows (**a**) segmental clustered ring non-mass enhancement in left upper outer quadrant and (**b**) stereotactic biopsy-related hematoma with thin marginal enhancement at the 1 o'clock direction of the right breast

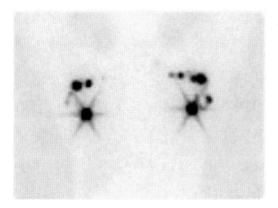

Fig. 88 Lymphoscintigraphy shows visualized sentinel lymph nodes in both axilla

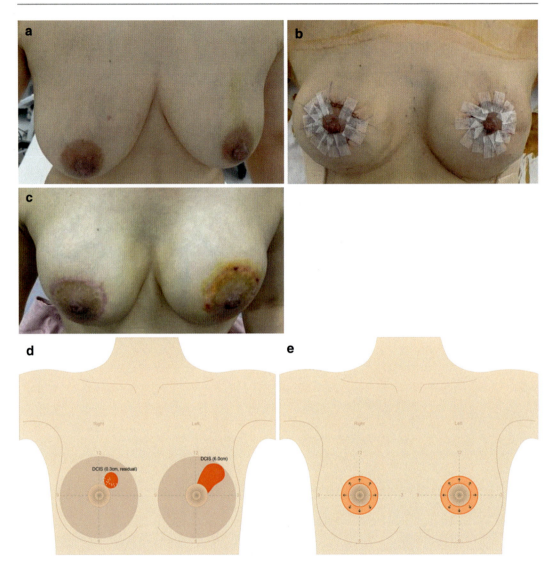

Fig. 89 (**a**, **d**) Preoperative, (**b**, **e**) immediate postoperative, and (**c**) late follow-up appearance

Carcinoma In Situ

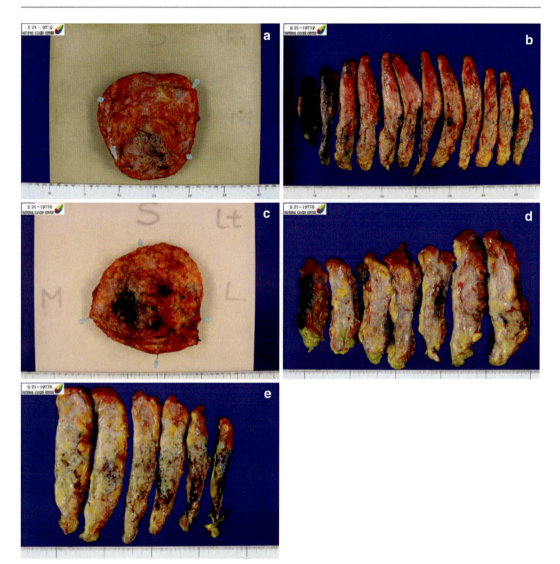

Fig. 90 (**a**, **b**) Gross pathology of right mastectomy specimen. (**c–e**) Gross pathology of left mastectomy specimen

20 Case 20

20.1 Patient History and Progress

Female/48 years old, pre-menopause.
Screen detected mass lesion on left breast 3 o'clock direction at first visit.
Pain on right breast at second visit.
No family history.
No comorbidities.
NGS: negative.

20.2 Important Radiologic Findings

See Figs. 91 and 92.

20.3 Courses of Treatment

First Operation + Tamoxifen 20 mg/day for 4 months.
Second Operation.

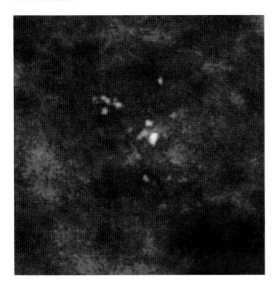

Fig. 91 Right magnification view shows grouped punctate or amorphous microcalcifications

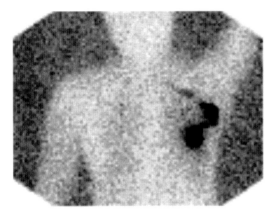

Fig. 92 Lymphoscintigraphy shows visualized sentinel lymph nodes in left axilla

20.3.1 Operation

First operation: Breast conserving surgery, sentinel lymph node biopsy (left).

Second operation: Skin sparing mastectomy with latissimus dorsi flap reconstruction (left).

Third operation: Excision (right).

Fourth operation: Wide excision (right) (Figs. 93 and 94).

20.3.2 Pathology Report

Left.

<First operation>

Invasive ductal Carcinoma, pathologic stage (AJCC 2010): pT1aN0(sn)

1. Size of invasive component: 0.5 cm (pT1a).
2. Size of intraductal component: 4.0 cm.
3. Histologic grade: 2/3 (tubule formation: 3/3, nuclear pleomorphism: 2/3, mitotic count: 1/3, 5/10HPF).
4. Intraductal component: present, intratumoral/extratumoral (90%) (nuclear grade: low, necrosis: absent, architectural pattern: solid and papillary, extensive intraductal component: present).
5. Skin: no involvement of tumor.
6. Surgical margins:
   (a) superior margin: 3 mm from atypical ductal hyperplasia (slide 1),
   (b) inferior margin: (see Note 1),
   (c) medial margin: (see Note 2),
   (d) lateral margin: 40 mm,
   (e) deep margin: positive for ductal carcinoma in situ (slide 9),
   (f) superficial margin: 3 mm.
7. Lymph nodes: no metastasis in seven axillary lymph nodes (pN0(sn)) (sentinel LN: 0/7, axillary LN: 0/0).
8. Vascular invasion: absent.
9. Lymphatic invasion: absent.
10. Tumor border: pushing.
11. Microcalcification: present, non-tumoral.

Note: 1. Atypical ductal hyperplasia is present only in the permanent section of Fro 3. The inferior margin of the lumpectomy specimen (slides 2, 5, 7, 9, and 11) is positive for ductal carcinoma in site 2. The medial margin of the lumpectomy specimen (slide 3) is close to ductal carcinoma in situ (1 mm) but this margin submitted for frozen diagnosis (Fro 4) is free of tumor.

	Result	Intensity	Positive %
Estrogen receptor	Strong (8/8)	3	>2/3
Progesterone receptor	Strong (8/8)	3	>2/3
C-erbB2	Negative (1+)		
Ki-67	Positive in 29% of tumor cells		

<Second operation>

Carcinoma In Situ

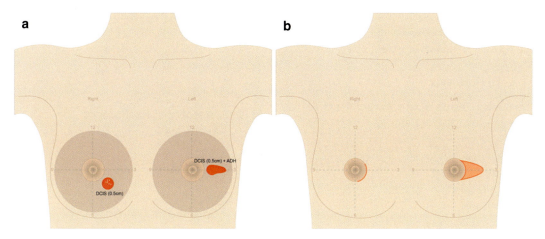

Fig. 93 (**a**) Preoperative, (**b**) immediate postoperative appearance

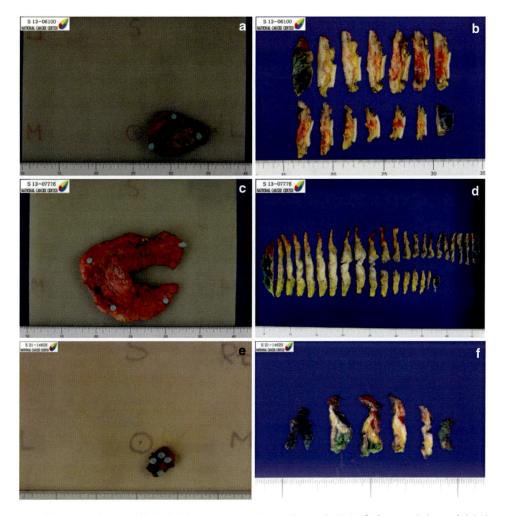

Fig. 94 (**a**, **b**) Gross pathology of left partial mastectomy specimen (first operation). (**c**, **d**) Gross pathology of left mastectomy specimen after breast conserving surgery (second operation). (**e**, **f**) Gross pathology of right breast excision specimen (third operation)

1. Atypical ductal hyperplasia, focal.
    (a) Post-lumpectomy status.
2. No residual tumor with foreign body reaction. Right.
    <Third operation>

Ductal carcinoma in situ, pathological TN category (AJCC 2017): pTis
1. Size of tumor: 0.5 cm (pTis).
2. Nuclear grade: low.
3. Necrosis: absent.
4. Architectural pattern: micropapillary/cribriform.
5. Skin: no involvement of tumor.
6. Surgical margins:
    (a) superior margin: 10 mm,
    (b) inferior margin: 10 mm,
    (c) medial margin: <1 mm from ductal carcinoma in situ (slide 6),
    (d) lateral margin: 5 mm,
    (e) deep margin: 2 mm,
    (f) superficial margin: 2 mm.
7. Microcalcification: present, tumoral/non-tumoral.

	Result	Intensity	Positive %
Estrogen receptor	Strong (8/8)	3	>2/3
Progesterone receptor	Strong (7/7)	3	>2/3
C-erbB2	Negative (0)		
Ki-67	Positive in <1% of tumor cells		

<Fourth operation>
No residual tumor with foreign body reaction.
1. Post-excision status.

21 Case 21

21.1 Patient History and Progress

Female/37 years old, pre-menopause.
Screen detected mass lesion on right breast 9 o'clock direction.
Outside result of biopsy: Right 9 o'clock, ductal carcinoma in situ.
No family history.

Thyroid papillary carcinoma: follow-up at outside hospital.
BRCA 1 and 2: not detected, POLE VUS (variant of uncertain).

21.2 Important Radiologic Findings

See Figs. 95, 96 and 97.

21.3 Courses of Treatment

Operation + Postoperative radiation therapy + Tamoxifen 20 mg/day for 5 years.

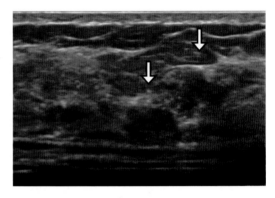

Fig. 95 US shows irregular hypoechoic masses with angular margin

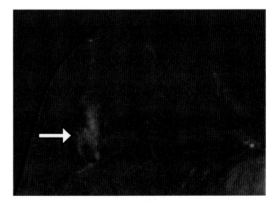

Fig. 96 MRI shows linear heterogeneous non-mass enhancement

21.3.1 Operation

Breast conserving surgery, sentinel lymph node biopsy (Figs. 98 and 99).

21.3.2 Pathology Report

Ductal carcinoma in situ, pathological TN category (AJCC 2017): pTisN0 (sn)

1. Size of tumor: 3.0 cm (pTis).
2. Nuclear grade: low.
3. Necrosis: absent.
4. Architectural pattern: papillary/micropapillary/cribriform/solid.
5. Skin: no involvement of tumor.
6. Surgical margins:
   (a) superior margin: 20 mm,
   (b) inferior margin: (see Note 1),
   (c) medial margin: (see Note 2),
   (d) lateral margin: 20 mm,
   (e) deep margin: <1 mm from ductal carcinoma in situ (slides 2 and 6),
   (f) superficial margin: <1 mm from ductal carcinoma in situ (slide 3).
7. Lymph nodes: no metastasis in two axillary lymph nodes (pN0(sn)) (sentinel LN: 0/2).
8. Microcalcification: present, tumoral/nontumoral.

   Note: 1. The inferior margin of the lumpectomy specimen (slide 9) is positive for ductal carcinoma in situ but this margin submitted for frozen diagnosis (Fro 2) is free of tumor.
   2. The medial margin of the lumpectomy specimen (slide 4) is close to ductal carcinoma in situ (2 mm) and atypical ductal hyperplasia is present only in the permanent section of Fro 3.

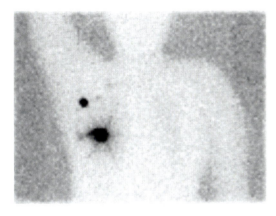

Fig. 97 Lymphoscintigraphy shows visualized sentinel lymph node in right axilla

	Result	Intensity	Positive %
Estrogen receptor	Strong (8/8)	3	>2/3
Progesterone receptor	Strong (8/8)	3	>2/3
C-erbB2	Negative (1+)		
Ki-67	Positive in 5% of tumor cells		

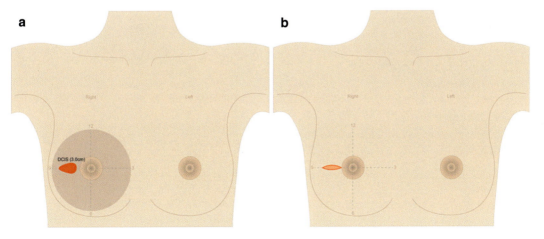

Fig. 98 (**a**) Preoperative, (**b**) immediate postoperative appearance

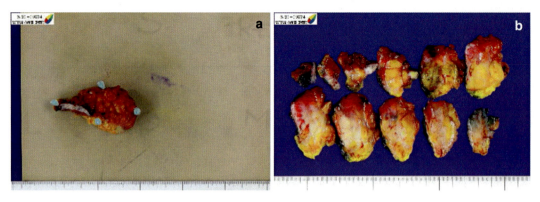

Fig. 99 (**a**, **b**) Gross pathology of right breast lumpectomy specimen. (**b**) The margins get marked and sliced with different colors on each direction

22 Case 22

22.1 Patient History and Progress

Female/57 years old, post-menopause.
 Visible detected redness on Left nipple.
 Outside result of biopsy: Paget's disease.
 Family history of breast cancer, sister at her 45 years old.
 No comorbidities.
 BRCA 1 and 2 mutation: Not detected.

22.2 Important Radiologic Findings

See Figs. 100, 101 and 102.

22.3 Courses of Treatment: Operation

22.3.1 Operation
Skin sparing mastectomy with immediate implant reconstruction, sentinel lymph node biopsy. (Figs. 103 and 104).

22.3.2 Pathology Report

Ductal carcinoma in situ, pathological TN category (AJCC 2017): pTis(Paget)N0(sn)
1. Size of tumor: 0.5 cm (pTis(Paget)).
2. Nuclear grade: high.
3. Necrosis: absent.
4. Architectural pattern: micropapillary.
5. Nipple: Paget disease with involvement of lactiferous duct.
6. Surgical margins: deep margin: 20 mm.
7. Lymph nodes: no metastasis in two axillary lymph nodes (pN0(sn)) (sentinel LN: 0/2).
8. Microcalcification: present, non-tumoral.

	Result	Intensity	Positive %
Estrogen receptor	Negative (0/8)	0	0
Progesterone receptor	Negative (0/8)	0	0
C-erbB2	Positive (3+)		
Ki-67	Positive in 14% of tumor cells		

Carcinoma In Situ

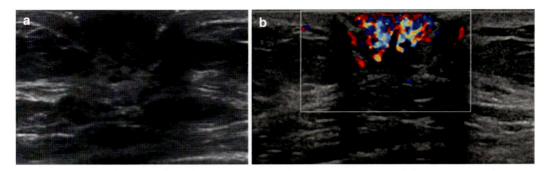

Fig. 100 (**a, b**) US shows mildly enlarged left nipple with increased vascularity

Fig. 101 MRI shows asymmetric strong enhancement and thickening of left nipple–areolar complex

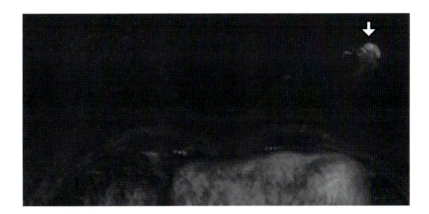

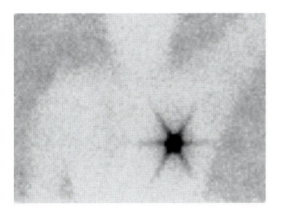

Fig. 102 Lymphoscintigraphy shows visualized sentinel lymph node in left axilla

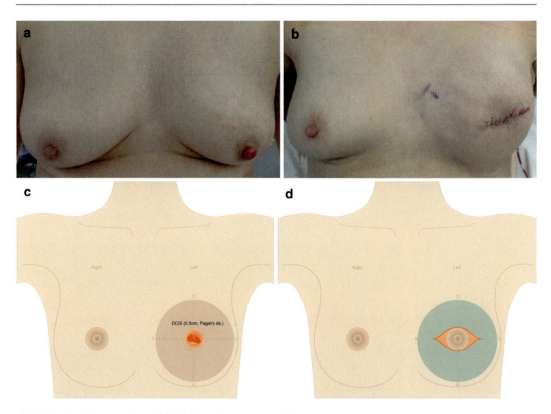

Fig. 103 (**a**, **c**) Preoperative and (**b**, **d**) immediate postoperative appearance

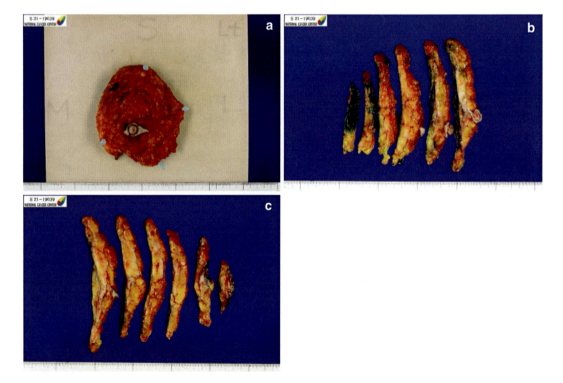

Fig. 104 (**a**) Gross pathology of left breast mastectomy specimen. (**b**, **c**) The margins get marked and sliced with different colors on each direction

23 Case 23

23.1 Patient History and Progress

Female/44 years old, pre-menopause.
Screen detected microcalcification on upper outer portion of right breast.
No family history.
No comorbidities.

23.2 Important Radiologic Findings

See Figs. 105 and 106.

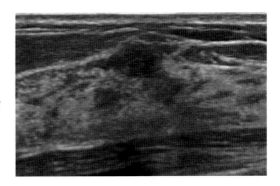

Fig. 106 US shows an irregular hypoechoic mass with angular margin at the corresponding area of the microcalcifications on mammography

23.3 Courses of Treatment: Operation

23.3.1 Operation
Excision (Figs. 107 and 108).

23.3.2 Pathology Report

Lobular carcinoma in situ, pathological TN category (AJCC 2017): pTis

1. Size of tumor: 0.5 cm (pTis).
2. Nuclear grade: low.
3. Necrosis: absent.
4. Architectural pattern: solid.
5. Skin: no involvement of tumor.
6. Surgical margins:
    (a) superior margin: <1 mm (slide 3),
    (b) inferior margin: 20 mm,
    (c) medial margin: 5 mm,
    (d) lateral margin: 5 mm,
    (e) deep margin: 10 mm,
    (f) superficial margin: 1 mm (slide 1).
7. Microcalcification: present, tumoral.

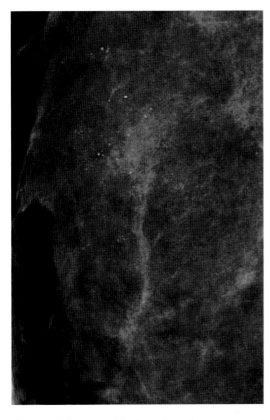

Fig. 105 Right magnification view shows segmental round or amorphous microcalcifications

	Result	Intensity	Positive %
Estrogen receptor	Strong (7/8)	3	1/3–2/3
Progesterone receptor	Strong (8/8)	3	>2/3
C-erbB2	Negative (1+)		
Ki-67	Positive in 7% of tumor cells		

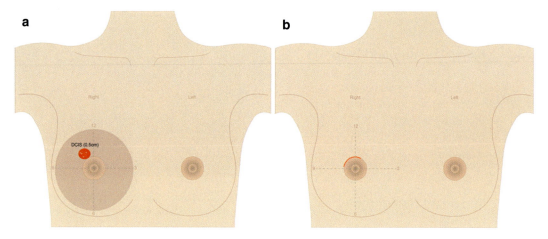

Fig. 107 (a) Preoperative and (b) immediate postoperative appearance

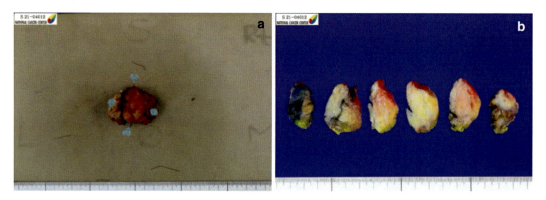

Fig. 108 (a) Gross pathology of right breast excision specimen. (b) The margins get marked and sliced with different colors on each direction

24 Case 24

24.1 Patient History and Progress

Female/42 years old, pre-menopause.

Screen detected mass lesion on left breast 2 o'clock direction.

Outside result of biopsy: Left breast 2 o'clock, fibroadenoma, favor lobular carcinoma in situ.

No family history.

S/P Retinal detachment operation 15 years ago.

24.2 Important Radiologic Findings

See Figs. 109, 110, 111.

24.3 Courses of Treatment: Operation

24.3.1 Operation

Breast conserving surgery (Fig 112 and 113).

Carcinoma In Situ

Fig. 109 Asymmetry was only seen on one view, the mediolateral oblique view

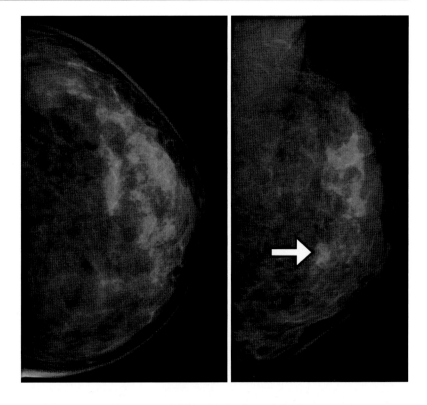

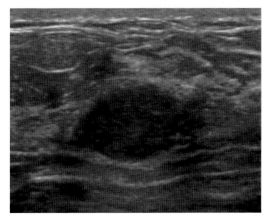

Fig. 110 US shows a microlobulated oval hypoechoic mass in left upper outer quadrant

24.3.2 Pathology Report

Lobular carcinoma in situ, pathological TN category (AJCC 2017): pTis
1. Size of tumor: 1.3 cm (pTis).
2. Nuclear grade: low.
3. Necrosis: absent.
4. Architectural pattern: solid.
5. Surgical margins:

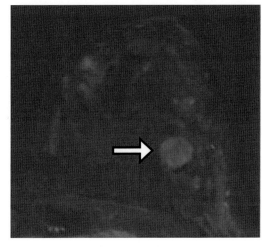

Fig. 111 MRI shows a circumscribed homogeneously enhancing mass at the 2 o'clock location of the left breast

   (a) superior margin: 11 mm,
   (b) inferior margin: 3 mm,
   (c) medial margin: 15 mm,
   (d) lateral margin: 15 mm,
   (e) deep margin: 2 mm,
   (f) superficial margin: 4 mm.
6. Microcalcification: absent.

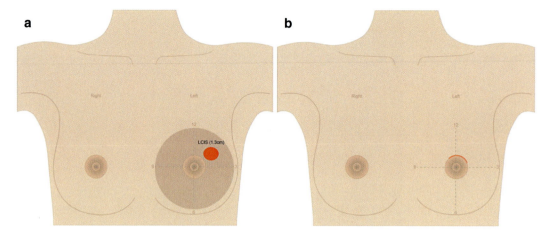

Fig. 112 (**a**) Preoperative and (**b**) immediate postoperative appearance

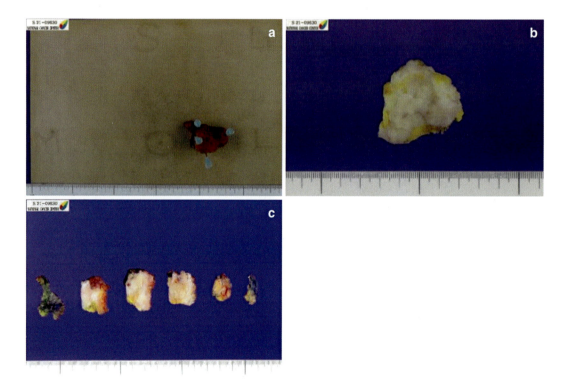

Fig. 113 (**a**) Gross pathology of left breast lumpectomy specimen. (**b**, **c**) The margins get marked and sliced with different colors on each direction

Carcinoma In Situ

	Result	Intensity	Positive %
Estrogen receptor	Strong (8/8)	3	>2/3
Progesterone receptor	Strong (8/8)	3	>2/3
C-erbB2	Equivocal (2+)		
Ki-67	Positive in 6% of tumor cells		

25 Case 25

25.1 Patient History and Progress

Female/52 years old, pre-menopause.

Screen detected mass lesion on left breast 1 o'clock direction.

Outside result of biopsy: Left breast 1 o'clock, ductal carcinoma in situ, r/o invasion.

No family history.

S/P Robotic cholecystectomy (GB stone).

BRCA 1 and 2: Not examination.

25.2 Important Radiologic Findings

See Figs. 114 and 115.

25.3 Courses of Treatment

Operation + Postoperative radiation therapy (Left) + Tamoxifen 20 mg/day for 5 years.

25.3.1 Operation
Both breast conserving surgery, sentinel lymph node biopsy (left) (Figs. 116 and 117).

25.3.2 Pathology Report
Right.

Lobular carcinoma in situ
1. Size of tumor: 0.3 cm.
2. Nuclear grade: low.
3. Necrosis: absent.
4. Architectural pattern: solid.
5. Skin: no involvement of tumor.

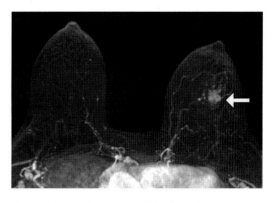

Fig. 114 MRI of a woman with known left breast cancer. MRI shows an irregular enhancing mass in the left breast (arrow). No signs of malignancy are present in the right breast. Right mammography and US were also negative (not shown). Left BCS and right reduction mammoplasty were performed. Pathology confirmed LCIS in the right breast

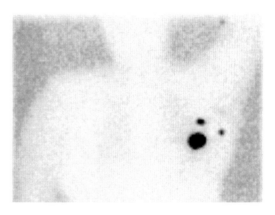

Fig. 115 Lymphoscintigraphy shows visualized sentinel lymph nodes in left axilla

6. Surgical margins:
   (a) superior margin: 2 mm,
   (b) inferior margin: 5 mm,
   (c) medial margin: 2 mm,
   (d) lateral margin: 2 mm,
   (e) deep margin: 2 mm,
   (f) superficial margin: 2 mm.
7. Microcalcification: present, tumoral/non-tumoral.
   Left.

Invasive ductal carcinoma, pathological TN category (AJCC 2017): pT1cN0(sn)
1. Size of invasive component: 1.5 cm (pT1c).
2. Size of intraductal component: 5.0 cm.

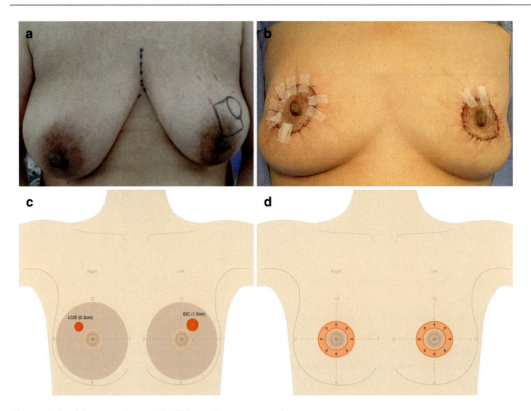

Fig. 116 (**a, c**) Preoperative and (**b, d**) immediate postoperative appearance

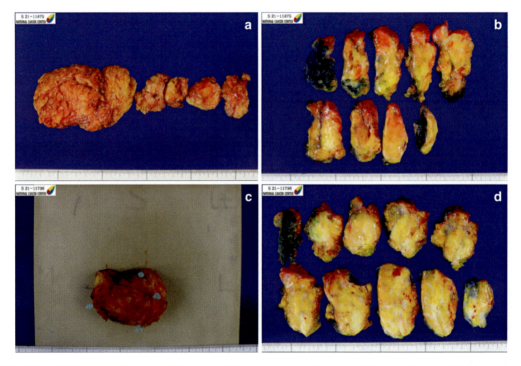

Fig 117 (**a, b**) Gross pathology of right breast partial mastectomy specimen. (**c, d**) Gross pathology of left breast partial mastectomy specimen

3. Histologic grade: 3/3 (tubule formation: 3/3, nuclear pleomorphism: 3/3, mitotic count: 3/3, 4/HPF).
4. Intraductal component: present, intratumoral/extratumoral (70%) (nuclear grade: high, necrosis: present, architectural pattern: cribriform/solid/comedo, extensive intraductal component: present).
5. Skin: no involvement of tumor.
6. Surgical margins:
   (a) superior margin: 5 mm,
   (b) inferior margin: 10 mm,
   (c) medial margin: 10 mm,
   (d) lateral margin: 10 mm,
   (e) deep margin: 2 mm,
   (f) superficial margin: <1 mm from ductal carcinoma in situ (slide 2).
7. Lymph nodes: no metastasis in one axillary lymph node (pN0(sn)) (sentinel LN: 0/1).
8. Arteriovenous invasion: absent.
9. Lymphovascular invasion: present, intratumoral.
10. Tumor border: infiltrative.
11. Microcalcification: present, tumoral/non-tumoral.

	Result	Intensity	Positive %
Estrogen receptor	Strong (7/8)	3	1/3–2/3
Progesterone receptor	Strong (7/8)	3	1/3–2/3
C-erbB2	Equivocal (2+)		
Ki-67	Positive in 25% of tumor cells		

26 Case 26

26.1 Patient History and Progress

Female/48 years old, pre-menopause.
Screen detected mass and microcalcification on upper portion of right breast.
No family history.
No comorbidities.

26.2 Important Radiologic Findings

See Figs. 118, 119 and 120.

26.3 Courses of Treatment

Operation + Tamoxifen 20 mg/day for 5 years.

26.3.1 Operation
Excision (Figs. 121 and 122).

26.3.2 Pathology Report
Lobular carcinoma in situ, pathological TN category (AJCC 2017): pTis
1. Size of tumor: up to 0.6 cm (pTis).
2. Nuclear grade: low.

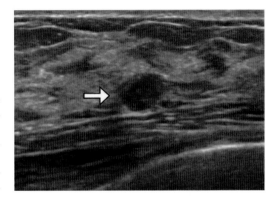

Fig. 118 Breast US shows an oval hypoechoic mass with partly microlobulated margins

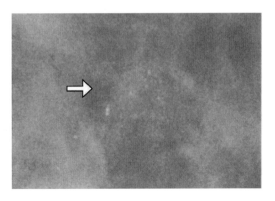

Fig. 119 Magnification view revealed grouped amorphous microcalcifications at the corresponding area of the mass

3. Necrosis: absent.
4. Architectural pattern: solid.
5. Surgical margins:

   (a) superior margin: 5 mm,
   (b) inferior margin: 5 mm,
   (c) medial margin: 10 mm,
   (d) lateral margin: 20 mm,
   (e) deep margin: 5 mm,
   (f) superficial margin: <1 mm from lobular carcinoma in situ (slide 2).
6. Microcalcification: absent.

	Result	Intensity	Positive %
Estrogen receptor	Intermediate (6/8)	2	1/3–2/3
Progesterone receptor	Strong (8/8)	3	>2/3
C-erbB2	Equivocal (2+)		
Ki-67	Positive in 4% of tumor cells		

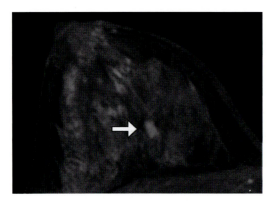

Fig. 120 MRI demonstrates an oval enhancing mass

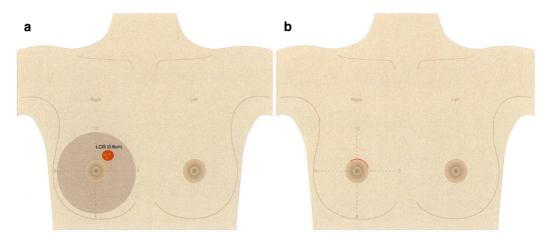

Fig. 121 (**a**) Preoperative and (**b**) immediate postoperative appearance

Carcinoma In Situ

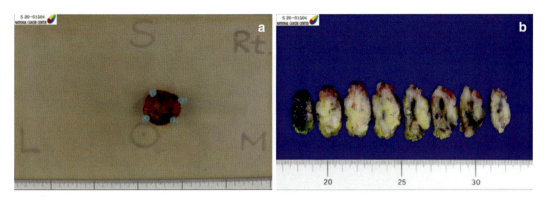

Fig. 122 (**a**) Gross pathology of right breast excision specimen. (**b**) The margins get marked and sliced with different colors on each direction

27 Case 27

27.1 Patient History and Progress

Female/50 years old, pre-menopause.

Screen detected mass lesion on left breast 2 o'clock direction.

Outside result of mammotome biopsy: Lobular carcinoma in situ.

No family history.

27.2 Important Radiologic Findings

See Figs. 123, 124 and 125.

27.3 Courses of Treatment

Operation + Tamoxifen 20 mg/day for 5 years.

27.3.1 Operation
Breast conserving surgery (Figs. 126 and 127).

27.3.2 Pathology Report

Lobular carcinoma in situ, pathological TN category (AJCC 2017): pTis
1. Size of tumor: 1.5 cm(pTis).
2. Nuclear grade: low.

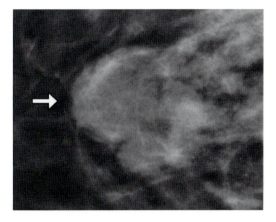

Fig. 123 Mammography shows an obscured mass

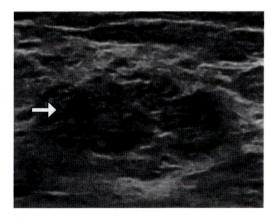

Fig. 124 US reveals an irregular hypoechoic mass. US-guided VAB = LCIS

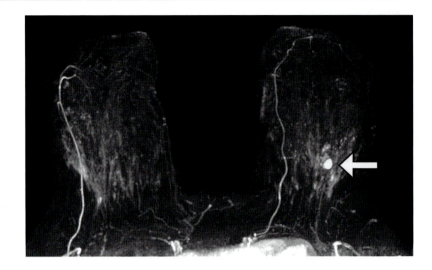

Fig. 125 MRI demonstrates an enhancing residual mass in the left breast

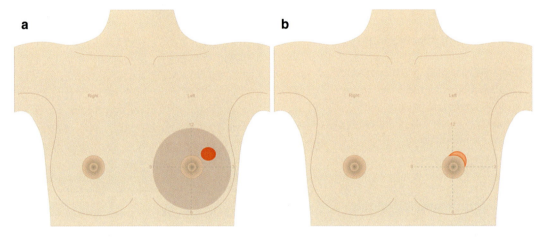

Fig. 126 (**a**) Preoperative and (**b**) immediate postoperative appearance

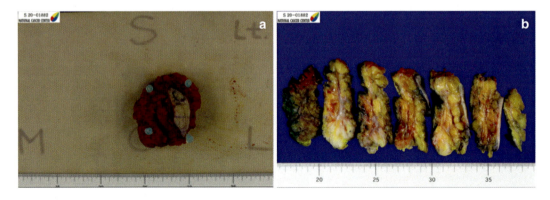

Fig. 127 (**a**) Gross pathology of left breast partial mastectomy specimen. (**b**) The margins get marked and sliced with different colors on each direction

3. Necrosis: absent.
4. Architectural pattern: solid.
5. Skin: no involvement of tumor.
6. Surgical margins:
   (a) superior margin: 50 mm,
   (b) inferior margin: (see Note 1),
   (c) medial margin: 5 mm,
   (d) lateral margin: 10 mm,
   (e) deep margin: positive for lobular carcinoma in situ (slide 1),
   (f) superficial margin: 5 mm.
7. Microcalcification: absent.

   Note: 1. The inferior margin of the lumpectomy specimen (slide 4) is close to lobular carcinoma in situ (<1 mm) but this margin submitted for frozen diagnosis (Fro 2) is free of tumor.

	Result	Intensity	Positive %
Estrogen receptor	Strong (7/8)	2	>2/3
Progesterone receptor	Strong (7/8)	2	>2/3
C-erbB2	Negative (0)		
Ki-67	Positive in 2% of tumor cells		

28 Case 28

28.1 Patient History and Progress

Female/50 years old, pre-menopause.

Screen detected microcalcification on upper outer portion of right breast.

Outside result of stereotactic excisional biopsy: Lobular carcinoma in situ.

No family history.

No comorbidities.

28.2 Important Radiologic Findings

See Figs. 128, 129 and 130.

28.3 Courses of Treatment

Operation + Tamoxifen 20 mg/day for 5 years.

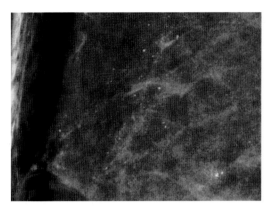

Fig. 128 Magnification view shows regional amorphous microcalcifications. Stereotactic VAB = LCIS

28.3.1 Operation

Breast conserving surgery (Figs. 131 and 132).

28.3.2 Pathology Report

Lobular carcinoma in situ, pathological TN category (AJCC 2017): pTis

1. Size of tumor: 0.7 cm (pTis).
2. Nuclear grade: low.
3. Necrosis: absent.
4. Architectural pattern: solid.
5. Skin: No involvement of tumor.
6. Surgical margins:
   (a) superior margin: (see Note),
   (b) inferior margin: 25 mm,
   (c) medial margin: 10 mm,
   (d) lateral margin: 20 mm,
   (e) deep margin: 5 mm,
   (f) superficial margin: 2 mm.
7. Microcalcification: absent.

   Note: 1. The superior margin of the lumpectomy specimen (slide 1) is close to lobular carcinoma in situ (1 mm) but this margin submitted for frozen diagnosis (Fro 1) is free of tumor.

	Result	Intensity	Positive %
Estrogen receptor	Intermediate (6/8)	1	>2/3
Progesterone receptor	Strong (7/8)	2	>2/3
C-erbB2	Negative (1+)		
Ki-67	Positive in 6% of tumor cells		

Fig. 129 Biopsy clip (white arrow) was inserted after stereotactic VAB. On MRI, note an artifact related to the VAB and inserted clip (black arrow)

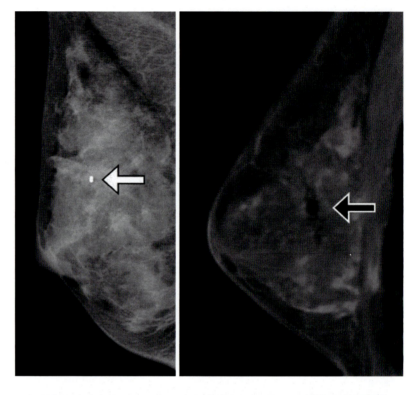

Fig. 130 MRI demonstrates mild BPE without definite abnormality

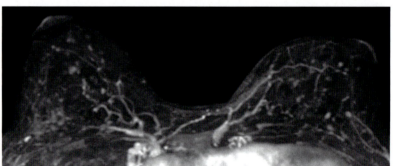

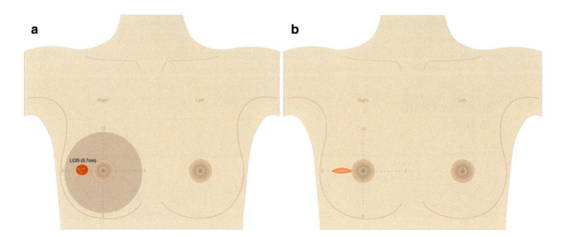

Fig. 131 (**a**) Preoperative and (**b**) immediate postoperative appearance

Carcinoma In Situ

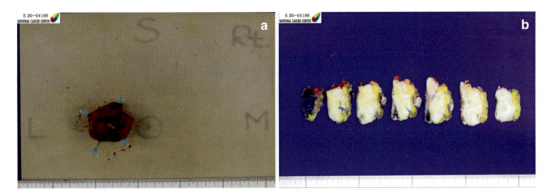

Fig. 132 (**a**) Gross pathology of right breast partial mastectomy specimen. (**b**) The margins get marked and sliced with different colors on each direction

29 Case 29

29.1 Patient History and Progress

Female/50 years old, post-menopause.

Screen detected mass lesion on left breast 2 o'clock direction.

Outside result of biopsy: Left breast 2 o'clock, invasive ductal carcinoma.

No family history.

No comorbidities.

BRCA 1 and 2 mutation: Not detected, MSH6 VUS (variant of uncertain).

29.2 Important Radiologic Findings

See Figs. 133, 134 and 135.

29.3 Courses of Treatment

Operation + Adjuvant chemotherapy #4 cycles (Doxorubicin and Cyclophosphamide) + Postoperative radiation therapy (both) + Letrozole 2.5 mg/day for 5 years.

29.3.1 Operation
Breast conserving surgery (left), sentinel lymph node biopsy (left), excision (right) (Figs. 136 and 137).

29.3.2 Pathology Report
Right.

Lobular carcinoma in situ, pathological TN category (AJCC 2017): pTis
1. Size of tumor: 2.5 cm (pTis).
2. Nuclear grade: low.
3. Necrosis: absent.
4. Architectural pattern: solid.
5. Surgical margins:
    (a) superior margin: (see Note 1),
    (b) inferior margin: (see Note 2),
    (c) medial margin: 5 mm,
    (d) lateral margin: positive for lobular carcinoma in situ (Fro 4) (see Note 3),
    (e) deep margin: <1 mm from lobular carcinoma in situ (slides 4 and 5),
    (f) superficial margin: 3 mm.
6. Microcalcification: present, tumoral/non-tumoral.

    Note: 1. The superior margin of the lumpectomy specimen (slide 2) is close to lobular carcinoma in situ (3 mm) but this margin submitted for frozen diagnosis (Fro 1) is free of tumor.
    2. The inferior margin of the lumpectomy specimen (slide 4) is close to lobular carcinoma in situ (<1 mm) but this margin submitted for frozen diagnosis (Fro 2) is free of tumor.
    3. Lobular carcinoma in situ is present only in the permanent section of Fro 4.

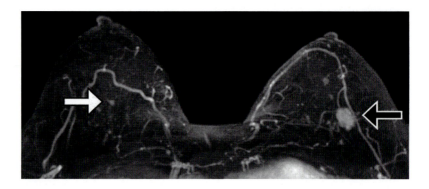

Fig. 133 MRI of a woman with known left breast cancer. MRI shows an enhancing malignant mass in the left breast (black arrow). An enhancing focus was seen in the right breast (white arrow)

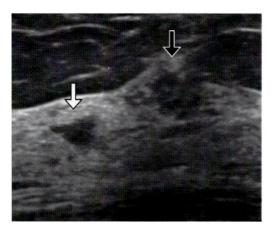

Fig. 134 On right breast US, a small irregular mass (white arrow) and another isoechoic lesion with indistinct margins (black arrow) were noted at the corresponding area of the enhancing focus on MRI. Excisional biopsy = LCIS

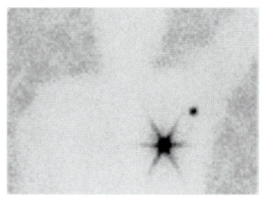

Fig. 135 Lymphoscintigraphy shows visualized sentinel lymph node in left axilla

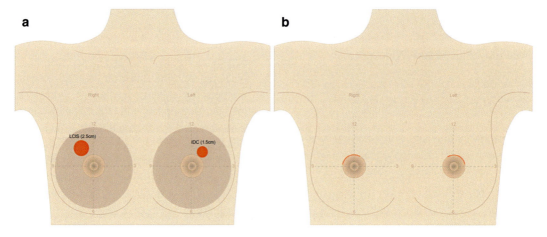

Fig. 136 (**a**) Preoperative and (**b**) immediate postoperative appearance

Carcinoma In Situ

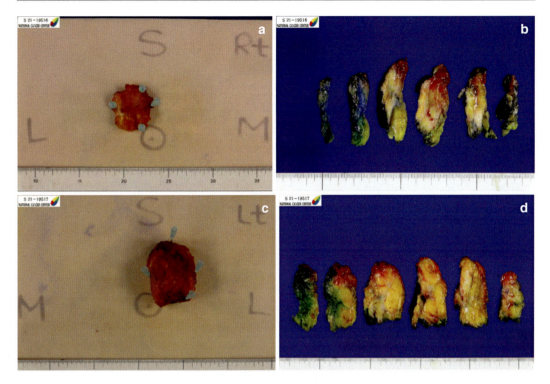

Fig. 137 (a, b) Gross pathology of right breast excision specimen. (c, d) Gross pathology of left breast partial mastectomy specimen

	Result	Intensity	Positive %
Estrogen receptor	Strong (8/8)	3	>2/3
Progesterone receptor	Intermediate (5/8)	3	1%–10%
C-erbB2	Negative (1+)		
Ki-67	Positive in 1% of tumor cells		

Left.

Invasive ductal carcinoma, pathological TN category (AJCC 2017): pT1cN0(sn)
1. Size of tumor: 1.5 cm (pT1c).
2. Histologic grade: 2/3 (tubule formation: 3/3, nuclear pleomorphism: 2/3, mitotic count: 2/3, 11/10HPF).
3. Intraductal component: present, intratumoral (20%) (nuclear grade: low, necrosis: present, architectural pattern: micropapillary/cribriform/solid/comedo, extensive intraductal component: absent).
4. Surgical margins:
   (a) superior margin: 20 mm,
   (b) inferior margin: 15 mm,
   (c) medial margin: 10 mm,
   (d) lateral margin: 10 mm,
   (e) deep margin: 8 mm,
   (f) superficial margin: 10 mm.
5. Lymph nodes: no metastasis in two axillary lymph nodes (pN0(sn)) (sentinel LN: 0/2).
6. Arteriovenous invasion: absent.
7. Lymphovascular invasion: present, intratumoral.
8. Tumor border: infiltrative.
9. Microcalcification: present, non-tumoral.

	Result	Intensity	Positive %
Estrogen receptor	Strong (8/8)	3	>2/3
Progesterone receptor	Negative (2/8)	1	<1%
C-erbB2	Negative (1+)		
Ki-67	Positive in 17% of tumor cells		

30 Case 30

30.1 Patient History and Progress

Female/60 years old, post-menopause.

Screen detected mass and microcalcification on left breast 10 o'clock direction.

Outside result of biopsy: Ductal carcinoma in situ.

No family history.

Claustrophobia, hypertension.

30.2 Important Radiologic Findings

Figs. 138, 139, 140 and 141.

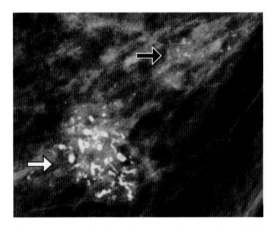

Fig. 138 Magnification view shows pleomorphic calcifications with (white arrow) and without (black arrow) mass formation

30.3 Courses of Treatment

Operation + Postoperative Radiation therapy.

30.3.1 Operation

Nipple–areolar complex sparing mastectomy with immediate implant reconstruction, sentinel lymph node biopsy (Figs. 142 and 143).

30.3.2 Pathology Report

Ductal carcinoma in situ, pathological TN category (AJCC 2017): pTisN0(sn)
1. Size of tumor: 2.0 cm (pTis).
2. Nuclear grade: high.
3. Necrosis: present.
4. Architectural pattern: micropapillary/cribriform/solid/comedo.
5. Skin: no involvement of tumor.
6. Surgical margins:
    (a) nipple margin: positive for ductal carcinoma in situ (Fro 4),
    (b) subareolar margin: positive for ductal carcinoma in situ (Fro 1),
    (c) deep margin: 2 mm,
    (d) superficial margin: 2 mm.
7. Lymph nodes: no metastasis in one axillary lymph node (pN0(sn)) (sentinel LN: 0/1).
8. Microcalcification: present, tumoral/non-tumoral.

Fig. 139 US demonstrates hypoechoic lesions with echogenic calcifications

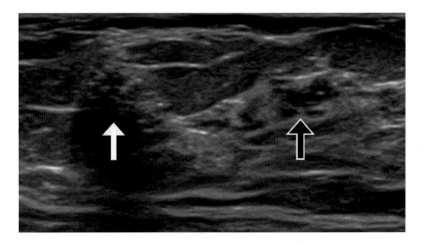

Carcinoma In Situ

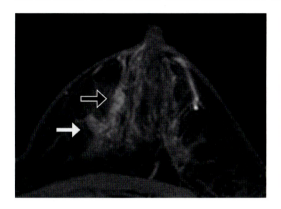

Fig. 140 MRI reveals segmental clustered ring non-mass enhancement

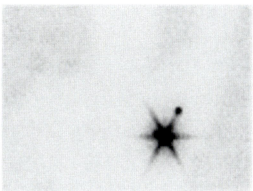

Fig. 141 Lymphoscintigraphy shows visualized sentinel lymph node in left axilla

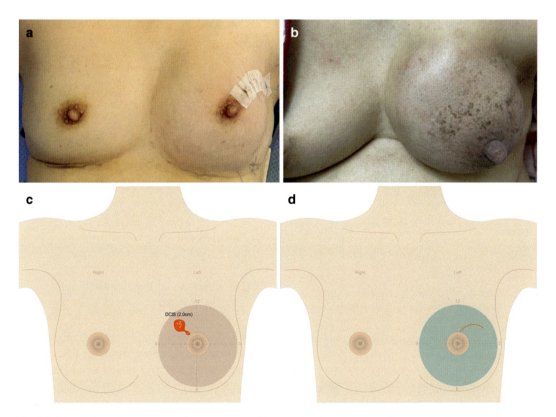

Fig. 142 (**a**, **d**) immediate postoperative appearance, (**c**) tumor location, (**b**) after adjuvant radiotherapy

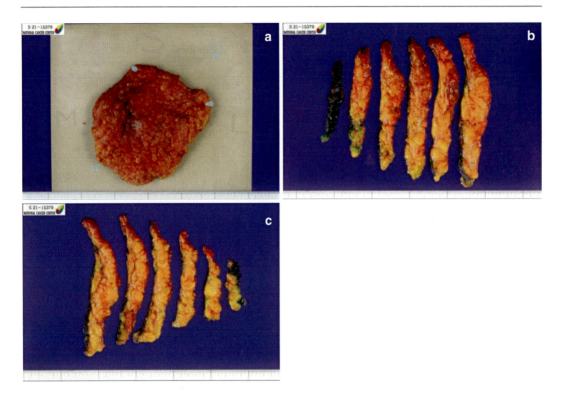

Fig. 143 (**a**) Gross pathology of left breast mastectomy specimen. (**b**, **c**) The margins get marked and sliced with different colors on each direction

	Result	Intensity	Positive %
Estrogen receptor	Strong (8/8)	3	>2/3
Progesterone receptor	Intermediate (5/8)	2	10%–1/3
C-erbB2	Positive (3+)		
Ki-67	Positive in 11% of tumor cells		

31 Case 31

31.1 Patient History and Progress

Female/31 years old, pre-menopause.
Screen detected calcification on left breast 11 o'clock direction.
Outside result of mammotome biopsy: Ductal carcinoma in situ.
No family history.
No comorbidities.
BRCA 1 and 2: Not detected.

31.2 Important Radiologic Findings

See Figs. 144 and 145.

31.3 Courses of Treatment: Operation

31.3.1 Operation
Nipple–areolar complex sparing mastectomy with immediate implant reconstruction (Figs. 146 and 147).

31.3.2 Pathology Report

Ductal carcinoma in situ, pathological TN category (AJCC 2017): pTis
1. Size of tumor: 2.0 cm (pTis).
2. Nuclear grade: low.
3. Necrosis: absent.
4. Architectural pattern: papillary/micropapillary/cribriform.

Carcinoma In Situ

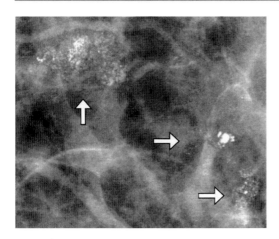

Fig. 144 Magnification view shows multiple groups of amorphous microcalcifications. Stereotactic VAB = DCIS

5. Skin: no involvement of tumor.
6. Surgical margins:
   (a) deep margin: 2 mm,
   (b) superficial margin: 2 mm.
7. Microcalcification: present, tumoral/non-tumoral.

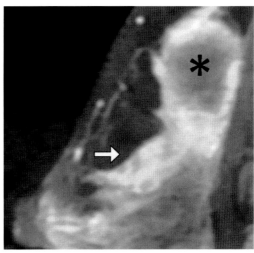

Fig. 145 MRI demonstrates segmental clustered ring non-mass enhancement (arrow). Note the biopsy-related hematoma (*)

	Result	Intensity	Positive %
Estrogen receptor	Strong (8/8)	3	>2/3
Progesterone receptor	Strong (8/8)	3	>2/3
C-erbB2	Equivocal (2+)		
Ki-67	Positive in 3% of tumor cells		

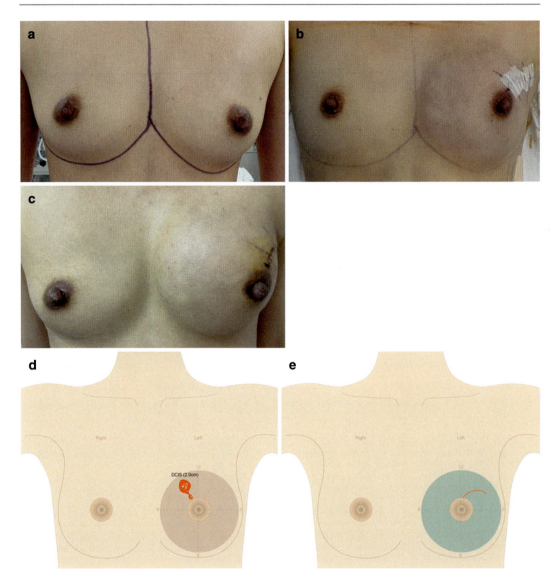

Fig. 146 (**a**, **d**) Preoperative, (**b**, **e**) immediate postoperative, and (**c**) late follow-up appearance

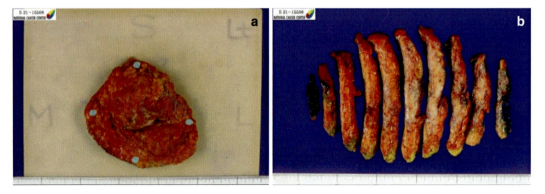

Fig. 147 (**a**) Gross pathology of left breast mastectomy specimen. (**b**) The margins get marked and sliced with different colors on each direction

32 Case 32

32.1 Patient History and Progress

Female/72 years old, post-menopause.

Screen detected mass lesion on right breast 8 o'clock direction.

Outside result of biopsy: Ductal carcinoma in situ.

No family history.
No comorbidities.

32.2 Important Radiologic Findings

See Figs. 148, 149 and 150.

32.3 Courses of Treatment

Operation + Postoperative radiation therapy.

32.3.1 Operation
Breast conserving surgery (Figs. 151 and 152).

32.3.2 Pathology Report

Ductal carcinoma in situ, pathological TN category (AJCC 2017): pTis
1. Size of tumor: 4.0 cm (pTis).
2. Nuclear grade: high.
3. Necrosis: present.
4. Architectural pattern: micropapillary/cribriform/comedo.

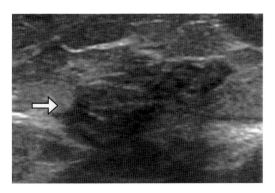

Fig. 149 US revealed an irregular mass at the corresponding area of the mass on mammography

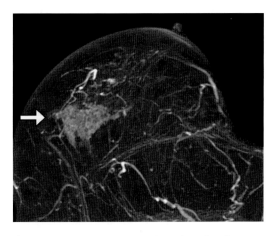

Fig. 150 MRI demonstrates an irregular enhancing mass

5. Skin: no involvement of tumor.
6. Surgical margins:
   (a) superior margin: 10 mm,
   (b) inferior margin: 10 mm,
   (c) medial margin: 40 mm,
   (d) lateral margin: 5 mm,
   (e) deep margin: 2 mm,
   (f) superficial margin: 2 mm.
7. Microcalcification: present, tumoral/non-tumoral.

	Result	Intensity	Positive %
Estrogen receptor	Negative (0/8)	0	0
Progesterone receptor	Negative (0/8)	0	0
C-erbB2	Equivocal (2+)		
Ki-67	Positive in 27% of tumor cells		

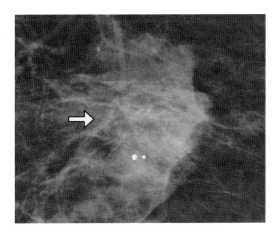

Fig. 148 Mammography shows an obscured mass

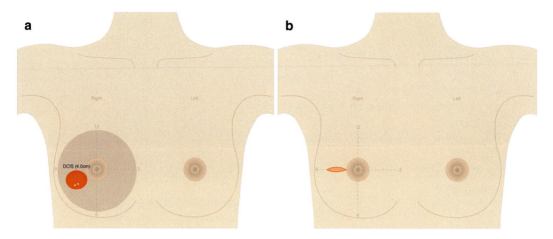

Fig. 151 (**a**) Preoperative, (**b**) immediate postoperative appearance

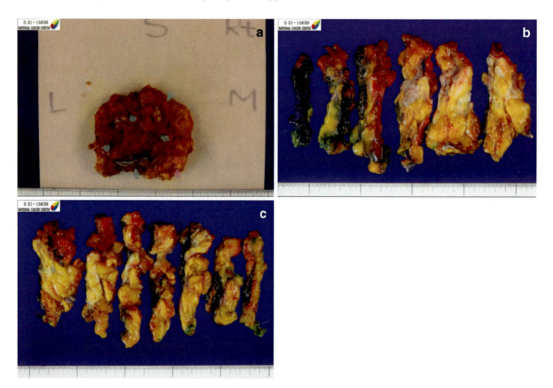

Fig. 152 (**a**) Gross pathology of right breast partial mastectomy specimen. (**b, c**) The margins get marked and sliced with different colors on each direction

33 Case 33

33.1 Patient History and Progress

Female/68 years old, post-menopause.
  Bloody nipple discharge from right breast.
  No family history.
  S/P Hysterectomy.

33.2 Important Radiologic Findings

See Figs. 153 and 154.

33.3 Courses of Treatment: Operation

33.3.1 Operation

First operation: Excision, second operation: Wide excision (Figs. 155 and 156).

33.3.2 Pathology Report

<First operation>

Ductal carcinoma in situ, pathological TN category (AJCC 2017): pTis

1. Size of tumor: 0.5 cm (pTis).
2. Nuclear grade: low.

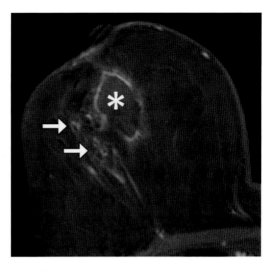

Fig. 154 MRI demonstrates regional heterogeneous non-mass enhancement adjacent to the postoperative fluid collection (*). Wide excision = ADH

3. Necrosis: absent.
4. Architectural pattern: papillary/cribriform.
5. Skin: no involvement of tumor.
6. Surgical margins:
   (a) superior margin: 10 mm,
   (b) inferior margin: 10 mm,
   (c) medial margin: 5 mm,
   (d) lateral margin: positive (Fro 5) (see Note),
   (e) deep margin: 2 mm,
   (f) superficial margin: 2 mm.
7. Microcalcification: present, tumoral/non-tumoral.

   Note: 1. Ductal carcinoma in situ is present only in the permanent section of Fro 5.

	Result	Intensity	Positive %
Estrogen receptor	Strong (8/8)	3	>2/3
Progesterone receptor	Strong (8/8)	3	>2/3
C-erbB2	Negative (0)		
Ki-67	Positive in 4% of tumor cells		

<Second operation>

Atypical ductal hyperplasia involving intraductal papilloma.

1. with a) foreign body reaction,
2. b) fat necrosis.
   (a) Post-excision status.

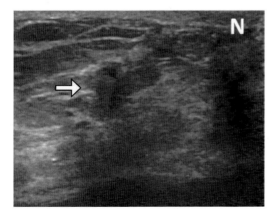

Fig. 153 This woman was presenting for evaluation of bloody nipple discharge. US showed an isoechoic mass with indistinct margins at the subareolar area. US biopsy yielded ADH. Followed surgical excision confirmed DCIS

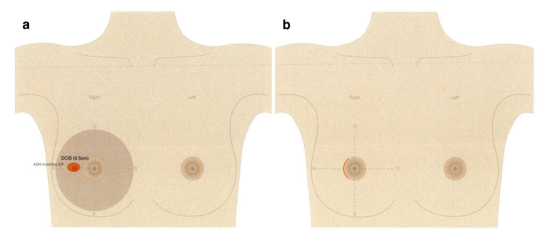

Fig. 155 (**a**) Preoperative, (**b**) immediate postoperative appearance

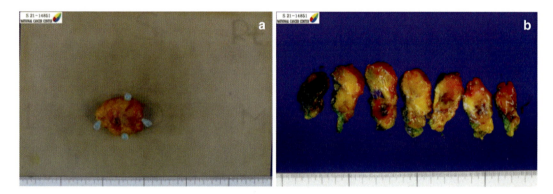

Fig. 156 (**a**) Gross pathology of right breast excision specimen (1st operation). (**b**) The margins get marked and sliced with different colors on each direction

34 Case 34

34.1 Patient History and Progress

Female/53 years old, pre-menopause.

Screen detected mass lesion on upper outer of right breast.

No family history.

S/P Total gastrectomy (gastric cancer), micropapillary thyroid carcinoma (follow-up).

BRCA 1 and 2: Not examination.

34.2 Important Radiologic Findings

See Figs. 157, 158, 159 and 160.

34.3 Courses of Treatment: Operation

34.3.1 Operation

First operation: Excision, second operation: Both excision (Figs. 161 and 162).

34.3.2 Pathology Report

<First operation>

Ductal carcinoma in situ, pathological TN category (AJCC 2017): pTis

1. Size of tumor: 0.5 cm (pTis).
2. Nuclear grade: low.
3. Necrosis: absent.
4. Architectural pattern: papillary/cribriform.
5. Surgical margins:

Carcinoma In Situ

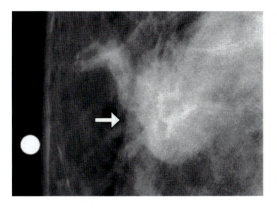

Fig. 157 This woman was presenting for evaluation of a palpable mass. A round BB marks the site of palpable finding on mammography

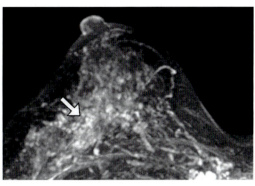

Fig. 159 MRI demonstrates marked BPE. Targeted US was advised for another focal non-mass enhancement

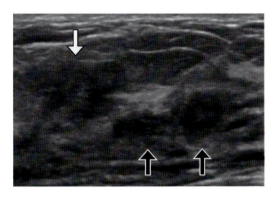

Fig. 158 US showed an irregular hypoechoic mass at the symptomatic area (white arrow). Other similar-appearing masses (black arrows) were seen near the palpable mass. US-guided core needle biopsy = intraductal papilloma. Surgical excision = DCIS

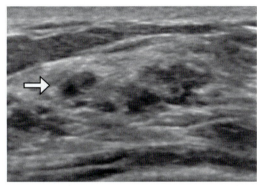

Fig. 160 MRI-directed US and core needle biopsy = intraductal papilloma. Surgical excision = LCIS

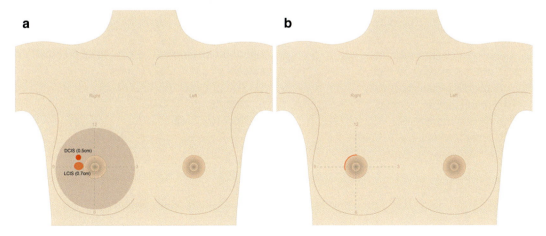

Fig. 161 (**a**) Preoperative, (**b**) immediate postoperative appearance

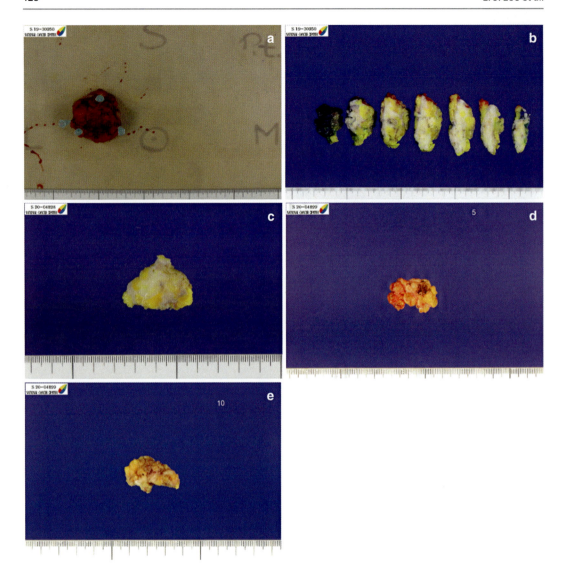

Fig. 162 (**a**, **b**) Gross pathology of right breast excision specimen (first operation). (**c**) Gross pathology of right breast excision specimen (second operation). (**d**, **e**) Gross pathology of left breast excision specimen (second operation)

- (a) superior margin: 15 mm,
- (b) inferior margin: 30 mm,
- (c) medial margin: 15 mm,
- (d) lateral margin: 15 mm,
- (e) deep margin: 8 mm,
- (f) superficial margin: 8 mm.
6. Microcalcification: absent.

<Second operation>
Right.

Lobular carcinoma in situ, pathological TN category (AJCC 2017): pTis

1. Size of tumor: 0.7 cm (pTis).
2. Nuclear grade: low.
3. Necrosis: absent.
4. Architectural pattern: solid.
5. Surgical margins: positive for lobular carcinoma in situ at the nearest resection margin (slide 1).
6. Microcalcification: absent.

Carcinoma In Situ

	Result	Intensity	Positive %
Estrogen receptor	Weak (4/8)	1	10%–1/3
Progesterone receptor	Weak (4/8)	1	10%–1/3
C-erbB2	Equivocal (2+)		
Ki-67	Positive in 3% of tumor cells		

Left.
Intraductal papilloma.

35 Case 35

35.1 Patient History and Progress

Female/59 years old, post-menopause.

Screen detected ductal dilatation on left breast 12 o'clock direction.

No family history.

S/P Hysterectomy and bilateral salpingo-oophorectomy, S/P total thyroidectomy (thyroid cancer), hypertension.

35.2 Important Radiologic Findings

See Figs. 163 and 164.

35.3 Courses of Treatment

Operation + Tamoxifen 20 mg/day for 5 years.

35.3.1 Operation
Breast conserving surgery (Figs. 165 and 166).

35.3.2 Pathology Report

Lobular carcinoma in situ, pathological TN category (AJCC 2017): pTis
1. Size of tumor: 0.5 cm (pTis).
2. Nuclear grade: low.
3. Necrosis: absent.
4. Architectural pattern: solid.
5. Skin: no involvement of tumor.
6. Surgical margins:
    (a) superior margin: 5 mm,

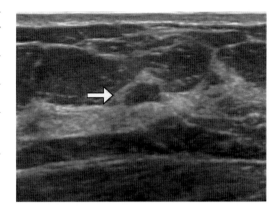

Fig. 163 This woman was referred for biopsy of a mass in the left breast. US showed an oval isoechoic mass. US-guided CNB = LCIS within FA

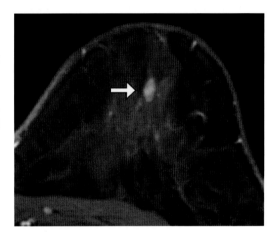

Fig. 164 MRI demonstrates an oval enhancing mass

  (b) inferior margin: 5 mm,
  (c) medial margin: 10 mm,
  (d) lateral margin: 10 mm,
  (e) deep margin: 2 mm,
  (f) superficial margin: 2 mm.
7. Microcalcification: present, tumoral/non-tumoral.

	Result	Intensity	Positive %
Estrogen receptor	Strong (7/8)	3	1/3–2/3
Progesterone receptor	Strong (7/8)	3	1/3–2/3
C-erbB2	Equivocal (2+)		
Ki-67	Positive in 2% of tumor cells		

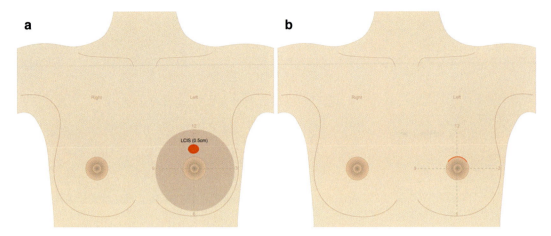

Fig. 165 (**a**) Preoperative, (**b**) immediate postoperative appearance

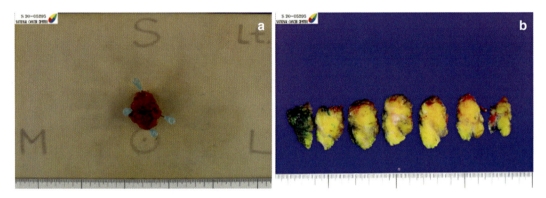

Fig. 166 (**a**) Gross pathology of left breast lumpectomy specimen. (**b**)The margins get marked and sliced with different colors on each direction

36 Case 36

36.1 Patient History and Progress

Female/47 years old, pre-menopause.

Screen detected mass lesion on right breast 11 o'clock direction.

No family history.

No comorbidities.

36.2 Important Radiologic Findings

See Figs. 167 and 168.

36.3 Courses of Treatment: Operation

36.3.1 Operation

Excision (Figs. 169 and 170).

36.3.2 Pathology Report

Lobular carcinoma in situ
1. Size of tumor: 0.5 cm.
2. Nuclear grade: low.
3. Necrosis: absent.
4. Architectural pattern: solid.
5. Skin: no involvement of tumor.
6. Surgical margins:
    (a) superior margin: 10 mm,
    (b) inferior margin: 5 mm,

Carcinoma In Situ

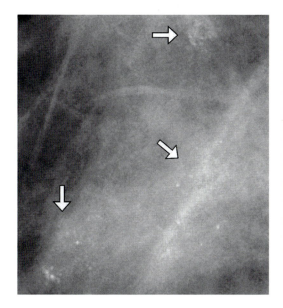

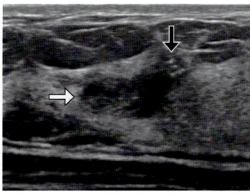

Fig. 168 US demonstrates an irregular hypoechoic mass (white arrow) with echogenic microcalcifications (black arrow)

Fig. 167 Magnification view shows multiple groups of amorphous microcalcifications

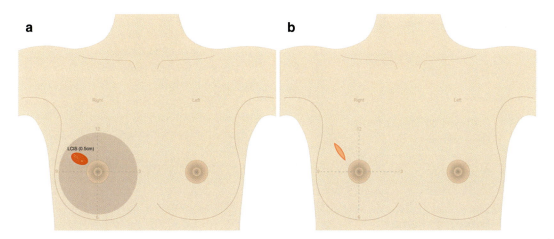

Fig. 169 (**a**) Preoperative, (**b**) immediate postoperative appearance

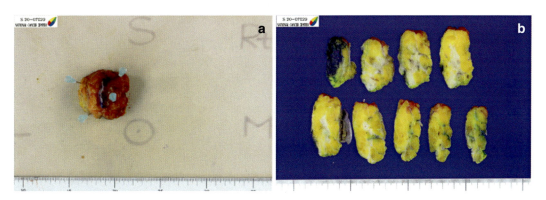

Fig. 170 (**a**) Gross pathology of right breast excision specimen. (**b**) The margins get marked and sliced with different colors on each direction

(c) medial margin: 20 mm,
(d) lateral margin: 10 mm,
(e) deep margin: 2 mm,
(f) superficial margin: 2 mm.
7. Microcalcification: present, tumoral/non-tumoral.

37 Case 37

37.1 Patient History and Progress

Female/46 years old, pre-menopause.

Screen detected mass lesion on left breast 12 o'clock direction.

Outside result of biopsy: Lobular carcinoma in situ.

No family history.

No comorbidities.

37.2 Important Radiologic Findings

See Figs. 171 and 172.

37.3 Courses of Treatment: Operation

37.3.1 Operation

Breast conserving surgery (Figs. 173 and 174).

37.3.2 Pathology Report

Lobular carcinoma in situ
1. Size of tumor: 2.0 cm.
2. Nuclear grade: low.

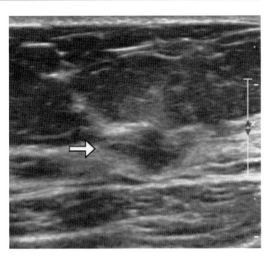

Fig. 171 US shows an irregular isoechoic mass in the left breast. US-guided CNB = LCIS

3. Necrosis: absent.
4. Architectural pattern: solid.
5. Skin: no involvement of tumor.
6. Surgical margins:
   (a) superior margin: positive (Fro 1),
   (b) inferior margin: 4 mm,
   (c) medial margin: positive (Fro 3),
   (d) lateral margin: positive (Fro 4),
   (e) deep margin: <1 mm (slide 6),
   (f) superficial margin: 10 mm.
7. Microcalcification: absent.

	Result	Intensity	Positive %
Estrogen receptor	Weak (4/8)	2	1–10%
Progesterone receptor	Weak (4/8)	2	1–10%
C-erbB2	Negative (1+)		
Ki-67	Positive in 8% of tumor cells		

Carcinoma In Situ

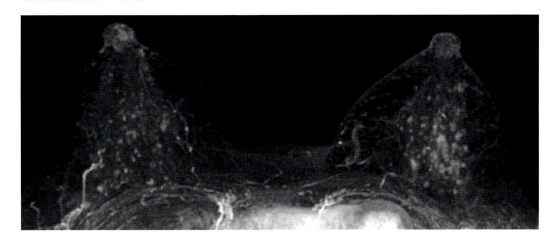

Fig. 172 MRI demonstrates mild BPE without definite abnormality

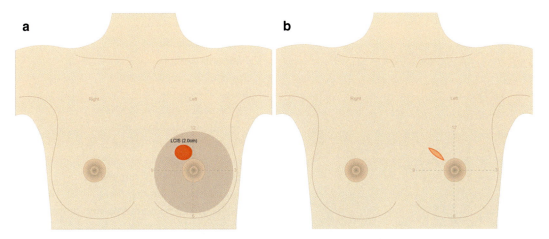

Fig. 173 (**a**) Preoperative, (**b**) immediate postoperative appearance

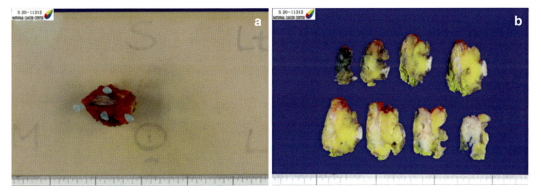

Fig. 174 (**a**) Gross pathology of left breast lumpectomy specimen. (**b**) The margins get marked and sliced with different colors on each direction

38 Case 38

38.1 Patient History and Progress

Female/51 years old, pre-menopause.

Screen detected mass and microcalcification on upper outer left breast.

No family history.

No comorbidities.

BRCA 1 and 2 mutation: Not detected, POLE VUS (variant of uncertain).

38.2 Important Radiologic Findings

See Figs. 175, 176, 177, 178 and 179.

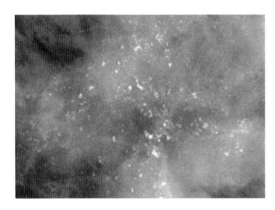

Fig. 175 Magnification view shows regional fine pleomorphic microcalcifications in the left breast

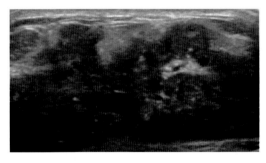

Fig. 176 US demonstrates irregular hypoechoic lesions with microcalcifications in the left breast. US-guided CNB = Microinvasive ductal carcinoma

38.3 Courses of Treatment

Neoadjuvant chemotherapy #6 cycles (Docetaxel and Carboplatin and Trastuzumab and Pertuzumab) + Operation + Postoperative radiation therapy + Tamoxifen 20 mg/day for 5 years + Trastuzumab for 1 year.

38.3.1 Operation

Both breast conserving surgery, sentinel lymph node biopsy (left) (Figs. 180 and 181).

38.3.2 Pathology Report

Right.

Lobular carcinoma in situ
1. Post-chemotherapy status.
2. Size of tumor: 1.5 cm.
3. Nuclear grade: low.
4. Necrosis: absent.
5. Architectural pattern: solid.
6. Surgical margins:
    (a) superior margin: (see note),
    (b) inferior margin: 4 mm,
    (c) medial margin: 20 mm,
    (d) lateral margin: (see note),
    (e) deep margin: <1 mm (MG2),
    (f) superficial margin: 2 mm.
7. Microcalcification: present, non-tumoral.

   Note: 1. The superior and lateral margins of the lumpectomy specimen (slides MG1and 5) are close to lobular carcinoma in situ (1 mm) but these margins submitted for frozen diagnosis (Fro 1 and Fro 4) are free of tumor.
Left.

Ductal carcinoma in situ
1. Post-chemotherapy status.
2. Size of tumor: up to 0.5 cm (ypTis).
3. Nuclear grade: high.
4. Necrosis: present.
5. Architectural pattern: papillary/cribriform/solid/comedo.
6. Skin: no involvement of tumor.
7. Surgical margins:
    (a) superior margin: 17 mm,
    (b) inferior margin: 10 mm,

Carcinoma In Situ

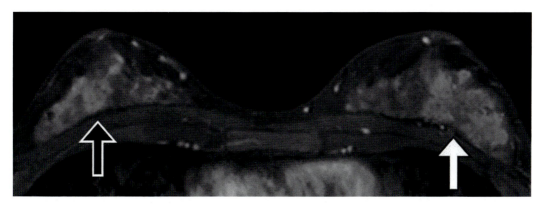

Fig. 177 MRI revealed clumped enhancement in the left breast (white arrow). Similar-appearing non-mass enhancement was concerning for contralateral breast malignancy (black arrow)

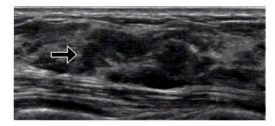

Fig. 178 MR-directed right breast US and biopsy = Mixed ductal carcinoma in situ and lobular carcinoma in situ. Right mammography was negative (not shown)

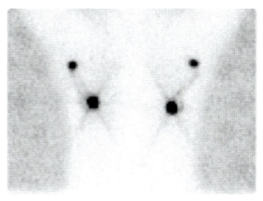

Fig. 179 Lymphoscintigraphy shows visualized sentinel lymph nodes in both axilla

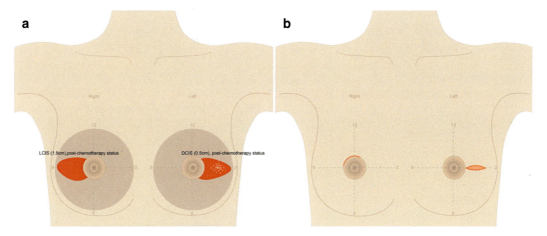

Fig. 180 (**a**) Preoperative, (**b**) immediate postoperative appearance

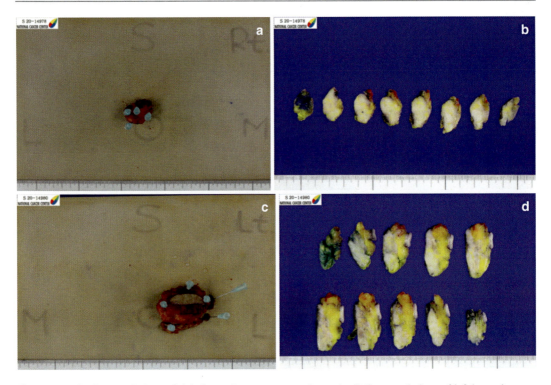

Fig. 181 (**a**, **b**) Gross pathology of right breast lumpectomy specimen. (**c**, **d**) Gross pathology of left breast lumpectomy specimen

    (c) medial margin: 40 mm,
    (d) lateral margin: 10 mm,
    (e) deep margin: 3 mm,
    (f) superficial margin: 14 mm.
8. Lymph nodes: no metastasis in five axillary lymph nodes (ypN0(sn)) (sentinel LN: 0/5).
9. Microcalcification: present.

	Result	Intensity	Positive %
Estrogen receptor	Negative (0/8)	0	0
Progesterone receptor	Negative (0/8)	0	0
C-erbB2	Positive (3+)		
Ki-67	Positive in 15% of tumor cells		

39 Case 39

39.1 Patient History and Progress

Female/47 years old, pre-menopause.
    Screen detected mass lesion on right breast 12 o'clock direction.

Outside result of biopsy: lobular carcinoma in situ.
No family history.
Hypertension.

39.2 Important Radiologic Findings

See Figs. 182 and 183.

39.3 Courses of Treatment

Operation + Tamoxifen 20 mg/day for 6 months.

39.3.1 Operation
Breast conserving surgery (Figs. 184 and 185).

39.3.2 Pathology Report
Lobular carcinoma in situ
1. Size of tumor: 2.0 cm.
2. Nuclear grade: low.
3. Necrosis: absent.

Carcinoma In Situ

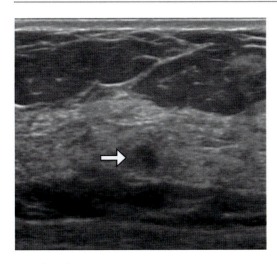

Fig. 182 US shows an isoechoic mass with non-parallel orientation and microlobulated margins. US-guided CNB = LCIS

4. Architectural pattern: solid.
5. Skin: no involvement of tumor.
6. Surgical margins:
   (a) superior margin: <1 mm (slide 2),
   (b) inferior margin: <1 mm (slide 5),
   (c) medial margin: 1 mm (slide 4),
   (d) lateral margin: <1 mm (slide 6),
   (e) deep margin: <1 mm (slide 3),
   (f) superficial margin: 2 mm.
7. Microcalcification: present, tumoral/non-tumoral.

	Result	Intensity	Positive %
Estrogen receptor	Strong (7/8)	3	1/3–2/3
Progesterone receptor	Strong (8/8)	3	>2/3
C-erbB2	Negative (1+)		
Ki-67	Positive in 6% of tumor cells		

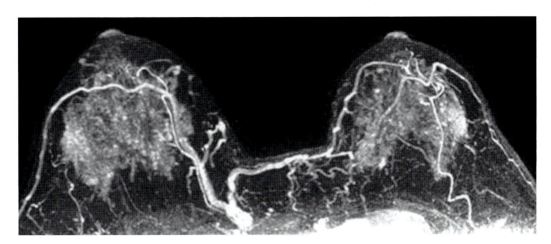

Fig. 183 MRI demonstrates marked BPE without discernible abnormality

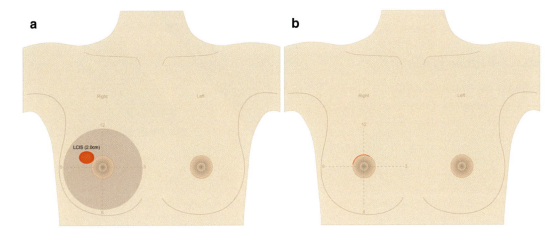

Fig. 184 (**a**) Preoperative, (**b**) immediate postoperative appearance

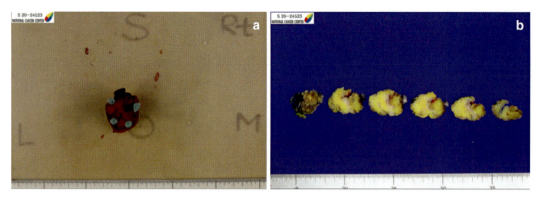

Fig. 185 (a) Gross pathology of right breast lumpectomy specimen. (b) The margins get marked and sliced with different colors on each direction

40 Case 40

40.1 Patient History and Progress

Female/47 years old, post-menopause.
Screen detected mass and microcalcification on right breast 10 o'clock direction.
No family history.
No comorbidities.

40.2 Important Radiologic Findings

See Figs. 186, 187 and 188.

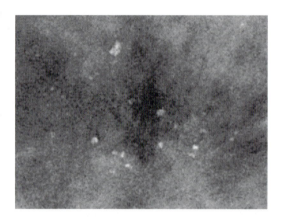

Fig. 186 Magnification view shows grouped fine pleomorphic microcalcifications

40.3 Courses of Treatment: Operation

40.3.1 Operation
Breast conserving surgery (Figs.189 and 190).

40.3.2 Pathology Report
Lobular carcinoma in situ
1. Post-stereotactic excision status.
2. Size of tumor: 1.0 cm, residual.
3. Nuclear grade: low.

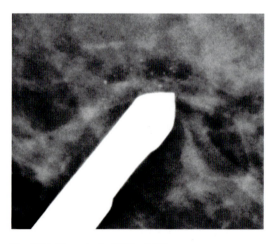

Fig. 187 Stereotactic VAB = LCIS

Carcinoma In Situ

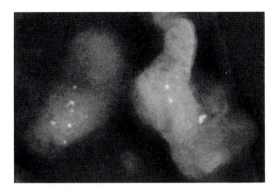

Fig. 188 Specimen radiograph confirms retrieval of the grouped microcalcifications

4. Necrosis: absent.
5. Architectural pattern: solid.
6. Skin: no involvement of tumor.
7. Surgical margins:
   (a) superior margin: 10 mm,
   (b) inferior margin: 10 mm,
   (c) medial margin: 10 mm,
   (d) lateral margin: 20 mm,
   (e) deep margin: 2 mm,
   (f) superficial margin: 2 mm.
8. Microcalcification: present, tumoral/non-tumoral.

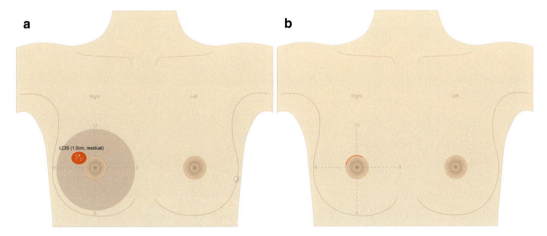

Fig. 189 (**a**) Preoperative, (**b**) immediate postoperative appearance

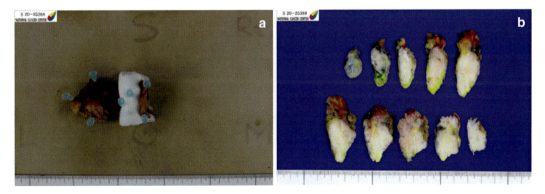

Fig. 190 (**a**) Gross pathology of right breast partial mastectomy specimen. (**b**) The margins get marked and sliced with different colors on each direction

	Result	Intensity	Positive %
Estrogen receptor	Strong (7/8)	3	1/3–2/3
Progesterone receptor	Negative (0/8)	0	0
C-erbB2	Equivocal (2+)		
Ki-67	Positive in 1% of tumor cells		

41 Case 41

41.1 Patient History and Progress

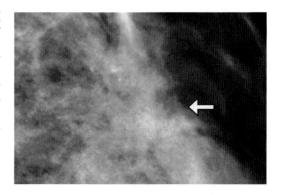

Fig. 191 Mammography shows an asymmetry with architectural distortion

Female/46 years old, pre-menopause.

Screen detected mass lesion on left breast 2 o'clock direction.

Outside result of biopsy: R/O Atypical ductal hyperplasia or ductal carcinoma in situ.

No family history.

No comorbidities.

41.2 Important Radiologic Findings

See Figs. 191, 192 and 193.

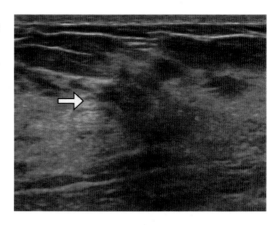

Fig. 192 On US, a heterogeneous lesion with indistinct margins was seen at the corresponding area of the mammographic abnormality. US-guided CNB = ADH, Excision = DCIS

41.3 Courses of Treatment

See Figs 194 and 195.

Operation + Tamoxifen 20 mg/day for 5 years.

41.3.1 Operation

First operation: Excision, second operation: Wide excision (Figs. 194 and 195).

41.3.2 Pathology Report
<First operation>

Ductal carcinoma in situ, pathological TN category (AJCC 2017): pTis
1. Size of tumor: 1.5 cm (pTis).
2. Nuclear grade: low.
3. Necrosis: absent.
4. Architectural pattern: solid.
5. Skin: no involvement of tumor.
6. Surgical margins:
    (a) superior margin: 5 mm,
    (b) inferior margin: 5 mm,
    (c) medial margin: <1 mm from ductal carcinoma in situ (slide 3),
    (d) lateral margin: 10 mm,
    (e) deep margin: 2 mm,
    (f) superficial margin: 2 mm.
7. Microcalcification: present, tumoral/non-tumoral.

	Result	Intensity	Positive %
Estrogen receptor	Strong (8/8)	3	>2/3
Progesterone receptor	Strong (8/8)	3	>2/3
C-erbB2	Negative (1+)		
Ki-67	Positive in 16% of tumor cells		

<Second operation>

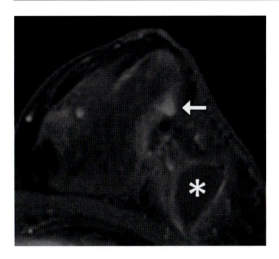

Fig. 193 MRI demonstrates a focal non-mass enhancement adjacent to the postoperative fluid collection (*). Wide excision = DCIS

Ductal carcinoma in situ
1. Post-excision status.
2. Size of tumor: 1.5 cm, residual.
3. Nuclear grade: low.
4. Necrosis: present.
5. Architectural pattern: cribriform/solid/comedo.
6. Skin: no involvement of tumor.
7. Surgical margins:
   (a) inferior margin: (see Note 1),
   (b) medial margin: (see Note 2).
8. Microcalcification: present, non-tumoral.

Note: 1. The inferior margin of the lumpectomy specimen (slides 2 and 3) is close to ductal carcinoma in situ (<1 mm) but this margin submitted for frozen diagnosis (Fro 1) is free of tumor.

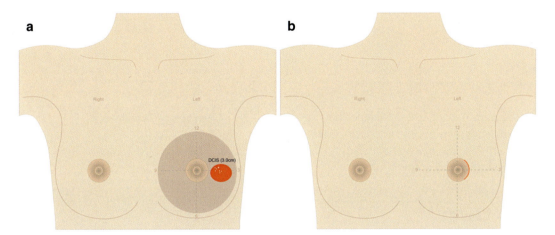

Fig. 194 (**a**) Preoperative, (**b**) immediate postoperative appearance

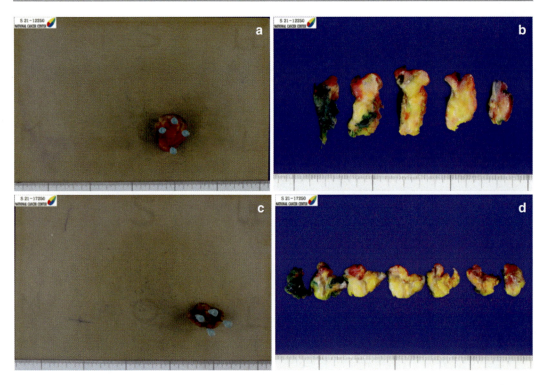

Fig. 195 (**a**, **b**) Gross pathology of left breast excision specimen (first operation). (**c**, **d**) Gross pathology of left breast wide excision specimen (second operation)

2. The medial margin of the lumpectomy specimen (slide 1) is positive for ductal carcinoma in situ but this margin submitted for frozen diagnosis (fro 2) is free of tumor.

42 Case 42

42.1 Patient History and Progress

Female/57 years old, post-menopause.

Screen detected microcalcification on left breast 6 o'clock direction.

Outside result of biopsy: Ductal carcinoma in situ.

No family history.

Diabetes mellitus.

42.2 Important Radiologic Findings

See Figs. 196, 197, 198 and 199.

42.3 Courses of Treatment

Operation + Postoperative radiation therapy.

42.3.1 Operation
Breast conserving surgery (Figs. 200 and 201).

42.3.2 Pathology Report

Ductal carcinoma in situ, pathological TN category (AJCC 2017): pTisNx
1. Size of tumor: 1.5 cm (pTis).
2. Nuclear grade: low.
3. Necrosis: absent.
4. Architectural pattern: papillary/cribriform.
5. Skin: no involvement of tumor.
6. Surgical margins:
    (a) superior margin: 10 mm,
    (b) inferior margin: 20 mm,
    (c) medial margin: 5 mm,
    (d) lateral margin: 5 mm,
    (e) deep margin: 2 mm,
    (f) superficial margin: 2 mm.

Carcinoma In Situ

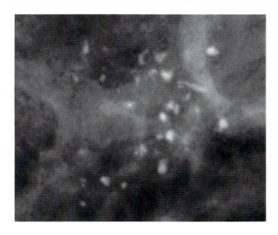

Fig. 196 Magnification view shows grouped fine pleomorphic microcalcifications

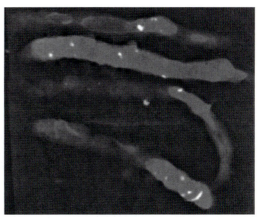

Fig. 198 Specimen radiograph confirms retrieval of representative microcalcifications

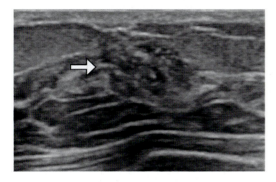

Fig. 197 US demonstrates a focal heterogeneous lesion with echogenic microcalcifications. US-guided CNB = DCIS

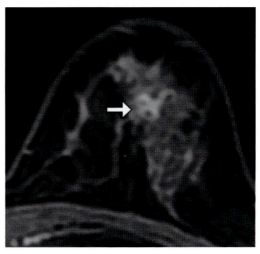

Fig. 199 MRI reveals focal clustered ring non-mass enhancement

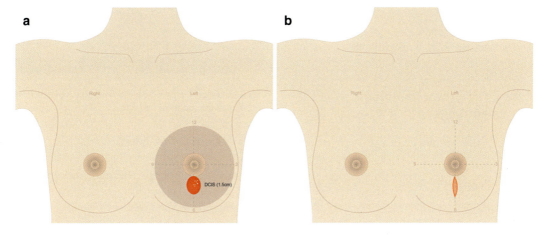

Fig. 200 (**a**) Preoperative, (**b**) immediate postoperative appearance

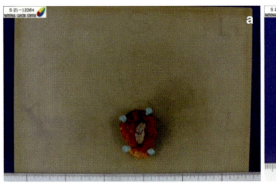
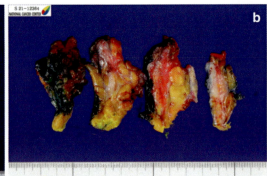

Fig. 201 (**a**) Gross pathology of left breast partial mastectomy specimen. (**b**) The margins get marked and sliced with different colors on each direction

7. Lymph nodes: not submitted (pNx).
8. Microcalcification: present, tumoral/non-tumoral.

	Result	Intensity	Positive %
Estrogen receptor	Strong (8/8)	3	>2/3
Progesterone receptor	Intermediate (5/8)	2	10%-1/3
C-erbB2	Negative (1+)		
Ki-67	Positive in 7% of tumor cells		

43 Case 43

43.1 Patient History and Progress

Female/67 years old, post-menopause.

Screen detected mass lesion on left breast 4 o'clock direction.

Outside result of biopsy: Ductal carcinoma in situ.

No family history.

Diabetes mellitus, hypertension.

43.2 Important Radiologic Findings

See Figs. 202, 203, 204 and 205.

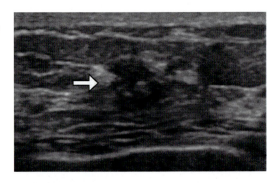

Fig. 202 Left breast US shows an isoechoic mass with microlobulated margins. US-guided CNB = DCIS

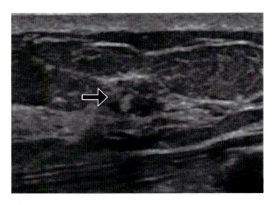

Fig. 203 Right breast US shows an isoechoic mass with microlobulated margins

43.3 Courses of Treatment

Operation + Postoperative radiation therapy (left).

Carcinoma In Situ

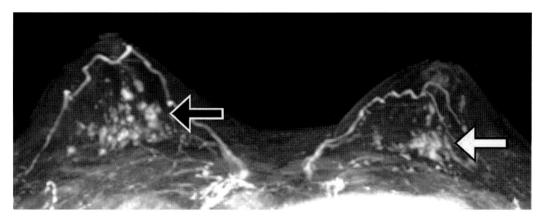

Fig. 204 MRI demonstrates moderate BPE with focal non-mass enhancements (arrows). Bilateral mammography was negative (not shown). Left BCS and right excisional biopsy were performed. Pathology confirmed LCIS in the right breast

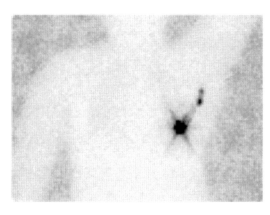

Fig. 205 Lymphoscintigraphy shows visualized sentinel lymph nodes in left axilla

43.3.1 Operation
Breast conserving surgery (left), sentinel lymph node biopsy (left), excision (right) (Figs. 206 and 207).

43.3.2 Pathology Report
Right.

Lobular carcinoma in situ
1. Size of tumor: 0.3 cm.
2. Nuclear grade: low.
3. Necrosis: absent.
4. Architectural pattern: solid.
5. Skin: no involvement of tumor.
6. Surgical margins:
    (a) superior margin: 5 mm,
    (b) inferior margin: 2 mm,
    (c) medial margin: 5 mm,
    (d) lateral margin: 5 mm,
    (e) deep margin: 2 mm,
    (f) superficial margin: 2 mm.
7. Microcalcification: present, tumoral/non-tumoral.
Left.

Ductal carcinoma in situ, pathological TN category (AJCC 2017): pTis
1. Size of tumor: 1.0 cm (pTis).
2. Nuclear grade: high.
3. Necrosis: present.
4. Architectural pattern: micropapillary/cribriform/comedo.
5. Skin: no involvement of tumor.
6. Surgical margins:
    (a) superior margin: 10 mm,
    (b) inferior margin: 10 mm,
    (c) medial margin: 10 mm,
    (d) lateral margin: 15 mm,
    (e) deep margin: 2 mm,
    (f) superficial margin: 2 mm.
7. Lymph nodes: no metastasis in one axillary lymph nodes (pN0(sn)) (sentinel LN: 0/1).
8. Microcalcification: present, tumoral/non-tumoral.

	Result	Intensity	Positive %
Estrogen receptor	Negative (0/8)	0	0
Progesterone receptor	Negative (0/8)	0	0
C-erbB2	Positive (3+)		
Ki-67	Positive in 8% of tumor cells		

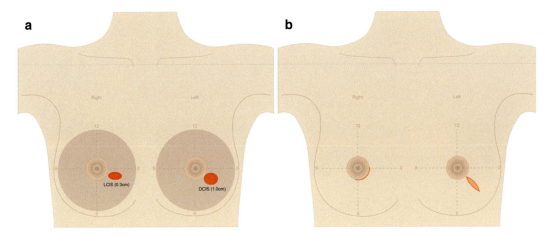

Fig. 206 (**a**) Preoperative, (**b**) immediate postoperative appearance

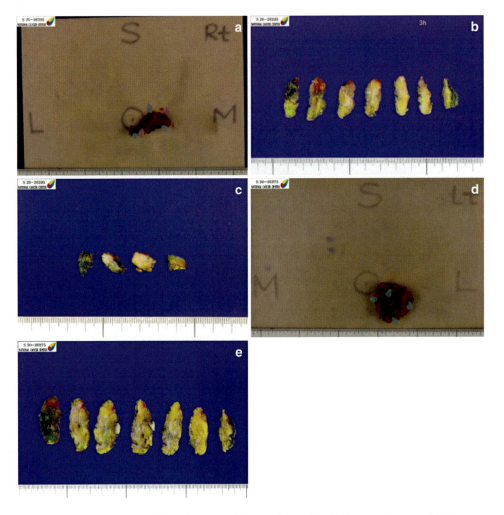

Fig. 207 (**a–c**) Gross pathology of right breast excision specimen. (**d**, **e**) Gross pathology of left lumpectomy specimen

Brief Overview of Breast Cancer Treatment

Ji Young You, Soojin Park, and Eun Sook Lee

1 Local Therapy: Surgery

1.1 History

In 1984, Halsted and Meyer reported the first radical mastectomy [1]. Under the concept that breast cancer metastasizes locally along the lymphatic vessels, the procedure removed the breast, the skin of the breast, the pectoralis major muscle, and the axillary lymph nodes. This technique became a technically feasible but not wholly effective local treatment for most breast cancers, especially advanced cases, found in the early twentieth century. However, many patients still had expired due to breast cancer metastasis after radical mastectomy, and it was found that about 25% of the breast cancer metastasis into the internal mammary lymph nodes. Therefore, in addition to the radical mastectomy, an extended radical mastectomy that included the internal mammary lymph nodes was

performed. However, even with that technique, the survival could not be extended, and the limits of the Halsted theory became clear. In 1948, Patey and Dyson [2] reported that many patients would continue to die of breast cancer after surgery unless effective breast cancer treatments could be developed. They designed a modified radical mastectomy that preserved the pectoralis major muscle. In the 1970s, radical mastectomy was the most commonly performed procedure, but oncologists acknowledged that local-segmental treatment alone could not completely prevent recurrence. In other words, the theory emerged that cancer cells had already spread throughout the body at the time of surgery, rather than being inadequately surgically resected. Fisher et al. found no difference in survival between patients who received postmastectomy radiation therapy and those who underwent radical mastectomy, according to the National Surgical Adjuvant Breast and Bowel Project (NSABP) B-04 study [3, 4]. They proposed that given the heterogeneous nature of malignant tissues, metastasis to surrounding organs can occur concurrently with systemic spread via lymphatic and blood vessels. This proposition marked a paradigm shift, underlining the significance of both local and systemic treatment modalities. Radiation therapy along with surgery plays a decisive role in reducing the scope of surgery in the local treatment of breast cancer. A mastectomy under the name quadrantectomy was first attempted by Veronesi [5]. In 1969, the World

J. Y. You (✉)
Division of Breast and Endocrine, Department of General Surgery, Korea University Medical Center, Seoul, Republic of Korea
e-mail: joliejean@korea.ac.kr

S. Park
Department of Surgery, Wonkwang University Sanbon Hospital, Gunpo, Republic of Korea

E. S. Lee
Center for Breast Cancer, National Cancer Center, Goyang, Kyonggi-do, Republic of Korea
e-mail: eslee@ncc.re.kr

© The Author(s), under exclusive license to Springer Nature Singapore Pte Ltd. 2023
E. S. Lee (ed.), *A Practical Guide to Breast Cancer Treatment*,
https://doi.org/10.1007/978-981-19-9044-1_4

Health Organization approved a clinical study of breast preservation surgery, and several prospective studies on breast preservation surgery were conducted. All those studies consistently reported no difference in survival between the group that received radiation therapy after breast preservation surgery and the group that underwent mastectomy [6]. Now that its safety has been proven, breast preservation surgery is accepted as the standard surgery for early-stage breast cancer and is undergone by many patients [7–12].

Axillary lymph node surgery is almost always performed during surgery for breast cancer. For patients with invasive breast cancer, the purpose of axillary lymph node surgery is the reduction of local recurrences and prolongation of survival, as well as obtaining disease information valuable to prognosis, selection of postoperative adjuvant chemotherapy, and staging. However, many patients suffer from complications and sequelae such as lymphedema. In addition, only about one-third of patients who underwent axillary lymph node dissection were reported to have lymph node metastases. As a result, new methods have emerged that are less invasive, have fewer complications, and provide appropriate treatment whether or not a patient has axillary lymph node metastases. The *sentinel lymph node* is the first lymph node that metastasizes through the lymph vessels. In 1977, Cabanas et al. used supervised lymphadenectomy for the first time for penile cancer [13]. In 1992, Morton et al. [14] began using it for lymphadenectomy of melanoma, laying the foundation for the theory. The sentinel lymph node biopsy was introduced to reduce possible complications during axillary lymphadenopathy in breast cancer. Based on the initial experience, Guiliano et al. conducted research to standardize monitored lymph node biopsies in breast cancer and announced that the monitoring lymph node detection rate was 93.5%, with a false negative rate of 0% and sensitivity and specificity of 100% [15, 16]. A significant difference in the incidence of complications was observed between the two procedures: a 3% incidence when only sentinel lymph node resection was performed, versus a 35% incidence when axillary lymph node dissection was conducted [17,

18]. However, no such difference was observed in terms of local recurrence. Presently, sentinel lymph node biopsies are extensively utilized to evaluate the metastatic status of lymph nodes [19–22].

1.2 Breast Surgery

1.2.1 Radical Mastectomy

1. Indications.
   (a) Breast cancer stage III or higher, a lesion fixed in the pectoralis major muscle that is resistant to chemotherapy or radiation therapy.
   (b) Inflammatory breast cancer that do not respond to chemotherapy or radiation therapy.
   (c) Advanced breast cancer with a fixed lesion in the pectoralis major that has recurred after a partial mastectomy.
   (d) A lesion fixed to the muscle and accompanied by a peripheral lesion near the clavicle and sternum.
2. Surgical technique.

   The skin incision takes an oval shape containing the primary lesion and the nipple–areola complex. At this time, it is better to lift the outer circumference of the breast to secure an appropriate boundary. If the diagnosis was previously confirmed by histological examination, it is advisable to include the biopsy site in the oval display if technically possible. The superior border of the resection is the inferior surface of the clavicle, the lateral border is the anterior surface of the latissimus dorsi, the medial border is the midline of the sternum, and the inferior border is the mammary fold over the extended tendon of the rectus abdominis.

   After retracting the skin flap, identify the insertion point of the pectoralis major muscle on the humerus. Subsequently, dissect the pectoralis major muscle towards its central and superior medial portions to expose the underlying pectoralis minor muscle. The pectoralis major muscle insertion to the humerus rotates inward after the incision. During the dissection, the pectoralis major nerve and blood vessels that enter the pectoralis major muscle are cut and ligated. Separation of the pectoralis major from the medial edge of the costosternal junction causes the pectoralis major and breast to emerge away from the chest wall. The pectoralis minor muscle is cut with the coracoid process of the scapula and then separated inwardly.

1.2.2 Modified Radical Mastectomy

1. Indication.

   It could be applied to patients diagnosed with breast cancer in the breast or axilla without tumor infiltration in the pectoralis major muscle or fascia.

2. Surgical technique.

   The techniques employed for anesthesia, surgical positioning, skin incision, and skin flap dissection in a modified radical mastectomy are similar to those used in a radical mastectomy. The Auchincloss method is used to pull the pectoralis minor muscle upward and medially for level I and level II axillary lymphadenopathy without removal of the pectoralis minor muscle. Using the Patty method, axillary lymph node dissection is performed by making an incision from near the origin of the pectoralis minor muscle to the region external to the pectoralis major nerve branch to remove the pectoralis minor muscle and level III lymph nodes.

1.2.3 Breast Conserving Surgery

1. Indications.

   Breast Conserving Surgery are commonly used techniques. If a mass is newly palpated, there is a negative or ectopic breast cancer on imaging study, or there is a shadow (microcalcification) on visual inspection that cannot be not touched, these techniques can be performed with an axillary lymphadenopathy for breast preservation. They are suitable for non-invasive or early stage breast cancer.

   These techniques may not include lesions in the dissected tissue. When dealing with a

tumor, it's essential to verify the cut surface using frozen section histology during surgery. Similarly, in the case of microcalcifications, the excised tissue must be confirmed via mammographic examination.

2. Surgical extent.

   For palpable masses, an incision is made directly on the skin above the mass, or an incision is made to include a portion of the skin above the mass. It is towed by the other hand and peeled off, but depending on the situation, 1–2 cm of normal surrounding tissue is usually removed. If the border is unclear, especially if the mass is close to the axillary tail side, it is better to pass through the pectoralis major fascia and remove some of the axillary subcutaneous fat.

   In the case of a mass shadow that cannot be touched or is suspected to be a microcalcification, it is advisable to preliminarily select the position under preoperative mastectomy, ultrasound guidance, or ultrasound guidance during surgery. The wire localization is placed at the suspicious lesion site, and the normal breast tissue around the lesion is excised based on the tip of the lead wire.

3. Surgical technique.

   The incision must be located within the mastectomy incision line because it can be enlarged by mastectomy after histologic examination. The most cosmetically effective incision is the circumareolar incision. The tumor excision extent contains 1–2 cm of normal surrounding tissue, excises the tumor, and bleeding control using electrocautery. The resected specimen is generally labeled with a knot, clip, or stain as cranio-caudal, medial-lateral, superficial-deep and then sent for a pathological examination or imaging.

1.2.4 Skin-Sparing Mastectomy

1. Indications.

   (a) AJCC (American Joint Committee on Cancers) stage 0, I, and II cancers for which a primary mastectomy is required and breast reconstruction can be performed immediately.

(b) Multicentric or multifocal lesions or with an extensive intraductal component of 25% or greater and tumor size that is significantly reduced after neoadjuvant therapy.

(c) A lesion significantly reduced in size after neoadjuvant therapy that is a T1 or partial T2 tumor located deep in the breast parenchyma.

Nipple–areolar complex (NAC) sparing mastectomy has also begun to improve the cosmetic effect. The risk of cancer cell infiltration or recurrence in the nipple–areola complex is an issue that requires consideration. Selecting target patients based on preoperative findings is very important. Patients with inflammatory breast cancer and stage III locally advanced breast cancer are generally not recommended for this surgery.

2. Surgical technique.

Several incision techniques are used: the peri-areolar incision, a separate dilated incision around the areola, a separate previous biopsy site incision, a modified oval incision that includes the nipple and areola area and the previous biopsy site, and an incision using the inframammary fold. Surgeons should carefully choose the type of skin incision, taking into account various factors. When performing a nipple–areola complex and skin-sparing mastectomy, a radial incision that minimizes the blockage of blood flow in the areola can be used. The first priority is that the tumor must be completely resected. The technique for removing the skin during a skin-sparing mastectomy, similar to a classical mastectomy, avoids the breast tissue and removes skin from the subcutaneous tissue and dermis to the surface of the superficial fascia. With the skin flap lifted, the breast tissue is detached from the chest wall together with the pectoralis major fascia from top to bottom. After the skin flap is completely lifted and most of the mastectomy is done, the breast is detached from the pectoralis major muscle and pulled outward to facilitate access

for sentinel lymph node biopsy or axillary lymph node dissection. It is necessary to remove as much breast tissue as possible and satisfy the two conditions so that necrosis does not occur in the remaining nipple. The best technique to use depends on the patient's skin thickness, areola size, presence or absence of inverted nipples, vascular distribution, breast size, age, and breast tightness. Surgeons must accumulate techniques through a lot of experience [23, 24].

3. Breast reconstruction.

Immediate breast reconstruction is performed by various methods depending on the characteristics of the patient. An artificial implant can be inserted, or the patient's own tissue can be used. For implant placement, a tissue expander is placed between the pectoralis major and pectoralis minor muscles under the resected breast to gradually increase the volume. Another method to make a breast that uses autologous tissue is a myocutaneous flap surgery. The skin and muscles are transferred from the patient's back (latissimus dorsi flap), lower abdomen (deep inferior epigastric artery perforator flap or transverse rectus myocutaneous flap), or buttocks or thighs [25–29].

4. Local recurrence.

When the indications are carefully selected, performing breast reconstruction immediately after a skin-sparing mastectomy has a better cosmetic effect than other options and has a similar local recurrence rate. Local recurrence is not difficult to detect because it recurs mostly on the chest wall. Therefore, skin-sparing mastectomy is oncologically safe and cosmetically superior to traditional mastectomy when performed selectively. There are not many reports of long-term follow-up for nipple–areola complex and skin-sparing mastectomy, and an excision of nipple–areola complex might be performed during surgery depending on the results of frozen section tests. Therefore, it is important to fully explain all the possibilities to the patient and proceed with surgery only after that consultation.

1.3 Axillary Lymph Node Surgery

1.3.1 Sentinel Lymph Node Biopsy and Intraoperative Evaluation of the Sentinel Lymph Node

1. Method using dye.

    Among the dyes, isosulfan blue is the most widely used. In combination with albumin, it selectively enters the lymph vessels and stains them and the sentinel lymph nodes blue. Methylene blue, indigo carmine, Paten blue V, indocyanine green, etc., have also been used and shown similar success rates. Among the methods for injecting dye for a sentinel lymph node biopsy, an intradermal injection around the areola is reported to have a higher detection rate of sentinel lymph nodes than a subcutaneous injection, intradermal injection, subareolar injection, or tumor site parenchymal injection. Some researchers argue that parenchymal injections around the tumor have a high detection rate. Gently massage the breast for about 5 min after injecting the dye to allow it to enter the lymph vessels well. Precise timekeeping is important because starting a biopsy too early after the injection might not result in staining, and waiting until too late to start could result in staining of non-sentinel lymph nodes with excessive stain. The time it takes for the dye to reach the sentinel lymph nodes becomes shorter as the tumor becomes closer to the axilla. It has been reported that massaging the breast after injection increases the sensitivity of finding the sentinel lymph nodes [30].

    After that, the clavipectoral fascia is found by making a 2–3-cm skin incision in front of the midaxillary line about 1 cm below the axillary hair line, and the axillary adipose tissue can be found. Look for stained lymph vessels in the area where the pectoral node is located along the margin of the pectoralis major muscle. If no lymph node is found there, look for lymph nodes at levels I and II, such as the external breast lymph node and the sub-shoulder central lymph node. All sentinel lymph nodes can only be found only by tracing both the proximal and distal parts of the stained lymph vessels and looking for the sentinel lymph nodes. After the sentinel lymph nodes are removed, the axilla should be re-examined, and any suspicious palpable lymph nodes should be removed and included in the sentinel lymph nodes. It is important to be careful not to cut or damage the stained lymph vessels because they play a role in the area where the sentinel lymph nodes can be found.

2. Method using radioactive isotopes.

    Among the radioactive isotopes, colloidal radioisotopes are most commonly used because they move quickly into the lymph vessels and are transported to the sentinel lymph nodes, where they remain long enough to be found during surgery.

    Currently, 99mTc-sulfur, 99mTc-human serum albumin, 99mTc-antimony sulfur colloid, 99mTc-dextran, 99mTc-tin, etc. are used. Other ideal radio colloids should be inexpensive, free from radiation exposure, and easy to handle. Radioactive isotopes can be injected around the tumor, subcutaneously, intradermally, subareolar, and around the areola, but many studies have shown that subareolar or around the areola injections are effective for sentinel lymph node detection. Preoperatively, sentinel lymph node locations can be determined by taking frontal and lateral lymphoscintigraphy images 15 min after injection. That also has the advantage of locating sentinel lymph nodes outside the axilla before surgery. Conversely, some reports indicate that it does not help the detection rate or false negative rate of the sentinel lymph nodes [31].

    Before starting surgery, a gamma-ray detector is used to confirm and display the exact locations of the sentinel lymph nodes. A minimal incision window is made at that location, and a gamma-ray detector is used to find hotspots with high radiation doses and remove those sentinel lymph nodes. There is no dispute that the stained lymph nodes should be considered as sentinel lymph nodes when dyes are used, but there is no standard for how many nodes should be considered sentinel lymph nodes when radioisotopes are used. One standard is that the absolute value of the radiation dose be 25 or more for 10 s, but another is that the radiation dose be 10 times or more than that of the surrounding tissue. Furthermore, once the sentinel lymph node with the highest radiation dose is excised, there is an increased risk of false negatives if the remaining lymph nodes, which exhibit a radiation dose of 10% or more of that value, are not removed by measuring the radiation dose as a sentinel lymph node. There is also a report that the standard can be lowered even further. Breast cancer usually shows the highest amount of metastasis to the sentinel lymph nodes with the highest radiation dose. But once metastasized tumor cells have completely replaced the lymph nodes, the lymph nodes might have very low or undetectable radiation doses, so all suspicious lymph nodes should be removed at the time of biopsy. The greater the number of sentinel lymph nodes resected, the higher the accuracy. According to the NSABP B-32 study, the false negative rate was 17.7% in one node, 10% in two nodes, 6.9% in three nodes, 3.3% in four nodes, and 1% in five nodes.

3. Combination of dyes and radioactive isotopes.

It has been reported that combining dyes and radioactive isotopes for sentinel lymph node biopsy increases the meaningful sentinel lymph node detection rate and average number of sentinel lymph nodes and lowers the false negative rate. Therefore, for surgeons who are not experienced with these procedures, it is easy to use both formulations together to shorten the learning curve [32].

4. Side effects and complications.

Isosulfan blue dyes rarely cause urticaria and anaphylaxis. The administration of steroids and antihistamines improves urticaria in a short time. Hypotensive anaphylaxis, however, requires aggressive and immediate treatment and 24-h intensive observation. In addition, the use of isosulfan blue during surgery can interfere with the measurement of intraoperative oxygen saturation by pulse oximetry, causing it to be measured as lower than the actual value. Other side effects that stain the epidermis can occur, but they usually disappear in a few weeks to a few months [17, 18].

It is well known that sentinel lymph node biopsy has fewer complications than axillary lymphadenectomy. When only the sentinel lymph node procedure is performed, effects such as postmastectomy pain syndrome, lymphedema, axillary pain, abnormal sensation in the surgical site, upper extremity movement on the affected side, cosmetic aspects of the axillary wound, postoperative wound infection, and seroma were held at satisfactory levels.

5. Sentinel lymph node evaluation.

With the advent of sentinel lymph nodes, a thorough and detailed examination of the axillary lymph nodes has become possible. According to the American Society of Pathology's draft recommended method, the sentinel lymph nodes are first cut in half in the longitudinal direction and then cut at intervals of 1.5–2 mm to make continuous sections [32]. It is recommended to make three sections for each block. If metastases are found, the pathologist should record whether they are macrometastases or micrometastases found by immunohistochemical staining or reverse transcription polymerase chain reactions. Due to controversy over the significance of sentinel lymph node metastases found by immunohistochemical staining, the American Pathology Society does not recommend the basic use of immunohistochemical staining.

According to the ACOSOG Z0010 trial, sentinel node metastases deemed positive by H&E staining had a significant effect on the 5-year overall survival rate, but sentinel node metastases deemed positive by immunohistochemical staining did not affect the survival rate. The clinical significance of micrometastasis is also still controversial. Some results show that micrometastases found by H&E staining indicate a difference in disease-free survival, but other reports persist that this is not [33, 34].

According to the seventh edition of the AJCC, isolated tumor cells or isolated clusters of tumor cells (ultra-micrometastases) are defined as a cell colony size of 0.2 mm or less, single tumor cells, or fewer than 200 colonies in a single histological cross-section, and they are classified as pN0.

1.3.2 Axillary Lymph Node Dissection

The presence or absence of axillary lymph node metastasis is one of the most important single prognostic factors in breast cancer. Axillary lymph node dissection is a local axillary treatment used to stage breast cancer and determine the direction of advanced treatment.

1. Indications.
   (a) A sentinel lymph node biopsy shows metastasis.
   (b) Contraindications for sentinel lymph node biopsy or if no sentinel lymph node is found.
   (c) Inflammatory breast cancer or surgery after neoadjuvant chemotherapy.
   (d) Cases of locoregional recurrence of axillary lymph nodes after sentinel lymph node resection.
2. Surgical anatomy.
   The axilla is divided into three levels, I, II, and III, depending on the positional relationship with the pectoralis minor muscle. Level I is the lateral portion of the pectoralis minor muscle, including the lateral border, and contains the lateral lymph nodes, the subscapularis, and the lateral axillary veins. Level II is situated between the lateral and medial borders of the pectoralis minor muscle, essentially just inferior to the pectoralis minor. This region is where the central lymph node group is located. The common axillary dissection involves a level I and II lymphadenectomy. Level III is the area inside the medial border of the pectoralis minor and contains the subclavian lymphoid group. Dissection is not generally considered except in cases in which the lymph nodes of level III are palpable, or when a level III dissection is required because metastasis to level I or II is clinically clear. Rotter's nodes mean the lymph nodes located between the pectoralis major and pectoralis minor.

3. Preoperative considerations and surgical steps.
   The patient's arms should be placed on the arm supports, with the affected arm at 90° or less, and the skin of the axilla is prepared for standard methods. From preparation for surgery until the end of surgery, the arm should not be hyperextended. It is important to place a pad on the arm struts to prevent shoulder dislocation and brachial plexus tension during surgery. To prevent infection, a wide range of antibiotics, including against Gram-positive bacteria, is given intravenously just before surgery. During anesthesia, avoid the use of long-acting muscle relaxants to make it easier to recognize the motor nerves during surgery.

   When performing a modified radical mastectomy, use the mastectomy line without a separate skin incision. In mastectomy, surgery is performed through a new axillary incision line. The anterior edge of the skin incision extends to the lateral aspect of the pectoralis major muscle, while the posterior edge reaches the anterior border of the latissimus dorsi muscle. In most cases, the incision is made parallel to the wrinkles of the skin, but in some cases, it can be made vertically or diagonally to the chest wall. The cutaneous flap is bordered by the axillary vein above, the chest wall below, the lateral edge of the pectoralis major muscle in the anterior, and the anterior edge of the distribution muscle in the posterior. At this time, attention should be paid to the external thoracic nerve that runs along the posterior side of the pectoralis major muscle and the internal thoracic nerve that runs in a Y shape on the inferolateral sides of the pectoralis major muscle.

   The surgeon dissects along the pectoralis minor muscle. When the axillary vein is identified, the fat layer covering it should be separated from top to bottom. At this time, thorough removal of the tissue around the vein induces lymphedema. When the axillary vein is exposed, the lower part of the vein is separated from the inside to the outside, and the upper part of the vein is not dissected. Rather than separating just below the vein, separating it at intervals of about 5 mm can prevent side holes from forming in the vein. When separating and ligating the branches of the axillary vein, the anterior thoracic branch of the axillary vein is ligated, and the thoracic vein just below is checked. Axillary lymph node dissection involves en bloc resection to prevent damage to the axillary lymphatic vessels and progresses in stages from medial to lateral. At this time, the thoracic neurovascular bundle is the first deep branch to be found. Detachment along the lateral and anterior sides of the latissimus dorsi muscle can prevent damage to the thoracodorsal nerve. The thoracodorsal nerve is located mainly inside the vein, slightly posterior, and can be pressed lightly to check the contraction of the latissimus dorsi muscles and the movement of the shoulder. Along with this, the long thoracic nerve must be found and preserved. The long thoracic nerve returns inferiorly and posteriorly along the thoracic wall from the fat layer at the intersection of the axillary vein and the thoracic wall, with the subscapular lymphatic group sample pulled downward and outward. Pressing it lightly allows the surgeon to check the movement of the serratus anterior. If it is not found along the chest wall, check that it is not pulled outward along the axillary tissue being exfoliated. If it has been pulled outward, it should be separated and placed on the chest wall. To safely preserve the long thoracic nerve, the surgeon should keep an eye on it and immediately dissect the anterior nerve, taking care not to dissect the inside of the nerve. Then, the surgeon dissects downward until the nerve enters the serratus anterior muscle, taking special care not to injure the nerves at this point because they run slightly outward just before entering the serratus anterior. It can be confirmed that the intercostal brachial nerve enters the chest wall through the third intercostal nerve during the separation of the long thoracic nerve. It runs about 1 cm below the axillary vein. Intermediate axillary adipose tissue is separated until the nerves are free. Preservation of the intercostal brachial nerve is not essential if the axilla is lymph node positive when viewed with the naked eye.

4. Postoperative management and complications.

When the 24-h drainage volume is 30 mL or less, the axillary drainage tube can be removed, and most of the time, it is removed 4–7 days after surgery. During this time, oral antibiotics are not usually required. Arm movements should begin the day after surgery and should be managed carefully until the range of movement returns to normal. Excessive exercise can increase drainage.

Lymphedema can appear at various times after surgery and must be diagnosed early in the condition and treated appropriately. Axillary cord syndrome, often known as Mondor's disease, involves a string of tender subcutaneous tissues extending from the lateral axilla to the upper and medial aspects of the arm, manifesting in a cord-like structure beneath the skin. It typically occurs 1–8 weeks after axillary dissection and appears when the axillary veins and lymphatic vessels were damaged proximally during surgery. It generally improves spontaneously and must be distinguished from lymphedema.

When the thoracic nerve is injured, the abduction of the arm is restricted, and when the long thoracic nerve is injured, the wing scapula and shoulders are affected. When the intercostobrachial nerve is injured, paresthesia of the upper medial part of the arm, axillary, and superior laterality of the chest appears. Complications such as upper arm movement range limitation can occur, but movement can be recovered by steady exercise and rehabilitation.

2 Local Therapy: Radiotherapy

2.1 History

Radiation began to be used in the treatment of cancer shortly after Roentgen discovered X-rays. Since then, radiation therapy has played an important role in improving the local remission rate and survival rate in breast cancer. Radiation therapy is also given to patients with distant metastases to relieve symptoms. After the Curie couple discovered a radioisotope called radium, radium needles were primarily used to treat breast cancer, but in the 1930s, low-energy external radiation therapy was used. However, much of the radiation from low-energy radiation therapy was absorbed into the skin and did not sufficiently irradiate the actual cancer tissue, which caused acute skin damage and chronic sequelae. In 1951, a radiation therapy device using cobalt was put into operation to reduce the amount of radiation absorbed by the skin. Thus, medical linear accelerators that generate high-energy X-rays and electron beams have been developed since the early 1950s, and they now play a major role in radiation therapy for breast cancer. Linear-accelerated radiotherapy equipment began to be used after the development of computer-based three-dimensional radiotherapy technology in the 1990s [35, 36]. Subsequently, intensity-modulated radiation therapy technology was developed, and now, respiratory gated radiation that treats patients according to their breathing has also been developed. Thanks to these advancements, side effects can be minimized and the target can be irradiated uniformly, thereby enhancing clinical effectiveness. In addition to radiation using electromagnetic waves such as X-rays and γ-rays, medium-particle radiotherapy devices for neutrons, protons, and carbon ions have also been developed, but they are still used in a limited manner for breast cancer. Recently, breast conserving surgery has become widespread, and radiation therapy is an important part of that breast cancer treatment. In recent years, the convenience and accessibility of radiation therapy have become the main concerns. Therefore, various methods for optimizing radiotherapy, such as reducing the number of sessions and performing partial radiotherapy, have been developed and tested [37–39].

2.2 Radiation Therapy After Breast-Conserving Surgery

2.2.1 Range of Radiation Therapy and Radiation Dose

The scope of radiation therapy for patients who undergo axillary lymph node dissection at the same time as breast conservation surgery includes the remaining total breast tissue, adjacent skin and subcutaneous tissue, and chest wall. It can be found by dividing up to 50 Gy over 25–28 days. The divided survey dose is thus 1.8–2 Gy and is administered once a day, 5 times a week. Subsequently, an electron beam is directed to the site of the surgical scar and previous tumor location, or brachytherapy is performed within the tissue. In some cases, additional irradiation is performed by three-dimensional modeling treatment using a photon beam and electron beam. Radiation therapy is usually available as outpatient treatment, and each treatment takes about 15 min. The total duration of radiation therapy is usually 6 weeks. If there is a tumor in the resection margin, the recurrence rate is high. In that situation, additional irradiation of 15–20 Gy is applied to the primary lesion site, for a total irradiation dose of 60–65 Gy. To evaluate the usefulness of additional irradiation, an EORTC study was conducted in patients with lesions of 3 cm or smaller and confirmed tumor-free excision. According to that study, 5-year survival did not change with additional radiation therapy of 16 Gy, but the local recurrence rate was significantly reduced. However, the researchers reported that the additional radiation had a negative effect on the cosmetic results [40, 41]. At the same time, the effect of an additional 10 Gy of irradiation was studied in France. That study reported that the local recurrence rate was significantly reduced without causing a difference in the cosmetic results [42].

The standard treatment to date has been radiation therapy to the whole breast, but partial treatment has been attempted in some studies. Holland et al. (1985) [43] reported that in the case of a tumor of 2 cm or smaller, the probability that a new tumor would be found at a site 2 cm or more away from the primary tumor was 28%. Therefore, they reported that the entire breast had to be treated. However, according to reports since 1990, most local recurrences occur around the surgical site, even when radiotherapy is not administered after surgery, and the recurrence rate in other lesions is not significantly different from the incidence of secondary tumors in the contralateral breast. This suggests the possible feasibility of partial treatment ([44, 45], Veronesi et al. [5]). Furthermore, such conservative treatment can be retried if cancer recurs in the breast after local treatment. Unlike whole breast therapy, partial treatment can be completed within 1 week using methods such as external radiation therapy, interstitial brachytherapy, balloon intracavitary brachytherapy, or low-energy radiation therapy. Therefore, it has the advantage of having little effect on the timing of systemic anticancer chemotherapy. Most studies conducted to date report that local recurrence rates and survival rates do not differ from those with existing treatments. However, the follow-up period is still short, so it is difficult to conclude the usefulness of partial radiotherapy.

2.2.2 Timing of Radiation Therapy

1. Timing of radiotherapy after surgery.

   It has never been established when radiation therapy should be started after surgery. It usually takes 4–6 weeks for the surgical scar to heal. Delaying radiation therapy for more than 8 weeks after surgery does not increase the local recurrence rate compared with radiation therapy given within 4 weeks after surgery. One study by Vujovic et al. reported that for axillary lymph node-negative patients, delaying radiation therapy for more than 16 weeks did not affect the local recurrence rate. However, that is not the case for patients aged 40 years or younger who have close resection margins (≤ 2 mm) or benign resection margins. In those cases, the local recurrence rate tended to increase, though not in a statistically significant way, when radiation therapy was given 8 or 12 weeks or more after surgery. In general, patients who are not eligible for systemic anticancer chemotherapy should receive radiation therapy within 8 weeks after surgery [46].

2. Timing of systemic chemotherapy and radiation therapy.

   For patients who are not eligible for systemic chemotherapy, radiation therapy begins after surgical scarring, generally 3–4 weeks after surgery. The order of treatment for patients who must receive both systemic che-

motherapy and radiation therapy is still controversial. An analysis of 11 studies with 1927 patients showed a high local recurrence rate of 16% in the group of patients who received chemotherapy first and radiation therapy later. The local recurrence rate in the group of patients who received radiation therapy first was 6% [47]. However, a large retrospective study reported that delaying radiation therapy did not increase local recurrence rates. A study of 718 axillary lymph node-positive patients reported no difference in the local recurrence rate between the group who received radiation therapy immediately after breast-conserving surgery and the group who received radiation therapy after 3 or 6 chemotherapy sessions.

2.2.3 Irradiation Method

The breast and surrounding tissues are irradiated through an internally and externally symmetrical tangential irradiation field. The treatment should be designed so that the whole target volume receives radiation in as uniform a dose as possible while minimizing the amount of lung tissue contained in the treatment area. When designing the internally and externally symmetrical tangential irradiation field, sufficiently treat the chest wall. At the same time, when treating lung tissue on the left side, the volume of radiation to which normal organs, such as the heart, are exposed should be minimized. Because the frequency of radiation pneumonia is proportional to the volume of exposed lung tissue, it is important to reduce the exposed area. Recently, 3-dimensional treatment plans using CT images to adjust the irradiation intensity have been proposed. Intensity-modulated radiation therapy, which irradiates tumors intensively, has been introduced, and makes it possible to reduce the amount of radiation applied to normal tissues.

It can also be helpful to fix the patient's body and induce postural changes to facilitate the setting of the radiation field. Various fixation devices are used to consistently maintain the patient's therapeutic posture for each fractionated irradiation. For breast treatment, low-density cradle-type fixing devices are commonly used.

2.3 Radiation Therapy After Radical Total Mastectomy

2.3.1 Indications

The local recurrence rate after radical mastectomy has been reported to be 9–36%, varying with the size of the primary lesion and the presence and degree of metastasis to the axillary lymph nodes. That is, in the absence of axillary lymph node metastasis, the local recurrence rate is only 5%, but in the presence of metastasis, the local recurrence rate is about 25%. The recurrence rate is about 10% with 3 or fewer lymph node metastases and 36% with 4 or more lymph node metastases. In patients with T1–2 breast cancer and lymph node metastasis (4 or more if the primary tumor is 2 cm or more), vascular lymphatic invasion of the tumor, or a primary tumor that is clinically palpable, the frequency of lymph node metastasis is significantly increased [48]. Therefore, patients with 4 or more lymph node metastases or other risk factors for recurrence should receive radiation therapy after mastectomy. For T3 and T4 tumors without lymph node metastases, radiation therapy is given after radical mastectomy, which reduces the local recurrence rate to 5%. Even when chemotherapy was performed as adjuvant therapy, local recurrence increased as the primary disease site and number of axillary lymph nodes affected became larger. Specifically, when the primary lesion is 5 cm or larger and 4 or more axillary lymph nodes have metastases, the local recurrence rate is reported to be 30% or more, so radiation therapy is absolutely necessary [49].

2.3.2 Method

Radiation therapy after radical mastectomy is usually split treatment once a day, 5 days a week, for about 5 weeks (25–28 sessions). A total dose of 45–50 Gy of radiation should be irradiated to the supraclavicular lymph node on the ipsilateral chest wall from which the tumor has been removed. According to the US Treatment Method Study [50], this irradiation dose has become universal, and it is the irradiation dose that is commonly prescribed in South Korea. The treatment area is based on the chest wall and some axillary lymph nodes. The supraclavicular lymph nodes on that side can also be included as dictated by the patient's risk factors. Because there is no evidence to recommend radiation therapy for internal mammary lymph nodes, it is performed only when lymph node metastases are clinically diagnosed by CT or MRI or confirmed by pathologic findings after surgery. Because recurrence often occurs in the skin or subcutaneous tissue within 3 cm above and below the wound site, it is necessary to ensure that the skin is exposed to a sufficient amount of radiation when the chest wall is irradiated. Treatment with electron beams ensures that the skin surface receives a high dose. When treating a tangential field using X-rays, the skin is covered with a tissue-equivalent substance for treatment. Because the depth varies depending on the anatomical position of the irradiation volume and major organs such as the lungs and heart are near the affected area, care must be taken to perform radiation therapy without complications.

2.4 Axillary Lymph Node Radiation Therapy

Axillary lymphadenopathy is performed to stage the disease, assess the risk, and prevent recurrence in the axillary lymph nodes. It is well known that the local control rate offered by surgery improves the survival rate, but side effects such as edema, pain, paresthesia, and restricted shoulder movement are problematic. For early-stage breast cancer, sentinel lymph node biopsy can significantly reduce these side effects. Furthermore, this procedure can provide similar outcomes to axillary lymph node dissection, while lowering the incidence of complications. The NSABP B-04 study at the Curie Institute demonstrated that axillary lymph node radiation therapy after breast conserving surgery had the same effect as lymphadenectomy, and many retrospective analyses have shown similar results [51]. If lymph node metastasis is confirmed by sentinel lymph node biopsy, further axillary lymph node dissection is performed. However, radiation therapy can be given instead of surgery to reduce lymphedema of the arm. Prospective studies, such as the AMAROS study, are underway to find the best treatment protocol. Some researchers have argued that if the sentinel lymph node are positive, radiation therapy could be a viable option if additional axillary lymphadenopathy is unlikely to change the chemotherapy treatment regimen [33, 39].

2.5 Breast Reconstruction and Radiation Therapy

Many women desire breast reconstruction after mastectomy. If patients have to undergo radiation therapy, they will face various problems and require close cooperation among specialists in breast surgery, orthopedics, and radiation oncology. Breast reconstruction uses artificial prostheses and autologous tissue. It can be performed at the time of the initial surgery or after a certain period of time, usually after radiation therapy. Immediate reconstruction has advantages in terms of skin sensation and cosmetology, but when radiation therapy is used, those advantages disappear, and it becomes difficult to establish a treatment plan. Geometric problems arise, especially for transplanted prostheses, and radiation is difficult without specially planned treatments, such as intensity-controlled radiation therapy. In many cases, fibrosis, constriction, etc., cause poor cosmetic results. Even when using autologous tissue, it is generally recommended to perform reconstruction after radiation therapy [23, 24].

2.6 Radiation Therapy for Palliative Purposes

Breast cancer patients, unlike other cancer patients, can survive for a long time even if they have a local recurrence or distant metastasis. To improve the patient's quality of life, long-term control of the pain, fractures, spinal cord compression, etc., that can be caused by distant metastases must be ensured. Extensive distant metastases can cause a short survival time, but metastasis confined to one organ, especially if the

time to metastasis is long, can permit long-term survival. Therefore, radiation therapy more aggressive than that required for short-term symptom-relieving radiation therapy, such as palliative radiation therapy for general cancer, is required.

3 Neoadjuvant Therapy

Neoadjuvant chemotherapy has two purposes: First, in patients (N2–3 or T4) who have difficulty with definitive surgery, it can induce a reaction in the tumor or metastasized lymph nodes that will facilitate local treatment such as surgery or radiation therapy. Second, in patients who can undergo definitive surgery (T3N1M0), it can make breast conserving possible. In addition, it has the advantage of revealing the susceptibility of the tumor to chemotherapy and, at least in theory, provides early treatment of micrometastases [52]. Most studies have shown similar clinical courses and prognoses with neoadjuvant chemotherapy and adjuvant chemotherapy, and both protocols are thus widely used as standard therapies. In addition, pathological complete remission (pCR) can be used as a prognostic factor for long-term survival. Whether adjuvant chemotherapy should be given before or after surgery depends on the stage, histology, hormone receptor, and HER2 receptor status of the invasive breast cancer. The choice must be made by comprehensively judging the state of expression and the possibility of breast preservation. Neoadjuvant chemotherapy can be performed for locally advanced breast cancer and (when surgery is possible) to reduce the surgical range for large breast cancers. Patient planning for advanced chemotherapy requires a core biopsy of the primary tumor. If axillary lymph node metastasis is clinically suspected, a biopsy or cell aspiration cytology of the lymph nodes is also recommended.

3.1 Chemotherapy

In principle, the drugs used for adjuvant chemotherapy can also be used for neoadjuvant chemotherapy. Combined therapy based on doxorubicin has mainly been performed, but since adjuvant chemotherapy including taxane showed superiority in the survival rate, taxane has also been used in neoadjuvant chemotherapy. Various other therapies have also been studied and reported better pCR rate. In the NSABP B-27 study of 2300 patients, pCR rates were higher in the group that received docetaxel after AC (doxorubicin, cyclophosphamide) than in the group that did not receive docetaxel (26% vs. 13%) [53]. In the Aberdeen study of 162 patients, the CVAP (cyclophosphamide, vincristine, doxorubicin, prednisolone) response group who received docetaxel after conversion had a higher pCR rate than the group who continued to receive CVAP therapy (34% vs. 16%). In the GEPARDUO study of 913 patients, AC (doxorubicin, cyclophosphamide) followed by DOC (docetaxel) sequential therapy had a better pathological complete remission rate than 2-week interval (dose dense) ADOC (doxorubicin, docetaxel) simultaneous combination therapy (14.3% vs. 7%) [54].

Following a neoadjuvant chemotherapy study with taxane, phase II or III studies on nanoparticle albumin-bound (nab)-paclitaxel were reported. The GeparSepto study compared epirubicin/cyclophosphamide (EC) administration after nab-paclitaxel or paclitaxel and found pCR rates of 38% and 29%, respectively [55]. In addition, after 4 years of follow-up, invasive disease-free survival was superior in the nab-paclitaxel group, though there was no difference in the overall survival rate. In contrast, the ETNA study did not show the superiority of nab-paclitaxel, with a pCR rate of 22.5% vs. 18.6% [56]. In different large studies, nab-paclitaxel did not show consistent results, but it did show a pCR rate similar to paclitaxel, so long-term follow-up results need to be collected.

In a study of the number of neoadjuvant chemotherapy treatments, the pCR rate with ED (epirubicin, docetaxel) was higher after 6 cycles than after 3 cycles. In the GeparTrio study of 2000 people, 2 doses of TAC (docetaxel, doxorubicin, cyclophosphamide) were administered first, and then 4 or 6 additional doses of TAC were administered to 1390 responders [57]. The study reported no differences in the pCR rate

between the two groups. The 2006 International Expert Panel recommendation is for a combination therapy that includes anthracycline or taxane to be administered at least 6 cycles for 4–6 months before surgery in eligible breast cancer patients.

The recent GeparQuinto study of 1509 patients given 4 cycles of EC (epirubicin, cyclophosphamide) therapy compared the addition of docetaxel monotherapy (EC-T), docetaxel + capecitabine combination therapy (EC-TX), and docetaxel → capecitabine sequential therapy (EC-T-X). It reported no difference in the pCR rate or breast-conserving surgery, so it is not recommended to increase the duration of anthracycline-taxane therapy or add capecitabine.

After completing 2–3 neoadjuvant chemotherapies, a clinical evaluation and response evaluation by imaging study must be performed. Then, the decision to continue the planned chemotherapy, switch to a new therapy, or administer local treatment must be made based on the results of those assessments. If trastuzumab or hormone therapy is indicated after surgery, it can be given in parallel with radiation therapy.

3.2 Endocrine Therapy

Studies of neoadjuvant endocrine therapy in premenopausal women who are hormone receptor positive are very restrictive. Reports have shown 3% complete pathological observation and 42% breast preservation from combination therapy with GnRH agonists and letrozole. According to several studies of neoadjuvant endocrine therapy in postmenopausal women, tamoxifen plus anastrozole, anastrozole alone, and letrozole monotherapy offer the best breast-conserving surgery and objective response rates [58]. Based on those studies, aromatase inhibitors are suitable neoadjuvant endocrine therapy for postmenopausal women with hormone receptor positive breast cancer. The appropriate duration of neoadjuvant endocrine therapy is 4–6 months, and co-administration of chemotherapy and aromatase inhibitors is not desirable. In addition, neoadjuvant therapy with a CDK4/6 inhibitor combined with endocrine therapy has recently been tested in clinical studies. According to the CORALLEEN phase 2 clinical study comparing 6 months of ribociclib + letrozole and prior endocrine therapy with doxorubicin/cyclophosphamide and paclitaxel, both therapies have the same low risk-of-relapse score [59].

4 Systemic Therapy: Adjuvant Setting

4.1 Chemotherapy

4.1.1 Adjuvant Chemotherapy

Adjuvant chemotherapy should be determined by the histological type of tumor, presence or absence of hormone receptor and HER2 overexpression, and lymph node metastasis. Chemotherapy and endocrine therapy should be given sequentially, not simultaneously. CMF and radiation therapy can be given at the same time, but except in special cases, all other chemotherapy is given prior to radiation therapy.

The first randomized studies of adjuvant chemotherapy in breast cancer demonstrated that adjuvant CMF chemotherapy significantly reduced the treatment failure rate. Four cycles of doxorubicin and cyclophosphamide have the same effect as six cycles of CMF chemotherapy. There is no benefit to be gained by increasing the dose of doxorubicin or cyclophosphamide above the standard dose. The comparison of 4 cycles of AC and 6 cycles of FEC for lymph node-negative breast cancer in the NSABP B-36 study found no difference in disease-free survival or overall survival between the two groups, but toxicity was higher with FEC therapy [60]. High-dose epirubicin-based CEF therapy for lymph node-positive breast cancer improved disease-free survival compared with CMF therapy [61]. The FASG-05 study comparing two epirubicin doses (high versus low doses) observed a significant improvement in survival with high-dose epirubicin-based CEF therapy [62].

Various studies have also been conducted on the role of taxane in adjuvant therapy. Sequential administration of docetaxel or paclitaxel for lymph node-positive breast cancer showed improved survival over FEC monotherapy. The addition of taxane to anthracycline-based therapy has been shown to improve the clinical course of lymph node-positive breast cancer and reduce the risk of recurrence in even high-risk lymph node-negative patients in several phase III studies [63]. The EBCTCG meta-analysis also showed a significant reduction in breast cancer related mortality with the addition of 4-cycle taxane to treatment with fixed doses of anthracyclines. The E1199 study by the Eastern Cooperative Oncology Group compared schedules of paclitaxel and docetaxel given after AC chemotherapy [64]. In a 12-year follow-up analysis, docetaxel therapy every 3 weeks showed a significant prolongation of disease-free survival compared with paclitaxel therapy every 3 weeks. Therefore, weekly paclitaxel or every 3-week docetaxel therapy is recommended for sequential administration after 4 cycles of AC [65]. The USON 9735 study compared docetaxel with cyclophosphamide (TC), doxorubicin, and cyclophosphamide (AC) and showed significantly longer disease-free survival with TC therapy. The CALGB 9741 study compared dose-intensive therapy with standard sequential chemotherapy and found that dose-dense therapy improved survival [66]. A meta-analysis also reported that dose-dense chemotherapy significantly improved both overall survival and disease-free survival. A meta-analysis restricted to clinical trials using equivalent doses demonstrated that dose-dense chemotherapy significantly improved survival without increasing chemotherapy-related side effects. In the meta-analysis results of 26 studies in EBCTCG, dose-dense chemotherapy significantly lowered the 10-year recurrence rate from 31.4% to 28.0% and lowered the 10-year breast cancer mortality rate from 21.3% to 18%, compared with the control group. From the viewpoint of improving the survival rate, dose-dense chemotherapy with prophylactic G-CSF assistance is preferred [67].

4.1.2 Chemotherapy in Elderly Patients

Chemotherapy may be recommended for all age groups younger than 70 years. The benefits of post-surgery chemotherapy are most pronounced in women younger than 50 and diminish with age above that. For patients older than 70, it is difficult to offer general clinical guidelines because clinical trial materials for adjuvant chemotherapy are rare. However, in the CALGB 49907 study, patients, especially those with ER-negative breast cancer, who were treated with capecitabine did more poorly than those who received AC or CMF standard therapy [68]. In other words, evidence suggests that it is better for older breast cancer patients to receive the same standard therapy as younger breast cancer patients. In a random-distribution open clinical trial comparing trastuzumab monotherapy with trastuzumab plus chemotherapy in patients aged 70–80 years with HER2-positive breast cancer who underwent surgical resection, 3-year disease-free survival was reported to be 85.9% in the trastuzumab monotherapy group and 93.8% in the trastuzumab/chemotherapy combination therapy group, demonstrating the noninferiority of trastuzumab monotherapy. Therefore, in principle, systemic adjuvant therapy for patients aged 70 years or older should be standard therapy, but decisions should be made individually in consideration of accompanying diseases and general condition.

4.1.3 Adjuvant Systemic Therapy for histology of Breast Cancer with Good Prognosis

For invasive cancer of good histological subtypes such as tubular carcinoma or mucinous carcinoma, adjuvant systemic therapy is not required in the absence of lymph node involvement or lymph node involvement of less than 2 mm when the tumor is less than 1 cm. With lymph node involvement less than 2 mm and a tumor of 1 cm or more and less than 3 cm, endocrine therapy can be considered if the hormone receptor is positive, and if the tumor is 3 cm or more, endocrine therapy should be performed irrespective of the hormone receptor status. The chemotherapy may be considered as an alternative to endocrine therapy when lymph node metastasis is 2 mm or greater, regardless of tumor size. If the hormone receptor is negative after retesting, chemotherapy based on common histological types can be considered [69, 70].

4.2 Endocrine Therapy

All breast cancer patients should be confirmed for ER and PR expression [71]. If one of them is positive, adjuvant endocrine therapy is given regardless of the patient's age, axillary lymph node metastasis, adjuvant chemotherapy, or HER2 overexpression. Adjuvant endocrine therapy may be omitted in some cases because the prognosis after surgery is very good if the size is 0.5 cm or less and there is no lymph node metastasis. However, in an ER-positive patient, adjuvant endocrine therapy is recommended because it reduces the risk of developing secondary cancer in the contralateral breast [72].

4.2.1 Endocrine Therapy for Breast Cancer in Premenopausal Women

For hormone receptor-positive premenopausal women, oral administration of 20 mg of tamoxifen daily is a priority, and the recommended duration of use is at least 5 years. The SOFT and TEXT trial found that the addition of ovarian suppression therapy to tamoxifen significantly improved disease-free survival and overall survival compared with the use of tamoxifen alone [73]. In addition, ovarian suppression therapy was used to induce menopause, and when an aromatase inhibitor was administered, the disease-free survival rate improved. Therefore, premenopausal women can undergo ovarian suppression therapy for 5 years with tamoxifen and aromatase inhibitors. Ovarian suppression therapy is more beneficial if anticancer treatment is required because of a high risk of recurrence or if the risk of other clinicopathological recurrence is high (35 years or younger, high tumor grade, N2 stage or higher, etc.). However, the decision must be made in consideration of the side effects that can occur due to ovarian suppression therapy and drug adaptability.

If tamoxifen is used for 5 years and menopause occurs, it can be replaced with an aromatase inhibitor and administered for another 5 years or more. Also, based on the ATLAS study, 10 years of endocrine therapy plus tamoxifen for another 5 years can be given with or without menopause. Because aromatase inhibitors are ineffective in women with ovarian action, serum LH, FSH, and estradiol (E2) concentrations should be checked every 3–6 months when considering aromatase inhibitor treatment in this group of patients.

When a GnRH agonist and an aromatase inhibitor are administered in combination to premenopausal patients, it has been reported that the administration of zoledronic acid significantly prolongs disease-free survival. It also delays bone density loss and helps to restore bone density after treatment is interrupted [74].

4.2.2 Endocrine Therapy for Breast Cancer in Postmenopausal Women

In general, the postmenopausal condition indicates one of the followings:

- Bilateral oophorectomy was performed.
- The patient is older than 60 years.
- The patient is younger than 60 years but has been amenorrheic (with FSH and E2 in the postmenopausal range) for at least 12 months without treatment with anticancer drugs (tamoxifen, etc.) or ovarian function suppressants.
- Among patients younger than 60 years who are taking tamoxifen and started adjuvant chemotherapy before menopause, when FSH and E2 were in the premenopausal range, menopause status after chemotherapy cannot be judged as amenorrhea. Therefore, treated amenorrheic patients can receive an aromatase inhibitor only if menopause is confirmed by regular follow-up of FSH and E2 levels [75, 76].

For postmenopausal patients with hormone receptor-positive breast cancer, we recommend upfront therapy as the initial adjuvant therapy. Initial administration of an aromatase inhibitor instead of tamoxifen for 5 years has been shown to reduce the risk of local recurrence, contralateral breast cancer development, and distant metastasis without affecting overall survival. In addition, after taking tamoxifen for 2–3 years, it can be changed to an aromatase inhibitor and administered for a total of 5 years (switch therapy as sequential with tamoxifen), or after tak-

ing tamoxifen for 5 years, the aromatase inhibitor can be used for 5 more years (extended therapy). Due to the absence of comparative studies determining the optimal duration of tamoxifen administration before initiating aromatase inhibitors, no specific duration can be recommended at this time. But patients who have been taking tamoxifen for 2–3 years are recommended to switch to an aromatase inhibitor. Based on the results of the ATLAS study, it is possible to use tamoxifen for 5 years and then administer the same drug for up to 10 years. However, no studies have yet shown whether either method is more effective than changing to an aromatase inhibitor. The decision between tamoxifen and aromatase inhibitors is best made in consultation with the patient, considering the benefits and potential side effects of each medication. Therefore, if aromatase inhibitors are contraindicated or unsuitable, tamoxifen is recommended for 5 years. Even in those cases, tamoxifen can be optionally used for 10 years [77].

Until now, it has not been recommended to maintain aromatase inhibitors for more than 5 years. Recently, a study of adjuvant endocrine therapies after surgery reported results from using an initial aromatase inhibitor for 5 years and then extending that therapy with an additional aromatase inhibitor for up to 10 years. Some results showed a tendency to improve disease-free survival, but the difference was not large, and no results showed an improvement in overall survival. However, given the results of studies showing the long-term recurrence potential of breast cancer and the effect of aromatase inhibitors in reducing secondary breast cancer, their use can be extended to 10 years in patients at high risk of recurrence. Other considerations are drug resistance and side effects [73].

To reduce the risk of osteoporosis, it is advisable to measure bone mineral density before using aromatase inhibitors. If necessary, appropriate physical exercise, calcium preparations, vitamin D, and zoledronic acid can be administered. The ABCSG-18 study reported that subcutaneous injections of denosumab

(60 mg every 6 months) in postmenopausal patients taking aromatase inhibitors as adjuvant endocrine therapy significantly delayed the development of clinical fractures [78].

4.2.3 CDK4/6 Inhibitor Combination Therapy as Adjuvant Therapy

In the MONARCHE study, patients diagnosed with hormone receptor-positive/HER2-negative breast cancer and having 4 or more lymph node metastasis or high risk with 1–3 lymph node metastasis were administered abemaciclib for a duration of 2 years alongside adjuvant endocrine therapy. The study reported that the drug combination improved the 2-year invasive disease-free survival rate from 88.7% with adjuvant endocrine therapy alone to 92.2%. In contrast, the PALLAS study, which added 2 years of palbociclib administration to adjuvant endocrine therapy in stage 2–3 patients, failed to show significant differences in 3-year invasive disease-free survival [79]. Although the MONARCHE study showed positive results, the follow-up period was relatively short, so we must wait for future long-term follow-up results [80]. Likewise, we have to wait to judge the results of the NATALEE research into ribociclib, another CDK4/6 inhibitor.

4.3 HER2-Targeted Therapy

Targeted treatment focuses on substances that play crucial roles in the development and progression of cancer, aiming to inhibit their actions and achieve therapeutic effects. As a general rule, targeted treatment is administered specifically to patients with identified targets, in contrast to conventional chemotherapy. This approach helps reduce side effects and enhances treatment efficacy. Targeted treatments are expected to play a major role in cancer treatment in the future. There are four human epidermal growth factor receptor (HER) families: epidermal growth factor receptor (EGFR), HER2, HER3, and HER4. These receptors are present throughout the cell membrane; are composed of extracellular, cell membrane, and intracellular regions; and have a morphological structure that transmits signals related to cell proliferation to the nucleus. GFR, HER3, and HER4, but not HER2,

possess a structure capable of specific binding to the extracellular ligand of the receptor. This ligand binding initiates the signal generation process and its transmission into the cell. EGFR, HER2, and HER4, but not HER3, possess a structure that activates the intracellular tyrosine kinase domain. Upon receptor dimerization, the phosphorylation of intracellular tyrosine kinase enzymes transmits the received signal into the nucleus. HER2 is expressed in 20–30% of all breast cancers and cannot bind to ligands, but it plays an important role in amplifying and transmitting the signals generated by forming dimers with other receptors. Therefore, much effort has been made to develop a therapeutic agent that can suppress the action of HER2 [81].

4.3.1 Trastuzumab

In current clinical practice, the representative HER2 inhibitor used in patients with HER2-overexpressing breast cancer is trastuzumab, a humanized monoclonal antibody that has four functions. First, by binding to the extracellular space of the HER2 receptor near the cell membrane and preventing it from shedding the extracellular space construct, it prevents signal activation via the remaining HER2 construct, p95 HER2. Second, it interferes with polymer formation between HER family receptors and suppresses signal transduction. Third, it induces antibody-dependent, cell-mediated cytotoxic effects. Fourth, the bound HER2 receptor is introduced into the cell to reduce the HER2 receptor. Trastuzumab is effective as a monologic in patients with HER2-overexpressing breast cancer. It also showed improved survival when used as a first-line treatment along with existing chemotherapeutic agents in patients with metastatic breast cancer [82]. Recent clinical studies have confirmed that trastuzumab improves disease-free survival and overall survival when used in combination or sequentially with existing chemotherapy drugs, even as postoperative adjuvant chemotherapy [83].

4.3.2 Lapatinib

Lapatinib is a low molecular-weight oral tyrosine kinase inhibitor that competitively binds to the intracellular ATP binding pockets of HER1 and HER2 and blocks receptor autophosphorylation. It regulates cell differentiation and survival by blocking receptor activity and blocking signal transduction of the MAPK and PI3K/AKT pathways below it [84]. Currently, lapatinib has been shown to have a therapeutic effect on breast cancer and is being applied clinically [85]. In particular, it is effective in the treatment of p95 HER2-active breast cancer in which the extracellular construct of the HER2 receptor is shed and does not respond to treatment with trastuzumab. Its role as a therapeutic agent for trastuzumab-resistant cancer is well known. Currently, large-scale clinical studies are underway on its usefulness as a first-line treatment for early-stage breast cancer and its usefulness as neoadjuvant chemotherapy.

4.3.3 Pertuzumab

Pertuzumab is a monoclonal antibody that binds to the binding site of trastuzumab (domain IV) and another site (domain II) and inhibits the HER2–HER3 disconjugate [86]. Trastuzumab suppresses ligand-independent HER2 signals, whereas pertuzumab suppresses ligand-dependent HER2 mediation signals and HER2–HER3 signals, which are heterodimerizations that send the strongest mitotic signaling [87]. Pertuzumab has limited efficacy as a monotherapy, but the results of the CLEOPATRA study show that it has a synergistic effect when used in combination with trastuzumab. The combination of trastuzumab and pertuzumab is currently being clinically applied, especially in trastuzumab-resistant patients [88].

4.3.4 Trastuzumab Emtansine (T-DM1)

T-DM1 combines trastuzumab with the anti-cancer drug DM1 (maytansine). After the trastuzumab portion of T-DM1 binds to HER2, the endocytosis of HER2–T-DM1 complex is occurred, where the DM1 portion is released by proteolytic degradation in lysosomes to exert an tumor-suppressive effect. DM1 is a maytansine derivative and is an anti-microtubule agent such as vinca alkaloid. It is clinically known to suppress mitosis 20–100 times more than vincristine.

The EMILIA study compared T-DM1 monotherapy with the lapatinib and capecitabine combination in HER2 overexpressing metastatic breast cancer previously treated with taxane and trastuzumab [89]. The excellent event-free and overall survival of the T-DM1 monotherapy group indicates its value as a second-line HER2 targeted treatment for patients with HER2-overexpressing breast cancer who have failed with trastuzumab. The ongoing MARIANNE study is intended to confirm the effect of T-DM1 as a first-line treatment, and if it succeeds in obtaining that result, T-DM1 might be the most effective target treatment for HER2 overexpressing metastatic breast cancer.

4.3.5 Pan-HER Inhibitors

Pan-HER inhibitors simultaneously block other EGFR family members, including HER2. Neratinib and afatinib are currently being studied as oral, irreversible, low molecular-weight substances that simultaneously block EGFR, HER2, and HER4 [90].

4.4 Immunotherapy

4.4.1 Antiangiogenic Agents

Angiogenesis is an essential step in tumor growth and metastasis that involves a variety of factors, including vascular endothelial growth factor (VEGF). Bevacizumab is a monoclonal antibody against VEGG-A. As a first-line treatment for HER2-negative breast cancer patients, the combination of paclitaxel and bevacizumab showed a significant improvement in event-free survival compared with paclitaxel monotherapy. It was approved in 2008 as a treatment for HER2-negative metastatic breast cancer. However, since then, some meta-analyses have shown no improvement in the survival rate, and it is found to have a low gain compared with its toxicity, such as hypertension, bleeding, and intestinal perforation. In 2011, the US FDA revoked its approval for the treatment of metastatic breast cancer. It is still approved for use with paclitaxel or capecitabine in Europe, but it is used in only a few patients because of its limited therapeutic effect, large side effects, and high price [91, 92].

Sunitinib and sorafenib were studied as multi-targeted tyrosine kinase inhibitors, including VEGFR. However, in HER2-negative metastatic breast cancer, sunitinib monotherapy was less effective than capecitabine monotherapy. There was no improvement in event-free survival compared with the monotherapy group when it was combined with docetaxel as the first-line treatment or administered as a combination therapy with capecitabine to previously treated HER2-negative metastatic breast cancer patients. Sorafenib in combination with capecitabine showed improved event-free survival in patients with advanced or metastatic HER2-negative breast cancer compared with capecitabine alone, but further research is needed.

4.4.2 PI3K/AKT/mTOR Pathway Inhibitors

The PI3K-AKT-mTOR pathway regulates cell proliferation and survival, making it a critical player in tumor development and progression [93]. It is also known to be associated with trastuzumab resistance and hormone therapy resistance [94]. Everolimus acts as an allosteric inhibitor of mTOR complex 1 with a rapamycin analog and suppresses tumors. As a clinical study to confirm the effects of everolimus, the BOLERO-1,2,3 trial was advanced, and the results were reported. In BOLERO-2, [95] the event-free survival rate of everolimus and exemestane combination therapy was significantly higher than that with exemestane monotherapy [96, 97]. The BOLERO-3 study compared vinorelbine, trastuzumab, and everolimus combination therapies with non-everolimus combinations in patients who failed with taxane and trastuzumab [98]. It found that the event-free survival rate was improved in the everolimus-using groups, but it was reported that the decision should be made in consideration of the toxicity of everolimus [99].

4.4.3 PARP Inhibitor

Poly-ADP-ribose polymerase (PARP) is one of the most well-known enzymes that maintain gene stability. PARP-1 activation is one of the early cellular reactions that occur when a DNA strand is destroyed, and if a DNA single strand is defective, it is detected and immediately recovered. The BRCA1,2 gene is responsible for repairing double-stranded DNA damage by means of homologous recombination. If a mutation in BRCA1 or BRCA2 causes a loss of its function, a PARP inhibitor can be used to induce DNA single-strand defects. In that situation, single-stranded DNA damage progresses from the replication process to double-stranded damage, which eventually leads to cell death due to chromosomal instability because repair using homologous recombination is difficult. There are many molecular pathological similarities between triple-negative breast cancer and BRCA-deficient breast cancer, suggesting that PARP inhibitors (olaparib, iniparib, etc.) could play a role as targeted therapeutic agents in triple-negative breast cancer [100].

4.5 Bone-Directed Therapy

Bone remodeling is the process by which bone is generated through osteoblasts and reabsorbed through osteoclasts. Osteoblasts secrete the RANK (receptor activator of nuclear factor kappa B) ligand (RANKL), which activates RANK in the cell membrane of the osteoclast precursor and activates osteoclasts. Integrin in the osteoclast membrane and proteins such as osteopontin secreted from osteoblasts interact with each other to activate osteoclasts. Osteoprotegerin secreted by bone lining cells binds to RANKL and inhibits RANK activity. Through this series of processes, balance is achieved between bone resorption (osteoblasts) and remodeling (osteoclasts). Cancer cells secrete substances that allow the stimuli necessary for their growth to occur and thus increase the activity of osteoclasts [101].

Bisphosphonate adjuvant therapy has shown the potential to reduce recurrence rates and improve survival, but it is difficult to apply to all patients. The therapeutic effect is good when it is used as an adjunct therapy in hormone treatment or anticancer treatment for female patients with early-stage breast cancer who have a low estrogen environment after menopause or whose ovarian function is suppressed. The mechanism of action of the bisphosphonates is to prevent bone resorption by activating osteoblasts and suppressing bone metabolism. Additionally, they contribute to reduced lifespan by inhibiting the replacement, adhesion, and activity of osteoclasts. Furthermore, they hinder the growth of macrophages responsible for generating osteoclasts, thereby curtailing the lifespan of osteoclasts. Indigestion is the most common side effect, and other side effects include heat sensation, arthralgia, myalgia, hypocalcemia, and decreased renal function. A pretreatment dental examination is essential as they can also cause osteonecrosis of the jaw [102].

References

1. Halsted WS. The results of operations for the cure of cancer of the breast performed at the Johns Hopkins hospital from June, 1889, to January, 1894. Ann Surg. 1894;20(5):497–555. https://doi.org/10.1097/00000658-189407000-00075.
2. Patey DH, Dyson WH. The prognosis of carcinoma of the breast in relation to the type of operation performed. Br J Cancer. 1948;2(1):7–13. https://doi.org/10.1038/bjc.1948.2.
3. Fisher B, Montague E, Redmond C, Deutsch M, Brown GR, Zauber A, et al. Findings from NSABP protocol no. B-04-comparison of radical mastectomy with alternative treatments for primary breast cancer. I. radiation compliance and its relation to treatment outcome. Cancer. 1980;46(1):1–13. https://doi.org/10.1002/1097-0142(19800701)46:1<1::aid-cncr2820460102>3.0.co;2-3.
4. Fisher B, Wolmark N, Redmond C, Deutsch M, Fisher ER. Findings from NSABP protocol no. B-04: comparison of radical mastectomy with alternative treatments. II. The clinical and biologic significance of medial-central breast cancers. Cancer. 1981;48(8):1863–72. https://doi.org/10.1002/1097-0142(19811015)48:8<1863::aid-cncr2820480825>3.0.co;2-u.
5. Veronesi U, Marubini E, Mariani L, Galimberti V, Luini A, Veronesi P, et al. Radiotherapy after breast-conserving surgery in small breast carcinoma: long-term results of a randomized trial. Ann Oncol. 2001;12(7):997–1003. https://doi.org/10.1023/a:1011136326943.
6. Veronesi U, Orecchia R, Luini A, Gatti G, Intra M, Zurrida S, et al. A preliminary report of intraoperative radiotherapy (IORT) in limited-stage breast cancers that are conservatively treated. Eur J Cancer.

2001;37(17):2178–83. https://doi.org/10.1016/s0959-8049(01)00285-4.
7. Veronesi U, Saccozzi R, Del Vecchio M, Banfi A, Clemente C, De Lena M, et al. Comparing radical mastectomy with quadrantectomy, axillary dissection, and radiotherapy in patients with small cancers of the breast. N Engl J Med. 1981;305(1):6–11. https://doi.org/10.1056/NEJM198107023050102.
8. Arriagada R, Le MG, Rochard F, Contesso G. Conservative treatment versus mastectomy in early breast cancer: patterns of failure with 15 years of follow-up data. Institut Gustave-Roussy Breast Cancer Group. J Clin Oncol. 1996;14(5):1558–64. https://doi.org/10.1200/JCO.1996.14.5.1558.
9. Blichert-Toft M, Rose C, Andersen JA, Overgaard M, Axelsson CK, Andersen KW, et al. Danish randomized trial comparing breast conservation therapy with mastectomy: six years of life-table analysis. Danish breast cancer cooperative group. J Natl Cancer Inst Monogr. 1992;11:19–25.
10. Fisher B, Anderson S, Bryant J, Margolese RG, Deutsch M, Fisher ER, et al. Twenty-year follow-up of a randomized trial comparing total mastectomy, lumpectomy, and lumpectomy plus irradiation for the treatment of invasive breast cancer. N Engl J Med. 2002;347(16):1233–41. https://doi.org/10.1056/NEJMoa022152.
11. Fisher B, Jeong JH, Anderson S, Bryant J, Fisher ER, Wolmark N. Twenty-five-year follow-up of a randomized trial comparing radical mastectomy, total mastectomy, and total mastectomy followed by irradiation. N Engl J Med. 2002;347(8):567–75. https://doi.org/10.1056/NEJMoa020128.
12. Jacobson JA, Danforth DN, Cowan KH, d'Angelo T, Steinberg SM, Pierce L, et al. Ten-year results of a comparison of conservation with mastectomy in the treatment of stage I and II breast cancer. N Engl J Med. 1995;332(14):907–11. https://doi.org/10.1056/NEJM199504063321402.
13. Cabanas RM. An approach for the treatment of penile carcinoma. Cancer. 1977;39(2):456–66. https://doi.org/10.1002/1097-0142(197702)39:2<456::aid-cncr2820390214>3.0.co;2-i.
14. Morton DL, Wen DR, Wong JH, Economou JS, Cagle LA, Storm FK, et al. Technical details of intraoperative lymphatic mapping for early stage melanoma. Arch Surg. 1992;127(4):392–9. https://doi.org/10.1001/archsurg.1992.01420040034005.
15. Giuliano AE, Haigh PI, Brennan MB, Hansen NM, Kelley MC, Ye W, et al. Prospective observational study of sentinel lymphadenectomy without further axillary dissection in patients with sentinel node-negative breast cancer. J Clin Oncol. 2000;18(13):2553–9. https://doi.org/10.1200/JCO.2000.18.13.2553.
16. Giuliano AE, Jones RC, Brennan M, Statman R. Sentinel lymphadenectomy in breast cancer. J Clin Oncol. 1997;15(6):2345–50. https://doi.org/10.1200/JCO.1997.15.6.2345.

17. Lucci A, McCall LM, Beitsch PD, Whitworth PW, Reintgen DS, Blumencranz PW, et al. Surgical complications associated with sentinel lymph node dissection (SLND) plus axillary lymph node dissection compared with SLND alone in the American college of surgeons oncology group trial Z0011. J Clin Oncol. 2007;25(24):3657–63. https://doi.org/10.1200/JCO.2006.07.4062.

18. Wilke LG, McCall LM, Posther KE, Whitworth PW, Reintgen DS, Leitch AM, et al. Surgical complications associated with sentinel lymph node biopsy: results from a prospective international cooperative group trial. Ann Surg Oncol. 2006;13(4):491–500. https://doi.org/10.1245/ASO.2006.05.013.

19. Schwartz GF, Guiliano AE, Veronesi U, Consensus CC. Proceeding of the consensus conference of the role of sentinel lymph node biopsy in carcinoma or the breast April 19-22, 2001, Philadelphia, PA, USA. Breast J. 2002;8(3):124–38. https://doi.org/10.1046/j.1524-4741.2002.08315.x.

20. Fisher B, Wolmark N, Bauer M, Redmond C, Gebhardt M. The accuracy of clinical nodal staging and of limited axillary dissection as a determinant of histologic nodal status in carcinoma of the breast. Surg Gynecol Obstet. 1981;152(6):765–72.

21. Kapteijn BA, Nieweg OE, Petersen JL, Rutgers EJ, Hart AA, van Dongen JA, et al. Identification and biopsy of the sentinel lymph node in breast cancer. Eur J Surg Oncol. 1998;24(5):427–30. https://doi.org/10.1016/s0748-7983(98)92372-1.

22. Rubio IT, Korourian S, Cowan C, Krag DN, Colvert M, Klimberg VS. Sentinel lymph node biopsy for staging breast cancer. Am J Surg. 1998;176(6):532–7. https://doi.org/10.1016/s0002-9610(98)00264-5.

23. Ho AL, Tyldesley S, Macadam SA, Lennox PA. Skin-sparing mastectomy and immediate autologous breast reconstruction in locally advanced breast cancer patients: a UBC perspective. Ann Surg Oncol. 2012;19(3):892–900. https://doi.org/10.1245/s10434-011-1989-4.

24. Meretoja TJ, Rasia S, von Smitten KA, Asko-Seljavaara SL, Kuokkanen HO, Jahkola TA. Late results of skin-sparing mastectomy followed by immediate breast reconstruction. Br J Surg. 2007;94(10):1220–5. https://doi.org/10.1002/bjs.5815.

25. Atisha D, Alderman AK, Lowery JC, Kuhn LE, Davis J, Wilkins EG. Prospective analysis of long-term psychosocial outcomes in breast reconstruction: two-year postoperative results from the Michigan breast reconstruction outcomes study. Ann Surg. 2008;247(6):1019–28. https://doi.org/10.1097/SLA.0b013e3181728a5c.

26. Cederna PS, Yates WR, Chang P, Cram AE, Ricciardelli EJ. Postmastectomy reconstruction: comparative analysis of the psychosocial, functional, and cosmetic effects of transverse rectus abdominis musculocutaneous flap versus breast implant reconstruction. Ann Plast Surg. 1995;35(5):458–68. https://doi.org/10.1097/00000637-199511000-00003.

27. Dean C, Chetty U, Forrest AP. Effects of immediate breast reconstruction on psychosocial morbidity after mastectomy. Lancet. 1983;1(8322):459–62. https://doi.org/10.1016/s0140-6736(83)91452-6.

28. Anderson BO, Masetti R, Silverstein MJ. Oncoplastic approaches to partial mastectomy: an overview of volume-displacement techniques. Lancet Oncol. 2005;6(3):145–57. https://doi.org/10.1016/S1470-2045(05)01765-1.

29. Spear SL, Bulan EJ, Venturi ML. Breast augmentation. Plast Reconstr Surg. 2006;118(7 Suppl):188S–96S; discussion 97S–98S. https://doi.org/10.1097/01.PRS.0000135945.02642.8B.

30. Kim T, Giuliano AE, Lyman GH. Lymphatic mapping and sentinel lymph node biopsy in early-stage breast carcinoma: a metaanalysis. Cancer. 2006;106(1):4–16. https://doi.org/10.1002/cncr.21568.

31. Martin RC II, Edwards MJ, Wong SL, Tuttle TM, Carlson DJ, Brown CM, et al. Practical guidelines for optimal gamma probe detection of sentinel lymph nodes in breast cancer: results of a multi-institutional study. For the University of Louisville Breast Cancer Study Group. Surgery. 2000;128(2):139–44. https://doi.org/10.1067/msy.2000.108064.

32. Lyman GH, Giuliano AE, Somerfield MR, Benson AB III, Bodurka DC, Burstein HJ, et al. American society of clinical oncology guideline recommendations for sentinel lymph node biopsy in early-stage breast cancer. J Clin Oncol. 2005;23(30):7703–20. https://doi.org/10.1200/JCO.2005.08.001.

33. Giuliano AE, Hunt KK, Ballman KV, Beitsch PD, Whitworth PW, Blumencranz PW, et al. Axillary dissection vs no axillary dissection in women with invasive breast cancer and sentinel node metastasis: a randomized clinical trial. JAMA. 2011;305(6):569–75. https://doi.org/10.1001/jama.2011.90.

34. Lee S, Kim EY, Kang SH, Kim SW, Kim SK, Kang KW, et al. Sentinel node identification rate, but not accuracy, is significantly decreased after pre-operative chemotherapy in axillary node-positive breast cancer patients. Breast Cancer Res Treat. 2007;102(3):283–8. https://doi.org/10.1007/s10549-006-9330-9.

35. Arthur DW, Vicini FA. Accelerated partial breast irradiation as a part of breast conservation therapy. J Clin Oncol. 2005;23(8):1726–35. https://doi.org/10.1200/JCO.2005.09.045.

36. Fisher B, Anderson S, Redmond CK, Wolmark N, Wickerham DL, Cronin WM. Reanalysis and results after 12 years of follow-up in a randomized clinical trial comparing total mastectomy with lumpectomy with or without irradiation in the treatment of breast cancer. N Engl J Med. 1995;333(22):1456–61. https://doi.org/10.1056/NEJM199511303332203.

37. Overgaard M, Hansen PS, Overgaard J, Rose C, Andersson M, Bach F, et al. Postoperative radiotherapy in high-risk premenopausal women with breast cancer who receive adjuvant chemotherapy. Danish Breast Cancer Cooperative Group 82b Trial. N Engl J Med. 1997;337(14):949–55. https://doi.org/10.1056/NEJM199710023371401.

38. Ragaz J, Olivotto IA, Spinelli JJ, Phillips N, Jackson SM, Wilson KS, et al. Locoregional radiation therapy in patients with high-risk breast cancer receiving adjuvant chemotherapy: 20-year results of the British Columbia randomized trial. J Natl Cancer Inst. 2005;97(2):116–26. https://doi.org/10.1093/jnci/djh297.

39. Veronesi U, Cascinelli N, Mariani L, Greco M, Saccozzi R, Luini A, et al. Twenty-year follow-up of a randomized study comparing breast-conserving surgery with radical mastectomy for early breast cancer. N Engl J Med. 2002;347(16):1227–32. https://doi.org/10.1056/NEJMoa0220989.

40. Bartelink H, Horiot JC, Poortmans P, Struikmans H, Van den Bogaert W, Barillot I, et al. Recurrence rates after treatment of breast cancer with standard radiotherapy with or without additional radiation. N Engl J Med. 2001;345(19):1378–87. https://doi.org/10.1056/NEJMoa010874.

41. Vrieling C, Collette L, Fourquet A, Hoogenraad WJ, Horiot JC, Jager JJ, et al. The influence of the boost in breast-conserving therapy on cosmetic outcome in the EORTC "boost versus no boost" trial. EORTC Radiotherapy and Breast Cancer Cooperative Groups. European Organization for Research and Treatment of Cancer. Int J Radiat Oncol Biol Phys. 1999;45(3):677–85. https://doi.org/10.1016/s0360-3016(99)00211-4.

42. Romestaing P, Lehingue Y, Carrie C, Coquard R, Montbarbon X, Ardiet JM, et al. Role of a 10-Gy boost in the conservative treatment of early breast cancer: results of a randomized clinical trial in Lyon, France. J Clin Oncol. 1997;15(3):963–8. https://doi.org/10.1200/JCO.1997.15.3.963.

43. Holland R, Veling SH, Mravunac M, Hendriks JH. Histologic multifocality of tis, T1-2 breast carcinomas. Implications for clinical trials of breast-conserving surgery. Cancer. 1985;56(5):979–90. https://doi.org/10.1002/1097-0142(19850901)56:5<979::aid-cncr2820560502>3.0.co;2-n.

44. Clark RM, Whelan T, Levine M, Roberts R, Willan A, McCulloch P, et al. Randomized clinical trial of breast irradiation following lumpectomy and axillary dissection for node-negative breast cancer: an update. Ontario Clinical Oncology Group. J Natl Cancer Inst. 1996;88(22):1659–64. https://doi.org/10.1093/jnci/88.22.1659.

45. Liljegren G, Holmberg L, Bergh J, Lindgren A, Tabar L, Nordgren H, et al. 10-year results after sector resection with or without postoperative radiotherapy for stage I breast cancer: a randomized trial. J Clin Oncol. 1999;17(8):2326–33. https://doi.org/10.1200/JCO.1999.17.8.2326.

46. Vujovic O, Cherian A, Yu E, Dar AR, Stitt L, Perera F. The effect of timing of radiotherapy after breast-conserving surgery in patients with positive or close resection margins, young age, and node-negative disease, with long term follow-up. Int J Radiat Oncol Biol Phys. 2006;66(3):687–90. https://doi.org/10.1016/j.ijrobp.2006.05.051.

47. Huang J, Barbera L, Brouwers M, Browman G, Mackillop WJ. Does delay in starting treatment affect the outcomes of radiotherapy? A systematic review. J Clin Oncol. 2003;21(3):555–63. https://doi.org/10.1200/JCO.2003.04.171.

48. Lee JH, Kim SH, Suh YJ, Shim BY, Kim HK. Predictors of axillary lymph node metastases (ALNM) in a Korean population with T1-2 breast carcinoma: triple negative breast cancer has a high incidence of ALNM irrespective of the tumor size. Cancer Res Treat. 2010;42(1):30–6. https://doi.org/10.4143/crt.2010.42.1.30.

49. Komoike Y, Akiyama F, Iino Y, Ikeda T, Akashi-Tanaka S, Ohsumi S, et al. Ipsilateral breast tumor recurrence (IBTR) after breast-conserving treatment for early breast cancer: risk factors and impact on distant metastases. Cancer. 2006;106(1):35–41. https://doi.org/10.1002/cncr.21551.

50. White N, Nosten F, Bjorkman A, Marsh K, Snow RW. WHO, the Global Fund, and medical malpractice in malaria treatment. Lancet. 2004;363(9415):1160. https://doi.org/10.1016/S0140-6736(04)15904-7.

51. Anderson SJ, Wapnir I, Dignam JJ, Fisher B, Mamounas EP, Jeong JH, et al. Prognosis after ipsilateral breast tumor recurrence and locoregional recurrences in patients treated by breast-conserving therapy in five National Surgical Adjuvant Breast and Bowel Project protocols of node-negative breast cancer. J Clin Oncol. 2009;27(15):2466–73. https://doi.org/10.1200/JCO.2008.19.8424.

52. Heys SD, Hutcheon AW, Sarkar TK, Ogston KN, Miller ID, Payne S, et al. Neoadjuvant docetaxel in breast cancer: 3-year survival results from the Aberdeen trial. Clin Breast Cancer. 2002;3(Suppl 2):S69–74. https://doi.org/10.3816/cbc.2002.s.015.

53. Mamounas EP. NSABP protocol B-27. Preoperative doxorubicin plus cyclophosphamide followed by preoperative or postoperative docetaxel. Oncology (Williston Park). 1997;11(6 Suppl 6):37–40.

54. von Minckwitz G, Raab G, Caputo A, Schutte M, Hilfrich J, Blohmer JU, et al. Doxorubicin with cyclophosphamide followed by docetaxel every 21 days compared with doxorubicin and docetaxel every 14 days as preoperative treatment in operable breast cancer: the GEPARDUO study of the German Breast Group. J Clin Oncol. 2005;23(12):2676–85. https://doi.org/10.1200/JCO.2005.05.078.

55. Untch M, Jackisch C, Schneeweiss A, Conrad B, Aktas B, Denkert C, et al. Nab-paclitaxel versus solvent-based paclitaxel in neoadjuvant chemotherapy for early breast cancer (GeparSepto-GBG 69): a randomised, phase 3 trial. Lancet Oncol. 2016;17(3):345–56. https://doi.org/10.1016/S1470-2045(15)00542-2.

56. Gianni L, Mansutti M, Anton A, Calvo L, Bisagni G, Bermejo B, et al. Comparing neoadjuvant nab-paclitaxel vs paclitaxel both followed by anthracycline regimens in women with ERBB2/HER2-negative breast cancer-the evaluating treatment with neoadjuvant abraxane (ETNA) trial: a randomized phase

3 clinical trial. JAMA Oncol. 2018;4(3):302–8. https://doi.org/10.1001/jamaoncol.2017.4612.

57. von Minckwitz G, Kummel S, Vogel P, Hanusch C, Eidtmann H, Hilfrich J, et al. Intensified neoadjuvant chemotherapy in early-responding breast cancer: phase III randomized GeparTrio study. J Natl Cancer Inst. 2008;100(8):552–62. https://doi.org/10.1093/jnci/djn089.

58. Nabholtz JM, Bonneterre J, Buzdar A, Robertson JF, Thurlimann B. Anastrozole (Arimidex) versus tamoxifen as first-line therapy for advanced breast cancer in postmenopausal women: survival analysis and updated safety results. Eur J Cancer. 2003;39(12):1684–9. https://doi.org/10.1016/s0959-8049(03)00326-5.

59. Prat A, Saura C, Pascual T, Hernando C, Munoz M, Pare L, et al. Ribociclib plus letrozole versus chemotherapy for postmenopausal women with hormone receptor-positive, HER2-negative, luminal B breast cancer (CORALLEEN): an open-label, multicentre, randomised, phase 2 trial. Lancet Oncol. 2020;21(1):33–43. https://doi.org/10.1016/S1470-2045(19)30786-7.

60. Geyer CE Jr, Bandos H, Rastogi P, Jacobs SA, Robidoux A, Fehrenbacher L, et al. Definitive results of a phase III adjuvant trial comparing six cycles of FEC-100 to four cycles of AC in women with operable node-negative breast cancer: the NSABP B-36 trial (NRG oncology). Breast Cancer Res Treat. 2022;193(3):555–64. https://doi.org/10.1007/s10549-021-06417-y.

61. Sugarman S, Wasserheit C, Hodgman E, Coglianese M, D'Alassandro A, Fornier M, et al. A pilot study of dose-dense adjuvant paclitaxel without growth factor support for women with early breast carcinoma. Breast Cancer Res Treat. 2009;115(3):609–12. https://doi.org/10.1007/s10549-008-0152-9.

62. Bonneterre J, Roche H, Kerbrat P, Bremond A, Fumoleau P, Namer M, et al. Epirubicin increases long-term survival in adjuvant chemotherapy of patients with poor-prognosis, node-positive, early breast cancer: 10-year follow-up results of the French adjuvant study group 05 randomized trial. J Clin Oncol. 2005;23(12):2686–93. https://doi.org/10.1200/JCO.2005.05.059.

63. Schneider BP, Zhao F, Wang M, Stearns V, Martino S, Jones V, et al. Neuropathy is not associated with clinical outcomes in patients receiving adjuvant taxane-containing therapy for operable breast cancer. J Clin Oncol. 2012;30(25):3051–7. https://doi.org/10.1200/JCO.2011.39.8446.

64. Adams S, Gray RJ, Demaria S, Goldstein L, Perez EA, Shulman LN, et al. Prognostic value of tumor-infiltrating lymphocytes in triple-negative breast cancers from two phase III randomized adjuvant breast cancer trials: ECOG 2197 and ECOG 1199. J Clin Oncol. 2014;32(27):2959–66. https://doi.org/10.1200/JCO.2013.55.0491.

65. Seidman AD, Berry D, Cirrincione C, Harris L, Muss H, Marcom PK, et al. Randomized phase III trial of weekly compared with every-3-weeks paclitaxel for metastatic breast cancer, with trastuzumab for all HER-2 overexpressors and random assignment to trastuzumab or not in HER-2 nonoverexpressors: final results of Cancer and Leukemia group B protocol 9840. J Clin Oncol. 2008;26(10):1642–9. https://doi.org/10.1200/JCO.2007.11.6699.

66. Zander AR, Schmoor C, Kroger N, Kruger W, Mobus V, Frickhofen N, et al. Randomized trial of high-dose adjuvant chemotherapy with autologous hematopoietic stem-cell support versus standard-dose chemotherapy in breast cancer patients with 10 or more positive lymph nodes: overall survival after 6 years of follow-up. Ann Oncol. 2008;19(6):1082–9. https://doi.org/10.1093/annonc/mdn023.

67. Early Breast Cancer Trialists' Collaborative G, Peto R, Davies C, Godwin J, Gray R, Pan HC, et al. Comparisons between different polychemotherapy regimens for early breast cancer: meta-analyses of long-term outcome among 100,000 women in 123 randomised trials. Lancet. 2012;379(9814):432–44. https://doi.org/10.1016/S0140-6736(11)61625-5.

68. Ruddy KJ, Pitcher BN, Archer LE, Cohen HJ, Winer EP, Hudis CA, et al. Persistence, adherence, and toxicity with oral CMF in older women with early-stage breast cancer (adherence companion study 60104 for CALGB 49907). Ann Oncol. 2012;23(12):3075–81. https://doi.org/10.1093/annonc/mds133.

69. Hortobagyi GN. Treatment of breast cancer. N Engl J Med. 1998;339(14):974–84. https://doi.org/10.1056/NEJM199810013391407.

70. Hayward J. Cancer of the breast. Treatment of the advanced disease. Br Med J. 1970;1(5707):469–71. https://doi.org/10.1136/bmj.2.5707.469.

71. Van Den Bemd GJ, Kuiper GG, Pols HA, Van Leeuwen JP. Distinct effects on the conformation of estrogen receptor alpha and beta by both the antiestrogens ICI 164,384 and ICI 182,780 leading to opposite effects on receptor stability. Biochem Biophys Res Commun. 1999;261(1):1–5. https://doi.org/10.1006/bbrc.1999.0864.

72. Kuiper GG, van den Bemd GJ, van Leeuwen JP. Estrogen receptor and the SERM concept. J Endocrinol Invest. 1999;22(8):594–603. https://doi.org/10.1007/BF03343616.

73. Regan MM, Pagani O, Fleming GF, Walley BA, Price KN, Rabaglio M, et al. Adjuvant treatment of premenopausal women with endocrine-responsive early breast cancer: design of the TEXT and SOFT trials. Breast. 2013;22(6):1094–100. https://doi.org/10.1016/j.breast.2013.08.009.

74. Jonat W, Kaufmann M, Sauerbrei W, Blamey R, Cuzick J, Namer M, et al. Goserelin versus cyclophosphamide, methotrexate, and fluorouracil as adjuvant therapy in premenopausal patients with node-positive breast cancer: the Zoladex early breast cancer research association study. J Clin Oncol. 2002;20(24):4628–35. https://doi.org/10.1200/JCO.2002.05.042.

75. Thurlimann B, Robertson JF, Nabholtz JM, Buzdar A, Bonneterre J, Arimidex Study G. Efficacy of tamoxifen following anastrozole ('Arimidex') compared with anastrozole following tamoxifen as first-line treatment for advanced breast cancer in postmenopausal women. Eur J Cancer. 2003;39(16):2310–7. https://doi.org/10.1016/s0959-8049(03)00602-6.

76. Piccart-Gebhart MJ, Burzykowski T, Buyse M, Sledge G, Carmichael J, Luck HJ, et al. Taxanes alone or in combination with anthracyclines as first-line therapy of patients with metastatic breast cancer. J Clin Oncol. 2008;26(12):1980–6. https://doi.org/10.1200/JCO.2007.10.8399.

77. Valsecchi ME, Recondo G, de la Vega M, Greco M, Recondo G, Diaz CE. Anti-hormonal therapies for premenopausal patients—what did we learn from the TEXT/SOFT trials? Rev Recent Clin Trials. 2015;10(2):90–100. https://doi.org/10.2174/157488 711002150714134611.

78. Gnant M, Pfeiler G, Dubsky PC, Hubalek M, Greil R, Jakesz R, et al. Adjuvant denosumab in breast cancer (ABCSG-18): a multicentre, randomised, double-blind, placebo-controlled trial. Lancet. 2015;386(9992):433–43. https://doi.org/10.1016/S0140-6736(15)60995-3.

79. Mayer EL, Dueck AC, Martin M, Rubovszky G, Burstein HJ, Bellet-Ezquerra M, et al. Palbociclib with adjuvant endocrine therapy in early breast cancer (PALLAS): interim analysis of a multicentre, open-label, randomised, phase 3 study. Lancet Oncol. 2021;22(2):212–22. https://doi.org/10.1016/S1470-2045(20)30642-2.

80. Johnston SRD, Harbeck N, Hegg R, Toi M, Martin M, Shao ZM, et al. Abemaciclib combined with endocrine therapy for the adjuvant treatment of HR+, HER2-, node-positive, high-risk, early breast cancer (monarchE). J Clin Oncol. 2020;38(34):3987–98. https://doi.org/10.1200/JCO.20.02514.

81. Yarden Y, Sliwkowski MX. Untangling the ErbB signalling network. Nat Rev Mol Cell Biol. 2001;2(2):127–37. https://doi.org/10.1038/35052073.

82. Joensuu H, Kellokumpu-Lehtinen PL, Bono P, Alanko T, Kataja V, Asola R, et al. Adjuvant docetaxel or vinorelbine with or without trastuzumab for breast cancer. N Engl J Med. 2006;354(8):809–20. https://doi.org/10.1056/NEJMoa053028.

83. Untch M, Rezai M, Loibl S, Fasching PA, Huober J, Tesch H, et al. Neoadjuvant treatment with trastuzumab in HER2-positive breast cancer: results from the GeparQuattro study. J Clin Oncol. 2010;28(12):2024–31. https://doi.org/10.1200/JCO.2009.23.8451.

84. Santen RJ, Song RX, McPherson R, Kumar R, Adam L, Jeng MH, et al. The role of mitogen-activated protein (MAP) kinase in breast cancer. J Steroid Biochem Mol Biol. 2002;80(2):239–56. https://doi.org/10.1016/s0960-0760(01)00189-3.

85. Moy B, Goss PE. Lapatinib-associated toxicity and practical management recommenda-

tions. Oncologist. 2007;12(7):756–65. https://doi.org/10.1634/theoncologist.12-7-756.

86. Agus DB, Gordon MS, Taylor C, Natale RB, Karlan B, Mendelson DS, et al. Phase I clinical study of pertuzumab, a novel HER dimerization inhibitor, in patients with advanced cancer. J Clin Oncol. 2005;23(11):2534–43. https://doi.org/10.1200/JCO.2005.03.184.

87. Holbro T, Beerli RR, Maurer F, Koziczak M, Barbas CF III, Hynes NE. The ErbB2/ErbB3 heterodimer functions as an oncogenic unit: ErbB2 requires ErbB3 to drive breast tumor cell proliferation. Proc Natl Acad Sci U S A. 2003;100(15):8933–8. https://doi.org/10.1073/pnas.1537685100.

88. Baselga J, Cortes J, Kim SB, Im SA, Hegg R, Im YH, et al. Pertuzumab plus trastuzumab plus docetaxel for metastatic breast cancer. N Engl J Med. 2012;366(2):109–19. https://doi.org/10.1056/NEJMoa1113216.

89. Baselga J, Bradbury I, Eidtmann H, Di Cosimo S, de Azambuja E, Aura C, et al. Lapatinib with trastuzumab for HER2-positive early breast cancer (NeoALTTO): a randomised, open-label, multicentre, phase 3 trial. Lancet. 2012;379(9816):633–40. https://doi.org/10.1016/S0140-6736(11)61847-3.

90. Twelves C, Trigo JM, Jones R, De Rosa F, Rakhit A, Fettner S, et al. Erlotinib in combination with capecitabine and docetaxel in patients with metastatic breast cancer: a dose-escalation study. Eur J Cancer. 2008;44(3):419–26. https://doi.org/10.1016/j.ejca.2007.12.011.

91. Thomas ES, Gomez HL, Li RK, Chung HC, Fein LE, Chan VF, et al. Ixabepilone plus capecitabine for metastatic breast cancer progressing after anthracycline and taxane treatment. J Clin Oncol. 2007;25(33):5210–7. https://doi.org/10.1200/JCO.2007.12.6557.

92. Thomas E, Tabernero J, Fornier M, Conte P, Fumoleau P, Lluch A, et al. Phase II clinical trial of ixabepilone (BMS-247550), an epothilone B analog, in patients with taxane-resistant metastatic breast cancer. J Clin Oncol. 2007;25(23):3399–406. https://doi.org/10.1200/JCO.2006.08.9102.

93. Serra V, Markman B, Scaltriti M, Eichhorn PJ, Valero V, Guzman M, et al. NVP-BEZ235, a dual PI3K/mTOR inhibitor, prevents PI3K signaling and inhibits the growth of cancer cells with activating PI3K mutations. Cancer Res. 2008;68(19):8022–30. https://doi.org/10.1158/0008-5472.CAN-08-1385.

94. Huang F, Reeves K, Han X, Fairchild C, Platero S, Wong TW, et al. Identification of candidate molecular markers predicting sensitivity in solid tumors to dasatinib: rationale for patient selection. Cancer Res. 2007;67(5):2226–38. https://doi.org/10.1158/0008-5472.CAN-06-3633.

95. Tabernero J, Rojo F, Calvo E, Burris H, Judson I, Hazell K, et al. Dose- and schedule-dependent inhibition of the mammalian target of rapamycin pathway with everolimus: a phase I tumor pharmacodynamic study in patients with advanced solid

tumors. J Clin Oncol. 2008;26(10):1603–10. https://doi.org/10.1200/JCO.2007.14.5482.

96. Diaby V, Adunlin G, Ali AA, Tawk R. Using quality-adjusted progression-free survival as an outcome measure to assess the benefits of cancer drugs in randomized-controlled trials: case of the BOLERO-2 trial. Breast Cancer Res Treat. 2014;146(3):669–73. https://doi.org/10.1007/s10549-014-3047-y.

97. Beaver JA, Park BH. The BOLERO-2 trial: the addition of everolimus to exemestane in the treatment of postmenopausal hormone receptor-positive advanced breast cancer. Future Oncol. 2012;8(6):651–7. https://doi.org/10.2217/fon.12.49.

98. Baselga J, Semiglazov V, van Dam P, Manikhas A, Bellet M, Mayordomo J, et al. Phase II randomized study of neoadjuvant everolimus plus letrozole compared with placebo plus letrozole in patients with estrogen receptor-positive breast cancer. J Clin Oncol. 2009;27(16):2630–7. https://doi.org/10.1200/JCO.2008.18.8391.

99. Morrow PK, Wulf GM, Ensor J, Booser DJ, Moore JA, Flores PR, et al. Phase I/II study of trastu-

zumab in combination with everolimus (RAD001) in patients with HER2-overexpressing metastatic breast cancer who progressed on trastuzumab-based therapy. J Clin Oncol. 2011;29(23):3126–32. https://doi.org/10.1200/JCO.2010.32.2321.

100. O'Shaughnessy J, Osborne C, Pippen JE, Yoffe M, Patt D, Rocha C, et al. Iniparib plus chemotherapy in metastatic triple-negative breast cancer. N Engl J Med. 2011;364(3):205–14. https://doi.org/10.1056/NEJMoa1011418.

101. Coleman RE, Rubens RD. The clinical course of bone metastases from breast cancer. Br J Cancer. 1987;55(1):61–6. https://doi.org/10.1038/bjc.1987.13.

102. Coscia M, Quaglino E, Iezzi M, Curcio C, Pantaleoni F, Riganti C, et al. Zoledronic acid repolarizes tumour-associated macrophages and inhibits mammary carcinogenesis by targeting the mevalonate pathway. J Cell Mol Med. 2010;14(12):2803–15. https://doi.org/10.1111/j.1582-4934.2009.00926.x.

HR(+) HER2(−) Breast Cancer

Yunju Kim, Bo Hwa Choi, Eun-Gyeong Lee,
Ji Young You, and Youngmi Kwon

1 Case 1

1.1 Patient History and Progress

Female/87 years old, post-menopause.

Screen detected mass lesion on left breast sub-areolar area.

No family history.

Hypertension, diabetes mellitus, arrhythmia, total knee replacement, cerebrovascular accident.

Y. Kim
Department of Pathology, National Cancer Center,
Goyang, Gyeonggi, Republic of Korea
e-mail: radkyj@ncc.re.kr

B. H. Choi
Division of Diagnostic Radiology, Center for Breast Cancer, National Cancer Center,
Goyang, Republic of Korea
e-mail: iawy82@ncc.re.kr

E.-G. Lee
Division of Surgery, Center for Breast Cancer,
National Cancer Center, Goyang, Republic of Korea
e-mail: bnf333@ncc.re.kr

J. Y. You
Division of Breast and Endocrine, Department of
General Surgery, Korea University Medical Center,
Seoul, Republic of Korea
e-mail: joliejean@korea.ac.kr

Y. Kwon (✉)
Department of Radiology, Center for Breast Cancer,
National Cancer Center, Goyang, Gyeonggi,
Republic of Korea
e-mail: ymk@ncc.re.kr

1.2 Important Radiologic Findings

See Figs. 1, 2 and 3.

1.3 Courses of Treatment

Operation + Letrozole 2.5 mg/day

1.3.1 Operation
Left total mastectomy, sentinel lymph node biopsy (Fig. 4).

1.3.2 Pathology Report
Invasive Ductal Carcinoma
Associated with encapsulated papillary carcinoma.

1. Size of tumor: 2.5 cm (pT2).
2. Histologic grade: 2/3 (tubule formation: 2/3, nuclear pleomorphism: 2/3, mitotic count: 2/3, 11/10 HPF).
3. Intraductal component: present, intratumoral/extratumoral (30%) (nuclear grade: low, necrosis: absent, architectural pattern: cribriform/solid, extensive intraductal component: present).
4. Skin and nipple: dermal involvement of tumor.
5. Surgical margins: deep margin: 7 mm.
6. Lymph nodes:
   (a) metastasis in one out of seven axillary lymph nodes (pN1mi) (sentinel LN: 1/7),

---

© The Author(s), under exclusive license to Springer Nature Singapore Pte Ltd. 2023
E. S. Lee (ed.), *A Practical Guide to Breast Cancer Treatment*,
https://doi.org/10.1007/978-981-19-9044-1_5

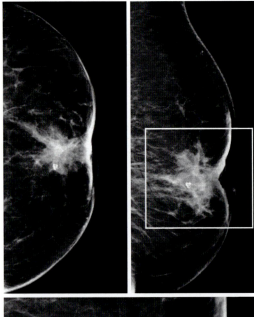

Fig. 1 Left mammography (Nov. 2020): an irregular mass with nipple retraction at subareolar area

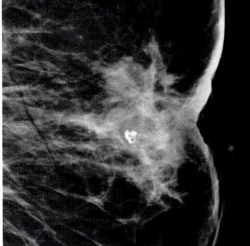

Fig. 2 Left breast US (Dec. 2020): a hypervascular irregular mass at subareolar area. US-CNB = IDC

    (b) perinodal extension: present,
    (c) size of metastatic carcinoma: 0.2 mm.
7. Arteriovenous invasion: present, peritumoral.
8. Lymphovascular invasion: present, peritumoral.
9. Tumor border: infiltrative.
10. Microcalcification: present, tumoral/non-tumoral.
11. Pathological TN category (AJCC 2017): pT2N1mi.

	Result	Intensity	Positive %
Estrogen receptor	Strong (8/8)	3	>2/3
Progesterone receptor	Strong (8/8)	3	>2/3
C-erbB2	Negative (1+)		
Ki-67	Positive in 4% of tumor cells		

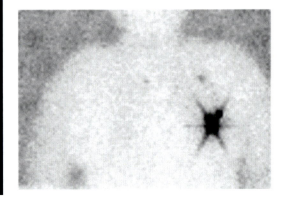

Fig. 3 Lymphoscintigraphy shows visualized sentinel lymph nodes in the left axilla

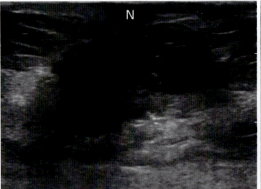

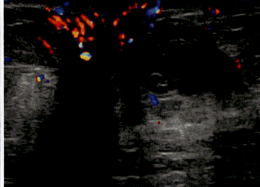

HR(+) HER2(−) Breast Cancer

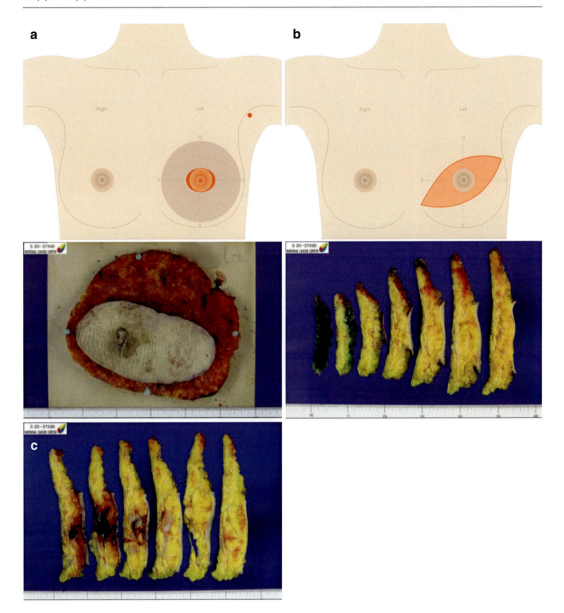

Fig. 4 (**a**) Gross pathology of mastectomy specimen. (**b, c**) The margins get marked and sliced with different colors on each direction

2 Case 2

2.1 Patient History and Progress

Female/61 years old, post-menopause.

Screen detected mass lesion on left breast 2 o'clock direction.

No family history.

Hepatitis B virus carrier, dyslipidemia.

2.2 Important Radiologic Findings

See Figs. 5, 6, 7 and 8.

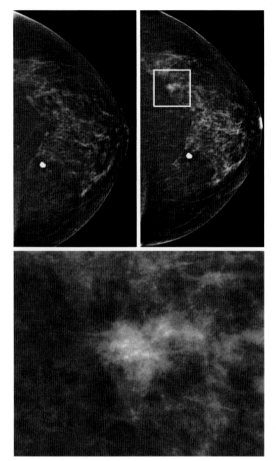

Fig. 5 Left CC mammography (Oct. 2018, Sept. 2020): negative finding in 2018. A developing asymmetry at outer breast in 2020

2.3 Courses of Treatment

Operation + Post-operative radiation therapy + Anastrozole 1 mg/day.

2.3.1 Operation

Left breast conserving surgery, sentinel lymph node biopsy (Fig. 9).

2.3.2 Pathology Report

Invasive Ductal Carcinoma
1. Size of tumor: 0.8 cm (pT1b).

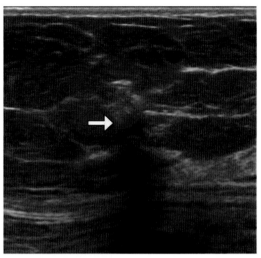

Fig. 6 Left breast US (Nov. 2020): a hypoechoic mass at upper outer quadrant. US-CNB = IDC

2. Histologic grade: 2/3 (tubule formation: 3/3, nuclear pleomorphism: 2/3, mitotic count: 2/3, 11/10 HPF).
3. Intraductal component: present, intratumoral/extratumoral (20%) (nuclear grade: low, necrosis: absent, architectural pattern: cribriform, extensive intraductal component: absent).
4. Skin: no involvement of tumor.
5. Surgical margins:
    (a) superior margin: 20 mm,
    (b) inferior margin: 15 mm,
    (c) medial margin: 20 mm,
    (d) lateral margin: 10 mm,
    (e) deep margin: 2 mm,
    (f) superficial margin: 2 mm.
6. Lymph nodes: no metastasis in one axillary lymph node (pN0(sn)) (sentinel LN: 0/1).
7. Arteriovenous invasion: absent.
8. Lymphovascular invasion: absent.
9. Tumor border: infiltrative.
10. Microcalcification: present, tumoral/non-tumoral.
11. Pathological TN category (AJCC 2017): pT1bN0(sn).

	Result	Intensity	Positive %
Estrogen receptor	Strong (8/8)	3	>2/3
Progesterone receptor	Strong (8/8)	3	>2/3
C-erbB2	Negative (0)		
Ki-67	Positive in 5% of tumor cells		

Fig. 7 Breast MRI (Dec. 2020): an irregular enhancing mass in the left breast

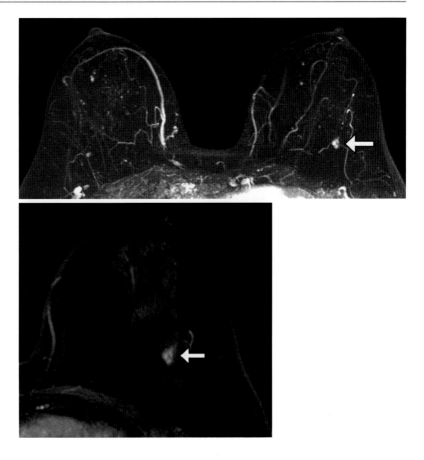

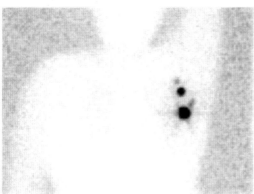

Fig. 8 Lymphoscintigraphy shows visualized sentinel lymph nodes in the left axilla

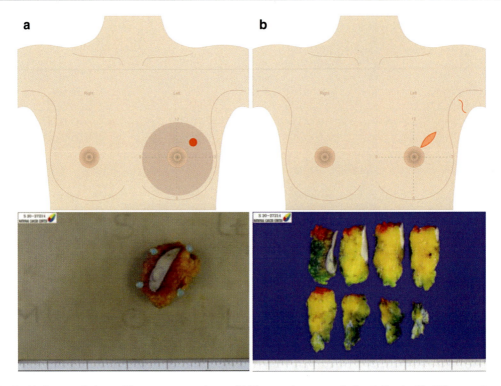

Fig. 9 (**a**) Gross pathology of lumpectomy specimen. (**b**) The margins get marked and sliced with different colors on each direction

3 Case 3

3.1 Patient History and Progress

Female/78 years old, post-menopause.
 Screen detected mass lesion on right breast 10 o'clock direction.
 No family history.
 L-spine disc herniation.

3.2 Important Radiologic Findings

See Figs. 10, 11, 12 and 13.

3.3 Courses of Treatment

Operation + Post-operative radiation therapy + Letrozole 2.5 mg/day.

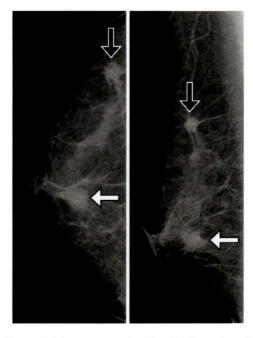

Fig. 10 Right mammography (Nov. 2020): two irregular masses at subareolar area (white arrow) and upper outer quadrant (black arrow)

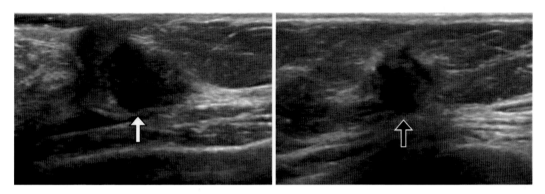

Fig. 11 Right breast US (Nov. 2020): two irregular masses at subareolar area (white arrow, US-CNB = IDC) and upper outer quadrant (black arrow, US-CNB = IDC)

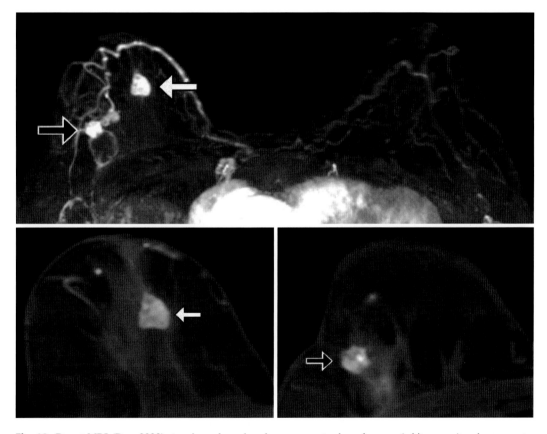

Fig. 12 Breast MRI (Dec. 2020): two irregular enhancing masses at subareolar area (white arrow) and upper outer quadrant (black arrow) of right breast

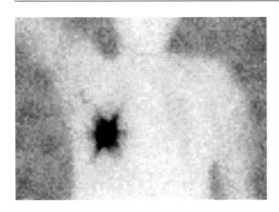

Fig. 13 Lymphoscintigraphy shows faintly visualized sentinel lymph nodes in the right axilla

3.3.1 Operation
Right breast conserving surgery, sentinel lymph node biopsy (Fig. 14).

3.3.2 Pathology Report
Breast, right 10 o'clock:

Invasive Ductal Carcinoma
1. Size of tumor: 0.9 cm.
2. Histologic grade: 2/3 (tubule formation: 3/3, nuclear pleomorphism: 2/3, mitotic count: 2/3, 11/10 HPF).
3. Intraductal component: present, intratumoral/extratumoral (5%) (nuclear grade: low, necrosis: absent, architectural pattern: cribriform, extensive intraductal component: absent).
4. Skin: no involvement of tumor.
5. Surgical margins:
   (a) superior margin: 10 mm,
   (b) inferior margin: 20 mm,
   (c) medial margin: 10 mm,
   (d) lateral margin: 10 mm (see note 1),
   (e) deep margin: 2 mm,
   (f) superficial margin: 2 mm.
6. Lymph nodes: no metastasis in three axillary lymph nodes (pN0(sn)) (sentinel LN: 0/1, non-sentinel LN: 0/2).
7. Arteriovenous invasion: absent.
8. Lymphovascular invasion: present, intratumoral.
9. Tumor border: infiltrative.
10. Microcalcification: present, tumoral/non-tumoral.

Breast, right subareolar:

Invasive Ductal Carcinoma
1. Size of tumor: 1.1 cm (pT1c).
2. Histologic grade: 2/3 (tubule formation: 3/3, nuclear pleomorphism: 2/3, mitotic count: 2/3, 11/10 HPF).
3. Intraductal component: present, intratumoral/extratumoral (10%) (nuclear grade: low, necrosis: absent, architectural pattern: cribriform, extensive intraductal component: absent).
4. Skin: no involvement of tumor.
5. Surgical margins:
   (a) superior margin: 10 mm,
   (b) inferior margin: (see note 2),
   (c) medial margin: 10 mm,
   (d) lateral margin: 10 mm,
   (e) deep margin: 1 mm from invasive ductal carcinoma (slide 9),
   (f) superficial margin: 2 mm.
6. Arteriovenous invasion: absent.
7. Lymphovascular invasion: present, intratumoral.
8. Tumor border: infiltrative.
9. Microcalcification: present, tumoral/non-tumoral.
10. Pathological TN category (AJCC 2017): pT1cN0(sn).

	Result	Intensity	Positive %
Estrogen receptor	Strong (7/8)	2	>2/3
Progesterone receptor	Weak (3/8)	1	1–10%
C-erbB2	Negative (1+)		
Ki-67	Positive in 4% of tumor cells		

HR(+) HER2(−) Breast Cancer

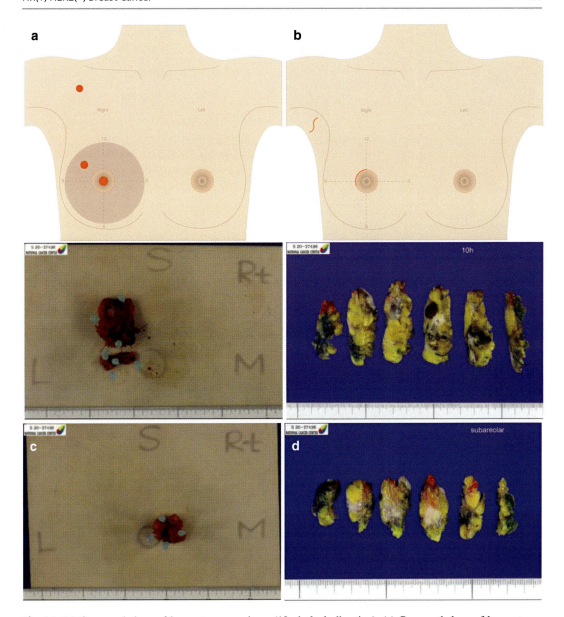

Fig. 14 (**a**) Gross pathology of lumpectomy specimen (10 o' clock direction). (**c**) Gross pathology of lumpectomy specimen (subareolar area). (**b, d**) The margins get marked and sliced with different colors on each direction

4 Case 4

4.1 Patient History and Progress

Female/57 years old, post-menopause.
 Screen detected mass lesion on right breast 10 o'clock direction.

No family history.
Dyslipidemia.

4.2 Important Radiologic Findings

See Figs. 15, 16, 17 and 18.

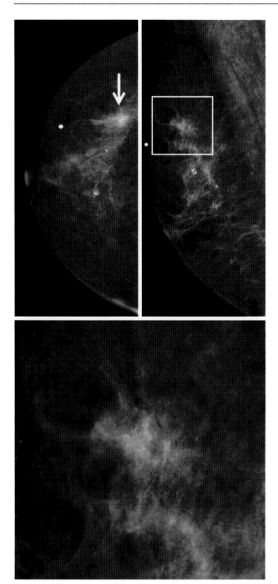

Fig. 15 Right mammography (Nov. 2020): a focal asymmetry at upper outer quadrant

4.3 Courses of Treatment

Operation + Post-operative radiation therapy + Letrozole 2.5 mg/day.

4.3.1 Operation

Right breast conserving surgery, sentinel lymph node biopsy (Fig. 19).

4.3.2 Pathology Report

Invasive Ductal Carcinoma
1. Size of tumor: 1.8 cm (pT1c).
2. Histologic grade: 2/3 (tubule formation: 3/3, nuclear pleomorphism: 3/3, mitotic count: 2/3, 17/10 HPF).
3. Intraductal component: present, intratumoral/extratumoral (10%) (nuclear grade: high, necrosis: present, architectural pattern: solid/comedo, extensive intraductal component: absent).
4. Skin: no involvement of tumor.
5. Surgical margins:
    (a) superior margin: 10 mm,
    (b) inferior margin: (see note),
    (c) medial margin: 10 mm,
    (d) lateral margin: 15 mm,
    (e) deep margin: 2 mm,
    (f) superficial margin: 2 mm.
6. Lymph nodes:
    (a) metastasis in one out of five axillary lymph nodes (pN1a(sn)) (sentinel LN: 1/1, axillary LN: 0/4),
    (b) perinodal extension: present,
    (c) size of metastatic carcinoma: 23 mm.
7. Arteriovenous invasion: absent.
8. Lymphovascular invasion: present, intratumoral.
9. Tumor border: infiltrative.
10. Microcalcification: present, tumoral/non-tumoral.
11. Pathological TN category (AJCC 2017): pT1cN1a(sn).

	Result	Intensity	Positive %
Estrogen receptor	Strong (8/8)	3	>2/3
Progesterone receptor	Negative (0/8)	0	0
C-erbB2	Equivocal (2+) (SISH negative)		
Ki-67	Positive in 6% of tumor cells		

HR(+) HER2(−) Breast Cancer

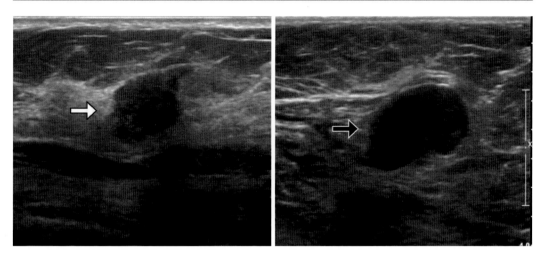

Fig. 16 Right breast US (Dec. 2020): an irregular hypoechoic mass at upper outer quadrant (white arrow, US-CNB = IDC). An enlarged lymph node at the right axillary fossa (black arrow)

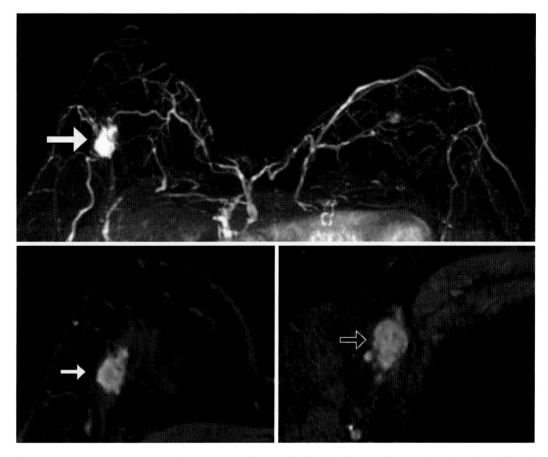

Fig. 17 Breast MRI (Dec. 2020): an irregular enhancing mass in the right breast (white arrow) and an enlarged lymph node at the right axillary fossa (black arrow)

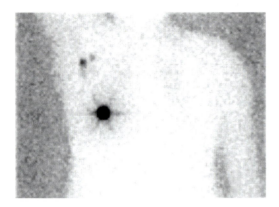

Fig. 18 Lymphoscintigraphy shows visualized sentinel lymph nodes in the right axilla

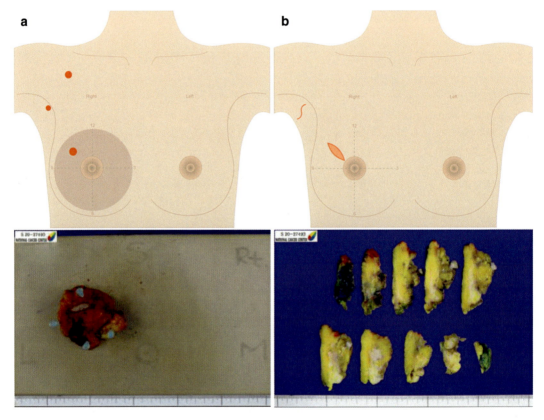

Fig. 19 (**a**) Gross pathology of lumpectomy specimen. (**b**) The margins get marked and sliced with different colors on each direction

5 Case 5

5.1 Patient History and Progress

Female/58 years old, post-menopause.
Screen detected mass lesion on right breast 4 o'clock direction.
No family history.
No comorbidities.

5.2 Important Radiologic Findings

See Figs. 20, 21, 22 and 23.

5.3 Courses of Treatment

Operation + Adjuvant chemotherapy (#4 cycles of docetaxel & cyclophosphamide) + Post-operative radiation therapy + Letrozole 2.5 mg/day.

5.3.1 Operation (1st, Dec. 2020)
Right breast conserving surgery, sentinel lymph node biopsy (Fig. 24).

5.3.2 Pathology Report
Invasive Ductal Carcinoma
1. Size of tumor: 2.1 cm (pT2).
2. Histologic grade: 2/3 (tubule formation: 3/3, nuclear pleomorphism: 2/3, mitotic count: 2/3, 14/10 HPF).
3. Intraductal component: present, intratumoral/extratumoral (20%) (nuclear grade: low, necrosis: present, architectural pattern: micropapillary/cribriform/comedo, extensive intraductal component: absent).
4. Skin: no involvement of tumor.
5. Surgical margins:
    (a) superior margin: (see note 2),
    (b) inferior margin: 5 mm,
    (c) medial margin: positive for invasive ductal carcinoma (Fro 6),
    (d) lateral margin: (see note 3),
    (e) deep margin: positive for invasive ductal carcinoma (slide 1),
    (f) superficial margin: 2 mm.
6. Lymph nodes:

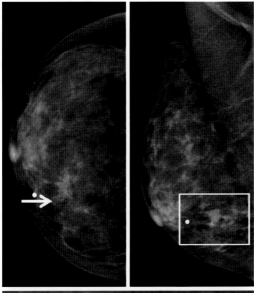

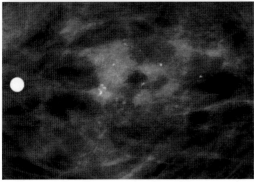

Fig. 20 Right mammography (Nov. 2020): a focal asymmetry with fine pleomorphic microcalcifications at lower inner quadrant

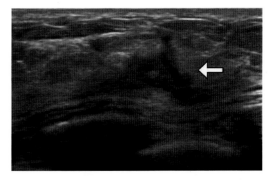

Fig. 21 Right breast US (Dec. 2020): an irregular hypoechoic mass. US-CNB = IDC with mucinous component

Fig. 22 Breast MRI (Dec. 2020): a focal non-mass enhancement in the right breast

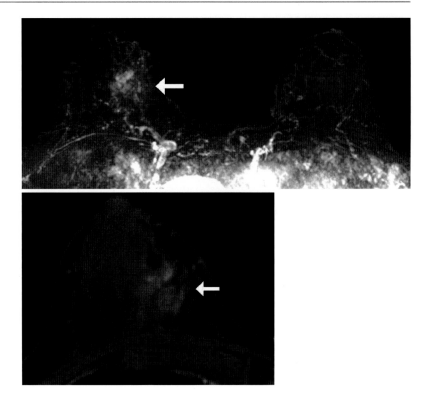

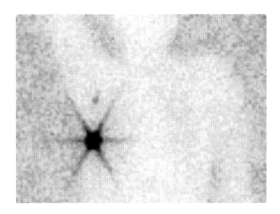

Fig. 23 Lymphoscintigraphy shows visualized sentinel lymph nodes in the right axilla

(a) metastasis in two out of three axillary lymph nodes (pN1a(sn)) (sentinel LN: 2/3),
(b) perinodal extension: absent,
(c) size of metastatic carcinoma: 2.5 mm.

7. Arteriovenous invasion: absent.
8. Lymphovascular invasion: present, intratumoral.
9. Tumor border: infiltrative.
10. Microcalcification: present, tumoral/non-tumoral.
11. Pathological TN category (AJCC 2017): pT2N1a(sn).

Note: 1. Micrometastasis is present in the frozen section of Fro 2.

2. The superior margin of the lumpectomy specimen (slide 6) is close to invasive ductal carcinoma (<1 mm) but this margin submitted for frozen diagnosis (Fro 4) is free of tumor.

3. The lateral margin of the lumpectomy specimen (slide 8) is close to invasive ductal carcinoma (<1 mm) but this margin submitted for frozen diagnosis (Fro 7) is free of tumor.

	Result	Intensity	Positive %
Estrogen receptor	Strong (7/8)	2	>2/3
Progesterone receptor	Negative (2/8)	1	<1%
C-erbB2	Negative (1+)		
Ki-67	Positive in 4% of tumor cells		

HR(+) HER2(−) Breast Cancer

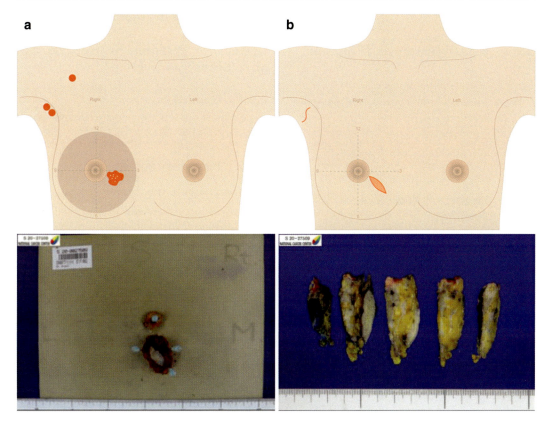

Fig. 24 (**a**) Gross pathology of lumpectomy specimen (black arrow). (**b**) The margins get marked and sliced with different colors on each direction

5.3.3 Operation (2nd, Jan. 2021)
Right breast wide excision (Fig. 25).

5.3.4 Pathology Report
Invasive Ductal Carcinoma
1. Post-lumpectomy status.
2. Size of tumor: 0.2 cm, residual.
3. Histologic grade: 2/3 (tubule formation: 3/3, nuclear pleomorphism: 2/3, mitotic count: 1/3).
4. Intraductal component: absent.
5. Surgical margins: 9 mm.
6. Arteriovenous invasion: absent.
7. Lymphovascular invasion: present, extratumoral.
8. Tumor border: infiltrative.
9. Microcalcification: present, non-tumoral.

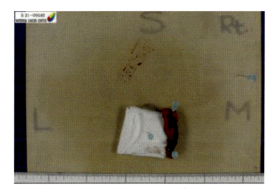

Fig. 25 Gross pathology of breast wide excision specimen

6 Case 6

6.1 Patient History and Progress

Female/51 years old, pre-menopause.
  Screen detected mass lesion on right breast 2 o'clock direction.
  No family history.
  S/P Thyroid benign mass, excision.

6.2 Important Radiologic Findings

See Figs. 26, 27, 28 and 29.

6.3 Courses of Treatment

Operation + Post-operative radiation therapy + Tamoxifen 20 mg/day.

6.3.1 Operation

Right breast conserving surgery, sentinel lymph node biopsy (Fig. 30).

6.3.2 Pathology Report

Invasive Ductal Carcinoma
1. Size of invasive component: 1.8 cm (pT1c).
2. Size of intraductal component: 4.0 cm.
3. Histologic grade: 2/3 (tubule formation: 3/3, nuclear pleomorphism: 2/3, mitotic count: 2/3, 11/10 HPF).
4. Intraductal component: present, intratumoral/extratumoral (60%) (nuclear grade: low, necrosis: present, architectural pattern: solid/comedo, extensive intraductal component: present).
5. Skin: no involvement of tumor.
6. Surgical margins:
    (a) superior margin: 5 mm,
    (b) inferior margin: 5 mm,
    (c) medial margin: 5 mm,
    (d) lateral margin: 5 mm,
    (e) deep margin: 2 mm,
    (f) superficial margin: 1 mm from ductal carcinoma in situ (slide 12).
7. Lymph nodes:

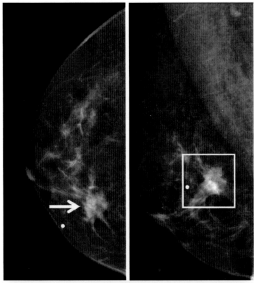

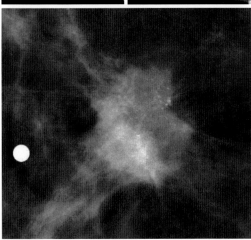

Fig. 26 Right mammography (Oct. 2020): a spiculated mass with microcalcifications at upper inner quadrant

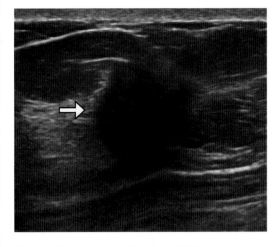

Fig. 27 Right breast US (Oct. 2020): an irregular hypoechoic mass (white arrow, US-CNB = IDC) with adjacent smaller masses (not shown)

Fig. 28 Breast MRI (Nov. 2020): an irregular enhancing mass (white arrow) with adjacent satellite lesions (black arrows) in the right breast

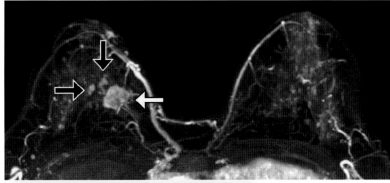

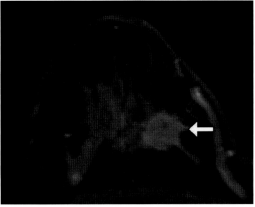

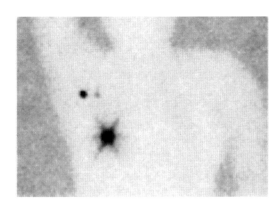

Fig. 29 Lymphoscintigraphy shows visualized sentinel lymph nodes in the right axilla

(a) metastasis in one out of four axillary lymph nodes (pN1a(sn)) (sentinel LN: 1/1, axillary LN: 0/3),
(b) perinodal extension: present,
(c) size of metastatic carcinoma: 7 mm.
8. Arteriovenous invasion: absent.
9. Lymphovascular invasion: present, intratumoral.
10. Tumor border: infiltrative.
11. Microcalcification: present, tumoral/non-tumoral.
12. Pathological TN category (AJCC 2017): pT1cN1a(sn).

	Result	Intensity	Positive %
Estrogen receptor	Intermediate (6/8)	2	1/3–2/3
Progesterone receptor	Intermediate (6/8)	2	1/3–2/3
C-erbB2	Negative (1+)		
Ki-67	Positive in 8% of tumor cells		

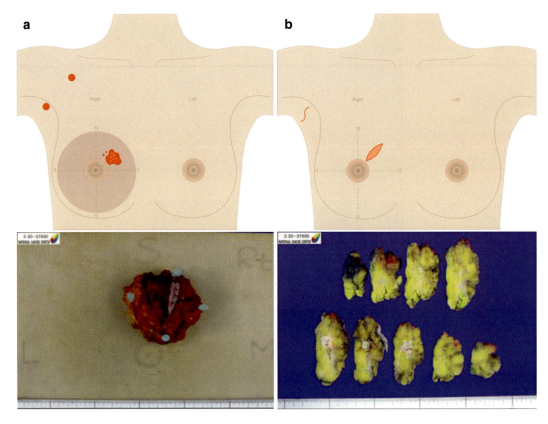

Fig. 30 (**a**) Gross pathology of lumpectomy specimen. (**b**) The margins get marked and sliced with different colors on each direction

7 Case 7

7.1 Patient History and Progress

Female/42 years old, pre-menopause.
  Screen detected mass lesion on left breast 2:30 and 3 o'clock direction.
  No family history.
  Depression.

7.2 Important Radiologic Findings

See Figs. 31, 32, 32, 33, 34 and 35.

7.3 Courses of Treatment

Operation + Post-operative radiation therapy + Tamoxifen 20 mg/day.

7.3.1 Operation

Left breast conserving surgery, sentinel lymph node biopsy (Fig. 36).

7.3.2 Pathology Report

Mucinous Carcinoma
1. Size of invasive component: 1.8 cm (pT1c).
2. Size of intraductal component: 3.0 cm.
3. Histologic grade: 2/3 (tubule formation: 3/3, nuclear pleomorphism: 2/3, mitotic count: 1/3, 6/10 HPF).

HR(+) HER2(−) Breast Cancer

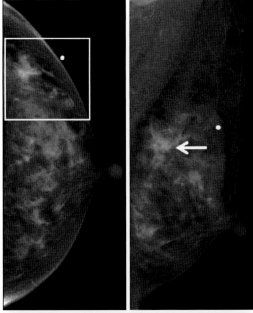

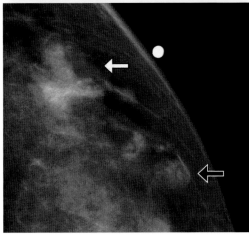

Fig. 31 Left mammography (Nov. 2020): an irregular palpable mass (white arrow) and another smaller mass (black arrow) at upper outer quadrant

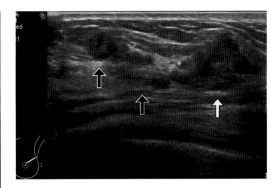

Fig. 32 Left breast US (Nov. 2020): an irregular mass (white arrow, US-CNB = Mucinous carcinoma) with adjacent smaller masses (black arrows)

4. Intraductal component: present, intratumoral/extratumoral (60%) (nuclear grade: low, necrosis: absent, architectural pattern: micropapillary/cribriform, extensive intraductal component: present).
5. Skin: no involvement of tumor.
6. Surgical margins:
    (a) superior margin: 10 mm,
    (b) inferior margin: (see note),
    (c) medial margin: 10 mm,
    (d) lateral margin: 5 mm,
    (e) deep margin: <1 mm from ductal carcinoma in situ (slide 9),
    (f) superficial margin: 2 mm.
7. Lymph nodes: no metastasis in six axillary lymph nodes (pN0(sn)) (sentinel LN: 0/2, non-sentinel LN: 0/4).
8. Arteriovenous invasion: absent.
9. Lymphovascular invasion: present, intratumoral.
10. Tumor border: infiltrative.
11. Microcalcification: present, tumoral/non-tumoral.
12. Pathological TN category (AJCC 2017): pT1cN0(sn).

Note: 1. The inferior margin of the lumpectomy specimen (slide 2) is close to ductal carcinoma in situ (3 mm) but this margin submitted for frozen diagnosis (Fro 2) is free of tumor.

	Result	Intensity	Positive %
Estrogen receptor	Strong (7/8)	2	>2/3
Progesterone receptor	Intermediate (6/8)	2	1/3–2/3
C-erbB2	Negative (1+)		
Ki-67	Positive in 5% of tumor cells		

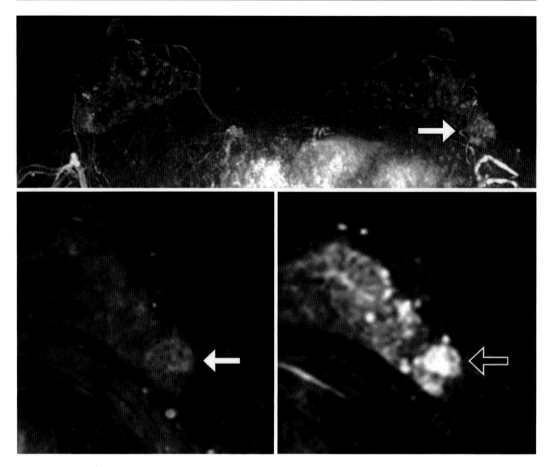

Fig. 33 Breast MRI (Nov. 2020): an enhancing mass (white arrow) with increased T2 signal intensity (black arrow) in the left breast

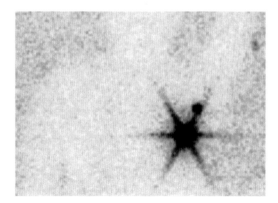

Fig. 34 Lymphoscintigraphy shows visualized sentinel lymph nodes in the left axilla

HR(+) HER2(−) Breast Cancer

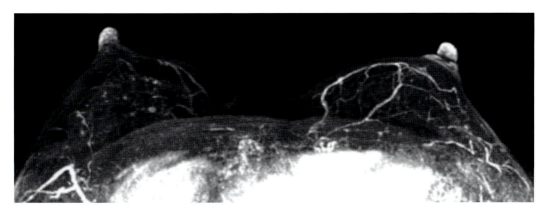

Fig. 35 Breast MRI for routine surveillance (Aug. 2021): no abnormal finding in both breasts

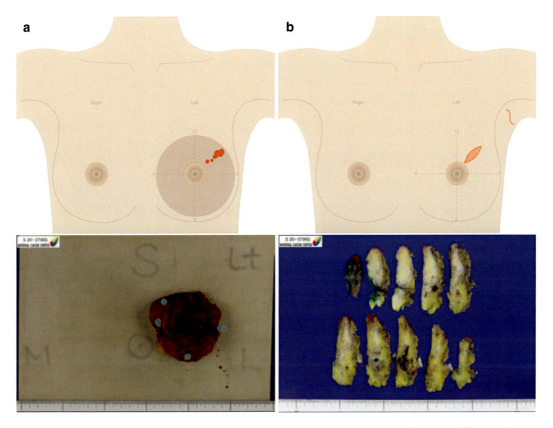

Fig. 36 (**a**) Gross pathology of lumpectomy specimen. (**b**) The margins get marked and sliced with different colors on each direction

8 Case 8

8.1 Patient History and Progress

Female/46 years old, pre-menopause.
Screen detected mass lesion on right breast 12 o'clock and left breast 2 o'clock direction.
No family history.
No comorbidities.
BRCA 1 and 2 mutation: not detected.

8.2 Important Radiologic Findings

See Figs. 37, 38, 39 and 40.

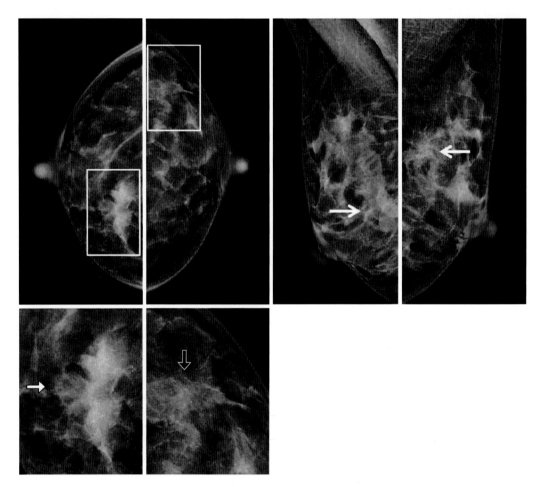

Fig. 37 Both mammography (Nov. 2020): irregular mass at upper inner quadrant of the right breast (white arrow) and upper outer quadrant of the left breast (black arrow)

HR(+) HER2(−) Breast Cancer

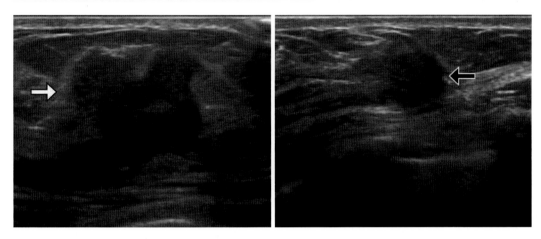

Fig. 38 Both breast US (Nov. 2020): irregular masses at upper inner quadrant of the right breast (white arrow) and upper outer quadrant of the left breast (black arrow). Both US-CNB = IDC

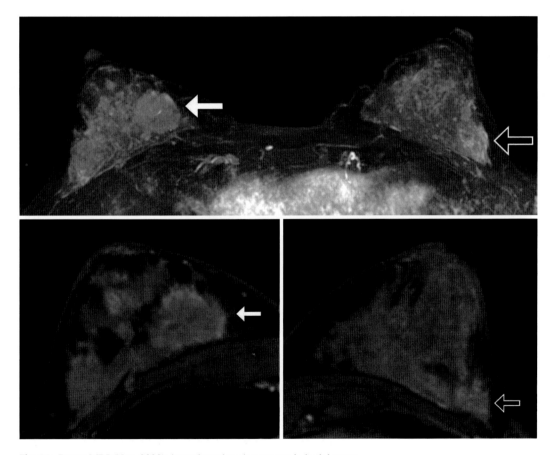

Fig. 39 Breast MRI (Nov. 2020): irregular enhancing masses in both breasts

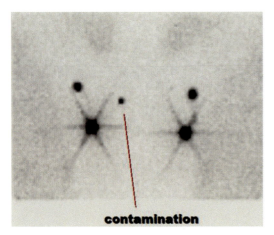

Fig. 40 Lymphoscintigraphy shows visualized sentinel lymph nodes in both axilla

8.3 Courses of Treatment

Operation + Post-operative radiation therapy + Tamoxifen 20 mg/day.

8.3.1 Operation
Right nipple–areolar complex sparing mastectomy, sentinel lymph node biopsy, Left nipple–areolar complex sparing mastectomy, sentinel lymph node biopsy (Figs. 41 and 42).

8.3.2 Pathology Report
[Right]

Invasive Ductal Carcinoma
1. Size of invasive component: 1.5 cm (pT1c).

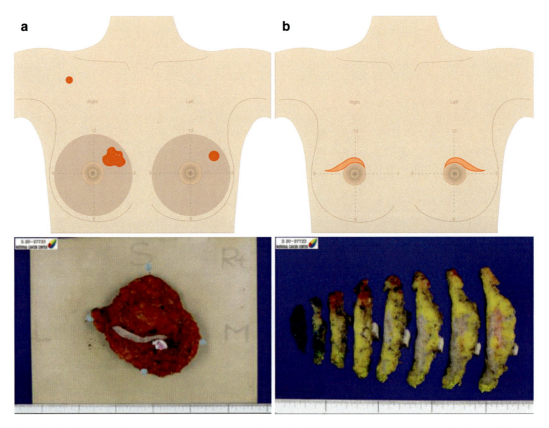

Fig. 41 (**a**) Gross pathology of right mastectomy specimen. (**b**, **c**) The margins get marked and sliced with different colors on each direction

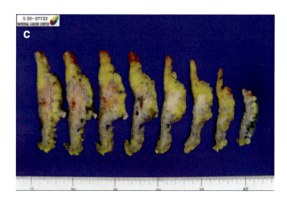

2. Size of intraductal component: 3.5 cm.
3. Histologic grade: 2/3 (tubule formation: 3/3, nuclear pleomorphism: 2/3, mitotic count: 2/3, 18/10 HPF).
4. Intraductal component: present, intratumoral/extratumoral (60%) (nuclear grade: low, necrosis: present, architectural pattern: micropapillary/cribriform/solid/comedo, extensive intraductal component: present).
5. Skin: no involvement of tumor.
6. Surgical margins:
    (a) nipple margin: positive for ductal carcinoma in situ (Fro 2),

Fig. 41 (continued)

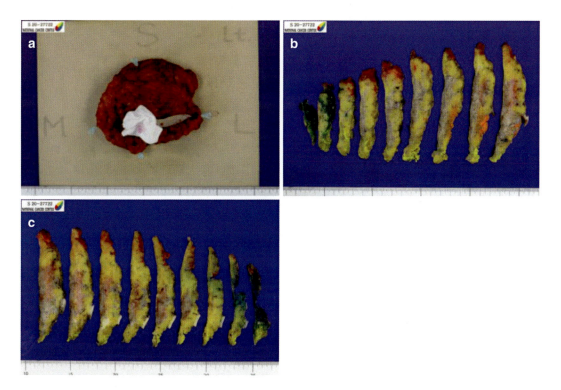

Fig. 42 (**a**) Gross pathology of left mastectomy specimen. (**b, c**) The margins get marked and sliced with different colors on each direction

(b) deep margin: <1 mm from ductal carcinoma in situ (slide 3),

(c) superficial margin: <1 mm from ductal carcinoma in situ (slide 5).

7. Lymph nodes: no metastasis in seven axillary lymph nodes (pN0) (sentinel LN: 0/1, nonsentinel LN: 0/6).

8. Arteriovenous invasion: absent.

9. Lymphovascular invasion: present, intratumoral.

10. Tumor border: infiltrative.

11. Microcalcification: present, tumoral/non-tumoral.

12. Pathological TN category (AJCC 2017): pT1cN0.

	Result	Intensity	Positive %
Estrogen receptor	Strong (7/8)	2	>2/3
Progesterone receptor	Strong (7/8)	2	>2/3
C-erbB2	Negative (1+)		
Ki-67	Positive in 26% of tumor cells		

[Left]

Invasive Ductal Carcinoma

1. Size of tumor: 1.5 cm (pT1c).

2. Histologic grade: 2/3 (tubule formation: 2/3, nuclear pleomorphism: 2/3, mitotic count: 2/3, 17/10 HPF).

3. Intraductal component: present, intratumoral/extratumoral (10%) (nuclear grade: low, necrosis: absent, architectural pattern: cribriform/solid, extensive intraductal component: absent).

4. Skin: no involvement of tumor.

5. Surgical margins:

(a) nipple margin: positive for ductal carcinoma in situ (Fro 1) (see note),

(b) deep margin: 1 mm from invasive ductal carcinoma (slide 1).

6. Lymph nodes: no metastasis in eight axillary lymph nodes (pN0) (sentinel LN: 0/3, nonsentinel LN: 0/5).

7. Arteriovenous invasion: absent.

8. Lymphovascular invasion: absent.

9. Tumor border: partly infiltrative.

10. Microcalcification: present, tumoral.

11. Pathological TN category (AJCC 2017): pT1cN0.

Note: 1. Ductal carcinoma in situ is present only in the permanent section of Fro 1

	Result	Intensity	Positive %
Estrogen receptor	Strong (8/8)	3	>2/3
Progesterone receptor	Strong (8/8)	3	>2/3
C-erbB2	Negative (0)		
Ki-67	Positive in 8% of tumor cells		

9 Case 9

9.1 Patient History and Progress

Female/55 years old, pre-menopause.

Self-detected palpable mass lesion on left breast 11 o'clock direction.

Family history of Prostate cancer, paternal uncle.

No comorbidities.

9.2 Important Radiologic Findings

See Figs. 43, 44, 45 and 46.

9.3 Courses of Treatment

Operation + Adjuvant chemotherapy (#4 cycles of docetaxel & cyclophosphamide) + Post-operative radiation therapy + Tamoxifen 20 mg/day.

9.3.1 Operation

Left breast conserving surgery, sentinel lymph node biopsy (Fig. 47).

HR(+) HER2(−) Breast Cancer

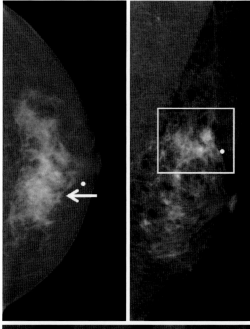

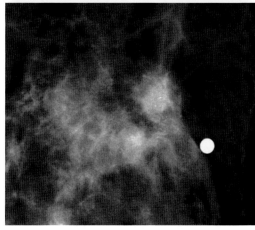

Fig. 43 Left mammography (Dec. 2020): an irregular mass with microcalcifications at upper inner quadrant

9.3.2 Pathology Report

Invasive Ductal Carcinoma

1. Size of tumor: 3.0 cm (pT2).
2. Histologic grade: 3/3 (tubule formation: 3/3, nuclear pleomorphism: 2/3, mitotic count: 3/3, 40/10 HPF).
3. Intraductal component: present, intratumoral/extratumoral (25%) (nuclear grade: high, necrosis: present, architectural pattern: solid/comedo, extensive intraductal component: present).
4. Skin: no involvement of tumor.
5. Surgical margins:

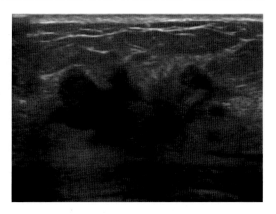

Fig. 44 Left breast US (Dec. 2020): an irregular hypoechoic mass with angular margins. US-CNB = IDC

(a) superior margin: (see note),
(b) inferior margin: 22 m,
(c) medial margin: 1 mm,
(d) lateral margin: 18 mm,
(e) deep margin: 3 mm,
(f) superficial margin: positive for ductal carcinoma in situ (slide 9).

6. Lymph nodes: no metastasis in two axillary lymph nodes (pN0(sn)) (sentinel LN: 0/2).
7. Arteriovenous invasion: absent.
8. Lymphovascular invasion: present, peritumoral.
9. Tumor border: pushing.
10. Microcalcification: present, tumoral/non-tumoral.
11. Pathological TN category (AJCC 2017): pT2N0(sn).

Intraductal Papilloma with Usual Ductal Hyperplasia

Note: 1. The superior margin of the lumpectomy specimen (slide 1) is close to ductal carcinoma in situ (<1 mm) but this margin submitted for frozen diagnosis (Fro 3) is free of tumor.

	Result	Intensity	Positive %
Estrogen receptor	Strong (7/8)	2	>2/3
Progesterone receptor	Weak (4/8)	2	1–10%
C-erbB2	Equivocal (2+) (SISH negative)		
Ki-67	Positive in 23% of tumor cells		

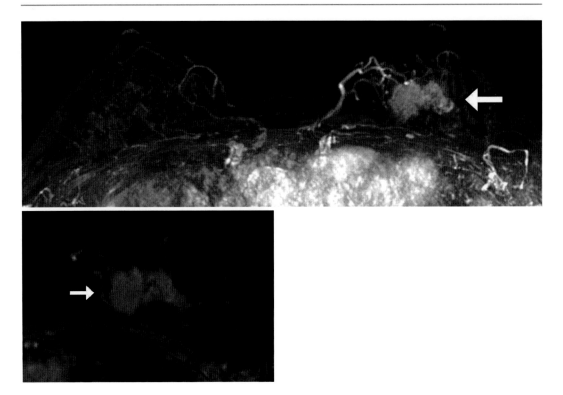

Fig. 45 Breast MRI (Dec. 2020): an irregular enhancing mass in the left breast

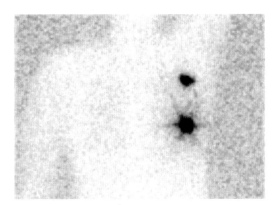

Fig. 46 Lymphoscintigraphy shows visualized sentinel lymph nodes in the left axilla

HR(+) HER2(−) Breast Cancer

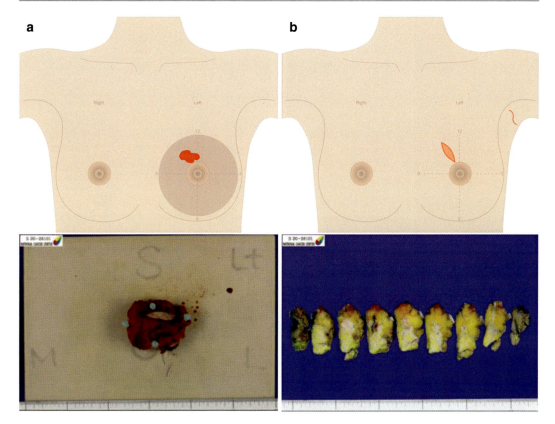

Fig. 47 (**a**) Gross pathology of lumpectomy specimen. (**b**) The margins get marked and sliced with different colors on each direction

10 Case 10

10.1 Patient History and Progress

Female/50 years old, pre-menopause.
　Screen detected mass lesion on left breast 12 o'clock direction.
　No family history.
　No comorbidities.

10.2 Important Radiologic Findings

See Figs. 48, 49, 50 and 51.

10.3 Courses of Treatment

Operation + Adjuvant chemotherapy (#4 cycles of docetaxel & cyclophosphamide) + Post-operative radiation therapy + Tamoxifen 20 mg/day.

10.3.1 Operation

Left breast conserving surgery, axillary lymph node dissection (Fig. 52).

10.3.2 Pathology Report

Invasive Ductal Carcinoma
1. Size of tumor: 2.7 cm (pT2).

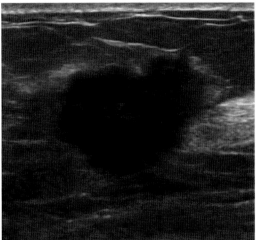

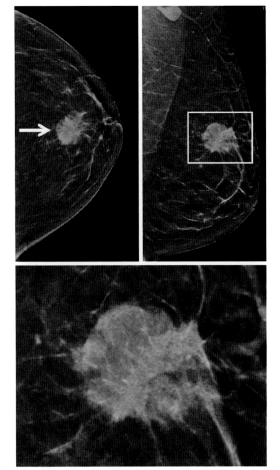

Fig. 48 Left mammography (Nov. 2020): an irregular hyperdense mass at upper center

Fig. 49 Left breast US (Nov. 2020): an irregular hypoechoic mass with spiculated margins. US-CNB = IDC

2. Histologic grade: 3/3 (tubule formation: 3/3, nuclear pleomorphism: 2/3, mitotic count: 3/3, 24/10 HPF).
3. Intraductal component: present, intratumoral/extratumoral (20%) (nuclear grade: high, necrosis: present, architectural pattern: cribriform/solid/comedo, extensive intraductal component: absent).
4. Skin: no involvement of tumor.
5. Surgical margins:
   (a) superior margin: 10 mm,
   (b) inferior margin: 30 mm,
   (c) medial margin: (see note),
   (d) lateral margin: 19 mm,
   (e) deep margin: 11 mm,
   (f) superficial margin: 2 mm.
6. Lymph nodes:
   (a) metastasis in one out of seventeen axillary lymph nodes (pN1a) (sentinel LN: 1/3, axillary LN: 0/14),
   (b) perinodal extension: absent,
   (c) size of metastatic carcinoma: 5 mm.
7. Arteriovenous invasion: absent.
8. Lymphovascular invasion: present, peritumoral.
9. Tumor border: pushing.
10. Microcalcification: absent.
11. Pathological TN category (AJCC 2017): pT2N1a.

Note: 1. The medial margin of the lumpectomy specimen (slide 7) is close to ductal carcinoma in situ (2 mm) but this margin submitted for frozen diagnosis (Fro 6) is free of tumor.

	Result	Intensity	Positive %
Estrogen receptor	Intermediate (6/8)	2	1/3–2/3
Progesterone receptor	Intermediate (6/8)	2	1/3–2/3
C-erbB2	Negative (1+)		
Ki-67	Positive in 19% of tumor cells		

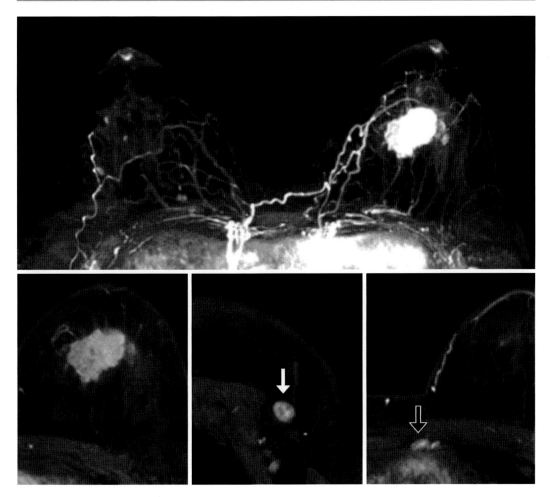

Fig. 50 Breast MRI (Dec. 2020): an irregular enhancing mass in the left breast. Enlarged lymph nodes at the left axilla (white arrow) and internal mammary chain (black arrow)

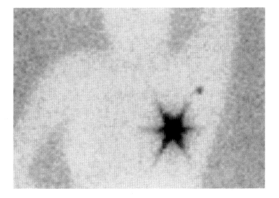

Fig. 51 Lymphoscintigraphy shows visualized sentinel lymph nodes in the left axilla

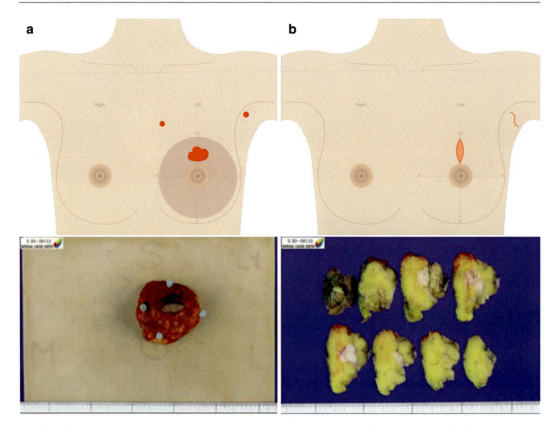

Fig. 52 (**a**) Gross pathology of lumpectomy specimen. (**b**) The margins get marked and sliced with different colors on each direction

11 Case 11

11.1 Patient History and Progress

Female/60 years old, post-menopause.
  Screen detected mass lesion on upper outer portion of left breast.
  No family history.
  Dyslipidemia.

11.2 Important Radiologic Findings

See Figs. 53, 54, 55 and 56.

11.3 Courses of Treatment

Operation + Adjuvant chemotherapy (#4 cycles of docetaxel & cyclophosphamide) + Post-operative radiation therapy + Letrozole 2.5 mg/day.

11.3.1 Operation
Left breast conserving surgery, sentinel lymph node biopsy (Fig. 57).

11.3.2 Pathology Report
Invasive Ductal Carcinoma
  1. Size of tumor: 2.5 cm (pT2).

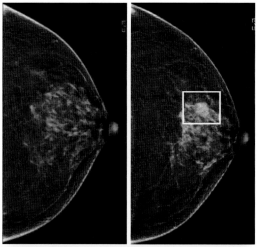

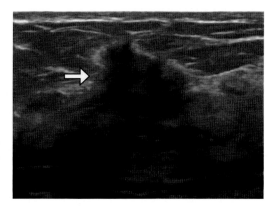

Fig. 54 Left breast US (Dec. 2020): an irregular hypoechoic mass at upper outer quadrant. US-CNB = IDC

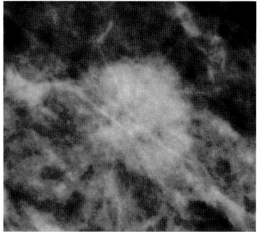

Fig. 53 Left CC mammography (Nov. 2016, Nov. 2020): negative finding in 2016. A new mass at the outer breast in 2020

2. Histologic grade: 3/3 (tubule formation: 3/3, nuclear pleomorphism: 2/3, mitotic count: 3/3, 29/10 HPF).
3. Intraductal component: present, intratumoral/extratumoral (10%) (nuclear grade: low, necrosis: absent, architectural pattern: cribriform, extensive intraductal component: absent).
4. Skin: no involvement of tumor.
5. Surgical margins:
   (a) superior margin: 5 mm,
   (b) inferior margin: 15 mm,
   (c) medial margin: 15 mm,
   (d) lateral margin: 25 mm,
   (e) deep margin: 10 mm,
   (f) superficial margin: positive for invasive ductal carcinoma (slide 3).
6. Lymph nodes:
   (a) metastasis in one out of four axillary lymph nodes (pN1a(sn)) (sentinel LN: 0/3, intramammary LN: 1/1),
   (b) perinodal extension: absent,
   (c) size of metastatic carcinoma: 3.5 mm.
7. Arteriovenous invasion: absent.
8. Lymphovascular invasion: absent.
9. Tumor border: infiltrative.
10. Microcalcification: present, non-tumoral.
11. Pathological TN category (AJCC 2017): pT2N1a(sn).

	Result	Intensity	Positive %
Estrogen receptor	Strong (7/8)	2	>2/3
Progesterone receptor	Intermediate (5/8)	2	10%–1/3
C-erbB2	Negative (0)		
Ki-67	Positive in 8% of tumor cells		

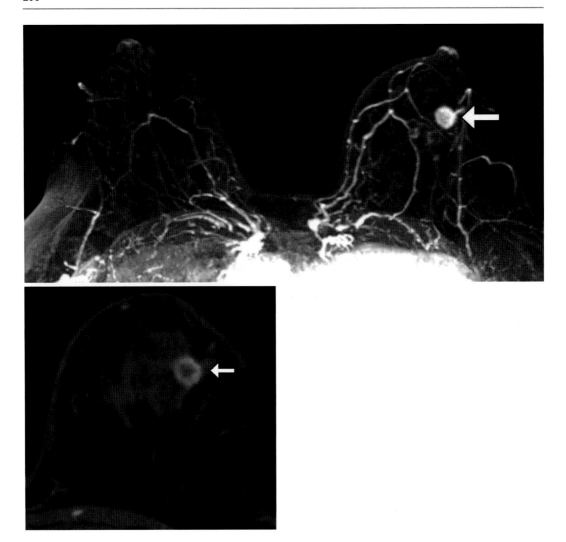

Fig. 55 Breast MRI (Dec. 2020): a rim-enhancing mass in the left breast

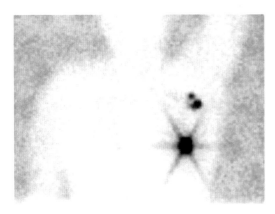

Fig. 56 Lymphoscintigraphy shows visualized sentinel lymph nodes in the left axilla

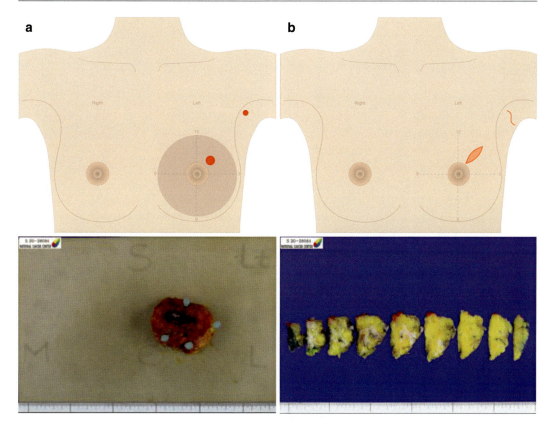

Fig. 57 (**a**) Gross pathology of lumpectomy specimen. (**b**) The margins get marked and sliced with different colors on each direction

12 Case 12

12.1 Patient History and Progress

Female/55 years old, pre-menopause.

Screen detected mass lesion on right breast 5 o'clock direction.

No family history.

S/P hysterectomy, dyslipidemia, diabetes mellitus, s/p cervical spine disc operation.

12.2 Important Radiologic Findings

See Figs. 58, 59, 60 and 61.

12.3 Courses of Treatment

Operation + Adjuvant chemotherapy (#4 cycles of docetaxel & cyclophosphamide) + Post-operative radiation therapy + Tamoxifen 20 mg/day.

12.3.1 Operation

Right breast conserving surgery, sentinel lymph node biopsy (Fig. 62).

12.3.2 Pathology Report

Invasive Ductal Carcinoma
1. Size of tumor: 2.3 cm (pT2).

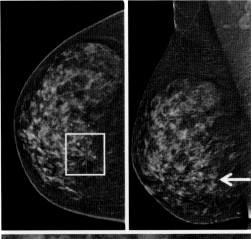

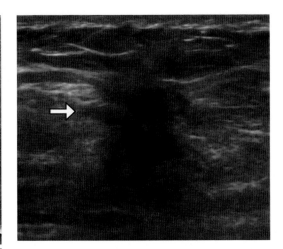

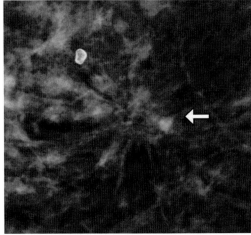

Fig. 58 Right mammography (Nov. 2020): a spiculated mass with architectural distortion at lower inner quadrant

Fig. 59 Right breast US (Dec. 2020): an irregular hypoechoic mass with non-parallel orientation. US-CNB = IDC

2. Histologic grade: 2/3 (tubule formation: 3/3, nuclear pleomorphism: 1/3, mitotic count: 1/3, 5/10 HPF).
3. Intraductal component: present, intratumoral/extratumoral (30%) (nuclear grade: low, necrosis: present, architectural pattern: solid, extensive intraductal component: present).
4. Skin: no involvement of tumor.
5. Surgical margins:
    (a) superior margin: 3 mm,
    (b) inferior margin: 17 mm,
    (c) medial margin: 10 mm,
    (d) lateral margin: <1 mm from ductal carcinoma in situ (slides 10 and 11),
    (e) deep margin: 5 mm,
    (f) superficial margin: positive for ductal carcinoma in situ (slide 8).
6. Lymph nodes: no metastasis in five axillary lymph nodes (pN0(sn)) (sentinel LN: 0/2, non-sentinel LN: 0/3).
7. Arteriovenous invasion: absent.
8. Lymphovascular invasion: present, peritumoral.
9. Tumor border: pushing.
10. Microcalcification: absent.
11. Pathological TN category (AJCC 2017): pT2N0(sn).

	Result	Intensity	Positive %
Estrogen receptor	Weak (4/8)	1	10%–1/3
Progesterone receptor	Intermediate (5/8)	2	10%–1/3
C-erbB2	Negative (0)		
Ki-67	Positive in 4% of tumor cells		

HR(+) HER2(−) Breast Cancer

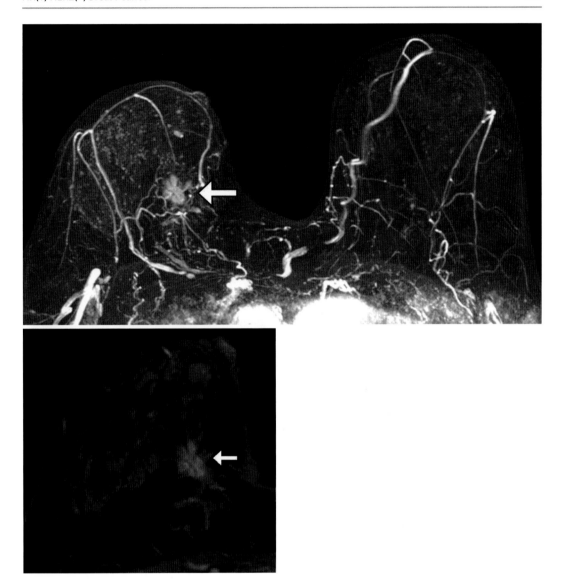

Fig. 60 Breast MRI (Dec. 2020): an irregular enhancing mass in the right breast

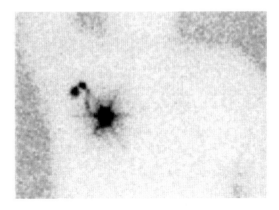

Fig. 61 Lymphoscintigraphy shows visualized sentinel lymph nodes in the right axilla

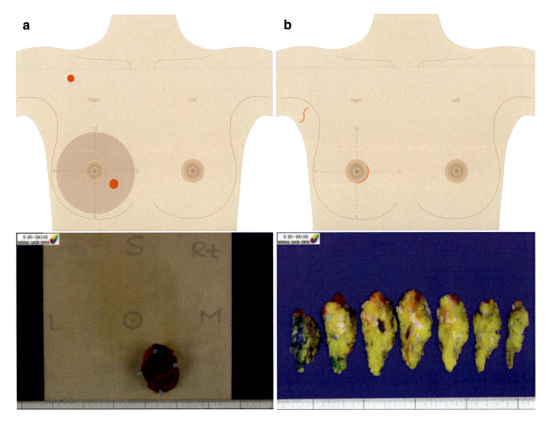

Fig. 62 (**a**) Gross pathology of lumpectomy specimen. (**b**) The margins get marked and sliced with different colors on each direction

13 Case 13

13.1 Patient History and Progress

Female/64 years old, post-menopause.
Screen detected mass lesion on left breast 10 o'clock direction.
No family history.
S/P Tuberculosis, S/P appendectomy.

13.2 Important Radiologic Findings

See Figs. 63, 64, 65 and 66.

13.3 Courses of Treatment

Operation + Adjuvant chemotherapy (#4 cycles of doxorubicin & cyclophosphamide followed by #4 cycles of docetaxel) + Postoperative radiation therapy + Letrozole 2.5 mg/day.

13.3.1 Operation
Left modified radical mastectomy (Fig. 67).

13.3.2 Pathology Report
Invasive Ductal Carcinoma
1. Size of tumor: 5.2 cm (pT3).

HR(+) HER2(−) Breast Cancer

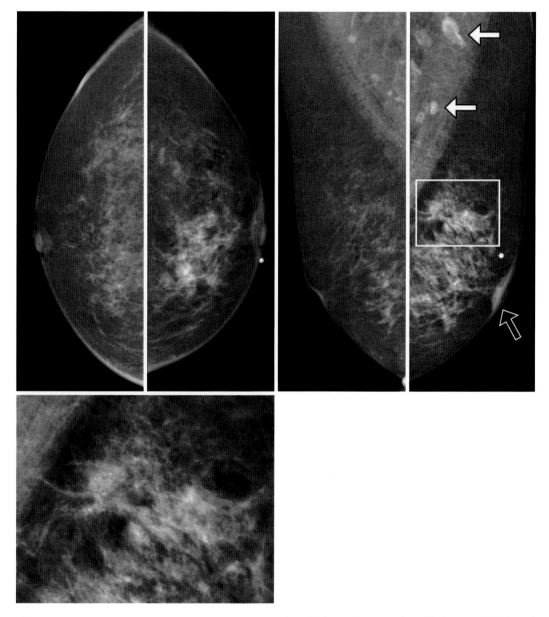

Fig. 63 Mammography (Nov. 2020): an irregular mass with microcalcifications at upper inner quadrant of the left breast. Associated global asymmetry and thickening of the nipple–areolar complex (black arrow). Enlarged lymph nodes at the left axilla (white arrows)

2. Histologic grade: 3/3 (tubule formation: 3/3, nuclear pleomorphism: 3/3, mitotic count: 2/3, 10/10 HPF).
3. Intraductal component: present, intratumoral (5%) (nuclear grade: high, necrosis: present, architectural pattern: solid/comedo, extensive intraductal component: absent).
4. Skin and nipple: dermal involvement of tumor.
5. Surgical margins: (see note).
   (a) deep margin: <1 mm from invasive ductal carcinoma (slide 3).
   (b) superficial margin: 2 mm.
6. Lymph nodes:

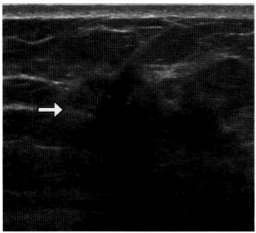

Fig. 64 Left breast US (Nov. 2020): an irregular hypoechoic mass with microcalcifications. US-CNB = IDC

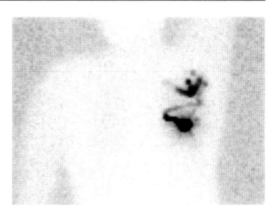

Fig. 66 Lymphoscintigraphy shows visualized sentinel lymph nodes in the left axilla

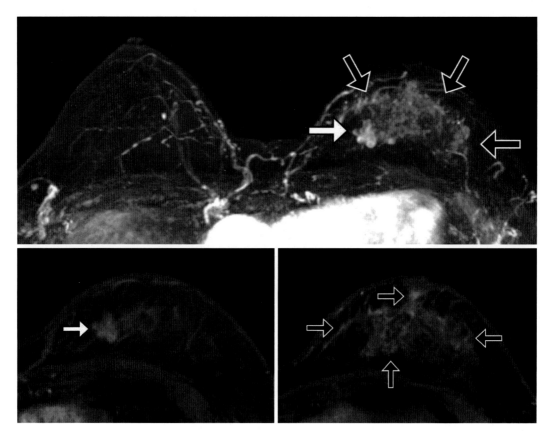

Fig. 65 Breast MRI (Dec. 2020): an irregular enhancing mass (white arrow) with diffuse non-mass enhancement (black arrows) in the left breast

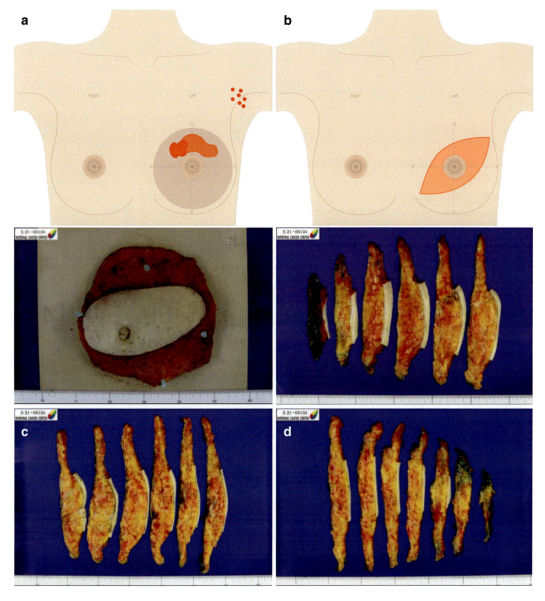

Fig. 67 (**a**) Gross pathology of mastectomy specimen. (**b**, **c** and **d**) The margins get marked and sliced with different colors on each direction

(a) metastasis in eight out of nine axillary lymph nodes (pN2a) (sentinel LN: 4/4, axillary LN: 4/5).
(b) perinodal extension: present.
(c) size of metastatic carcinoma: 11 mm.
7. Arteriovenous invasion: absent.
8. Lymphovascular invasion: present, intratumoral.
9. Tumor border: infiltrative.
10. Microcalcification: present, tumoral.
11. Pathological TN category (AJCC 2017): pT3N2a.

Note: 1. The medial border of the mastectomy specimen (slide 10) is close to invasive ductal carcinoma (<1 mm).

	Result	Intensity	Positive %
Estrogen receptor	Strong (8/8)	3	>2/3
Progesterone receptor	Intermediate (6/8)	2	1/3–2/3
C-erbB2	Negative (1+)		
Ki-67	Positive in 26% of tumor cells		

14 Case 14

14.1 Patient History and Progress

Female/43 years old, pre-menopause.
Screen detected mass lesion on left breast 1 and 3 o'clock direction.
No family history.
No comorbidities.

14.2 Important Radiologic Findings

See Figs. 68, 69, 70, 71 and 72.

14.3 Courses of Treatment

Neoadjuvant therapy (Palbociclib 125 mg/day & tamoxifen 20 mg/day with goserelin) + Operation + Post-operative radiation therapy + Letrozole 2.5 mg/day with goserelin.

14.3.1 Operation
Left breast conserving surgery, sentinel lymph node biopsy (Fig. 73).

14.3.2 Pathology Report
Mucinous Carcinoma
1. Post-chemotherapy status.
2. Size of tumor: 2.0 cm (ypT1c).
3. Histologic grade: 2/3 (tubule formation: 3/3, nuclear pleomorphism: 2/3, mitotic count: 1/3, 6/10 HPF).

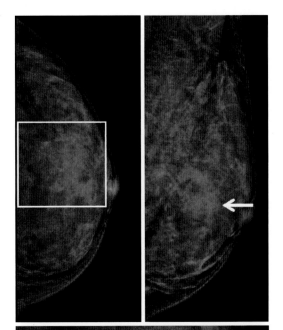

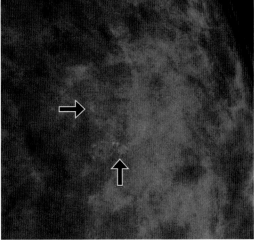

Fig. 68 Left mammography (Dec. 2020): a focal asymmetry with microcalcifications (black arrows) at outer subareolar area

HR(+) HER2(−) Breast Cancer

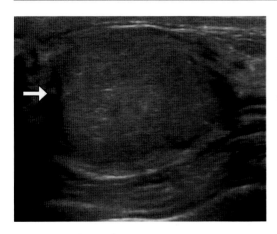

Fig. 69 Left breast US (Dec. 2020): an oval isoechoic mass with microcalcifications. US-CNB = IDC with mucinous component

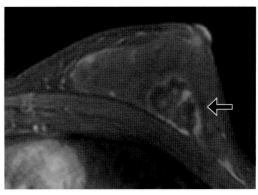

Fig. 71 Post-NAC breast MRI (June 2021): decreased tumor burden after NAC

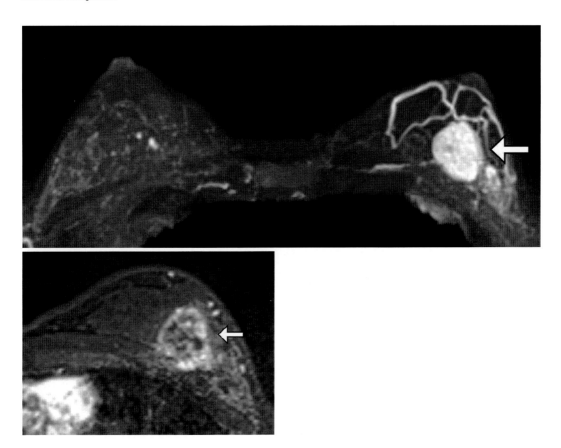

Fig. 70 Breast MRI (Dec. 2020): a rim-enhancing mass in the left breast

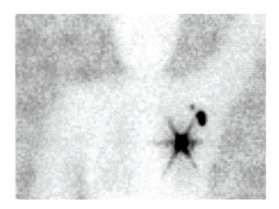

Fig. 72 Lymphoscintigraphy shows visualized sentinel lymph nodes in the left axilla

4. Intraductal component: present, intratumoral/extratumoral (30%) (nuclear grade: low, necrosis: absent, architectural pattern: cribriform/solid, extensive intraductal component: present).
5. Skin: no involvement of tumor.
6. Surgical margins:
    (a) superior margin: 5 mm.
    (b) inferior margin: (see note 1).
    (c) medial margin: (see note 2).
    (d) lateral margin: (see note 3).
    (e) deep margin: <1 mm from mucinous carcinoma (slide 1).
    (f) superficial margin: <1 mm from mucinous carcinoma (slide 1).

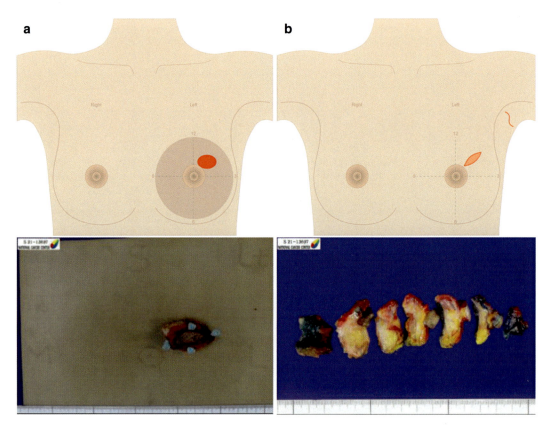

Fig. 73 (**a**) Gross pathology of lumpectomy specimen. (**b**) The margins get marked and sliced with different colors on each direction

HR(+) HER2(−) Breast Cancer

7. Lymph nodes: no metastasis in three axillary lymph nodes (ypN0(sn)) (sentinel LN: 0/3).
8. Arteriovenous invasion: absent.
9. Lymphovascular invasion: absent.
10. Tumor border: infiltrative.
11. Microcalcification: present, tumoral/non-tumoral.
12. Pathological TN category (AJCC 2017): ypT1cN0(sn).

  Note: 1. The inferior margin of the lumpectomy specimen (slide 4) is close to mucinous carcinoma (<1 mm) but this margin submitted for frozen diagnosis (Fro 3) is free of tumor.

2. The medial margin of the lumpectomy specimen (slide 3) is close to mucinous carcinoma (1 mm) but this margin submitted for frozen diagnosis (Fro 4) is free of tumor.
3. The lateral margin of the lumpectomy specimen (slide 7) is close to ductal carcinoma in situ (<1 mm) but this margin submitted for frozen diagnosis (Fro 11) is free of tumor.

	Result	Intensity	Positive %
Estrogen receptor	Strong (8/8)	3	>2/3
Progesterone receptor	Strong (8/8)	3	>2/3
C-erbB2	Negative (0)		
Ki-67	Positive in 3% of tumor cells		

15 Case 15

15.1 Patient History and Progress

Female/58 years old, post-menopause.

Screen detected mass lesion on left breast 12 o'clock direction.

No family history.

Hypertension, dyslipidemia, s/p transobturator tape for stress urinary incontinence.

15.2 Important Radiologic Findings

See Figs. 74, 75, 76 and 77.

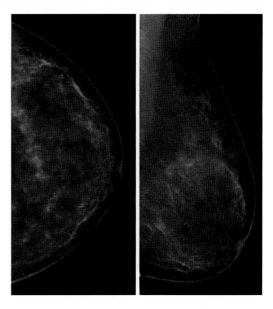

Fig. 74 Left mammography (Dec. 2020): negative finding

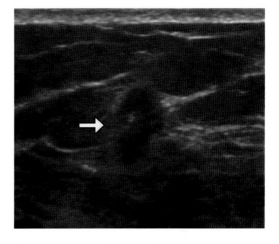

Fig. 75 Left breast US (Dec. 2020): a hypoechoic mass with non-parallel orientation at upper outer quadrant. US-CNB = IDC

15.3 Courses of Treatment

Operation + Post-operative radiation therapy + Anastrozole 1 mg/day.

15.3.1 Operation
Left breast conserving surgery, sentinel lymph node biopsy (Fig. 78).

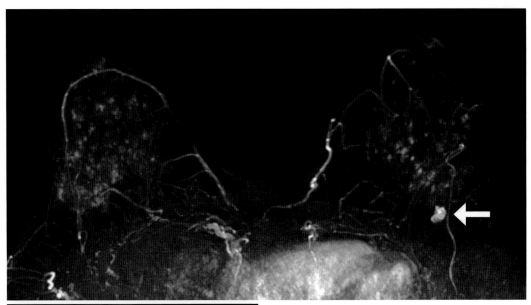
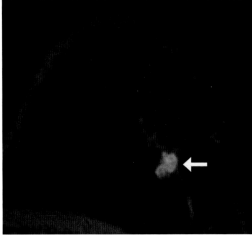

Fig. 76 Breast MRI (Dec. 2020): an irregular enhancing mass in the left breast

15.3.2 Pathology Report

Invasive Ductal Carcinoma
1. Size of tumor: 0.9 cm (pT1b).
2. Histologic grade: 2/3 (tubule formation: 2/3, nuclear pleomorphism: 2/3, mitotic count: 2/3, 10/10 HPF).
3. Intraductal component: absent.
4. Skin: no involvement of tumor.
5. Surgical margins:
   (a) superior margin: 35 mm.
   (b) inferior margin: 10 mm.
   (c) medial margin: 15 mm.
   (d) lateral margin: 5 mm.
   (e) deep margin: 12 mm.
   (f) superficial margin: 4 mm.
6. Lymph nodes: no metastasis in two axillary lymph nodes (pN0(sn)) (sentinel LN: 0/2).
7. Arteriovenous invasion: absent.
8. Lymphovascular invasion: absent.
9. Tumor border: infiltrative.
10. Microcalcification: present, tumoral/non-tumoral.
11. Pathological TN category (AJCC 2017): pT1bN0(sn).

HR(+) HER2(−) Breast Cancer

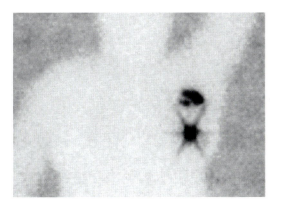

Fig. 77 Lymphoscintigraphy shows visualized sentinel lymph nodes in the left axilla

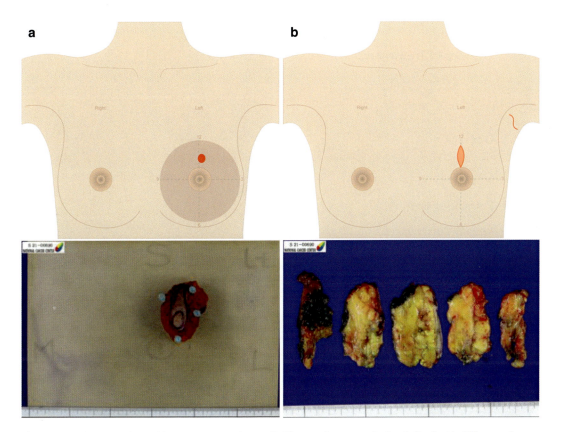

Fig. 78 (a) Gross pathology of lumpectomy specimen. (b) The margins get marked and sliced with different colors on each direction

	Result	Intensity	Positive %
Estrogen receptor	Strong (8/8)	3	>2/3
Progesterone receptor	Intermediate (5/8)	2	10%–1/3
C-erbB2	Negative (1+)		
Ki-67	Positive in 19% of tumor cells		

16 Case 16

16.1 Patient History and Progress

Female/51 years old, peri-menopause.
Screen detected mass lesion on left breast 2 o'clock direction.
No family history.
No comorbidities.

16.2 Important Radiologic Findings

See Figs. 79, 80, 81 and 82.

16.3 Courses of Treatment

Operation + Post-operative radiation therapy + Tamoxifen 20 mg/day.

16.3.1 Operation
Left breast conserving surgery, sentinel lymph node biopsy (Fig. 83).

16.3.2 Pathology Report
Invasive Ductal Carcinoma
1. Post-mammotome excision status.
2. Size of tumor: 0.6 cm, residual.
3. Histologic grade: 2/3 (tubule formation: 3/3, nuclear pleomorphism: 2/3, mitotic count: 1/3, 1/10 HPF).
4. Intraductal component: present, intratumoral/extratumoral (40%) (nuclear grade: low, necrosis: absent, architectural pattern: cribriform/solid, extensive intraductal component: present).
5. Skin: no involvement of tumor.
6. Surgical margins:
   (a) superior margin: 20 mm.
   (b) inferior margin: (see note).
   (c) medial margin: 10 mm.
   (d) lateral margin: 15 mm.
   (e) deep margin: positive for ductal carcinoma in situ (slide 6).

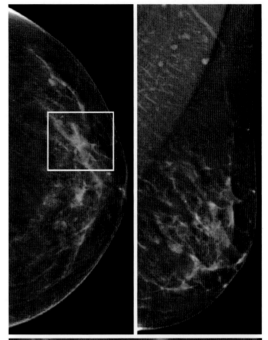
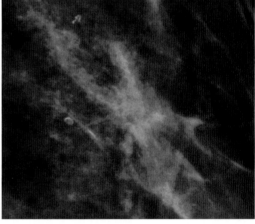

Fig. 79 Left mammography (Oct. 2020): one-view asymmetry at outer breast. Outside US-VABE = IDC (no available image)

   (f) superficial margin: 15 mm.
7. Lymph nodes: no metastasis in three axillary lymph nodes (pN0(sn)) (sentinel LN: 0/2, non-sentinel LN: 0/1).
8. Arteriovenous invasion: absent.
9. Lymphovascular invasion: absent.
10. Tumor border: infiltrative.
11. Microcalcification: present, non-tumoral.

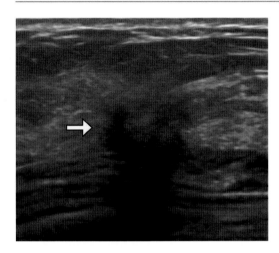

Note: 1. The inferior margin of the lumpectomy specimen (slide 6) is close to ductal carcinoma in situ (<1 mm) but this margin submitted for frozen diagnosis (Fro 7) is free of tumor.

	Result	Intensity	Positive %
Estrogen receptor	Strong (8/8)	3	>2/3
Progesterone receptor	Intermediate (6/8)	1	>2/3
C-erbB2	Negative (1+)		
Ki-67	Positive in 3% of tumor cells		

Fig. 80 Left breast US (Dec. 2020): an irregular hypoechoic area at the VABE site

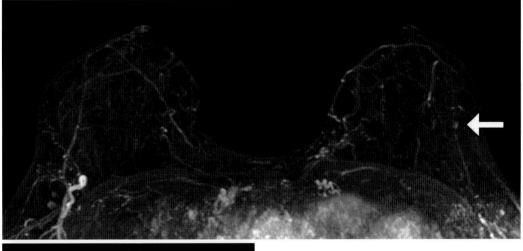

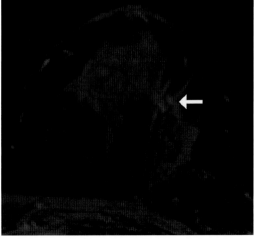

Fig. 81 Breast MRI (Dec. 2020): some enhancing foci at the VABE site

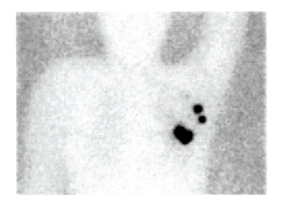

Fig. 82 Lymphoscintigraphy shows visualized sentinel lymph nodes in the left axilla

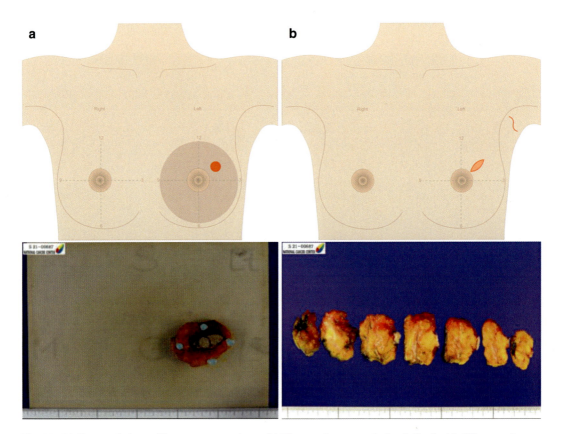

Fig. 83 (**a**) Gross pathology of lumpectomy specimen. (**b**) The margins get marked and sliced with different colors on each direction

17 Case 17

17.1 Patient History and Progress

Female/50 years old, peri-menopause.
Screen detected mass lesion on left breast 4 o'clock direction.
No family history.
S/P Lumbar spine disc herniation operation, s/p pain block in lumbar spine.
S/p hormone replacement due to amenorrhea.

17.2 Important Radiologic Findings

See Figs. 84, 85, 86 and 87.

17.3 Courses of Treatment

Operation + Post-operative radiation therapy + Tamoxifen 20 mg/day.

17.3.1 Operation

Left breast conserving surgery, sentinel lymph node biopsy (Fig. 88).

17.3.2 Pathology Report

Invasive Ductal Carcinoma
1. Size of invasive component: 0.4 cm (pT1a).
2. Size of intraductal component: 3.0 cm.
3. Histologic grade: 2/3 (tubule formation: 3/3, nuclear pleomorphism: 2/3, mitotic count: 1/3, 1/10 HPF).
4. Intraductal component: present, extratumoral (80%) (nuclear grade: low, necrosis: absent, architectural pattern: cribriform/solid, extensive intraductal component: present).
5. Skin: no involvement of tumor.
6. Surgical margins:
    (a) superior margin: 5 mm.
    (b) inferior margin: (see note 1).
    (c) medial margin: 5 mm.
    (d) lateral margin: (see note 2).
    (e) deep margin: 1 mm from invasive ductal carcinoma (slide 5).
    (f) superficial margin: 3 mm.
7. Lymph nodes: no metastasis in one axillary lymph node (pN0(i+)(sn)) (see note 3) (sentinel LN: 0/1).
8. Arteriovenous invasion: absent.
9. Lymphovascular invasion: absent.
10. Tumor border: infiltrative.
11. Microcalcification: present, non-tumoral.
12. Pathological TN category (AJCC 2017): pT1aN0(i+)(sn).

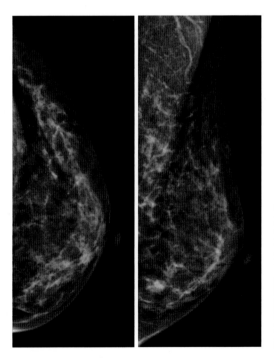

Fig. 84 Left mammography, MLO view (Dec. 2020): negative finding

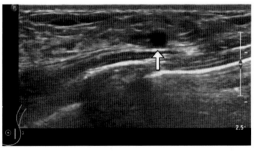

Fig. 85 Left breast US (Dec. 2020): a small hypoechoic mass at lower outer quadrant. US-CNB = IDC

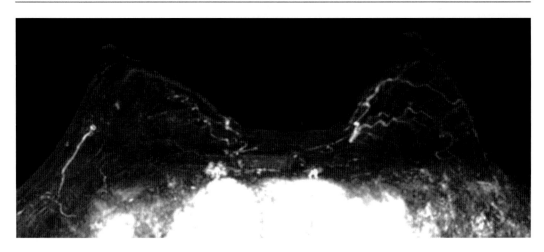

Fig. 86 Breast MRI (Dec. 2020): no suspicious finding in both breasts

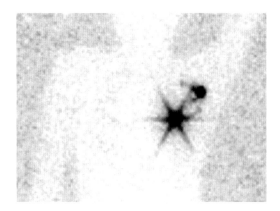

Fig. 87 Lymphoscintigraphy shows visualized sentinel lymph nodes in the left axilla

Note: 1. The inferior margin of the lumpectomy specimen (slide 3) is close to ductal carcinoma in situ (2 mm) but this margin submitted for frozen diagnosis (Fro 4) is free of tumor.
2. The lateral margin of the lumpectomy specimen (slide 5) is close to invasive ductal carcinoma (1 mm) but this margin submitted for frozen diagnosis (Fro 4) is free of tumor.
3. A few isolated tumor cells are present only in the permanent section of Fro 5.

	Result	Intensity	Positive %
Estrogen receptor	Strong (8/8)	3	>2/3
Progesterone receptor	Weak (4/8)	1	10%–1/3
C-erbB2	Negative (0)		
Ki-67	Positive in 1% of tumor cells		

HR(+) HER2(−) Breast Cancer

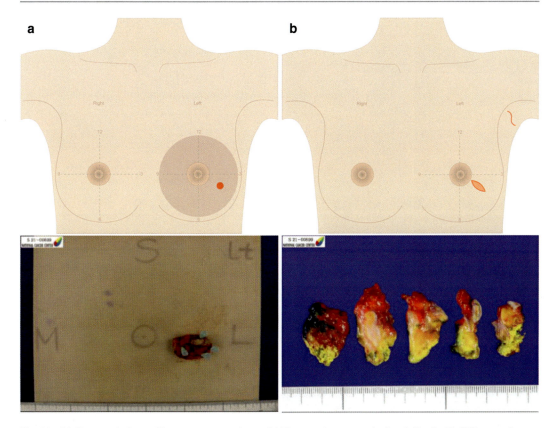

Fig. 88 (**a**) Gross pathology of lumpectomy specimen. (**b**) The margins get marked and sliced with different colors on each direction

18   Case 18

18.1   Patient History and Progress

Female/61 years old, post-menopause.

Screen detected microcalcification of upper outer portion on left breast.

No family history.

S/P unilateral salpingo-oophorectomy, s/p hysterectomy, Hypertension.

18.2   Important Radiologic Findings

See Figs. 89, 90, 91, 92, 93, 94, 95 and 96.

18.3   Courses of Treatment

Operation (1st & 2nd, Aug. 2010) + Postoperative radiation therapy + Tamoxifen 20 mg/day.

Operation (3rd, Jan. 2021) + Adjuvant chemotherapy (docetaxel & cyclophosphamide) + Letrozole 2.5 mg/day.

18.3.1   Operation (1st, Aug. 2010)
Left breast excision (Fig. 97).

18.3.2   Pathology Report
Ductal Carcinoma in Situ
1. Size of tumor: 0.5 cm (pTis).

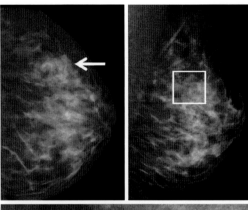

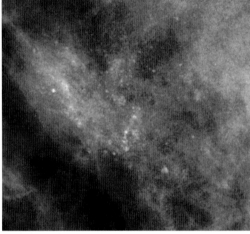

Fig. 89 Left mammography (July 2010): regional amorphous microcalcifications at upper outer quadrant

2. Nuclear grade: low.
3. Necrosis: present.
4. Architectural pattern: cribriform and comedo.
5. Surgical margins:
    (a) superior margin: 30 mm.
    (b) inferior margin: positive (slide 3).
    (c) medial margin: 10 mm.
    (d) lateral margin: 10 mm.
    (e) deep margin: 2 mm.
6. Microcalcification: present, tumoral/non-tumoral.
7. Pathologic stage (AJCC 2010): pTis.

Flat Epithelial Atypia
- With microcalcification.

	Result	Intensity	Positive %
Estrogen receptor	Strong (7/7)	3	>2/3
Progesterone receptor	Strong (6/7)	3	1/3–2/3
C-erbB2	Equivocal (2+)		
Ki-67	Positive in 1% of tumor cells		

18.3.3 Operation (2nd, Aug. 2010)
Left breast conserving surgery, sentinel lymph node biopsy (Fig. 98).

18.3.4 Pathology Report
No residual carcinoma.
1. Post-excisional biopsy status.
2. Lymph nodes: no metastasis in five axillary lymph nodes (pN0) (sentinel LN: 0/2, axillary LN: 0/3).
3. Additional pathologic findings: Flat atypia with microcalcification.

18.3.5 Operation (3rd, Jan. 2021)
Left total mastectomy, sentinel lymph node biopsy, right total mastectomy (Figs. 99 and 100).

18.3.6 Pathology Report
[Right]

1. Fibroadenoma
2. Sclerosing adenosis with microcalcification.

[Left]

Invasive Ductal Carcinoma
1. Post-lumpectomy status.
2. Size of tumor: 2.0 cm (rpT1c).

HR(+) HER2(−) Breast Cancer

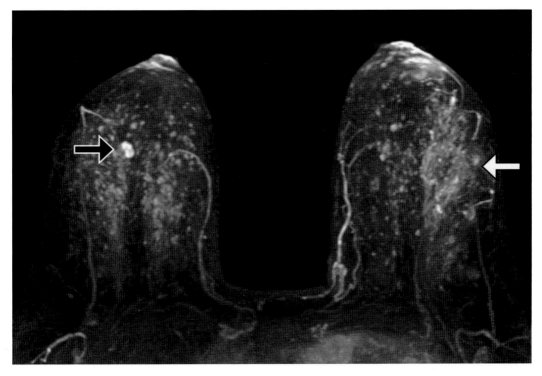

Fig. 90 Breast MRI (Aug. 2010): regional non-mass enhancement at the operative site (white arrow). A benign appearing mass in the right breast (black arrow)

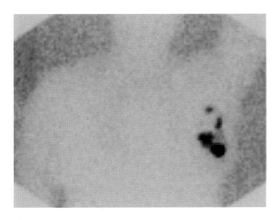

Fig. 91 Lymphoscintigraphy shows visualized sentinel lymph nodes in the left axilla (Aug. 2010)

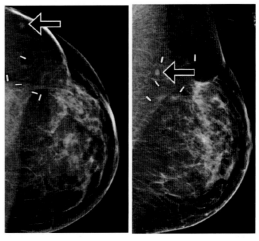

Fig. 92 Left mammography (Nov. 2011): post-operative change at upper outer quadrant. An intramammary lymph node at upper outer quadrant (black arrow)

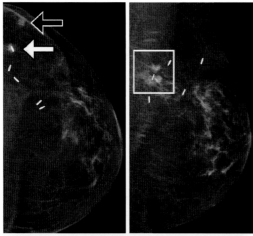

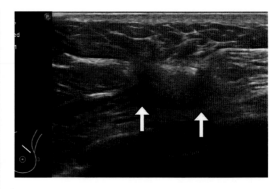

Fig. 94 Left breast US (Nov. 2020): two masses with non-parallel orientation. US-CNB = IDC

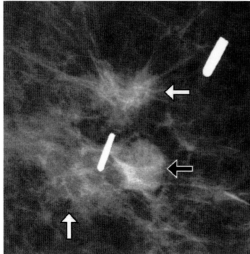

Fig. 93 Left mammography (Nov. 2020): newly developed irregular masses at the operative site (white arrows). No change in the benign intramammary lymph node (black arrow)

3. Histologic grade: 2/3 (tubule formation: 3/3, nuclear pleomorphism: 2/3, mitotic count: 1/3, 3/10 HPF).
4. Intraductal component: present, intratumoral (5%) (nuclear grade: low, necrosis: absent, architectural pattern: solid, extensive intraductal component: absent).
5. Skin and nipple: no involvement of tumor.
6. Surgical margins:
   (a) deep margin: 3 mm.
   (b) superficial margin: 2 mm.
7. Lymph nodes: no metastasis in two axillary lymph nodes (rpN0(sn)) (axillary LN: 0/2).
8. Arteriovenous invasion: present, intratumoral.
9. Lymphovascular invasion: present, intratumoral/peritumoral.
10. Tumor border: infiltrative.
11. Microcalcification: present, tumoral.
12. Pathological TN category (AJCC 2017): rpT1cN0(sn).

	Result	Intensity	Positive %
Estrogen receptor	Strong (8/8)	3	>2/3
Progesterone receptor	Intermediate (5/8)	3	1–10%
C-erbB2	Negative (0)		
Ki-67	Positive in 8% of tumor cells		

HR(+) HER2(−) Breast Cancer

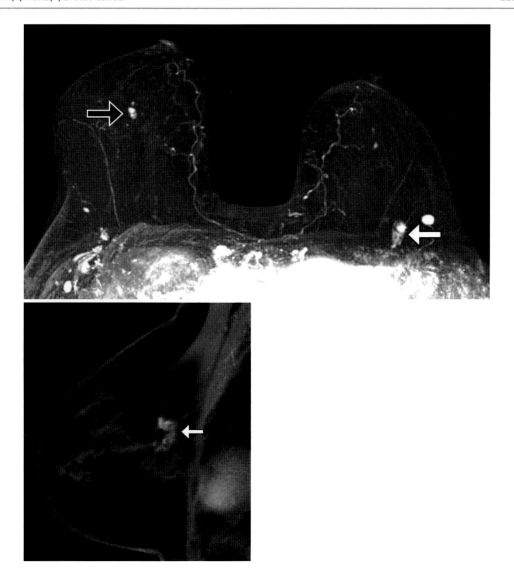

Fig. 95 Breast MRI (Nov. 2020): an irregular enhancing mass in the left breast (white arrow). No change of a benign appearing mass in the right breast (black arrow)

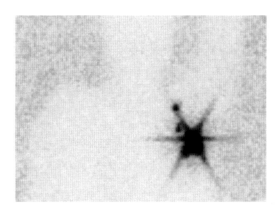

Fig. 96 Lymphoscintigraphy shows visualized sentinel lymph nodes in the left axilla (Jan. 2021)

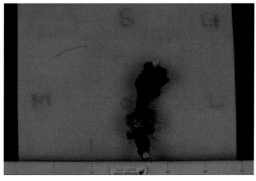

Fig. 97 Gross pathology of breast excision specimen

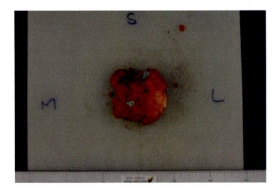

Fig. 98 Gross pathology of lumpectomy specimen

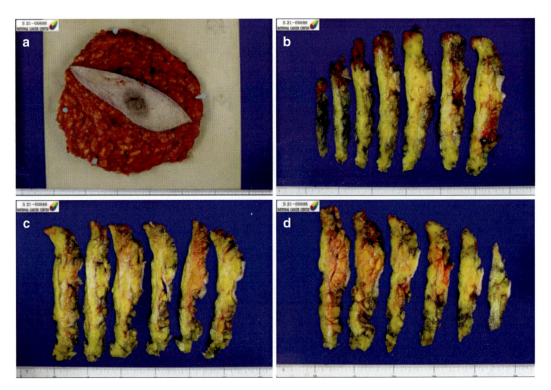

Fig. 99 (**a**) Gross pathology of right mastectomy specimen. (**b, c** and **d**) The margins get marked and sliced with different colors on each direction

HR(+) HER2(−) Breast Cancer

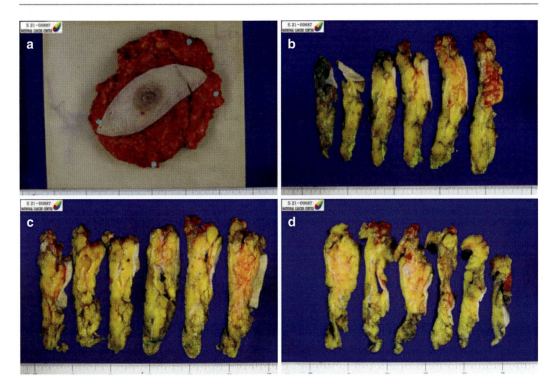

Fig. 100 (**a**) Gross pathology of left mastectomy specimen. (**b**, **c** and **d**) The margins get marked and sliced with different colors on each direction

19 Case 19

19.1 Patient History and Progress

Female/43 years old, pre-menopause.
Screen detected mass lesion of lower inner on left breast.
No family history.
No comorbidities.

19.2 Important Radiologic Findings

See Figs. 101, 102, 103, 104 and 105.

19.3 Courses of Treatment

Operation + Tamoxifen 20 mg/day with leuprolide acetate.

19.3.1 Operation

Left nipple–areolar complex sparing mastectomy with immediate implant reconstruction, sentinel lymph node biopsy (Figs. 106 and 107).

19.3.2 Pathology Report

Invasive Ductal Carcinoma
1. Size of tumor: 1.7 cm and 0.5 cm (pT1c(2)).
2. Histologic grade: 2/3 (tubule formation: 3/3, nuclear pleomorphism: 2/3, mitotic count: 2/3, 11/10 HPF).
3. Intraductal component: present, intratumoral/extratumoral (20%) (nuclear grade: low, necrosis: present, architectural pattern: cribriform/solid/comedo, extensive intraductal component: present).
4. Skin: no involvement of tumor.
5. Surgical margins:
   (a) deep margin: 2 mm.
   (b) superficial margin: 2 mm.

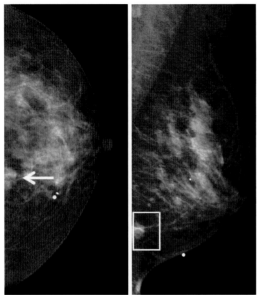

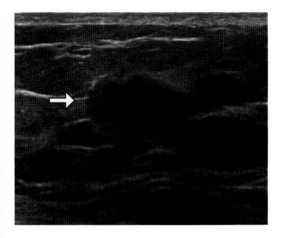

Fig. 102 Left breast US (Jan. 2021): a hypoechoic mass with angular margins at lower inner quadrant. US-CNB = IDC

6. Lymph nodes: no metastasis in one axillary lymph node (pN0(sn)) (sentinel LN: 0/1).
7. Arteriovenous invasion: absent.
8. Lymphovascular invasion: present, intratumoral.
9. Tumor border: infiltrative.
10. Microcalcification: present, tumoral/non-tumoral.
11. Pathological TN category (AJCC 2017): pT1c(2)N0(sn).

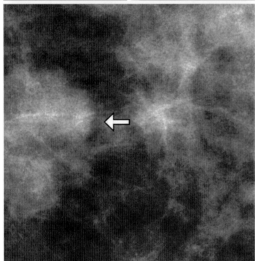

Fig. 101 Left mammography (Jan. 2021): an irregular mass at lower inner quadrant

	Result	Intensity	Positive %
Estrogen receptor	Strong (8/8)	3	>2/3
Progesterone receptor	Strong (8/8)	3	>2/3
C-erbB2	Equivocal (2+) (SISH negative)		
Ki-67	Positive in 9% of tumor cells		

HR(+) HER2(−) Breast Cancer

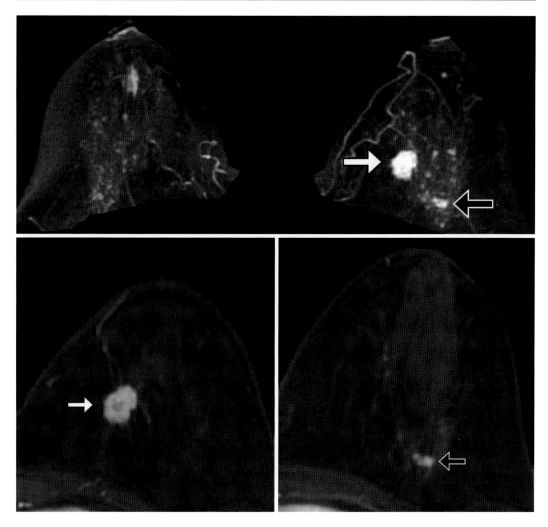

Fig. 103 Breast MRI (Jan. 2021): an irregular enhancing mass at lower inner quadrant of the left breast (white arrow, proven IDC). Another irregular enhancing mass at the lower outer quadrant of the left breast (black arrow)

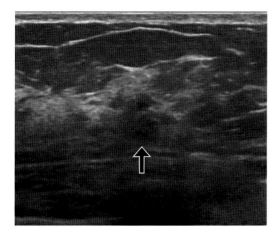

Fig. 104 MRI-directed left breast US (Jan. 2021): a hypoechoic mass with non-parallel orientation at lower outer quadrant. US-CNB = IDC

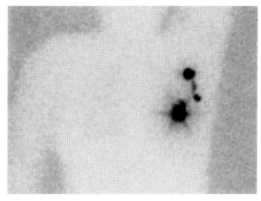

Fig. 105 Lymphoscintigraphy shows visualized sentinel lymph nodes in the left axilla

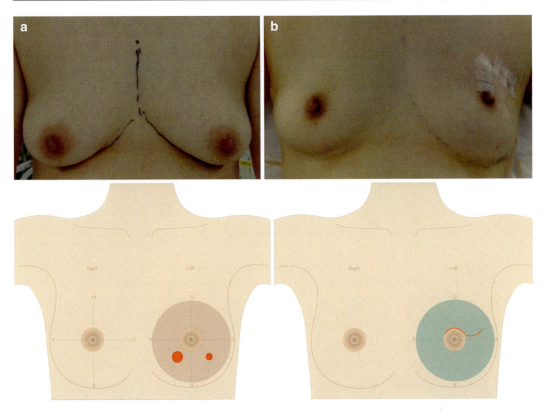

Fig. 106 (**a**) Preoperative and (**b**) immediate post-operative appearance

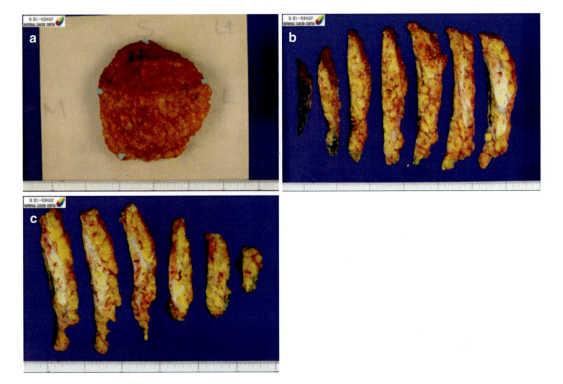

Fig. 107 (**a**) Gross pathology of mastectomy specimen. (**b, c**) The margins get marked and sliced with different colors on each direction

20 Case 20

20.1 Patient History and Progress

Female/49 years old, pre-menopause.
Screen detected mass lesion on left breast 2 o'clock direction.
No family history.
S/P Tuberculosis, S/P duodenal adenoma excision.

20.2 Important Radiologic Findings

See Figs. 108, 109, 110, 111 and 112.

20.3 Courses of Treatment

Operation + Post-operative radiation therapy + Tamoxifen 20 mg/day.

20.3.1 Operation
Left breast conserving surgery, sentinel lymph node biopsy (Fig. 113).

20.3.2 Pathology Report
Invasive Ductal Carcinoma
1. Size of tumor: 0.9 cm (pT1b).
2. Histologic grade: 1/3 (tubule formation: 2/3, nuclear pleomorphism: 2/3, mitotic count: 1/3, 1/10 HPF).
3. Intraductal component: present, intratumoral/extratumoral (40%) (nuclear grade: low, necrosis: absent, architectural pattern: micropapillary/cribriform/solid/comedo, extensive intraductal component: present).
4. Skin: no involvement of tumor.
5. Surgical margins:
    (a) superior margin: 15 mm.
    (b) inferior margin: 20 mm.
    (c) medial margin: 15 mm.
    (d) lateral margin: 5 mm.
    (e) deep margin: 5 mm.
    (f) superficial margin: 3 mm.

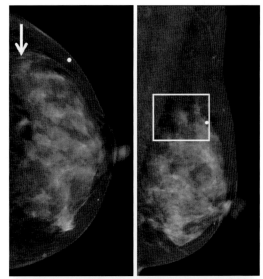

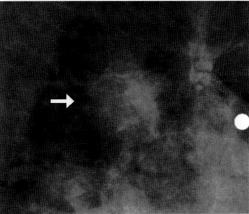

Fig. 108 Left mammography (Nov. 2020): an irregular mass at upper outer quadrant

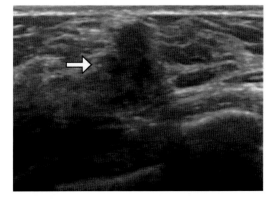

Fig. 109 Left breast US (Nov. 2020): an irregular mass with non-parallel orientation. US-CNB = IDC

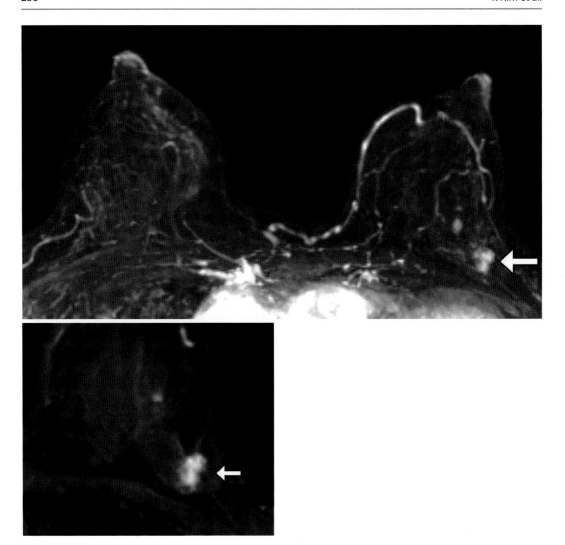

Fig. 110 Breast MRI (Nov. 2021): an irregular enhancing mass in the left breast

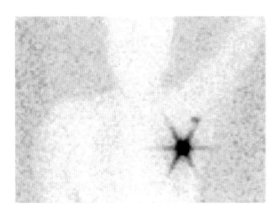

Fig. 111 Lymphoscintigraphy shows visualized sentinel lymph nodes in the left axilla

6. Lymph nodes: no metastasis in six axillary lymph nodes (pN0(sn)) (sentinel LN: 0/3, non-sentinel LN: 0/3).
7. Arteriovenous invasion: absent.
8. Lymphovascular invasion: absent.
9. Tumor border: infiltrative.
10. Microcalcification: present, tumoral/non-tumoral.
11. Pathological TN category (AJCC 2017): pT1bN0(sn).

    Note: 1. Atypical ductal hyperplasia is present in the permanent section of Fro 1.

HR(+) HER2(−) Breast Cancer

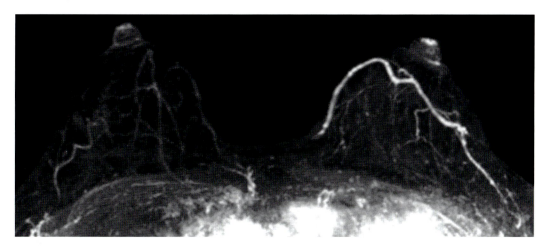

Fig. 112 Breast MRI for routine surveillance (Oct. 2021): No abnormal finding in both breasts

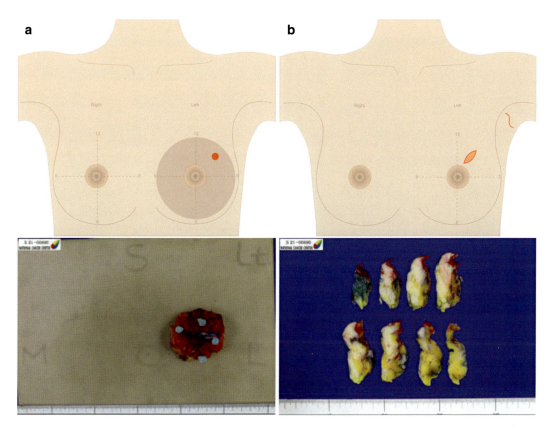

Fig. 113 (**a**) Gross pathology of lumpectomy specimen. (**b**) The margins get marked and sliced with different colors on each direction

	Result	Intensity	Positive %
Estrogen receptor	Intermediate (6/8)	1	>2/3
Progesterone receptor	Intermediate (6/8)	2	1/3–2/3
C-erbB2	Equivocal (2+)		
Ki-67	Positive in 21% of tumor cells		
SISH	Negative		

21 Case 21

21.1 Patient History and Progress

Female/78 years old, post-menopause.
Screen detected mass lesion on left breast 12 o'clock direction.
No family history.
Hypertension, s/p hysterectomy.

21.2 Important Radiologic Findings

See Figs. 114, 115, 116 and 117.

21.3 Courses of Treatment

Operation + Post-operative radiation therapy + Letrozole 2.5 mg/day.

21.3.1 Operation (1st, Dec. 2020)
Left breast conserving surgery (Fig. 118).

21.3.2 Pathology Report

Invasive Ductal Carcinoma
1. Size of tumor: 1.2 cm (pT1c).
2. Histologic grade: 2/3 (tubule formation: 3/3, nuclear pleomorphism: 2/3, mitotic count: 2/3, 11/10 HPF).
3. Intraductal component: present, intratumoral/extratumoral (20%) (nuclear grade: low, necrosis: present, architectural pattern: solid/comedo, extensive intraductal component: absent).
4. Skin: no involvement of tumor.
5. Surgical margins:
    (a) superior margin: 5 mm.
    (b) inferior margin: 20 mm.
    (c) medial margin: 10 mm.
    (d) lateral margin: 20 mm.
    (e) deep margin: 2 mm.
    (f) superficial margin: 2 mm.
6. Arteriovenous invasion: absent.
7. Lymphovascular invasion: present, intratumoral.
8. Tumor border: infiltrative.

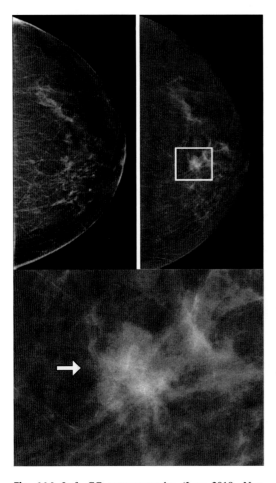

Fig. 114 Left CC mammography (June 2019, Nov. 2020): negative finding in 2019. A new mass at the central breast in 2020

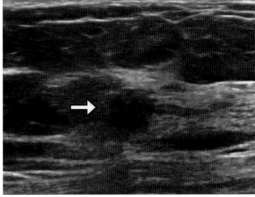

Fig. 115 Left breast US (Nov. 2020): a hypoechoic mass with microlobulated margins at 12 o'clock direction. Outside US-CNB = DCIS

HR(+) HER2(−) Breast Cancer

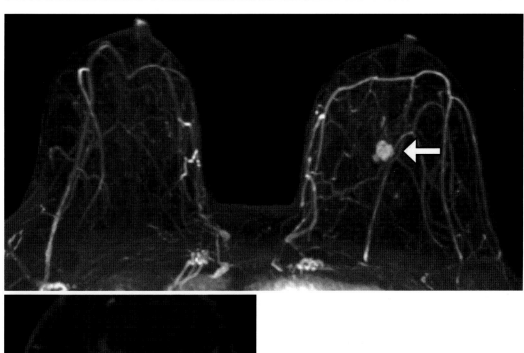

Fig. 116 Breast MRI (Nov. 2020): an irregular enhancing mass in the left breast

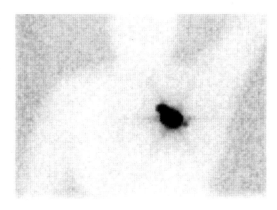

Fig. 117 Lymphoscintigraphy shows visualized sentinel lymph nodes in the left lateral breast

9. Microcalcification: present, tumoral/non-tumoral.
10. Pathological TN category (AJCC 2017): pT1c.

	Result	Intensity	Positive %
Estrogen receptor	Intermediate (6/8)	3	10%–1/3
Progesterone receptor	Strong (7/8)	3	1/3–2/3
C-erbB2	Negative (0)		
Ki-67	Positive in 2% of tumor cells		

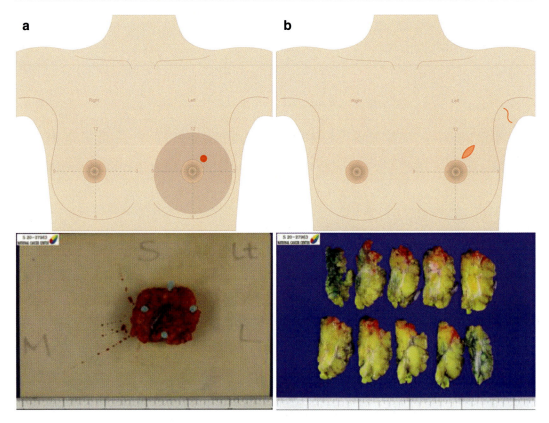

Fig. 118 (**a**) Gross pathology of lumpectomy specimen. (**b**) The margins get marked and sliced with different colors on each direction

21.3.3 Operation (2nd, Jan. 2021)
Left sentinel lymph node biopsy.

21.3.4 Pathology Report
No metastasis in two axillary lymph nodes
1. Post-lumpectomy status.

22 Case 22

22.1 Patient History and Progress

Female/61 years old, post-menopause.
　Screen detected mass lesion on entire left breast.
　No family history.
　Diabetes mellitus, Spinal stenosis.

22.2 Important Radiologic Findings

See Figs. 119, 120, 121, 122, 123 and 124.

22.3 Courses of Treatment

Neoadjuvant chemotherapy (#4 cycles of doxorubicin & cyclophosphamide followed by #4 cycles of docetaxel) + Operation + Postoperative radiation therapy + Letrozole 2.5 mg/day.

22.3.1 Operation
Left modified radical mastectomy (Fig. 125).

HR(+) HER2(−) Breast Cancer

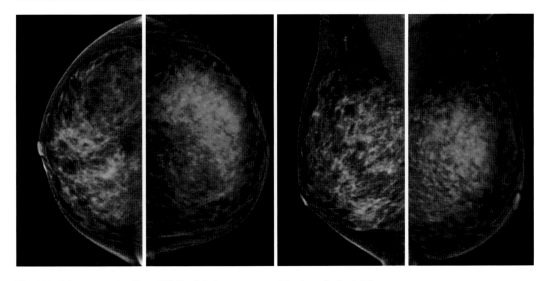

Fig. 119 Mammography (June 2020): global asymmetry with edema in the left breast

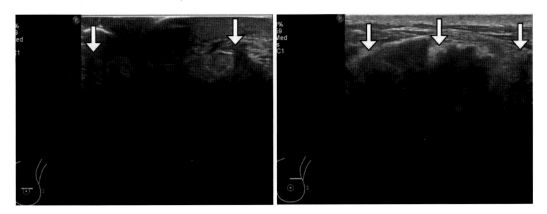

Fig. 120 Left breast US (July 2020): irregular hypoechoic lesion with posterior acoustic shadowing involving the entire left breast (partly shown). US-CNB = IDC

22.3.2 Pathology Report

Invasive Micropapillary Carcinoma
1. Post-chemotherapy status.
2. Size of tumor: 11.0 cm (ypT3).
3. Histologic grade: 2/3 (tubule formation: 3/3, nuclear pleomorphism: 2/3, mitotic count: 1/3, 2/10HPF).
4. Intraductal component: absent.
5. Skin and nipple: dermal involvement of tumor.
6. Surgical margins:
   (a) deep margin: positive for invasive carcinoma (slide 1).
   (b) superficial margin: positive for invasive carcinoma (slide 4).
7. Lymph nodes:
   (a) metastasis in nine out of nine axillary lymph nodes (ypN2a).
   (b) perinodal extension: present.
   (c) size of metastatic carcinoma: 6 mm.
8. Arteriovenous invasion: present, peritumoral.
9. Lymphovascular invasion: present, peritumoral.
10. Tumor border: infiltrative.

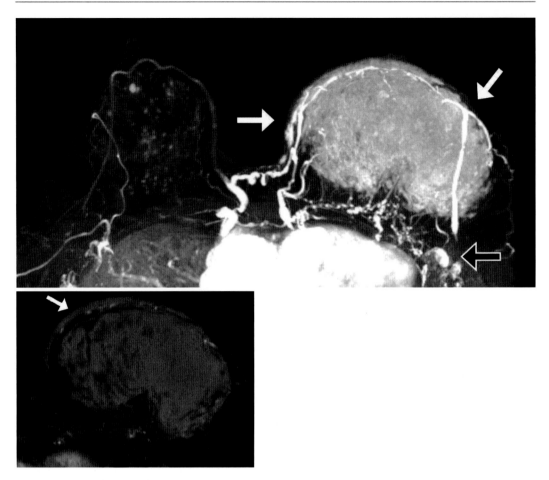

Fig. 121 Breast MRI (Aug. 2020): diffuse non-mass enhancement with involvement of the skin. Enlarged lymph nodes at the left axilla (black arrow)

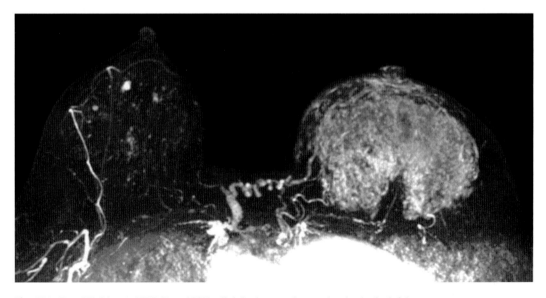

Fig. 122 Post-NAC breast MRI (Dec. 2020): slightly decreased tumor burden in the left breast

HR(+) HER2(−) Breast Cancer

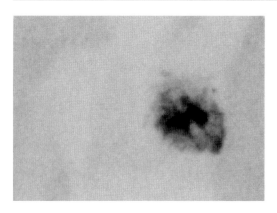

Fig. 123 Lymphoscintigraphy shows visualized sentinel lymph nodes in the left axilla

11. Microcalcification: present, tumoral/non-tumoral.
12. Pathological TN category (AJCC 2017): ypT3N2a.

	Result	Intensity	Positive %
Estrogen receptor	Strong (8/8)	3	>2/3
Progesterone receptor	Negative (2/8)	1	<1%
C-erbB2	Equivocal (2+) (SISH negative)		
Ki-67	Positive in 14% of tumor cells		

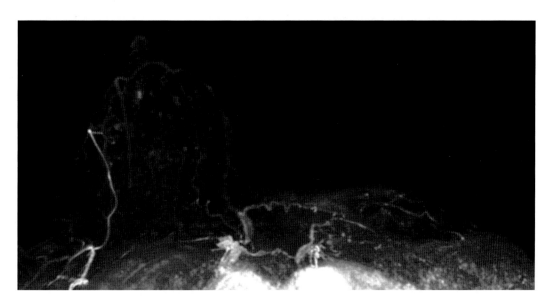

Fig. 124 Breast MRI for routine surveillance (July 2021): no abnormal finding in right breast and anterior left chest wall

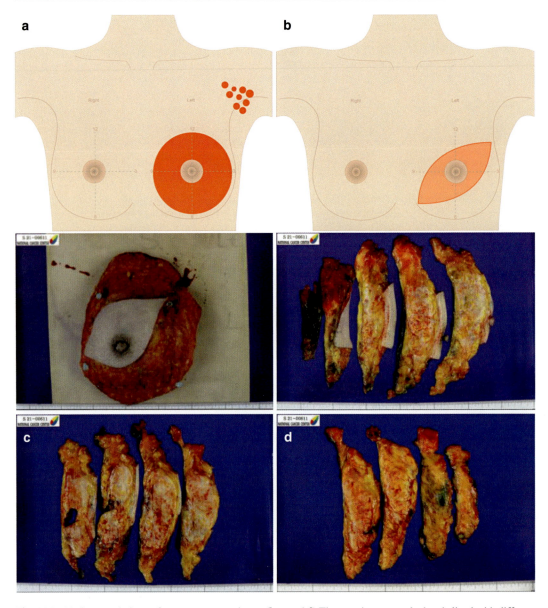

Fig. 125 (**a**) Gross pathology of mastectomy specimen. (**b, c** and **d**) The margins get marked and sliced with different colors on each direction

23 Case 23

23.1 Patient History and Progress

Female/53 years old, post-menopause.

Screen detected mass lesion on right breast 7 o'clock direction.

Family history of breast cancer, younger sister.

Diabetes mellitus, s/p right thyroidectomy (thyroid cancer), s/p cholecystectomy, s/p hysterectomy.

BRCA 1 and 2 mutation: Not detected.

23.2 Important Radiologic Findings

See Figs. 126, 127, 128, 129 and 130.

HR(+) HER2(−) Breast Cancer

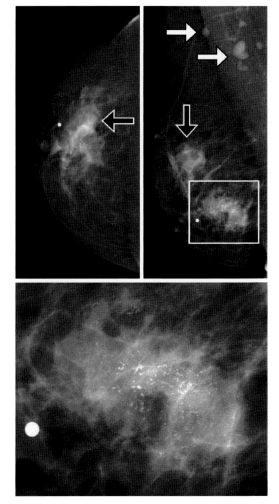

Fig. 126 Right mammography (July 2020): an irregular mass with microcalcifications at lower center. Another oval mass at the upper outer quadrant (black arrow). Multiple enlarged lymph nodes at the right axilla (white arrows)

23.3 Courses of Treatment

Neoadjuvant chemotherapy (#4 cycles of doxorubicin & cyclophosphamide followed by #4 cycles of docetaxel) + Operation + Postoperative radiation therapy + Letrozole 2.5 mg/day.

23.3.1 Operation
Right breast conserving surgery, sentinel lymph node biopsy (Fig. 131).

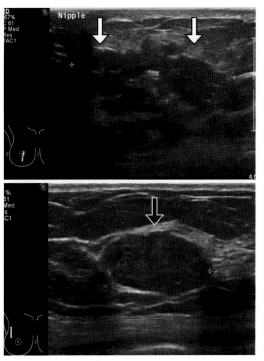

Fig. 127 Right breast US (July 2020): an irregular hypoechoic mass with microcalcifications at lower center (white arrows, US-CNB = IDC). Another oval isoechoic mass at the upper outer quadrant (black arrow)

23.3.2 Pathology Report
1. Microinvasive ductal carcinoma
   (a) Post-chemotherapy status.
   (b) Size of invasive component: <0.1 cm (ypT1mi).
   (c) Size of intraductal component: 1.5 cm.
   (d) Histologic grade: 3/3 (tubule formation: 3/3, nuclear pleomorphism: 3/3, mitotic count: 2/3, 10/10 HPF)
   (e) Intraductal component: present, intratumoral/extratumoral (99%) (nuclear grade: high, necrosis: present, architectural pattern: solid/comedo, extensive intraductal component: present).
   (f) Skin: no involvement of tumor.
   (g) Surgical margins:
   - superior margin: 10 mm.
   - inferior margin: (see note).
   - medial margin: 5 mm.
   - lateral margin: 10 mm.

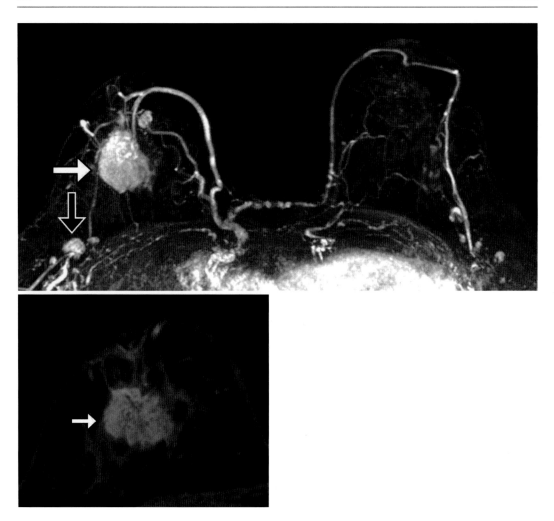

Fig. 128 Breast MRI (July 2020): an irregular enhancing mass in the right breast (white arrow). Enlarged lymph node at the right axilla (black arrow)

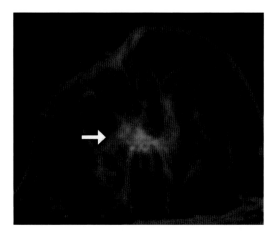

Fig. 129 Post-NAC breast MRI (Dec. 2020): Decreased size of the tumor after NAC

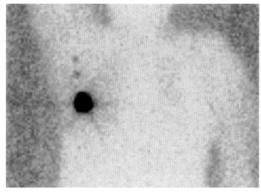

Fig. 130 Lymphoscintigraphy shows visualized sentinel lymph nodes in the right axilla

HR(+) HER2(−) Breast Cancer

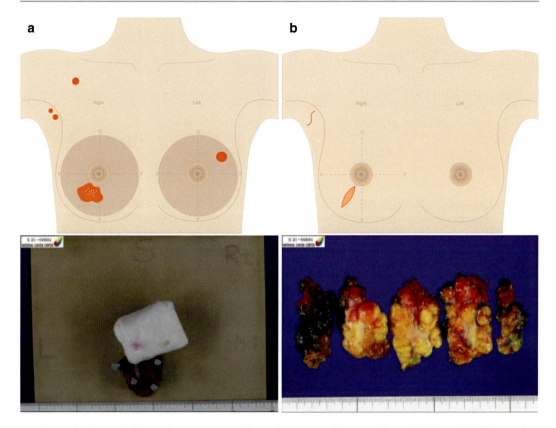

Fig. 131 (**a**) Gross pathology of lumpectomy specimen. (**b**) The margins get marked and sliced with different colors on each direction

- deep margin: <1 mm from ductal carcinoma in situ (slide 1).
- superficial margin: 5 mm.
(h) Lymph nodes: no metastasis in three axillary lymph nodes (ypN0(sn)) (sentinel LN: 0/1, axillary LN: 0/2)
(i) Arteriovenous invasion: absent.
(j) Lymphovascular invasion: absent.
(k) Tumor border: infiltrative.
(l) Microcalcification: present, tumoral/non-tumoral.

(m) Pathological TN category (AJCC 2017): ypT1miN0(sn).
2. Intraductal papilloma with usual ductal hyperplasia.
3. Fibroadenoma.
4. Complex sclerosing lesion.

Note: 1. The inferior margin of the lumpectomy specimen (slide 7) is close to ductal carcinoma in situ (2 mm) but this margin submitted for frozen diagnosis (Fro 4) is free of tumor.

	Result	Intensity	Positive %
Estrogen receptor	Strong (7/8)	3	1/3–2/3
Progesterone receptor	Weak (3/8)	1	1–10%
C-erbB2	Negative (1+)		
Ki-67	Positive in 15% of tumor cells		

24 Case 24

24.1 Patient History and Progress

Female/45 years old, pre-menopause.
Screen detected mass lesion on right breast 9 o'clock direction and right axillary LN.
No family history.
No comorbidities.

24.2 Important Radiologic Findings

See Figs. 132, 133, 134, 135 and 136.

24.3 Courses of Treatment

Neoadjuvant chemotherapy (#4 cycles of doxorubicin & cyclophosphamide followed by #4 cycles of docetaxel) & letrozole 2.5 mg/day with leuprolide acetate + Operation + Postoperative radiation therapy.

24.3.1 Operation (1st, Jan. 2021)
Right breast conserving surgery, axillary lymph node dissection (Fig. 137).

24.3.2 Pathology Report
Invasive Ductal Carcinoma
1. Post-chemotherapy status.
2. Size of tumor: 2.0 cm (ypT1c).
3. Histologic grade: 2/3 (tubule formation: 3/3, nuclear pleomorphism: 2/3, mitotic count: 1/3, 1/10 HPF)
4. Intraductal component: present, intratumoral/extratumoral (5%) (nuclear grade: low, necrosis: absent, architectural pattern: solid, extensive intraductal component: absent).

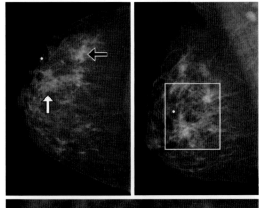
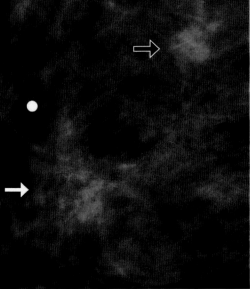

Fig. 132 Breast MRI (July 2020): an irregular enhancing mass in the right breast (white arrow). Enlarged lymph node at the right axilla (black arrow)

5. Skin: no involvement of tumor.
6. Surgical margins:
    (a) superior margin: positive for ductal carcinoma in situ (Fro 1) (see note).
    (b) inferior margin: 10 mm.
    (c) medial margin: 10 mm.

HR(+) HER2(−) Breast Cancer

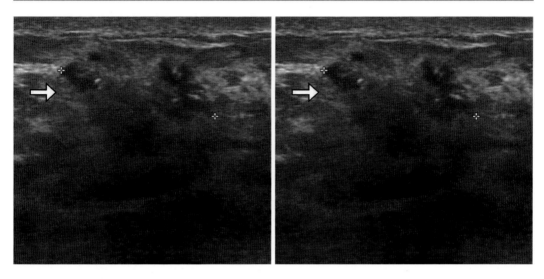

Fig. 133 Right breast US (June 2020): an irregular mass with microcalcifications at outer center (white arrow, US-CNB = IDC). Another irregular mass at the lower outer quadrant (black arrow)

- (d) lateral margin: positive for invasive ductal carcinoma (Fro 4).
- (e) deep margin: 5 mm.
- (f) superficial margin: 3 mm.
7. Lymph nodes:
   - (a) metastasis in five out of twelve axillary lymph nodes (ypN2a) (sentinel LN: 3/3, axillary LN: 2/9)
   - (b) perinodal extension: present.
   - (c) size of metastatic carcinoma: 6 mm.
8. Arteriovenous invasion: absent.
9. Lymphovascular invasion: present, intratumoral.
10. Tumor border: infiltrative.
11. Microcalcification: present, tumoral/non-tumoral.
12. Pathological TN category (AJCC 2017): ypT1cN2a.

Note: 1. Ductal carcinoma in situ is present only in the permanent section of Fro 1.

	Result	Intensity	Positive %
Estrogen receptor	Strong (8/8)	3	>2/3
Progesterone receptor	Weak (3/8)	1	1–10%
C-erbB2	Equivocal (2+) (SISH equivocal)		
Ki-67	Positive in 1% of tumor cells		

24.3.3 Operation (2nd, Feb. 2021)
Right breast wide excision (Fig. 138).

24.3.4 Pathology Report
No residual tumor with foreign body reaction.
1. Post-lumpectomy status.

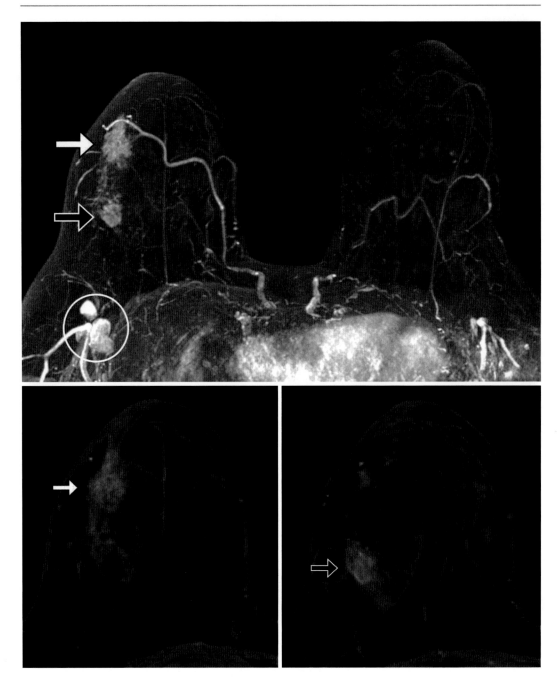

Fig. 134 Breast MRI (June 2020): two irregular enhancing masses in the right breast. Multiple enlarged lymph nodes at the right axilla (circle, US-CNB = Metastatic ductal carcinoma)

HR(+) HER2(−) Breast Cancer

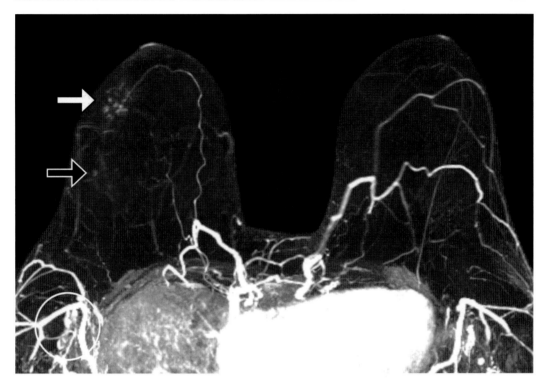

Fig. 135 Post-NAC breast MRI (Jan. 2021): decreased size of the tumors and lymph nodes after NAC

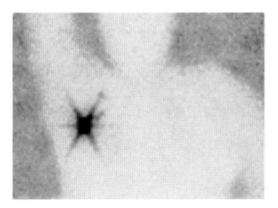

Fig. 136 Lymphoscintigraphy shows visualized sentinel lymph nodes in the right axilla

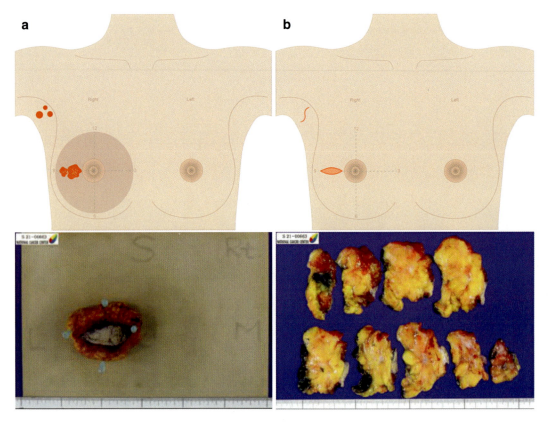

Fig. 137 (**a**) Gross pathology of lumpectomy specimen. (**b**) The margins get marked and sliced with different colors on each direction

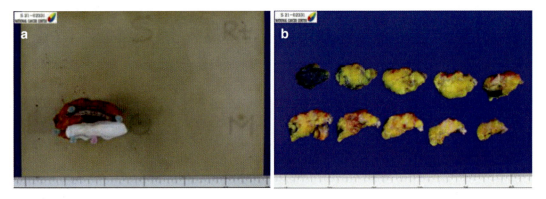

Fig. 138 (**a**) Gross pathology of breast wide excision specimen. (**b**) The margins get marked and sliced with different colors on each direction

25 Case 25

25.1 Patient History and Progress

Female/61 years old, post-menopause.
Screen detected mass lesion on left breast 12 o'clock direction and left axillary LN.
No family history.
No comorbidities.

25.2 Important Radiologic Findings

See Figs. 139, 140, 141, 142 and 143.

25.3 Courses of Treatment

Neoadjuvant therapy (giredestrant 30 mg/day with palbociclib 100 mg/day) + Operation + Adjuvant chemotherapy (#4 cycles of doxorubicin & cyclophosphamide followed by #4 cycles of docetaxel) + Post-operative radiation therapy + Letrozole 2.5 mg/day.

25.3.1 Operation
Left breast conserving surgery, axillary lymph node dissection (Fig. 144).

25.3.2 Pathology Report
Invasive Ductal Carcinoma
1. Post-chemotherapy status.
2. Size of tumor: 1.8 cm (ypT1c).
3. Histologic grade: 2/3 (tubule formation: 3/3, nuclear pleomorphism: 2/3, mitotic count: 2/3, 11/10 HPF)
4. Intraductal component: present, intratumoral/extratumoral (5%) (nuclear grade: low, necrosis: present, architectural pattern: solid/comedo, extensive intraductal component: absent).
5. Skin: no involvement of tumor.
6. Surgical margins:
   (a) superior margin: 20 mm.

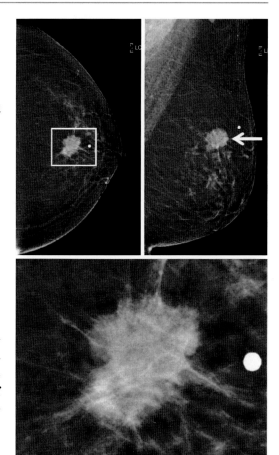

Fig. 139 Left mammography (Dec. 2020): an irregular mass with spiculated margins at upper center

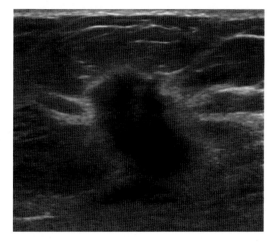

Fig. 140 Left breast US (Dec. 2020): an irregular hypoechoic mass with angular margins. US-CNB = IDC

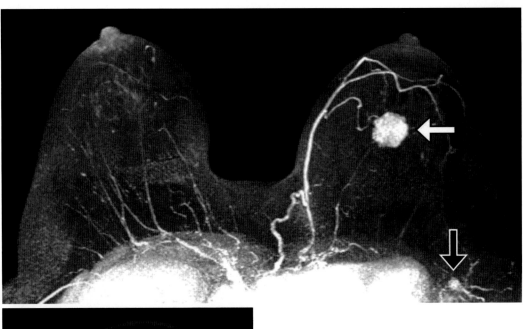
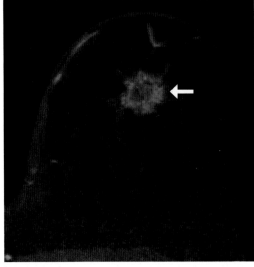

Fig. 141 Breast MRI (Dec. 2020): an irregular enhancing mass in the left breast (white arrow). Mildly enlarged lymph node at the left axilla (black arrow, US-CNB = Metastatic ductal carcinoma)

    (b) inferior margin: 10 mm.
    (c) medial margin: 10 mm.
    (d) lateral margin: 10 mm.
    (e) deep margin: 2 mm.
    (f) superficial margin: 2 mm.
7. Lymph nodes:
    (a) metastasis in eight out of twelve axillary lymph nodes (ypN2a) (sentinel LN: 2/2, axillary LN: 6/10)
    (b) perinodal extension: present.
    (c) size of metastatic carcinoma: 5 mm.
8. Arteriovenous invasion: absent.
9. Lymphovascular invasion: present, intratumoral.
10. Tumor border: infiltrative.
11. Microcalcification: present, tumoral/non-tumoral.
12. Pathological TN category (AJCC 2017): ypT1cN2a.

HR(+) HER2(−) Breast Cancer

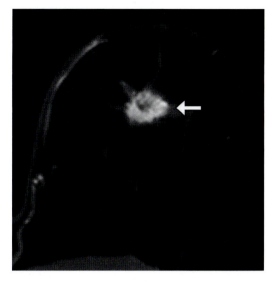

Fig. 142 Post-NAC breast MRI (June 2021): decreased volume of the tumor after NAC

Fig. 143 Lymphoscintigraphy shows faintly visualized sentinel lymph nodes in the left axilla

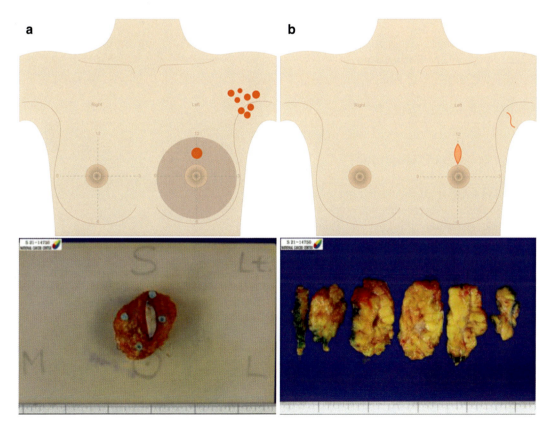

Fig. 144 (**a**) Gross pathology of lumpectomy specimen. (**b**) The margins get marked and sliced with different colors on each direction

	Result	Intensity	Positive %
Estrogen receptor	Intermediate (6/8)	2	1/3–2/3
Progesterone receptor	Negative (0/8)	0	0
C-erbB2	Negative (0)		
Ki-67	Positive in 43% of tumor cells		

26 Case 26

26.1 Patient History and Progress

Female/48 years old, pre-menopause.
Screen detected mass lesion on left breast 1 o'clock direction.
Family history of breast cancer, maternal aunt.
No comorbidities.
BRCA 1 and 2 mutation: Not detected.

26.2 Important Radiologic Findings

See Figs. 145, 146, 147 and 148.

26.3 Courses of Treatment

Operation + Adjuvant chemotherapy (#4 cycles of doxorubicin & cyclophosphamide) + Post-operative radiation therapy + Tamoxifen 20 mg/day.

26.3.1 Operation
Left breast conserving surgery, sentinel lymph node biopsy (Fig. 149).

26.3.2 Pathology Report
Invasive Ductal Carcinoma
1. Size of tumor: 1.7 cm (pT1c).
2. Histologic grade: 2/3 (tubule formation: 3/3, nuclear pleomorphism: 2/3, mitotic count: 1/3, 2/10 HPF)

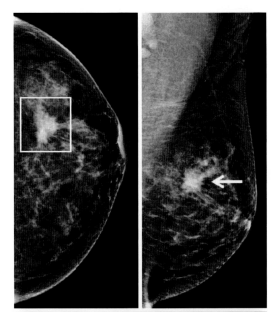
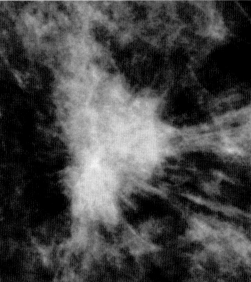

Fig. 145 Left mammography (Dec. 2020): an irregular mass with spiculated margins at upper outer quadrant

3. Intraductal component: present, intratumoral (5%) (nuclear grade: low, necrosis: absent, architectural pattern: solid, extensive intraductal component: absent).
4. Skin: no involvement of tumor.
5. Surgical margins:
   (a) superior margin: 25 mm.

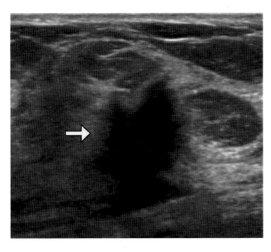

Fig. 146 Left breast US (Dec. 2020): an irregular hypoechoic mass with non-parallel orientation. US-CNB = IDC

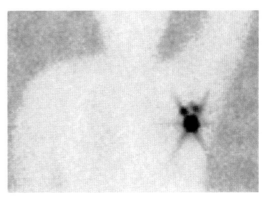

Fig. 148 Lymphoscintigraphy shows visualized sentinel lymph nodes in the left axilla

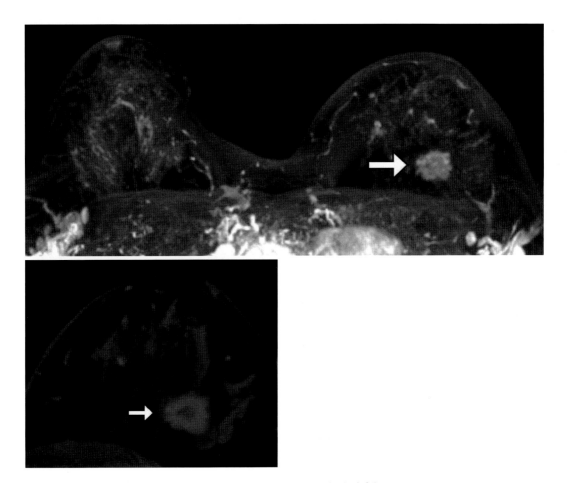

Fig. 147 Breast MRI (Dec. 2020): an irregular rim-enhancing mass in the left breast

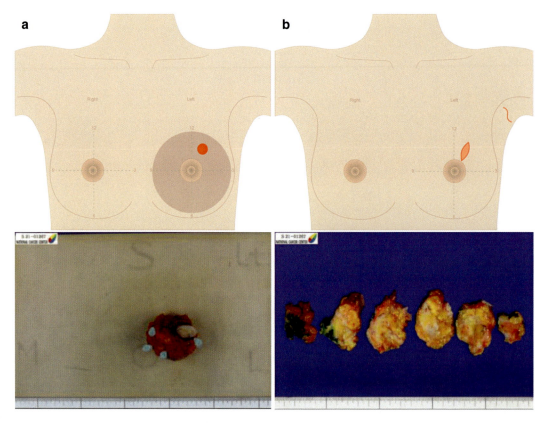

Fig. 149 (a) Gross pathology of lumpectomy specimen. (b) The margins get marked and sliced with different colors on each direction

  (b) inferior margin: 6 mm.
  (c) medial margin: 10 mm.
  (d) lateral margin: 15 mm.
  (e) deep margin: 8 mm.
  (f) superficial margin: 15 mm.
6. Lymph nodes: no metastasis in two axillary lymph nodes (pN0(sn)) (sentinel LN: 0/2)
7. Arteriovenous invasion: absent.
8. Lymphovascular invasion: absent.
9. Tumor border: infiltrative.
10. Microcalcification: present, tumoral/non-tumoral.
11. Pathological TN category (AJCC 2017): pT1cN0(sn).

	Result	Intensity	Positive %
Estrogen receptor	Strong (7/8)	2	>2/3
Progesterone receptor	Strong (8/8)	3	>2/3
C-erbB2	Negative (0)		

	Result	Intensity	Positive %
Ki-67	Positive in 62% of tumor cells		

27 Case 27

27.1 Patient History and Progress

Female/60 years old, post-menopause.
Screen detected mass lesion on left breast 10 o'clock direction.
No family history.
No comorbidities.

27.2 Important Radiologic Findings

See Figs. 150, 151, 152 and 153.

HR(+) HER2(−) Breast Cancer

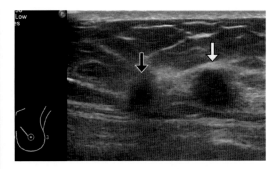

Fig. 151 Left breast US (Dec. 2020): two hypoechoic masses with spiculated margins. US-CNB = IDC

27.3.1 Operation (1st, Jan. 2021)

Left breast conserving surgery, sentinel lymph node biopsy (Fig. 154).

27.3.2 Pathology Report

Invasive Ductal Carcinoma

1. Size of tumor: 2.1 cm (pT2).
2. Histologic grade: 2/3 (tubule formation: 3/3, nuclear pleomorphism: 2/3, mitotic count: 1/3, 3/10 HPF)
3. Intraductal component: present, intratumoral/extratumoral (50%) (nuclear grade: low, necrosis: present, architectural pattern: cribriform/solid/comedo, extensive intraductal component: present).
4. Surgical margins:
   (a) superior margin: positive for ductal carcinoma in situ (Fro 1) (see note 1).
   (b) inferior margin: 25 mm.
   (c) medial margin: (see note 2).
   (d) lateral margin: 15 mm.
   (e) deep margin: <1 mm from invasive ductal carcinoma (slide 7).
   (f) superficial margin: <1 mm from invasive ductal carcinoma (slide 6).
5. Lymph nodes: no metastasis in one axillary lymph node (pN0(sn)) (sentinel LN: 0/1)
6. Arteriovenous invasion: absent.
7. Lymphovascular invasion: absent.
8. Tumor border: infiltrative.
9. Microcalcification: present, tumoral.
10. Pathological TN category (AJCC 2017): pT2N0(sn).

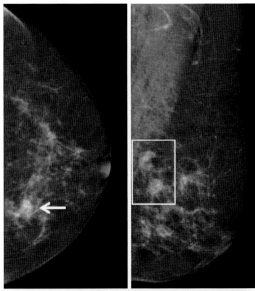

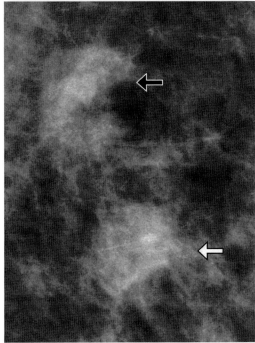

Fig. 150 Left mammography (Dec. 2020): two irregular masses at upper inner quadrant

27.3 Courses of Treatment

Operation + Post-operative radiation therapy + Anastrozole 1 mg/day.

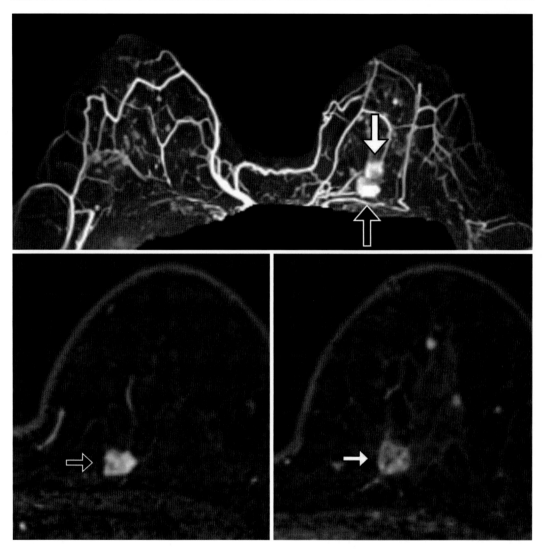

Fig. 152 Breast MRI (Dec. 2020): two irregular enhancing masses in the left breast

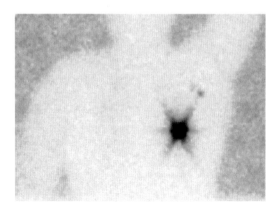

Fig. 153 Lymphoscintigraphy shows visualized sentinel lymph nodes in the left axilla

Intraductal Papilloma

Note: 1. Ductal carcinoma in situ is present only in the permanent section of Fro 1.

The medial margin of the lumpectomy specimen (slide 9) is positive for ductal carcinoma in situ but this margin submitted for frozen diagnosis (Fro 3) is free of tumor

	Result	Intensity	Positive %
Estrogen receptor	Strong (8/8)	3	>2/3
Progesterone receptor	Intermediate (6/8)	2	1/3–2/3
C-erbB2	Negative (1+)		
Ki-67	Positive in 44% of tumor cells		

HR(+) HER2(−) Breast Cancer

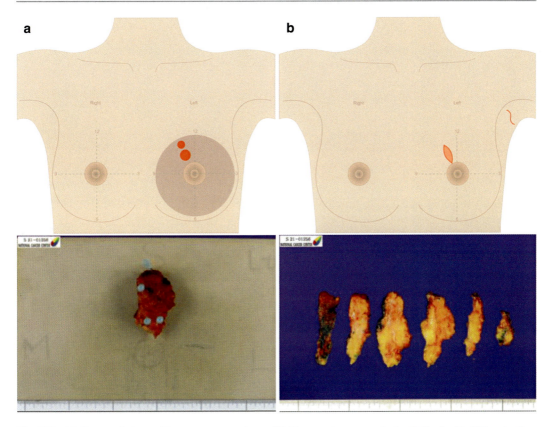

Fig. 154 (**a**) Gross pathology of lumpectomy specimen. (**b**) The margins get marked and sliced with different colors on each direction

27.3.3 Operation (2nd, Feb. 2021)
Left breast wide excision.

27.3.4 Pathology Report
No residual tumor with foreign body reaction.

1. Post-lumpectomy status.

---

28 Case 28

28.1 Patient History and Progress

Female/72 years old, post-menopause.
 Screen detected mass lesion on right breast 8 o'clock direction.
 No family history.
 S/p cholecystectomy, hypertension.

28.2 Important Radiologic Findings

See Figs. 155, 156, 157 and 158.

28.3 Courses of Treatment

Operation + Post-operative radiation therapy + Letrozole 2.5 mg/day with palbociclib 100 mg/day.

28.3.1 Operation
Right breast conserving surgery, sentinel lymph node biopsy (Fig. 159).

28.3.2 Pathology Report

Invasive Ductal Carcinoma
1. Size of tumor: 2.9 cm (pT2).
2. Histologic grade: 2/3 (tubule formation: 3/3, nuclear pleomorphism: 2/3, mitotic count: 1/3, 3/10 HPF)
3. Intraductal component: present, intratumoral/extratumoral (5%) (nuclear grade: low, necrosis: absent, architectural pattern: cribriform/solid, extensive intraductal component: absent).
4. Skin: no involvement of tumor.

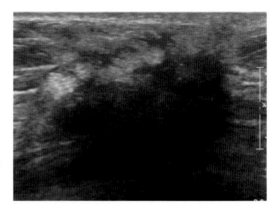

Fig. 156 Right breast US (Dec. 2020): an irregular hypoechoic mass. US-CNB = IDC

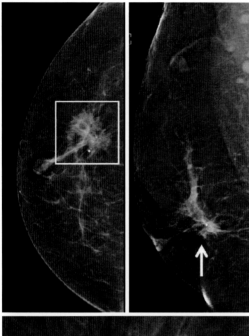

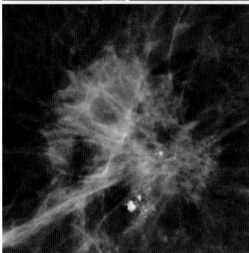

Fig. 155 Right mammography (Oct. 2020): an irregular mass with microcalcifications at lower outer quadrant

5. Surgical margins:
    (a) superior margin: 15 mm.
    (b) inferior margin: 6 mm.
    (c) medial margin: 10 mm.
    (d) lateral margin: 10 mm.
    (e) deep margin: 5 mm.
    (f) superficial margin: 2 mm.
6. Lymph nodes:
    (a) metastasis in two out of two axillary lymph nodes (pN1a(sn)) (see note) (sentinel LN: 1/1, axillary LN: 1/1)
    (b) perinodal extension: present.
    (c) size of metastatic carcinoma: 6 mm.
7. Arteriovenous invasion: absent.
8. Lymphovascular invasion: present, intratumoral.
9. Tumor border: infiltrative.
10. Microcalcification: present, tumoral.
11. Pathological TN category (AJCC 2017): pT2N1a(sn).

Note: 1. Micrometastasis is present only in the permanent section of Fro 1.

	Result	Intensity	Positive %
Estrogen receptor	Strong (8/8)	3	>2/3
Progesterone receptor	Intermediate (6/8)	2	1/3–2/3
C-erbB2	Negative (1+)		
Ki-67	Positive in 9% of tumor cells		

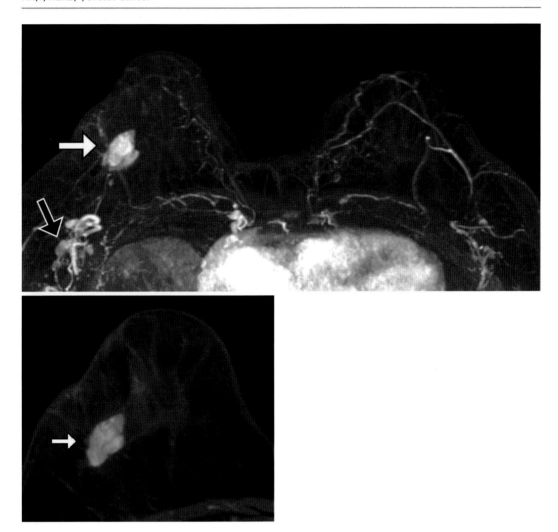

Fig. 157 Breast MRI (Dec. 2020): an irregular enhancing mass in the right breast (white arrow). Enlarged lymph nodes at the right axilla (black arrow)

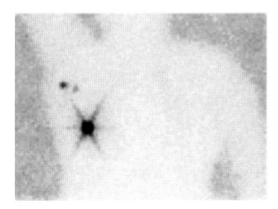

Fig. 158 Lymphoscintigraphy shows visualized sentinel lymph nodes in the right axilla

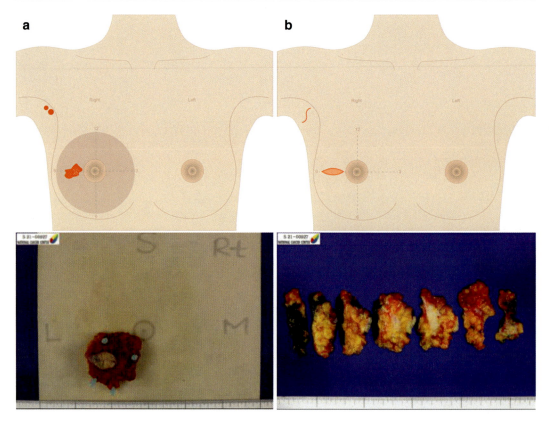

Fig. 159 (**a**) Gross pathology of lumpectomy specimen. (**b**) The margins get marked and sliced with different colors on each direction

29　Case 29

29.1　Patient History and Progress

Female/80 years old, post-menopause.

Screen detected mass lesion on left breast 10 o'clock direction.

No family history.

S/P hysterectomy, hypertension, s/p left cerebral infarction, s/p transient ischemic attack.

29.2　Important Radiologic Findings

See Figs. 160, 161, 162 and 163.

29.3　Courses of Treatment

Operation + Post-operative radiation therapy + Letrozole 2.5 mg/day.

HR(+) HER2(−) Breast Cancer

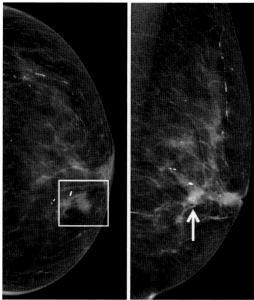

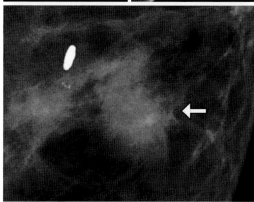

Fig. 160 Left mammography (Dec. 2020): an irregular mass at upper inner quadrant

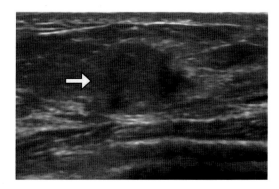

Fig. 161 Left breast US (Dec. 2020): an irregular isoechoic mass with angular margins. US-CNB = Mucinous carcinoma

29.3.1 Operation

Left breast conserving surgery, sentinel lymph node biopsy (Fig. 164).

29.3.2 Pathology Report

Invasive ductal carcinoma with mucinous component associated with mucocele-like lesion.

1. Size of tumor: 0.8 cm (pT1b).
2. Histologic grade: 2/3 (tubule formation: 3/3, nuclear pleomorphism: 2/3, mitotic count: 1/3, 1/10 HPF)
3. Intraductal component: absent.
4. Skin: no involvement of tumor.
5. Surgical margins:
    (a) superior margin: 20 mm.
    (b) inferior margin: 10 mm.
    (c) medial margin: 15 mm.
    (d) lateral margin: 15 mm.
    (e) deep margin: 10 mm.
    (f) superficial margin: 5 mm.
6. Lymph nodes: no metastasis in two axillary lymph nodes (pN0(sn)) (sentinel LN: 0/2, non-sentinel LN: 0/0)
7. Arteriovenous invasion: absent.
8. Lymphovascular invasion: absent.
9. Tumor border: infiltrative.
10. Microcalcification: present, non-tumoral.
11. Pathological TN category (AJCC 2017): pT1bN0(sn).

	Result	Intensity	Positive %
Estrogen receptor	Strong (8/8)	3	>2/3
Progesterone receptor	Strong (8/8)	3	>2/3
C-erbB2	Negative (0)		
Ki-67	Positive in 4% of tumor cells		

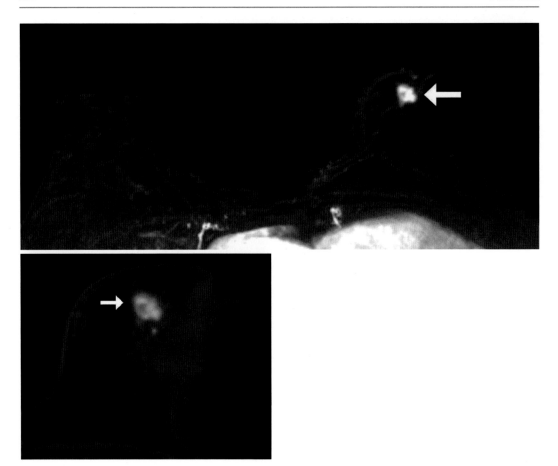

Fig. 162 Breast MRI (Dec. 2020): an irregular enhancing mass in the left breast

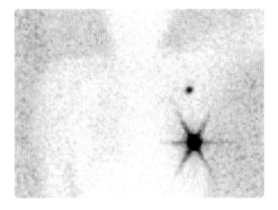

Fig. 163 Lymphoscintigraphy shows visualized sentinel lymph nodes in the left axilla

HR(+) HER2(−) Breast Cancer

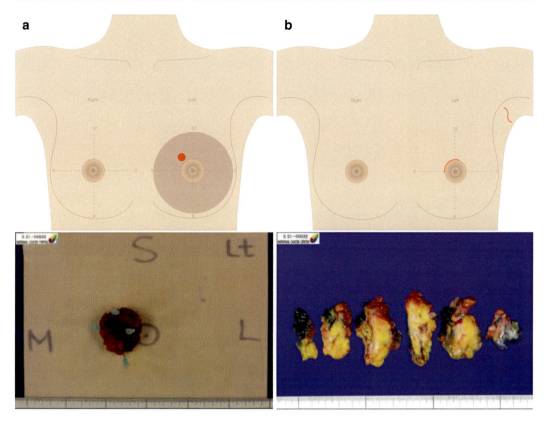

Fig. 164 (**a**) Gross pathology of lumpectomy specimen. (**b**) The margins get marked and sliced with different colors on each direction

30 Case 30

30.1 Patient History and Progress

Female/63 years old, post-menopause.

Screen detected mass lesion on left breast 4 o'clock direction.

No family history.

s/p Left optic nerve palsy, hypertension, s/p right rotator cuff tear operation.

30.2 Important Radiologic Findings

See Figs. 165, 166, 167 and 168.

30.3 Courses of Treatment

Operation + Post-operative radiation therapy + Letrozole 2.5 mg/day.

30.3.1 Operation
Left breast conserving surgery, sentinel lymph node biopsy (Fig. 169).

30.3.2 Pathology Report
Invasive Ductal Carcinoma
1. Size of tumor: 1.1 cm (pT1c).
2. Histologic grade: 2/3 (tubule formation: 3/3, nuclear pleomorphism: 2/3, mitotic count: 1/3, 6/10 HPF)

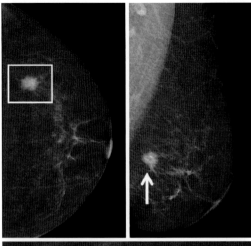

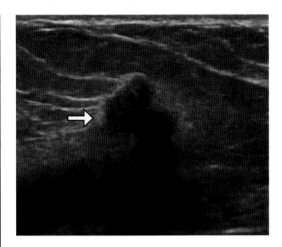

Fig. 166 Left breast US (Dec. 2020): an irregular hypoechoic mass with non-parallel orientation. US-CNB = IDC

5. Surgical margins:
   (a) superior margin: 15 mm.
   (b) inferior margin: 15 mm.
   (c) medial margin: 10 mm.
   (d) lateral margin: 15 mm.
   (e) deep margin: 3 mm.
   (f) superficial margin: 15 mm.
6. Lymph nodes: no metastasis in one axillary lymph node (pN0(i+)(sn)) (see note) (sentinel LN: 0/1, non-sentinel LN: 0/0)
7. Arteriovenous invasion: absent.
8. Lymphovascular invasion: present, intratumoral.
9. Tumor border: infiltrative.
10. Microcalcification: present, non-tumoral.
11. Pathological TN category (AJCC 2017): pT1cN0(i+)(sn).

Note: 1. A few isolated tumor cells are present only in the permanent section of Fro 1 for immunohistochemical staining.

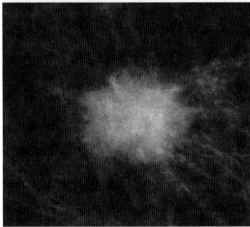

Fig. 165 Left mammography (Dec. 2020): an irregular mass with spiculated margins at lower outer quadrant

3. Intraductal component: present, intratumoral/extratumoral (10%) (nuclear grade: low, necrosis: absent, architectural pattern: cribriform/solid, extensive intraductal component: absent).
4. Skin: no involvement of tumor.

	Result	Intensity	Positive %
Estrogen receptor	Strong (8/8)	3	>2/3
Progesterone receptor	Strong (7/8)	2	>2/3
C-erbB2	Negative (1+)		
Ki-67	Positive in 11% of tumor cells		

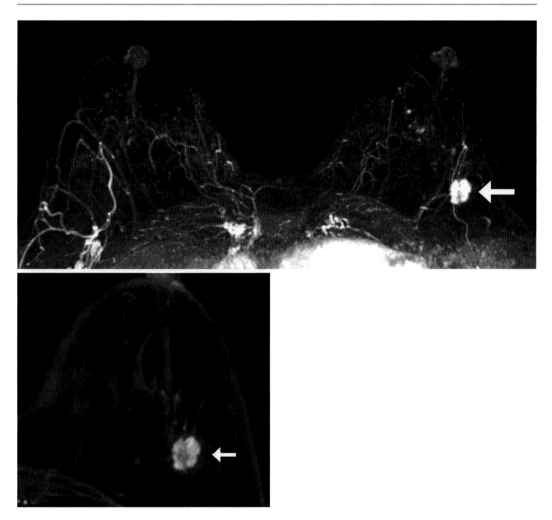

Fig. 167 Breast MRI (Dec. 2020): an irregular enhancing mass in the left breast

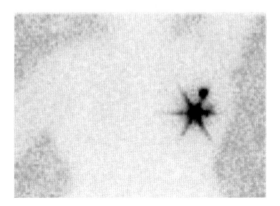

Fig. 168 Lymphoscintigraphy shows visualized sentinel lymph nodes in the left axilla

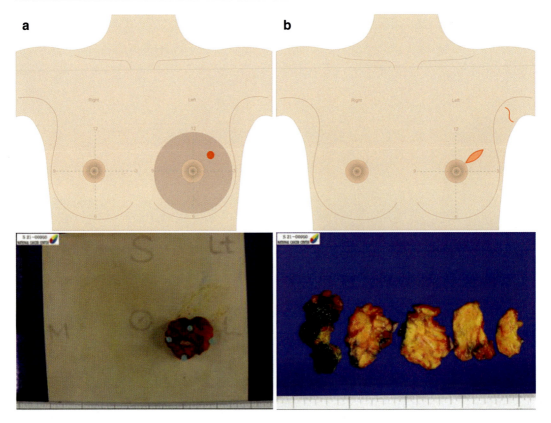

Fig. 169 (**a**) Gross pathology of lumpectomy specimen. (**b**) The margins get marked and sliced with different colors on each direction

31   Case 31

31.1   Patient History and Progress

Female/65 years old, post-menopause.

Screen detected mass lesion on right breast 6 o'clock direction.

Family history of breast cancer, older sister, niece.

S/P Hysterectomy and salpingo-oophorectomy.

BRCA 1 exon 9-13 deletion, exon 2-6 deletion.

31.2   Important Radiologic Findings

See Figs. 170, 171, 172 and 173.

31.3   Courses of Treatment

Operation + Adjuvant chemotherapy (#4 cycles of docetaxel & cyclophosphamide) + Post-operative radiation therapy + Letrozole 2.5 mg/day.

31.3.1   Operation

Right breast conserving surgery, sentinel lymph node biopsy (Fig. 174).

31.3.2   Pathology Report

Invasive Ductal Carcinoma
1. Size of tumor: 2.2 cm (pT2).
2. Histologic grade: 2/3 (tubule formation: 3/3, nuclear pleomorphism: 2/3, mitotic count: 2/3, 10/10 HPF)
3. Intraductal component: present, intratumoral/extratumoral (5%) (nuclear grade:

HR(+) HER2(−) Breast Cancer

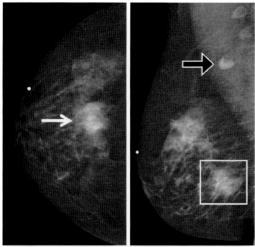

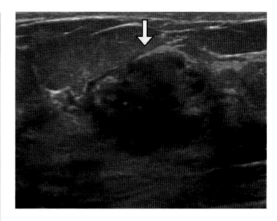

Fig. 171 Right breast US (Dec. 2020): an irregular hypoechoic mass. US-CNB = IDC

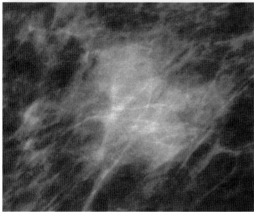

Fig. 170 Right mammography (Dec. 2020): an irregular mass at lower outer quadrant. A lymph node with cortical thickening at the right axilla (black arrow)

high, necrosis: absent, architectural pattern: cribriform/solid, extensive intraductal component: absent).
4. Skin: no involvement of tumor.

5. Surgical margins:
   (a) superior margin: 30 mm.
   (b) inferior margin: 40 mm.
   (c) medial margin: 10 mm.
   (d) lateral margin: 10 mm.
   (e) deep margin: <1 mm from invasive ductal carcinoma (slide 2).
   (f) superficial margin: 5 mm.
6. Lymph nodes:
   (a) metastasis in one out of four axillary lymph nodes (pN1a(sn)) (sentinel LN: 1/1, axillary LN: 0/3)
   (b) perinodal extension: present.
   (c) size of metastatic carcinoma: 10 mm.
7. Arteriovenous invasion: absent.
8. Lymphovascular invasion: present, intratumoral.
9. Tumor border: infiltrative.
10. Microcalcification: absent.
11. Pathological TN category (AJCC 2017): pT2N1a(sn).

	Result	Intensity	Positive %
Estrogen receptor	Strong (8/8)	3	>2/3
Progesterone receptor	Negative (1/8) IDC	1	<1%
	Strong (8/8) DCIS	3	>2/3
C-erbB2	Equivocal (2+) (SISH negative)		
Ki-67	Positive in 43% of tumor cells		

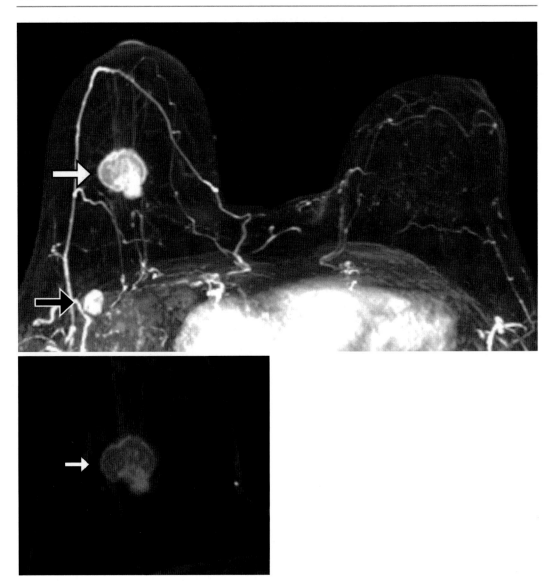

Fig. 172 Breast MRI (Dec. 2020): an irregular enhancing mass in the right breast (white arrow). An enlarged lymph node at the right axilla (black arrow)

HR(+) HER2(−) Breast Cancer

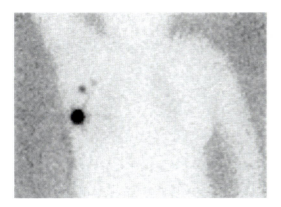

Fig. 173 Lymphoscintigraphy shows visualized sentinel lymph nodes in the right axilla

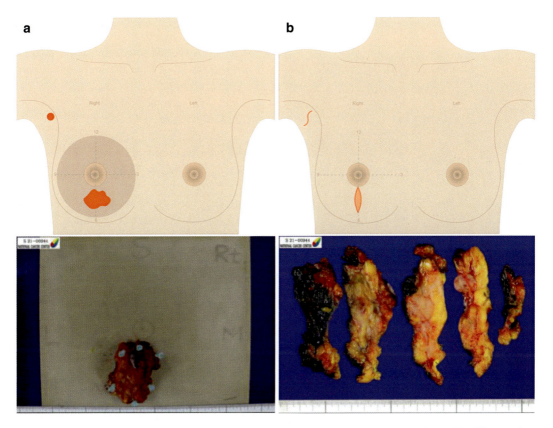

Fig. 174 (**a**) Gross pathology of lumpectomy specimen. (**b**) The margins get marked and sliced with different colors on each direction

32 Case 32

32.1 Patient History and Progress

Female/70 years old, post-menopause.
Screen detected mass lesion on right breast 10 o'clock direction.
No family history.
Hypertension, s/p bronchiectasis, s/p left hip arthroplasty.

32.2 Important Radiologic Findings

See Figs. 175, 176, 177 and 178.

32.3 Courses of Treatment

Operation + Post-operative radiation therapy + Letrozole 2.5 mg/day.

32.3.1 Operation
Right breast conserving surgery, sentinel lymph node biopsy (Fig. 179).

32.3.2 Pathology Report
Invasive Ductal Carcinoma
1. Size of tumor: 2.0 cm (pT1c).
2. Histologic grade: 2/3 (tubule formation: 3/3, nuclear pleomorphism: 2/3, mitotic count: 1/3, 1/10 HPF)
3. Intraductal component: present, intratumoral/extratumoral (5%) (nuclear grade: low, necrosis: absent, architectural pattern: cribriform/solid, extensive intraductal component: absent).
4. Skin: no involvement of tumor.
5. Surgical margins:
    (a) superior margin: 20 mm.
    (b) inferior margin: 40 mm.
    (c) medial margin: 15 mm.
    (d) lateral margin: 20 mm.
    (e) deep margin: 5 mm.
    (f) superficial margin: 10 mm.
6. Lymph nodes: no metastasis in one axillary lymph node (pN0(sn)) (sentinel LN: 0/1, non-sentinel LN: 0/0)

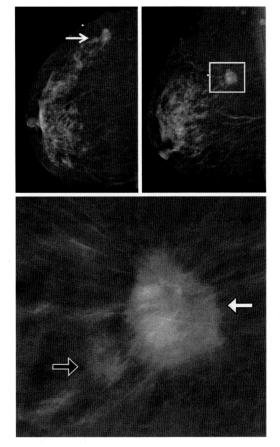

Fig. 175 Right mammography (Dec. 2020): a spiculated mass (white arrow) with an adjacent smaller mass (black arrow) at upper outer quadrant

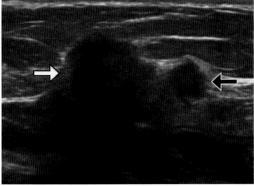

Fig. 176 Right breast US (Dec. 2020): two irregular hypoechoic masses. US-CNB = IDC

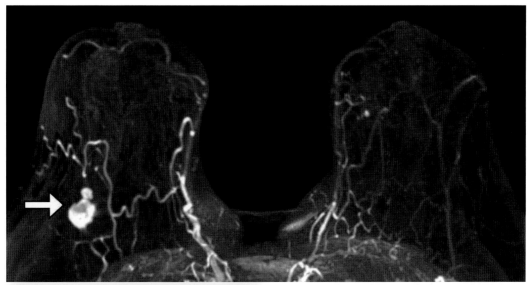

Fig. 177 Breast MRI (Dec. 2020): a bilobed rim-enhancing mass in the right breast

7. Arteriovenous invasion: absent.
8. Lymphovascular invasion: present, intratumoral.
9. Tumor border: infiltrative.
10. Microcalcification: present, non-tumoral.
11. Pathological TN category (AJCC 2017): pT1cN0(sn).

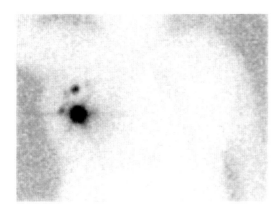

Fig. 178 Lymphoscintigraphy shows visualized sentinel lymph nodes in the right axilla

	Result	Intensity	Positive %
Estrogen receptor	Strong (8/8)	3	>2/3
Progesterone receptor	Strong (8/8)	3	>2/3
C-erbB2	Negative (0)		
Ki-67	Positive in 9% of tumor cells		

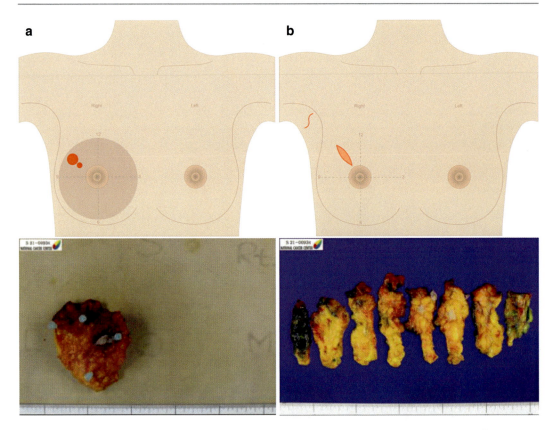

Fig. 179 (**a**) Gross pathology of lumpectomy specimen. (**b**) The margins get marked and sliced with different colors on each direction

33 Case 33

33.1 Patient History and Progress

Female/42 years old, pre-menopause.
   Screen detected mass lesion on left breast 12 o'clock direction.
   No family history.
   Restless legs.

33.2 Important Radiologic Findings

See Figs. 180, 181, 182, 183 and 184.

33.3 Courses of Treatment

Operation + Post-operative radiation therapy + Tamoxifen 20 mg/day.

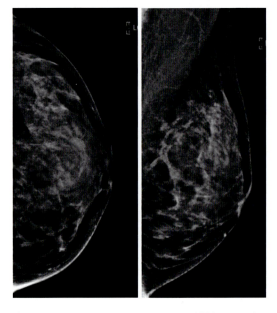

Fig. 180 Left mammography (Dec. 2020): negative finding

HR(+) HER2(−) Breast Cancer

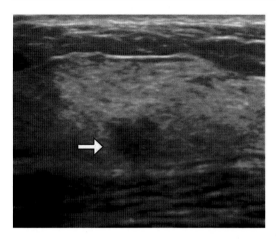

Fig. 181 Left breast US (Dec. 2020): an irregular mass with microlobulated margins at 12 o'clock direction. US-CNB = IDC

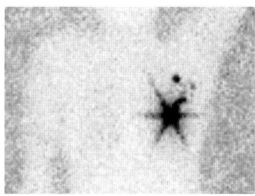

Fig. 183 Lymphoscintigraphy shows visualized sentinel lymph nodes in the left axilla

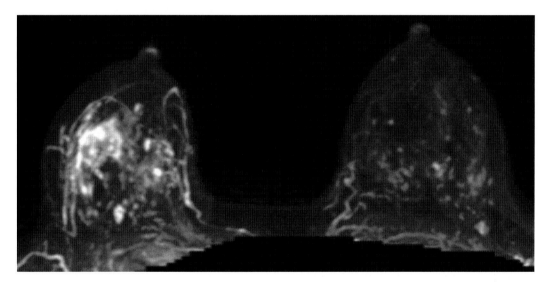

Fig. 182 Breast MRI (Dec. 2020): no discernible suspicious finding in both breasts

33.3.1 Operation
Left breast conserving surgery, sentinel lymph node biopsy (Fig. 185).

33.3.2 Pathology Report
Invasive Ductal Carcinoma
1. Size of invasive component: 0.4 cm (pT1a).
2. Size of intraductal component: 1.3 cm.
3. Histologic grade: 1/3 (tubule formation: 2/3, nuclear pleomorphism: 2/3, mitotic count: 1/3, 1/10 HPF)
4. Intraductal component: present, intratumoral/extratumoral (70%) (nuclear grade: low, necrosis: absent, architectural pattern: micropapillary/cribriform, extensive intraductal component: present).
5. Skin: no involvement of tumor.

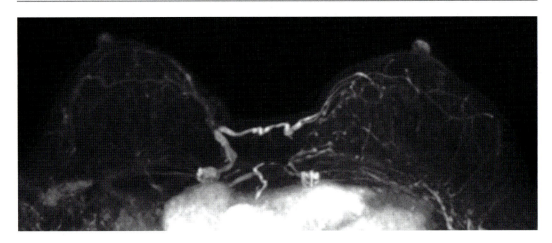

Fig. 184 Breast MRI for routine surveillance (Feb. 2022): no abnormal finding in both breasts

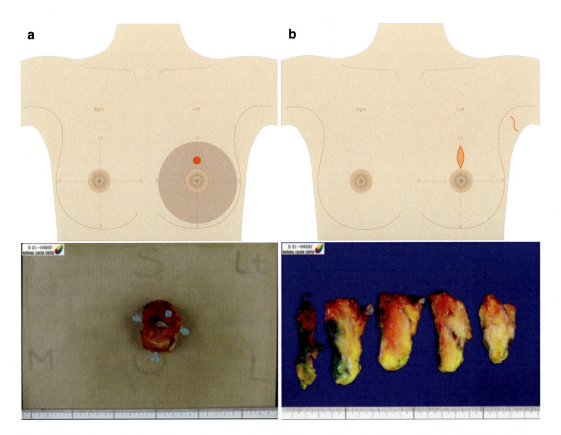

Fig. 185 (**a**) Gross pathology of lumpectomy specimen. (**b**) The margins get marked and sliced with different colors on each direction

6. Surgical margins:
    (a) superior margin: 25 mm.
    (b) inferior margin: 20 mm.
    (c) medial margin: 15 mm.
    (d) lateral margin: 10 mm.
    (e) deep margin: 3 mm.
    (f) superficial margin: 5 mm.

7. Lymph nodes: no metastasis in three axillary lymph nodes (pN0(sn)) (sentinel LN: 0/1, axillary LN: 0/2)
8. Arteriovenous invasion: absent.
9. Lymphovascular invasion: absent.
10. Tumor border: infiltrative.
11. Microcalcification: absent.
12. Pathological TN category (AJCC 2017): pT1aN0(sn).

	Result	Intensity	Positive %
Estrogen receptor	Strong (7/8)	3	>2/3
Progesterone receptor	Strong (8/8)	3	>2/3
C-erbB2	Negative (1+)		
Ki-67	Positive in 5% of tumor cells		

34 Case 34

34.1 Patient History and Progress

Female/43 years old, pre-menopause.
 Screen for high risk for breast cancer.
 Family history of breast cancer, mother.
 Pancreatic cancer, maternal uncle.
 No comorbidities.
 BRCA 1 mutation carrier.

34.2 Important Radiologic Findings

See Figs. 186, 187, 188 and 189.

34.3 Courses of Treatment

34.3.1 Operation

Right nipple–areolar complex sparing mastectomy with immediate implant reconstruction, sentinel lymph node biopsy, left nipple–areolar complex sparing mastectomy with immediate implant reconstruction (Figs. 190, 191 and 192).

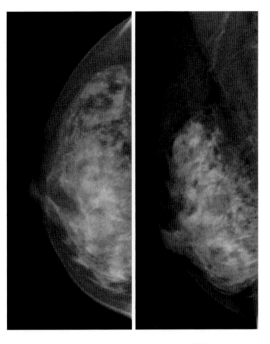

Fig. 186 Right mammography (Dec. 2020): negative finding

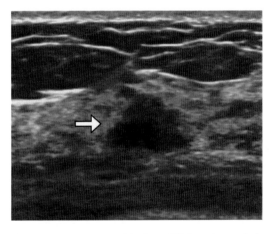

Fig. 187 Right breast US (Dec. 2020): a hypoechoic mass with microlobulated margins at upper outer quadrant. US-CNB = IDC

34.3.2 Pathology Report

[Right]

Invasive Ductal Carcinoma
1. Size of tumor: 1.8 cm (pT1c).
2. Histologic grade: 3/3 (tubule formation: 3/3, nuclear pleomorphism: 3/3, mitotic count: 2/3, 11/10 HPF)

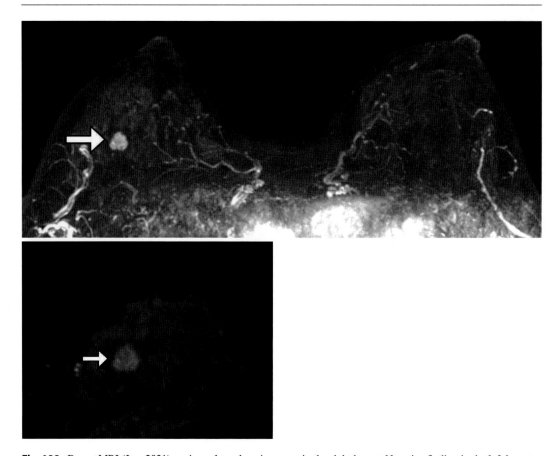

Fig. 188 Breast MRI (Jan. 2021): an irregular enhancing mass in the right breast. Negative finding in the left breast

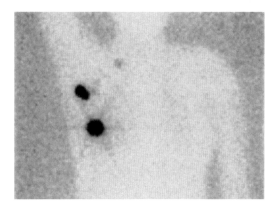

Fig. 189 Lymphoscintigraphy shows visualized sentinel lymph nodes in the right axilla

3. Intraductal component: present, intratumoral/extratumoral (10%) (nuclear grade: high, necrosis: absent, architectural pattern: cribriform/solid, extensive intraductal component: absent).
4. Skin: no involvement of tumor.
5. Surgical margins:
   (a) deep margin: <1 mm from ductal carcinoma in situ (slide 1).
   (b) superficial margin: 5 mm.
6. Lymph nodes: no metastasis in one axillary lymph node (pN0(sn)) (sentinel LN: 0/1)
7. Arteriovenous invasion: absent.

HR(+) HER2(−) Breast Cancer

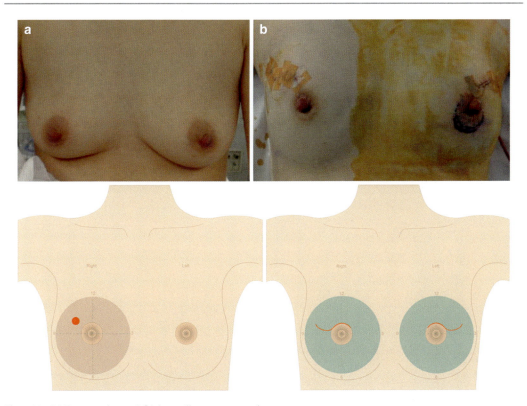

Fig. 190 (**a**) Preoperative and (**b**) immediate post-operative appearance

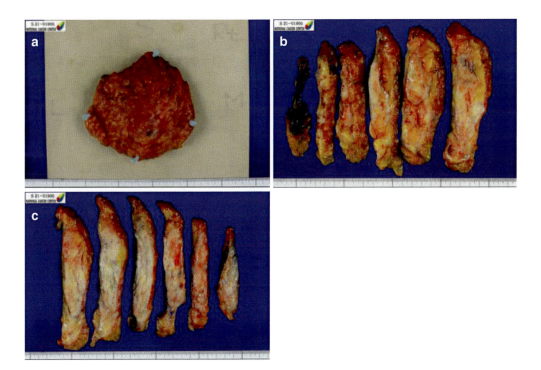

Fig. 191 (**a**) Gross pathology of right mastectomy specimen. (**b** and **c**) The margins get marked and sliced with different colors on each direction

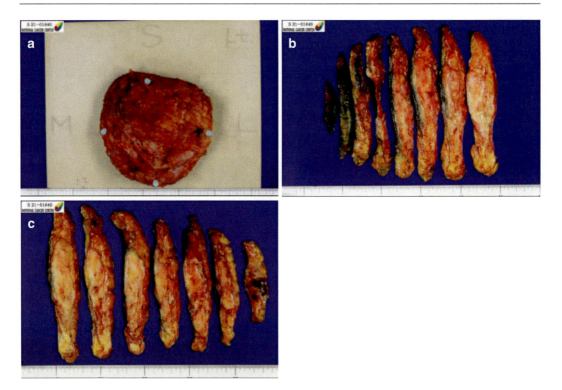

Fig. 192 (**a**) Gross pathology of left mastectomy specimen. (**b** and **c**) The margins get marked and sliced with different colors on each direction

8. Lymphovascular invasion: present, intratumoral.
9. Tumor border: infiltrative.
10. Microcalcification: present, tumoral/non-tumoral.
11. Pathological TN category (AJCC 2017): pT1cN0(sn).

	Result	Intensity	Positive %
Estrogen receptor	Strong (8/8)	3	>2/3
Progesterone receptor	Strong (8/8)	3	>2/3
C-erbB2	Equivocal (2+) (SISH negative)		
Ki-67	Positive in 14% of tumor cells		

[Left]
Fibrocystic change.

35 Case 35

35.1 Patient History and Progress

Female/48 years old, pre-menopause.
Screen detected mass lesion on left breast 4 o'clock direction.
Family history of breast cancer, maternal aunt.
No comorbidities.
BRCA 1 and 2 mutation: no examination.

35.2 Important Radiologic Findings

See Figs. 193, 194, 195, 196 and 197.

HR(+) HER2(−) Breast Cancer

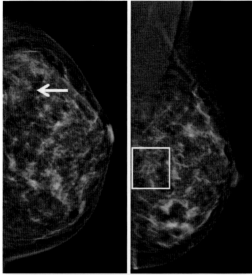

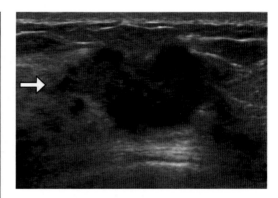

Fig. 194 Left breast US (Feb. 2021): an irregular hypoechoic mass with angular margins. US-CNB = IDC

35.3.1 Operation

Left breast conserving surgery, sentinel lymph node biopsy (Fig. 198).

35.3.2 Pathology Report

Invasive Ductal Carcinoma
1. Post-chemotherapy status.
2. Size of tumor: 1.1 cm (ypT1c).
3. Histologic grade: 2/3 (tubule formation: 3/3, nuclear pleomorphism: 2/3, mitotic count: 2/3, 11/10 HPF)
4. Intraductal component: present, intratumoral/extratumoral (50%) (nuclear grade: low, necrosis: present, architectural pattern: cribriform/solid/comedo, extensive intraductal component: present).
5. Skin: no involvement of tumor.
6. Surgical margins:
    (a) superior margin: 15 mm.
    (b) inferior margin: 15 mm.
    (c) medial margin: 10 mm.
    (d) lateral margin: 10 mm.
    (e) deep margin: 2 mm.
    (f) superficial margin: 2 mm.
7. Lymph nodes:
    (a) metastasis in two out of five axillary lymph nodes (ypN1a(sn)) (sentinel LN: 2/2, axillary LN: 0/3)

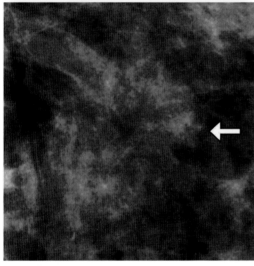

Fig. 193 Left mammography (Jan. 2021): a focal asymmetry at lower outer quadrant

35.3 Courses of Treatment

Operation + Adjuvant chemotherapy (#4 cycles of docetaxel & cyclophosphamide) + Post-operative radiation therapy + Tamoxifen 20 mg/day.

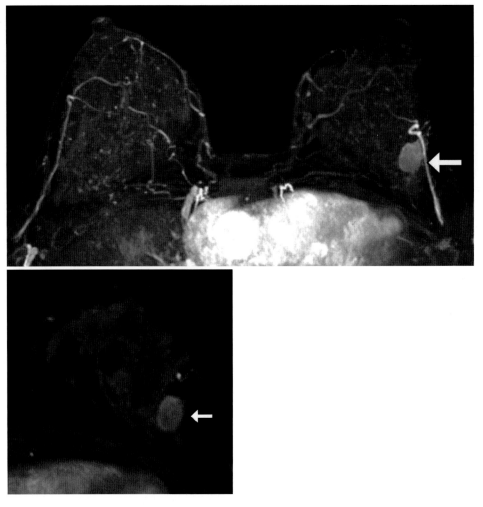

Fig. 195 Breast MRI (Feb. 2021): an oval enhancing mass with irregular margins in the left breast

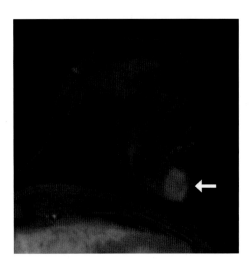

Fig. 196 Post-NAC breast MRI (June 2021): minimally decreased volume of the tumor after NAC

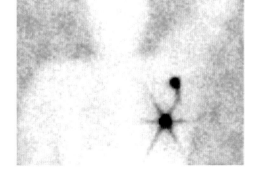

Fig. 197 Lymphoscintigraphy shows visualized sentinel lymph nodes in the left axilla

HR(+) HER2(−) Breast Cancer

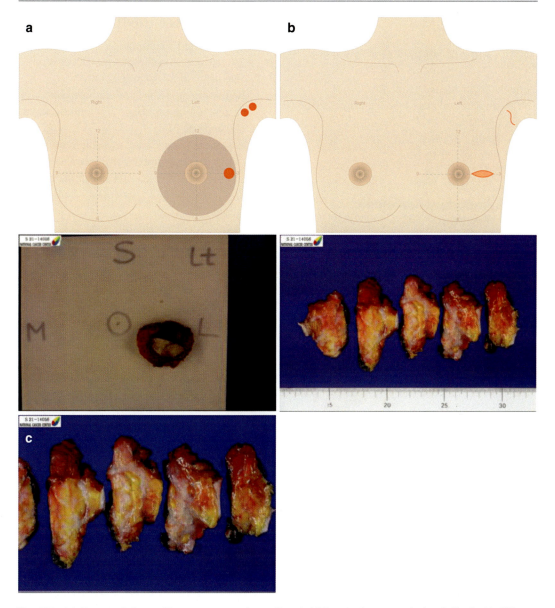

Fig. 198 (**a**) Gross pathology of lumpectomy specimen. (**b** and **c**) The margins get marked and sliced with different colors on each direction

    (b) perinodal extension: absent.
    (c) size of metastatic carcinoma: 6 mm.
8. Arteriovenous invasion: absent.
9. Lymphovascular invasion: present, intratumoral.
10. Tumor border: infiltrative.
11. Microcalcification: present, tumoral/non-tumoral.
12. Pathological TN category (AJCC 2017): ypT1cN1a(sn).

	Result	Intensity	Positive %
Estrogen receptor	Strong (7/8)	2	>2/3
Progesterone receptor	Strong (8/8)	3	>2/3
C-erbB2	Negative (1+)		
Ki-67	Positive in 8% of tumor cells		

36 Case 36

36.1 Patient History and Progress

Female/50 years old, pre-menopause.
Screen detected mass lesion on right breast 10 o'clock direction.
No family history.
s/p endometrial curettage.

36.2 Important Radiologic Findings

See Figs. 199, 200, 201, 202 and 203.

36.3 Courses of Treatment

Operation + Post-operative radiation therapy + Tamoxifen 20 mg/day.

36.3.1 Operation
Right breast conserving surgery, sentinel lymph node biopsy (Fig. 204).

36.3.2 Pathology Report

Invasive Ductal Carcinoma
- Associated with complex sclerosing lesion.
  1. Size of tumor: 0.9 cm (pT1b).
  2. Histologic grade: 1/3 (tubule formation: 2/3, nuclear pleomorphism: 2/3, mitotic count: 1/3, 6/10 HPF)
  3. Intraductal component: present, intratumoral (40%) (nuclear grade: low, necrosis: absent, architectural pattern: micropapillary/cribriform, extensive intraductal component: present).
  4. Skin: no involvement of tumor.
  5. Surgical margins:
     (a) superior margin: 10 mm.
     (b) inferior margin: 25 mm.
     (c) medial margin: 10 mm.
     (d) lateral margin: 20 mm.
     (e) deep margin: <1 mm from invasive ductal carcinoma (slide 1).
     (f) superficial margin: 5 mm.
  6. Lymph nodes: no metastasis in two axillary lymph nodes (pN0(sn)) (sentinel LN: 0/1, non-sentinel LN: 0/1)
  7. Arteriovenous invasion: absent.

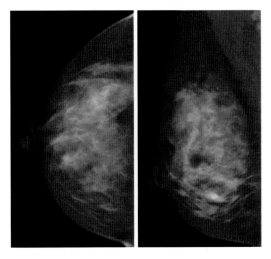

Fig. 199 Right mammography (Dec. 2020): negative finding

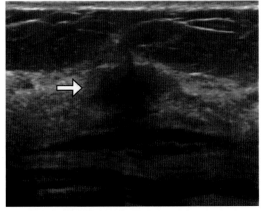

Fig. 200 Right breast US (Dec. 2020): an irregular hypoechoic mass with angular margins at upper outer quadrant. US-CNB = IDC

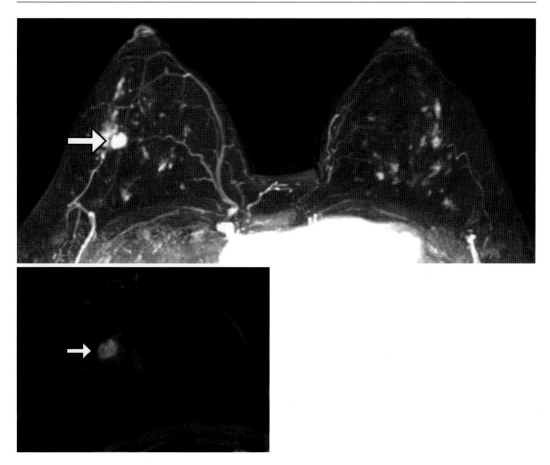

Fig. 201 Breast MRI (Jan. 2021): an enhancing mass with irregular margins in the right breast

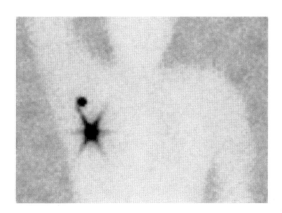

Fig. 202 Lymphoscintigraphy shows visualized sentinel lymph nodes in the right axilla

8. Lymphovascular invasion: absent.
9. Tumor border: infiltrative.
10. Microcalcification: present, tumoral/non-tumoral.
11. Pathological TN category (AJCC 2017): pT1bN0(sn).

	Result	Intensity	Positive %
Estrogen receptor	Strong (7/8)	3	1/3–2/3
Progesterone receptor	Strong (7/8)	3	1/3–2/3
C-erbB2	Negative (1+)		
Ki-67	Positive in 9% of tumor cells		

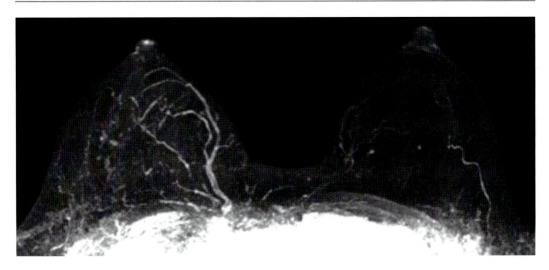

Fig. 203 Breast MRI for routine surveillance (Feb. 2022): no abnormal finding in both breasts

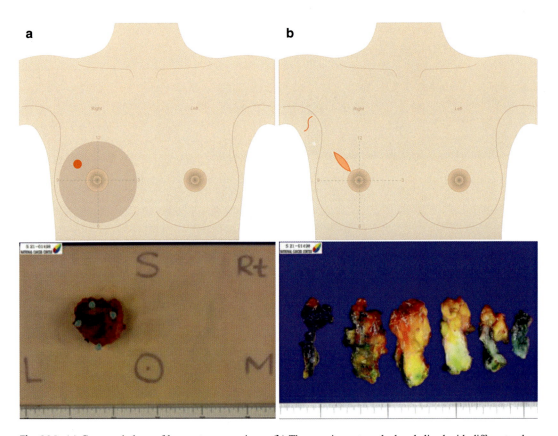

Fig. 204 (**a**) Gross pathology of lumpectomy specimen. (**b**) The margins get marked and sliced with different colors on each direction

37 Case 37

37.1 Patient History and Progress

Female/43 years old, pre-menopause.
Screen detected mass lesion on right breast 4–5 o'clock direction.
No family history.
Hypertension, s/p Lumbar spine disc operation.

37.2 Important Radiologic Findings

See Figs. 205, 206, 207 and 208.

37.3 Courses of Treatment

Operation + Adjuvant chemotherapy (#4 cycles of docetaxel & cyclophosphamide) + Post-operative radiation therapy + Tamoxifen 20 mg/day.

37.3.1 Operation
Left breast conserving surgery, sentinel lymph node biopsy (Fig. 209).

37.3.2 Pathology Report
Invasive Ductal Carcinoma
1. Size of tumor: 2.5 cm (pT2).
2. Histologic grade: 3/3 (tubule formation: 3/3, nuclear pleomorphism: 3/3, mitotic count: 2/3, 13/10 HPF)
3. Intraductal component: present, intratumoral/extratumoral (40%) (nuclear grade: high, necrosis: present, architectural pattern: cribriform/solid/comedo, extensive intraductal component: present).
4. Skin: no involvement of tumor.
5. Surgical margins:
   (a) superior margin: 10 mm.
   (b) inferior margin: 15 mm.
   (c) medial margin: 10 mm.
   (d) lateral margin: (see note).
   (e) deep margin: 4 mm.
   (f) superficial margin: <1 mm from ductal carcinoma in situ (slide 8).

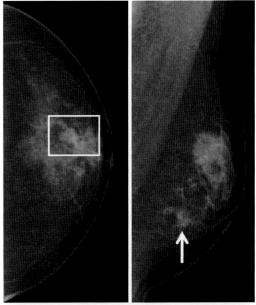

Fig. 205 Left mammography (Dec. 2020): a focal asymmetry with fine pleomorphic microcalcifications at lower outer quadrant

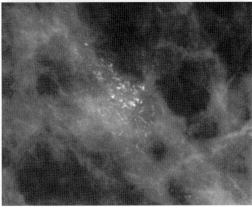

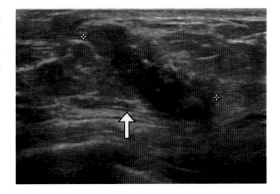

Fig. 206 Left breast US (Jan. 2021): an irregular hypoechoic mass with microcalcifications. US-CNB = IDC

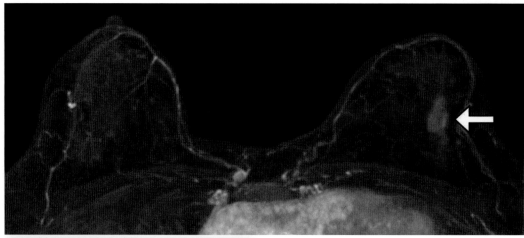

Fig. 207 Breast MRI (Jan. 2021): an irregular enhancing mass in the left breast

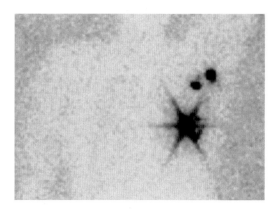

Fig. 208 Lymphoscintigraphy shows visualized sentinel lymph nodes in the left axilla

6. Lymph nodes: no metastasis in four axillary lymph nodes (pN0(sn)) (sentinel LN: 0/4)
7. Arteriovenous invasion: absent.
8. Lymphovascular invasion: present, intratumoral.
9. Tumor border: infiltrative.
10. Microcalcification: present, tumoral/non-tumoral.
11. Pathological TN category (AJCC 2017): pT2N0(sn).

Note: 1. The lateral margin of the lumpectomy specimen (slide 6) is close to ductal carcinoma in situ (<1 mm) but this margin submitted for frozen diagnosis (Fro 9) is free of tumor.

HR(+) HER2(−) Breast Cancer

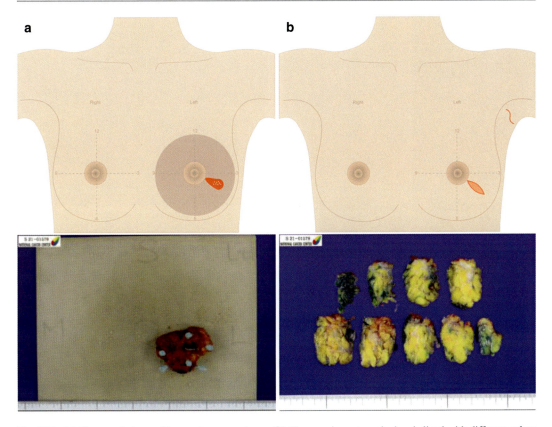

Fig. 209 (a) Gross pathology of lumpectomy specimen. (b) The margins get marked and sliced with different colors on each direction

	Result	Intensity	Positive %
Estrogen receptor	Strong (7/8)	2	>2/3
Progesterone receptor	Intermediate (6/8)	3	10%–1/3
C-erbB2	Negative (1+) IDC Positive (3+) DCIS		
Ki-67	Positive in 47% of tumor cells		

38 Case 38

38.1 Patient History and Progress

Female/57 years old, post-menopause.

Screen detected mass lesion on left breast 2 o'clock direction.

No family history.

Diabetes mellitus, dyslipidemia, s/p cataract operation.

38.2 Important Radiologic Findings

See Figs. 210, 211, 212, 213 and 214.

38.3 Courses of Treatment

Operation + Post-operative radiation therapy + Letrozole 2.5 mg/day.

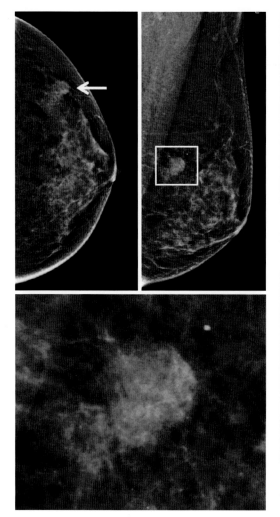

Fig. 210 Left mammography (Nov. 2020): an irregular hyperdense mass at outer center

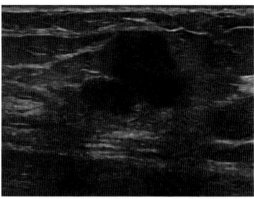

Fig. 211 Left breast US (Nov. 2020): a circumscribed hypoechoic mass. Outside US-VABE = IDC

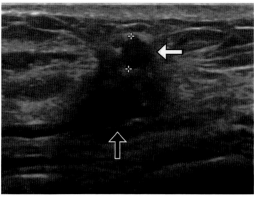

Fig. 212 Left breast US (Jan. 2021): post-VABE changes (black arrow) with a residual mass (white arrow)

38.3.1 Operation

Left breast conserving surgery, sentinel lymph node biopsy (Fig. 215).

38.3.2 Pathology Report

Invasive Ductal Carcinoma
1. Post-mammotome excision status.
2. Size of tumor: 0.5 cm, residual.
3. Histologic grade: 2/3 (tubule formation: 3/3, nuclear pleomorphism: 2/3, mitotic count: 1/3, 3/10 HPF)
4. Intraductal component: present, extratumoral (60%) (nuclear grade: low, necrosis: present, architectural pattern: cribriform/comedo, extensive intraductal component: present).
5. Skin: no involvement of tumor.
6. Surgical margins:
    (a) superior margin: 20 mm.
    (b) inferior margin: 7 mm.
    (c) medial margin: 15 mm.
    (d) lateral margin: 10 mm.
    (e) deep margin: 2 mm.
    (f) superficial margin: 5 mm.
7. Lymph nodes: no metastasis in one axillary lymph node (pN0(sn)) (sentinel LN: 0/1)

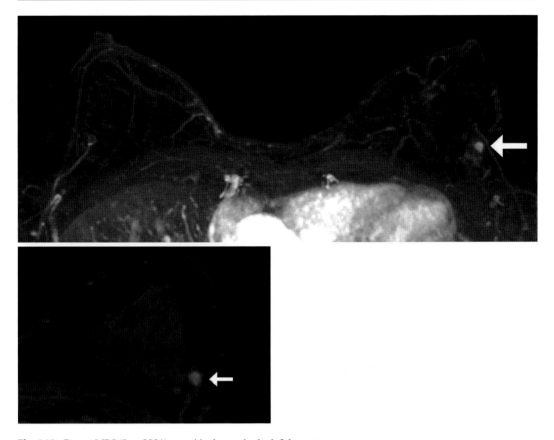

Fig. 213 Breast MRI (Jan. 2021): a residual mass in the left breast

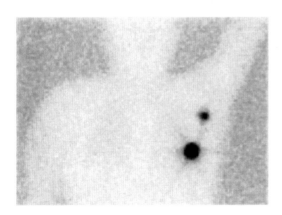

Fig. 214 Lymphoscintigraphy shows visualized sentinel lymph nodes in the left axilla

8. Arteriovenous invasion: absent.
9. Lymphovascular invasion: absent.
10. Tumor border: infiltrative.
11. Microcalcification: present, non-tumoral.

	Result	Intensity	Positive %
Estrogen receptor	Strong (7/8)	2	>2/3
Progesterone receptor	Weak (3/8)	1	1–10%
C-erbB2	Negative (1+)		
Ki-67	Positive in 19% of tumor cells		

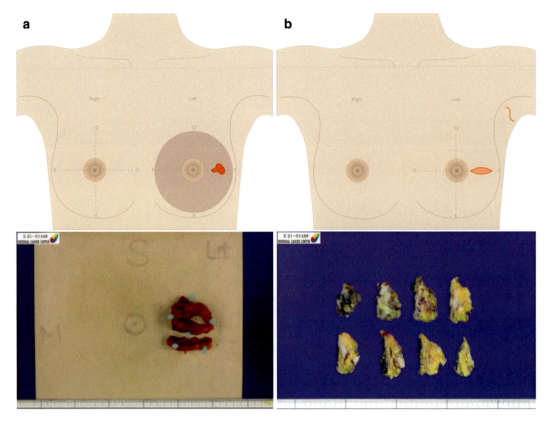

Fig. 215 (**a**) Gross pathology of lumpectomy specimen. (**b**) The margins get marked and sliced with different colors on each direction

39 Case 39

39.1 Patient History and Progress

Female/47 years old, pre-menopause.
Screen detected mass lesion on right breast 11 o'clock direction.
No family history.
No comorbidities.

39.2 Important Radiologic Findings

See Figs. 216, 217, 218 and 219.

39.3 Courses of Treatment

Operation + Adjuvant chemotherapy (#4 cycles of docetaxel & cyclophosphamide) + Tamoxifen 20 mg/day.

39.3.1 Operation
Right nipple–areolar complex sparing mastectomy with immediate implant reconstruction, left breast mass excision (Figs. 220, 221 and 222).

39.3.2 Pathology Report
[Right]

Invasive Lobular Carcinoma
1. Size of tumor: 2.5 cm (pT2).

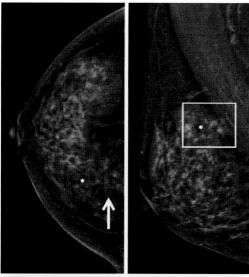

Fig. 216 Right mammography (Feb. 2021): a focal asymmetry at upper inner quadrant

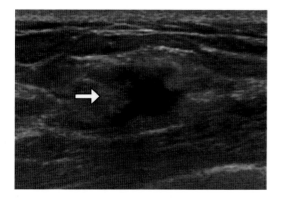

Fig. 217 Right breast US (Feb. 2021): an irregular hypoechoic mass with angular margins. US-CNB = IDC

2. Histologic grade: 2/3 (tubule formation: 3/3, nuclear pleomorphism: 2/3, mitotic count: 1/3, 6/10 HPF)
3. In situ component: present, intratumoral/extratumoral (70%).
4. Skin: no involvement of tumor.
5. Surgical margins: (see note).
    (a) deep margin: <1 mm from invasive lobular carcinoma (slides 1 and 9).
    (b) superficial margin: <1 mm from invasive lobular carcinoma (slide 1).
6. Lymph nodes: no metastasis in one axillary lymph node (pN0(sn)) (sentinel LN: 0/1)
7. Arteriovenous invasion: absent.
8. Lymphovascular invasion: absent.
9. Tumor border: infiltrative.
10. Microcalcification: present, tumoral/non-tumoral.
11. Pathological TN category (AJCC 2017): pT2N0(sn).

    Note: 1. Lobular carcinoma in situ is present only in the permanent sections of Fro 9 and Fro 10.

	Result	Intensity	Positive %
Estrogen receptor	Strong (8/8)	3	>2/3
Progesterone receptor	Strong (8/8)	3	>2/3
C-erbB2	Equivocal (2+) (SISH negative)		
Ki-67	Positive in 5% of tumor cells		

[Left]
Intraductal papilloma.

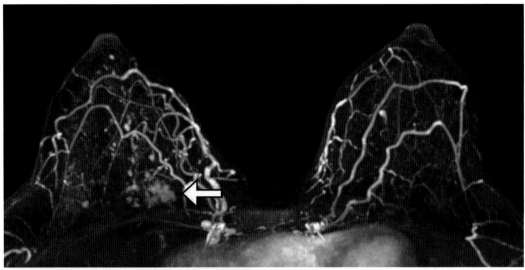
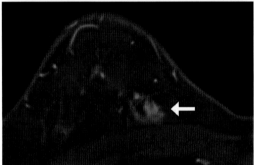

Fig. 218 Breast MRI (Feb. 2021): an irregular enhancing mass in the right breast

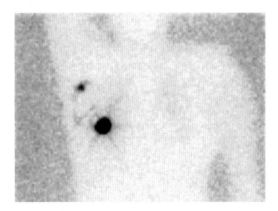

Fig. 219 Lymphoscintigraphy shows visualized sentinel lymph nodes in the right axilla

HR(+) HER2(−) Breast Cancer

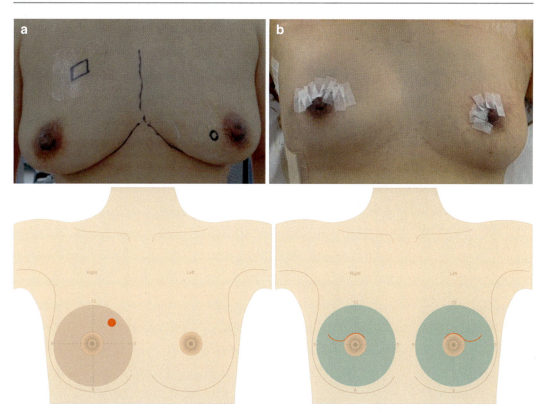

Fig. 220 (**a**) Preoperative and (**b**) immediate post-operative appearance

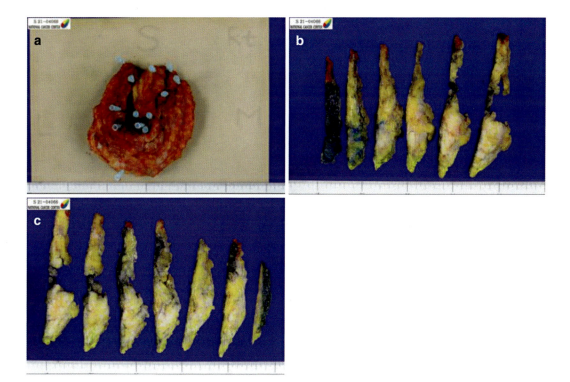

Fig. 221 (**a**) Gross pathology of right mastectomy specimen. (**b** and **c**) The margins get marked and sliced with different colors on each direction

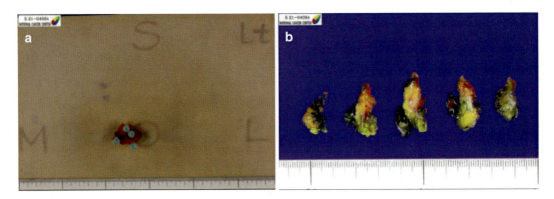

Fig. 222 (**a**) Gross pathology of left breast mass excision specimen. (**b**) The margins get marked and sliced with different colors on each direction

HR(+) HER2(+) Breast Cancer

Soojin Park, Ran Song, Yunju Kim, Bo Hwa Choi,
Eun Sook Lee, Chan Wha Lee, and Eun-Gyeong Lee

1 Case 1

1.1 Patient History and Progress

Female/47 years old, pre-menopause.

Screen detected mass lesion on left breast 5 o'clock direction.

No family history.

No comorbidities.

S. Park
Department of Surgery, Wonkwang University
Sanbon Hospital, Gunpo, Republic of Korea

R. Song · E.-G. Lee (✉)
Division of Surgery, Center for Breast Cancer,
National Cancer Center, Goyang, Republic of Korea
e-mail: thdfks37@ncc.re.kr; bnf333@ncc.re.kr

Y. Kim
Department of Pathology, National Cancer Center,
Goyang, Gyeonggi, Republic of Korea
e-mail: radkyj@ncc.re.kr

B. H. Choi · C. W. Lee
Division of Diagnostic Radiology, Center for Breast
Cancer, National Cancer Center,
Goyang, Republic of Korea
e-mail: iawy82@ncc.re.kr; cwlee@ncc.re.kr

E. S. Lee
Center for Breast Cancer, National Cancer Center,
Goyang, Kyonggi-do, Republic of Korea
e-mail: eslee@ncc.re.kr

1.2 Important Radiologic Findings

See Figs. 1, 2, 3, 4, 5 and 6.

1.3 Courses of Treatment

Neoadjuvant chemotherapy (#6 cycles of docetaxel and carboplatin and trastuzumab and pertuzumab) + Operation + Postoperative radiation therapy + Tamoxifen 20 mg/day.

Operation: Left breast conserving surgery, sentinel lymph node biopsy (Fig. 7).

1.3.1 Pathology Report

Invasive Ductal Carcinoma
1. Post-chemotherapy status.
2. Size of invasive component: 0.2 cm (pT1a).
3. Size of intraductal component: 1.0 cm.
4. Histologic grade:1/3 (tubule formation: 2/3, nuclear pleomorphism: 2/3, mitotic count: 1/3, 4/10 HPF).
5. Intraductal component: present, extratumoral (99%) (nuclear grade: high, necrosis: present, architectural pattern: cribriform/solid/comedo, extensive intraductal component: present).
6. Surgical margins:

© The Author(s), under exclusive license to Springer Nature Singapore Pte Ltd. 2023
E. S. Lee (ed.), *A Practical Guide to Breast Cancer Treatment*,
https://doi.org/10.1007/978-981-19-9044-1_6

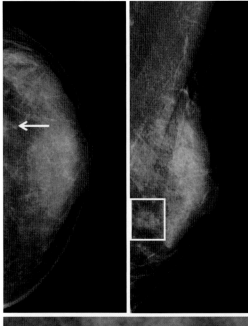

Fig. 1 Left mammography (Dec. 2020): an irregular mass with microcalcifications at lower outer quadrant

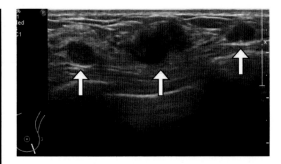

Fig. 2 Left breast US (Dec. 2020): multiple hypoechoic masses at lower outer quadrant. US-CNB = IDC

(a) superior margin: 18 mm,
(b) inferior margin: 17 mm,
(c) medial margin: 10 mm,
(d) lateral margin: 10 mm,
(e) deep margin: 4 mm,
(f) superficial margin: 14 mm.
7. Lymph nodes:
   (a) metastasis in one out of five axillary lymph nodes (ypN1mi(sn)) (sentinel LN: 1/5),
   (b) perinodal extension: absent,
   (c) size of metastatic carcinoma: 1 mm.
8. Arteriovenous invasion: absent.
9. Lymphovascular invasion: absent.
10. Tumor border: infiltrative.
11. Microcalcification: present, non-tumoral.
12. Pathological TN category (AJCC 2017): ypT1aN1mi(sn).

	Result	Intensity	Positive %
Estrogen receptor	Strong (8/8)	3	>2/3
Progesterone receptor	Strong (7/8)	3	1/3-2/3
C-erbB2	Equivocal (2+)		
Ki-67	Positive in 1% of tumor cells		

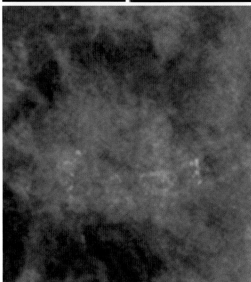

HR(+) HER2(+) Breast Cancer 301

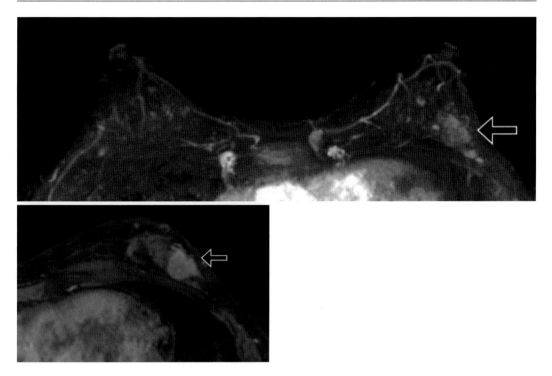

Fig. 3 Breast MRI (Dec. 2020): an irregular enhancing mass in the left breast

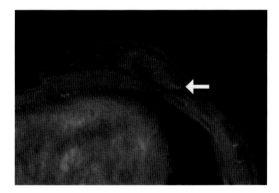

Fig. 4 Post-NAC breast MRI (May 2021): a residual enhancing focus after NAC

Fig. 5 PET-CT shows (**a**) a hypermetabolic mass in the left lower outer breast (mSUV = 9.9) and (**b**) hypermetabolic lymph node in the left axilla level I (mSUV = 3.7)

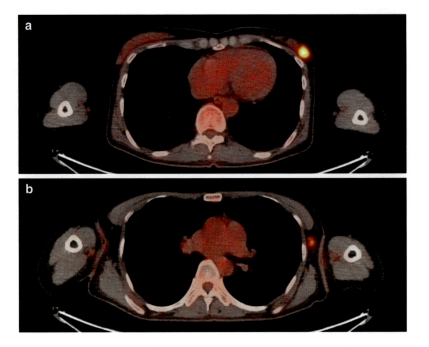

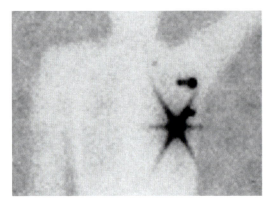

Fig. 6 Lymphoscintigraphy shows visualized sentinel lymph nodes in the left axilla

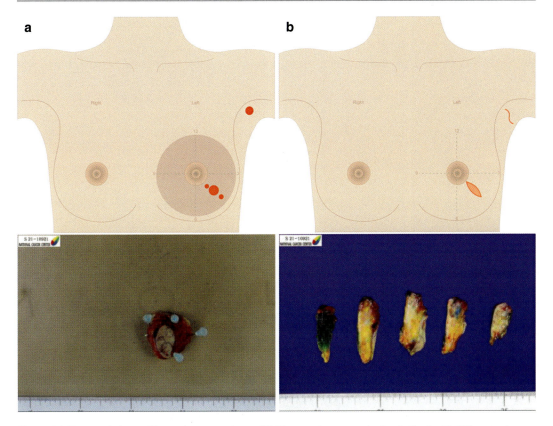

Fig. 7 (**a**) Gross pathology of lumpectomy specimen. (**b**) The margins get marked and sliced with different colors on each direction

2 Case 2

2.1 Patient History and Progress

Female/42 years old, pre-menopause.
Screen detected mass lesion on left breast 1:30 and 2 o'clock direction.
No family history.
S/P Cervical spine disc operation.

2.2 Important Radiologic Findings

See Figs. 8, 9, 10 and 11.

2.3 Courses of Treatment

Neoadjuvant chemotherapy (#6 cycles of docetaxel and carboplatin and trastuzumab and pertuzumab) + Operation + Post-operative radiation therapy + Trastuzumab emtansine + Tamoxifen 20 mg/day.

Operation: Left breast conserving surgery, sentinel lymph node biopsy (Fig. 12).

2.3.1 Pathology Report
1. Microinvasive ductal carcinoma.
    (a) Post-chemotherapy status.
    (b) Size of tumor: <0.1 cm (ypT1mi).

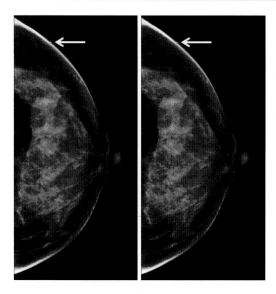

Fig. 8 Left mammography (Dec. 2020): no discernible focal lesion at the palpable area at upper outer quadrant

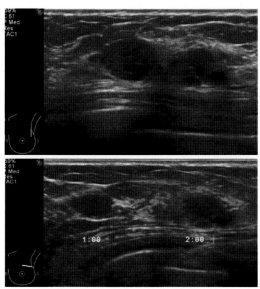

Fig. 9 Left breast US (Jan. 2021): multiple masses with microlobulated margins at upper outer quadrant. US-CNB = IDC

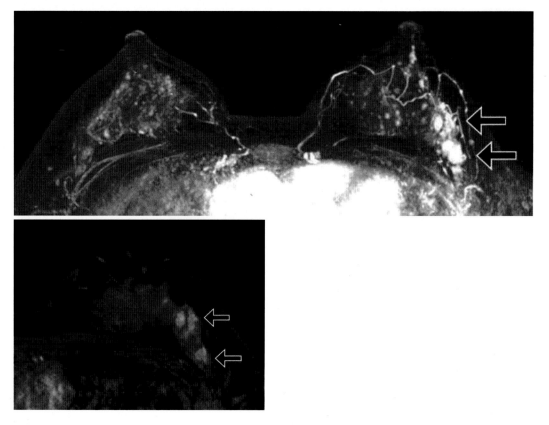

Fig. 10 Breast MRI (Jan. 2021): multiple enhancing masses in the left breast

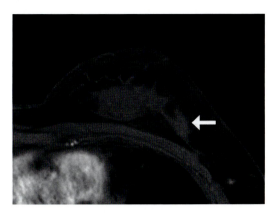

Fig. 11 Post-NAC breast MRI (May 2021): no residual enhancing lesion after NAC

(c) Histologic grade: 2/3 (tubule formation: 3/3, nuclear pleomorphism: 2/3, mitotic count: 2/3, 11/10 HPF).
(d) Intraductal component: absent.
(e) Skin: no involvement of tumor.
(f) Surgical margins:
   - superior margin: 2 mm from microinvasive ductal carcinoma (Fro 6),
   - inferior margin: 30 mm,
   - medial margin: >10 mm,
   - lateral margin: >10 mm,
   - deep margin: 2 mm,
   - superficial margin: 2 mm.

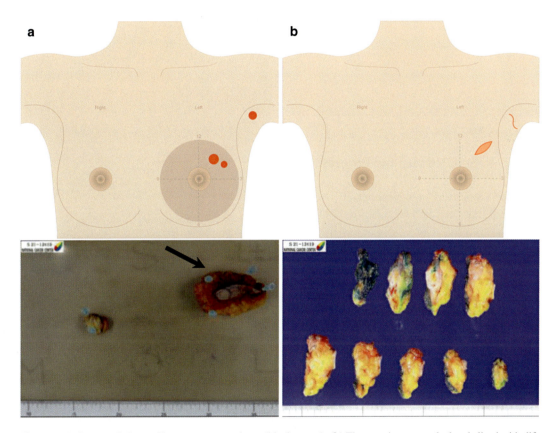

Fig. 12 (**a**) Gross pathology of lumpectomy specimen (black arrow). (**b**) The margins get marked and sliced with different colors on each direction

(g) Lymph nodes: no metastasis in two axillary lymph nodes (ypN0(sn)) (sentinel LN: 0/2).
(h) Arteriovenous invasion: absent.
(i) Lymphovascular invasion: absent.
(j) Tumor border: infiltrative.
(k) Microcalcification: present, tumoral/non-tumoral.
(l) Pathological TN category (AJCC 2017): ypT1miN0(sn).
(m) Related slides:
2. Sclerosing adenosis with microcalcification.

	Result	Intensity	Positive %
Estrogen receptor	Strong (8/8)	3	>2/3
Progesterone receptor	Negative (0/8)	0	0
C-erbB2	Equivocal (2+)		
Ki-67	Positive in 2% of tumor cells		

3 Case 3

3.1 Patient History and Progress

Female/58 years old, post-menopause.
Screen detected mass lesion on right breast 7 o'clock direction.
No family history.
Dyslipidemia.

3.2 Important Radiologic Findings

See Figs. 13, 14, 15, 16 and 17.

3.3 Courses of Treatment

Operation + Adjuvant chemotherapy (#4 cycles of doxorubicin and cyclophosphamide) + Post-operative radiation therapy + Trastuzumab + Letrozole 2.5 mg/day.

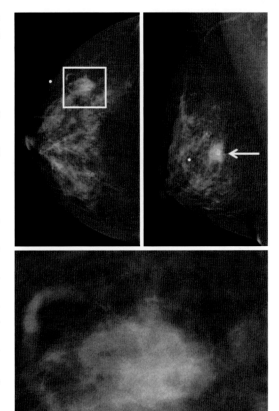

Fig. 13 Right mammography (Dec. 2020): an irregular mass at lower outer quadrant

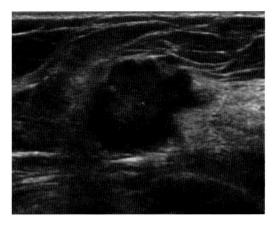

Fig. 14 Right breast US (Dec. 2020): an irregular hypoechoic mass. US-CNB = IDC

HR(+) HER2(+) Breast Cancer

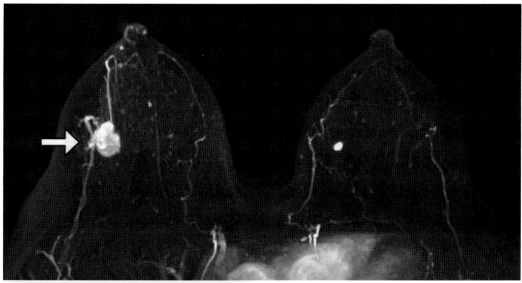

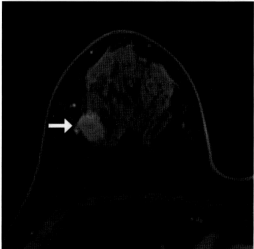

Fig. 15 Breast MRI (Jan. 2021): an irregular enhancing mass in the right breast

Operation: Right breast conserving surgery, sentinel lymph node biopsy (Fig. 18).

3.3.1 Pathology Report

Invasive Ductal Carcinoma
1. Size of tumor: 1.8 cm (pT1c).
2. Histologic grade: 3/3 (tubule formation: 3/3, nuclear pleomorphism: 3/3, mitotic count: 2/3, 10/10 HPF).
3. Intraductal component: present, intratumoral/extratumoral (10%) (nuclear grade: high, necrosis: present, architectural pattern: solid/comedo, extensive intraductal component: absent).
4. Skin: no involvement of tumor.
5. Surgical margins:
    (a) superior margin: 10 mm,
    (b) inferior margin: (see note),
    (c) medial margin: 5 mm,
    (d) lateral margin: 10 mm,
    (e) deep margin: 2 mm,
    (f) superficial margin: 4 mm.

6. Lymph nodes: no metastasis in one axillary lymph node (pN0(sn)) (sentinel LN: 0/1).
7. Arteriovenous invasion: absent.
8. Lymphovascular invasion: absent.
9. Tumor border: infiltrative.
10. Microcalcification: present, tumoral/non-tumoral.
11. Pathological TN category (AJCC 2017): pT1cN0(sn).

Note: 1. The inferior margin of the lumpectomy specimen (slides 3 and 4) is close to ductal carcinoma in situ (2 mm) but this margin submitted for frozen diagnosis (Fro 2) is free of tumor.

	Result	Intensity	Positive %
Estrogen receptor	Strong (7/8)	2	>2/3
Progesterone receptor	Intermediate (6/8)	2	1/3–2/3
C-erbB2	Equivocal (2+)		
Ki-67	Positive in 43% of tumor cells		
SISH	Positive		

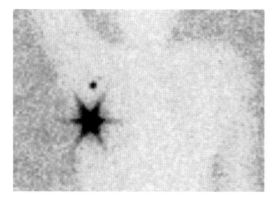

Fig. 16 Lymphoscintigraphy shows visualized sentinel lymph nodes in the right axilla

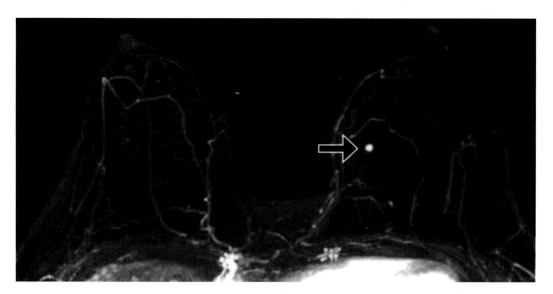

Fig. 17 Breast MRI for routine surveillance (Apr. 2022): no abnormal finding in the right breast. No change of the benign appearing mass in the left breast (black arrow)

HR(+) HER2(+) Breast Cancer

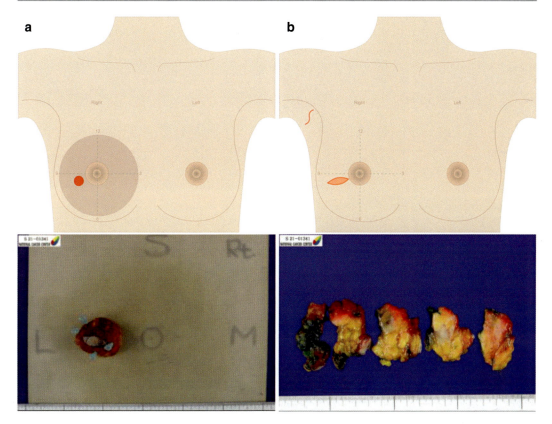

Fig. 18 (**a**) Gross pathology of lumpectomy specimen. (**b**) The margins get marked and sliced with different colors on each direction

4 Case 4

4.1 Patient History and Progress

Female/56 years old, post-menopause.

Screen detected mass lesion on right breast 12 o'clock direction.

No family history.

S/P Thyroid radiofrequency ablation.

4.2 Important Radiologic Findings

See Figs. 19, 20, 21 and 22.

4.3 Courses of Treatment

Operation + Adjuvant chemotherapy (#4 cycles of doxorubicin and cyclophosphamide) + Post-operative radiation therapy + Letrozole 2.5 mg/day.

Operation: Right breast conserving surgery, sentinel lymph node biopsy (Fig. 23).

4.3.1 Pathology Report

Invasive Ductal Carcinoma
1. Size of tumor: 0.6 cm (pT1b).
2. Histologic grade: 3/3 (tubule formation: 3/3, nuclear pleomorphism: 3/3, mitotic count: 2/3, 10/10 HPF).

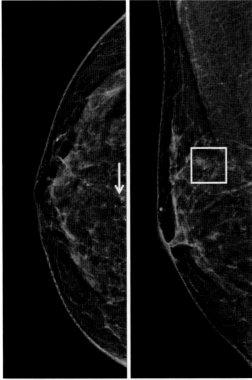

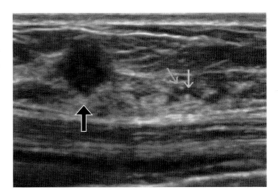

Fig. 20 Right breast US (Dec. 2020): a hypoechoic mass with non-parallel orientation (black arrow) and adjacent microcalcifications (white arrows). US-CNB = IDC

cribriform/comedo, extensive intraductal component: present).
4. Skin: no involvement of tumor.
5. Surgical margins:
   (a) superior margin: 10 mm,
   (b) inferior margin: 5 mm,
   (c) medial margin: 15 mm,
   (d) lateral margin: 25 mm,
   (e) deep margin: 1.5 mm from ductal carcinoma in situ (slide 3),
   (f) superficial margin: 8 mm.
6. Lymph nodes: no metastasis in two axillary lymph nodes (pN0(sn)) (sentinel LN: 0/2).
7. Arteriovenous invasion: absent.
8. Lymphovascular invasion: absent.
9. Tumor border: infiltrative.
10. Microcalcification: present, tumoral/non-tumoral.
11. Pathological TN category (AJCC 2017): pT1bN0(sn).

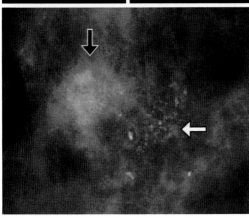

Fig. 19 Right mammography (Dec. 2020): grouped fine-pleomorphic microcalcifications (white arrow) and an asymmetry (black arrow) at upper center

3. Intraductal component: present, extratumoral (50%) (nuclear grade: high, necrosis: present, architectural pattern: micropapillary/

	Result	Intensity	Positive %
Estrogen receptor	Strong (8/8)	3	>2/3
Progesterone receptor	Intermediate (5/8)	2	10% to 1/3
C-erbB2	Positive (3+)		
Ki-67	Positive in 27% of tumor cells		

HR(+) HER2(+) Breast Cancer

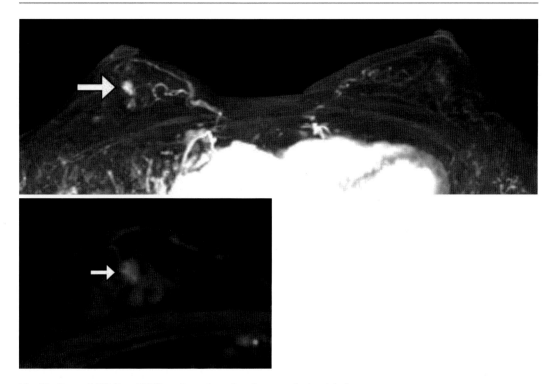

Fig. 21 Breast MRI (Jan. 2021): an irregular enhancing mass in the right breast

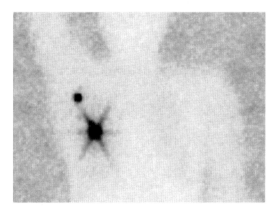

Fig. 22 Lymphoscintigraphy shows visualized sentinel lymph nodes in the right axilla

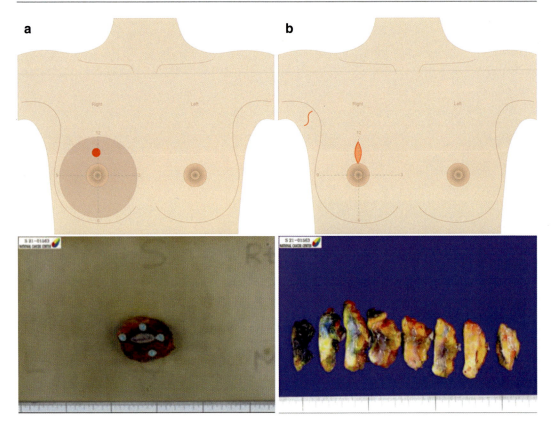

Fig. 23 (**a**) Gross pathology of lumpectomy specimen. (**b**) The margins get marked and sliced with different colors on each direction

5 Case 5

5.1 Patient History and Progress

Female/53 years old, peri-menopause.

Screen detected mass lesion on right breast 12 o'clock direction.

No family history.

Hypothyroidism, dyslipidemia, s/p cold knife conization of cervix.

5.2 Important Radiologic Findings

See Figs. 24, 25, 26 and 27.

5.3 Courses of Treatment

Operation + Adjuvant chemotherapy (#4 cycles of docetaxel and cyclophosphamide) + Post-operative radiation therapy + Trastuzumab + Tamoxifen 20 mg/day.

Operation: Right breast conserving surgery, sentinel lymph node biopsy (Fig. 28).

5.3.1 Pathology Report

Invasive Ductal Carcinoma
1. Size of tumor: 1.5 cm (pT1c).
2. Histologic grade: 3/3 (tubule formation: 3/3, nuclear pleomorphism: 3/3, mitotic count: 3/3, 3/HPF).

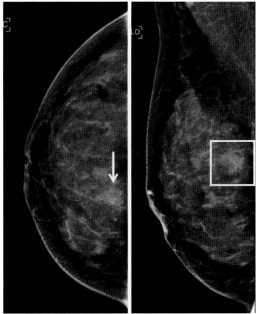

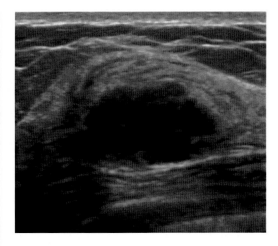

Fig. 25 Right breast US (Jan. 2021): a hypoechoic mass with microlobulated margins. US-CNB = IDC

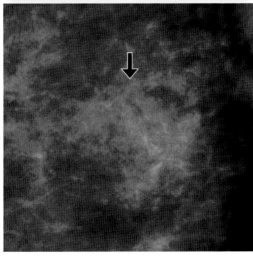

Fig. 24 Right mammography (Jan. 2021): a focal asymmetry at upper inner quadrant

3. Intraductal component: present, intratumoral/extratumoral (20%) (nuclear grade: high, necrosis: present, architectural pattern: solid/comedo, extensive intraductal component: present).
4. Skin: no involvement of tumor.
5. Surgical margins:
   (a) superior margin: 10 mm,
   (b) inferior margin: (see note),
   (c) medial margin: 5 mm,
   (d) lateral margin: (see note),
   (e) deep margin: <1 mm from invasive ductal carcinoma (slide 4),
   (f) superficial margin: 2 mm.
6. Lymph nodes: no metastasis in one axillary lymph node (pN0(sn)) (sentinel LN: 0/1).
7. Arteriovenous invasion: absent.
8. Lymphovascular invasion: present, intratumoral.
9. Tumor border: infiltrative.
10. Microcalcification: present, tumoral/non-tumoral.
11. Pathological TN category (AJCC 2017): pT1cN0(sn).

Note: 1. The inferior and lateral margins of the lumpectomy specimen (slides 9 and 10, respectively) are close to ductal carcinoma in situ (<1 mm) but these margins submitted for frozen diagnosis (Fro 3 and Fro 5, respectively) are free of tumor.

	Result	Intensity	Positive %
Estrogen receptor	Strong (8/8)	3	>2/3
Progesterone receptor	Intermediate (6/8)	3	10%-1/3
C-erbB2	Equivocal (2+)		
Ki-67	Positive in 39% of tumor cells		
SISH	Positive		

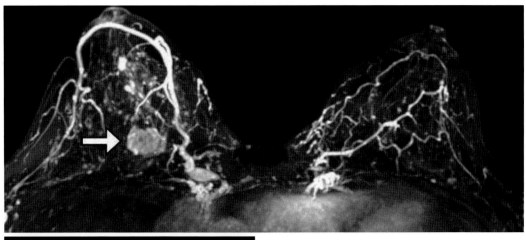
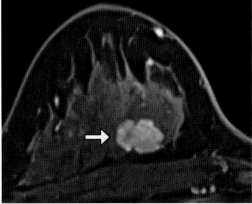

Fig. 26 Breast MRI (Jan. 2021): an irregular enhancing mass in the right breast

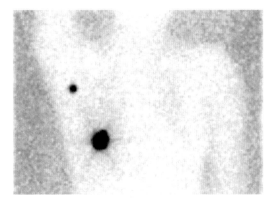

Fig. 27 Lymphoscintigraphy shows visualized sentinel lymph nodes in the right axilla

HR(+) HER2(+) Breast Cancer

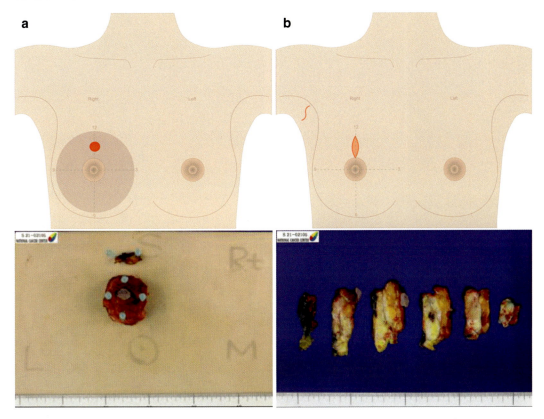

Fig. 28 (**a**) Gross pathology of lumpectomy specimen. (**b**) The margins get marked and sliced with different colors on each direction

6 Case 6

6.1 Patient History and Progress

Female/42 years old, pre-menopause.
   Screen detected mass lesion on right breast 12 o'clock direction.
   No family history.
   Hypertension.

6.2 Important Radiologic Findings

See Figs. 29, 30, 31, 32, 33 and 34.

6.3 Courses of Treatment

Operation + Adjuvant chemotherapy (#4 cycles of doxorubicin and cyclophosphamide) + Post-operative radiation therapy + Trastuzumab + Tamoxifen 20 mg/day.
   Operation: Left breast conserving surgery, sentinel lymph node biopsy (Fig. 35).

6.3.1 Pathology Report
1. Invasive ductal carcinoma.
    (a) Size of tumor: 1.5 cm (pT1c).
    (b) Histologic grade: 3/3 (tubule formation: 3/3, nuclear pleomorphism: 3/3, mitotic count: 3/3, 5/HPF).

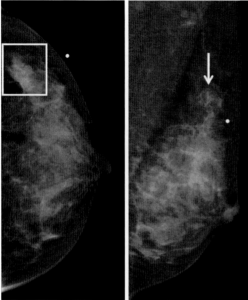

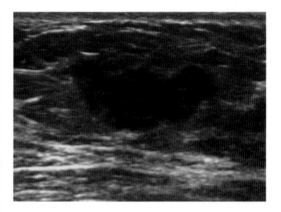

Fig. 30 Left breast US (Dec. 2020): an irregular hypoechoic mass. US-CNB = IDC

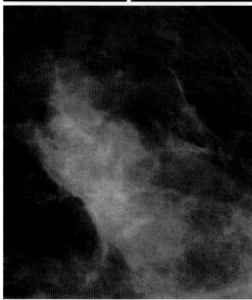

Fig. 29 Left mammography (Dec. 2020): an obscured mass at upper outer quadrant

(c) Intraductal component: present, intratumoral/extratumoral (10%) (nuclear grade: high, necrosis: present, architectural pattern: solid/comedo, extensive intraductal component: absent).

(d) Skin: no involvement of tumor.
(e) Surgical margins:
- superior margin: 10 mm,
- inferior margin: 10 mm,
- medial margin: 20 mm,
- lateral margin: 10 mm,
- deep margin: 2 mm,
- superficial margin: 2 mm.

(f) Lymph nodes: no metastasis in seven axillary lymph nodes (pN0) (sentinel LN: 0/4, non-sentinel LN: 0/3).
(g) Arteriovenous invasion: absent.
(h) Lymphovascular invasion: absent.
(i) Tumor border: infiltrative.
(j) Microcalcification: present, tumoral/non-tumoral.
(k) Pathological TN category (AJCC 2017): pT1cN0.

2. Intraductal papilloma with (1) myoepithelial hyperplasia usual ductal hyperplasia.

	Result	Intensity	Positive %
Estrogen receptor	Strong (7/8)	3	1/3-2/3
Progesterone receptor	Strong (8/8)	3	>2/3
C-erbB2	Positive (3+)		
Ki-67	Positive in 52% of tumor cells		

HR(+) HER2(+) Breast Cancer

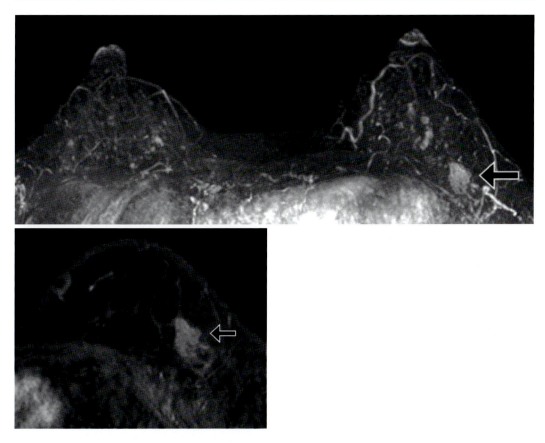

Fig. 31 Breast MRI (Dec. 2020): an irregular enhancing mass in the left breast

Fig. 32 PET-CT shows (**a**) a hypermetabolic mass in the left upper outer breast (mSUV = 4.8) and (**b**) there was no enlarged hypermetabolic lymph node in the left axilla

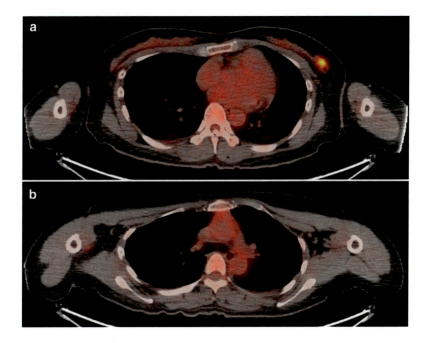

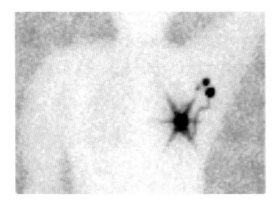

Fig. 33 Lymphoscintigraphy shows visualized sentinel lymph nodes in the left axilla

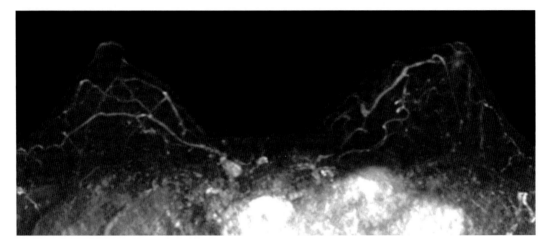

Fig. 34 Breast MRI for routine surveillance (Feb. 2022): no abnormal finding in both breasts

HR(+) HER2(+) Breast Cancer

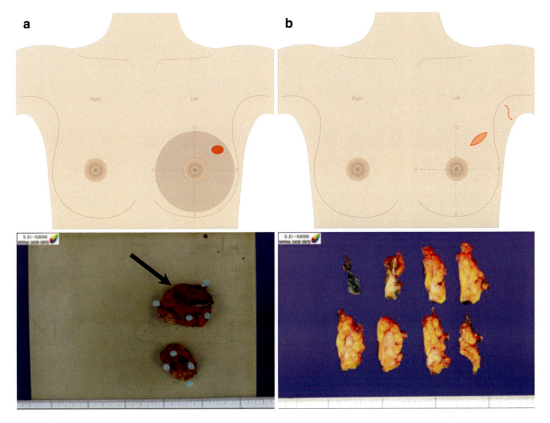

Fig. 35 (**a**) Gross pathology of lumpectomy specimen. (**b**) The margins get marked and sliced with different colors on each direction

7 Case 7

7.1 Patient History and Progress

Female/50 years old, pre-menopause.

Screen detected mass lesion on left breast 3 o'clock direction.

No family history.

Paroxysmal supraventricular tachycardia, s/p atrial septal defect closure.

S/P thyroid lobectomy (thyroid cancer).

7.2 Important Radiologic Findings

See Figs. 36, 37, 38, 39, 40 and 41.

7.3 Courses of Treatment

Neoadjuvant chemotherapy (#6 cycles of docetaxel and carboplatin and trastuzumab and pertuzumab) + Operation + Post-operative radiation therapy + Trastuzumab emtansine + Tamoxifen 20 mg/day.

Operation: Left breast conserving surgery, sentinel lymph node biopsy (Fig. 42).

7.3.1 Pathology Report

Invasive Ductal Carcinoma
1. Post-chemotherapy status.
2. Size of tumor: 1.1 cm (ypT1c).
3. Histologic grade: 2/3 (tubule formation: 3/3, nuclear pleomorphism: 2/3, mitotic count: 1/3, 6/10 HPF).

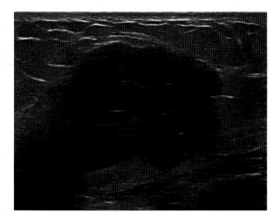

Fig. 37 Left breast US (Sep. 2020): an irregular hypoechoic mass. US-CNB = IDC

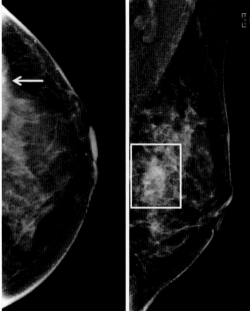

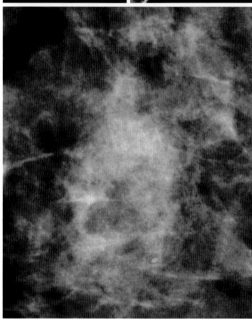

Fig. 36 Left mammography (Aug. 2020): a focal asymmetry at outer breast

4. Intraductal component: present, intratumoral/extratumoral (30%) (nuclear grade: high, necrosis: absent, architectural pattern: solid, extensive intraductal component: present).
5. Skin: no involvement of tumor.
6. Surgical margins:
   (a) superior margin: 10 mm,
   (b) inferior margin: (see note),
   (c) medial margin: 10 mm,
   (d) lateral margin: 5 mm,
   (e) deep margin: 2 mm,
   (f) superficial margin: 2 mm.
7. Lymph nodes: no metastasis in 13 axillary lymph nodes (ypN0) (sentinel LN: 0/3, axillary LN: 0/10).
8. Arteriovenous invasion: absent.
9. Lymphovascular invasion: present, intratumoral.
10. Tumor border: infiltrative.
11. Microcalcification: present, tumoral/non-tumoral.
12. Pathological TN category (AJCC 2017): ypT1cN0.

Note: 1. The inferior margin of the lumpectomy specimen (slide 7) is close to ductal carcinoma in situ (<1 mm) but this margin submitted for frozen diagnosis (Fro 2) is free of tumor.

	Result	Intensity	Positive %
Estrogen receptor	Strong (8/8)	3	>2/3
Progesterone receptor	Strong (8/8)	3	>2/3
C-erbB2	Positive (3+)		
Ki-67	Positive in 6% of tumor cells		

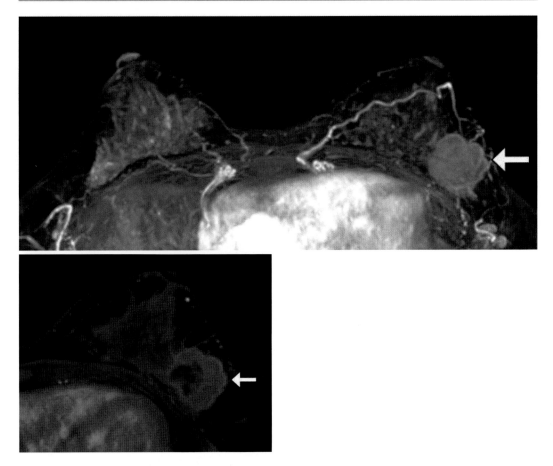

Fig. 38 Breast MRI (Sep. 2020): an enhancing mass with central necrosis in the left breast

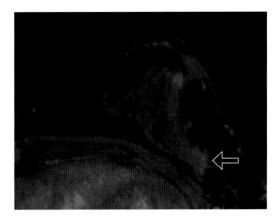

Fig. 39 Post-NAC breast MRI (Feb. 2021): a residual focal non-mass enhancement after NAC

Fig. 40 PET-CT shows (**a**) a hypermetabolic mass in the left outer breast (mSUV = 8.6) and (**b**) mild hypermetabolic enlarged lymph nodes with fatty hilum in the left axilla level I–II (mSUV = 2.3)

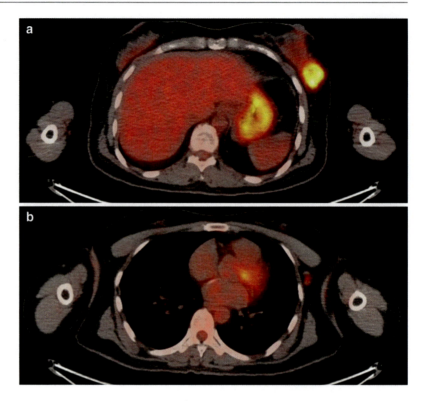

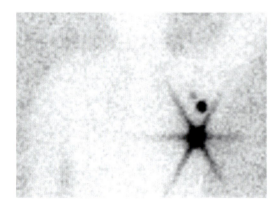

Fig. 41 Lymphoscintigraphy shows visualized sentinel lymph nodes in the left axilla

HR(+) HER2(+) Breast Cancer   323

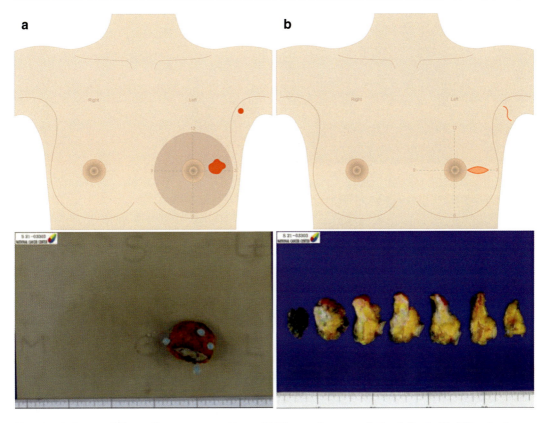

Fig. 42 (**a**) Gross pathology of lumpectomy specimen. (**b**) The margins get marked and sliced with different colors on each direction

8 Case 8

8.1 Patient History and Progress

Female/61 years old, post-menopause.

Screen detected mass lesion on right breast 9 o'clock direction.

No family history.

Hypertension, s/p cholecystectomy, arrhythmia.

8.2 Important Radiologic Findings

See Figs. 43, 44, 45 and 46.

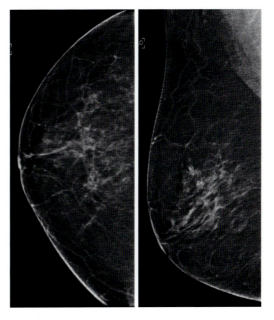

Fig. 43 Right mammography (Dec. 2020): negative finding

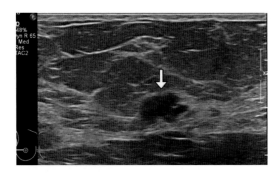

Fig. 44 Right breast US (Jan. 2021): an irregular hypoechoic mass at 9 o'clock direction. Outside US-CNB = ADH. Excision = IDC

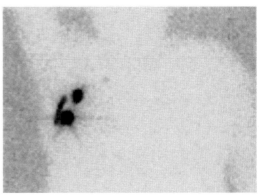

Fig. 45 Lymphoscintigraphy shows visualized sentinel lymph nodes in the left axilla

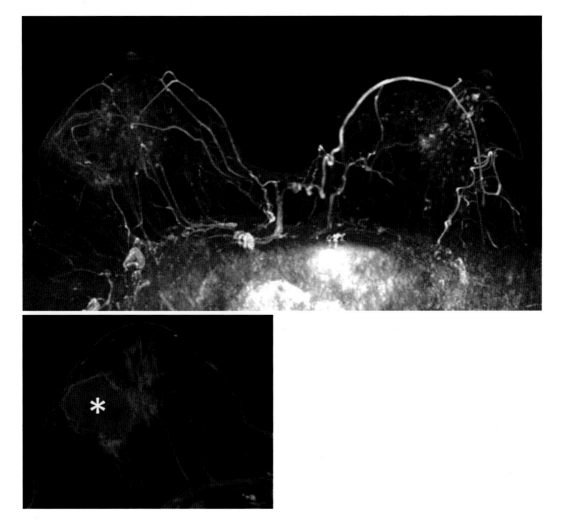

Fig. 46 Breast MRI (Mar. 2021): post-operative fluid collection (*) without the residual suspicious enhancing lesion

8.3 Courses of Treatment

Operation + Adjuvant chemotherapy (#4 cycles of doxorubicin and cyclophosphamide) + Post-operative radiation therapy + Trastuzumab + Letrozole 2.5 mg/day.

Operation: Right breast conserving surgery, sentinel lymph node biopsy (Fig. 47).

8.3.1 Pathology Report
1. No residual tumor with foreign body reaction.
   (a) Post-excision status.
   (b) Lymph nodes: no metastasis in one axillary lymph node (pN0(sn)) (sentinel LN: 0/1).
2. Intraductal papilloma.

	Result	Intensity	Positive %
Estrogen receptor	Strong (8/8)	3	>2/3
Progesterone receptor	Weak (4/8)	2	1–10%
C-erbB2	Positive (3+)		
Ki-67	Positive in 29% of tumor cells		

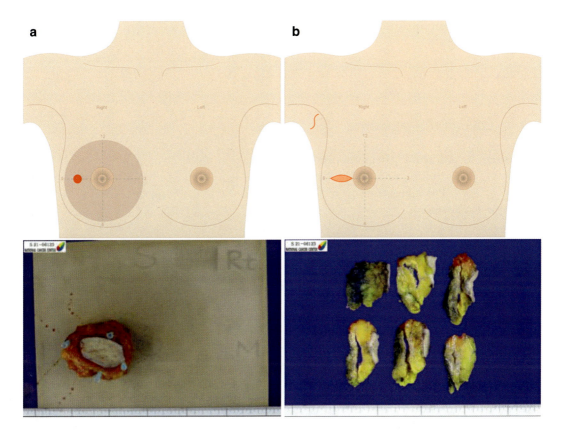

Fig. 47 (a) Gross pathology of lumpectomy specimen. (b) The margins get marked and sliced with different colors on each direction

9 Case 9

9.1 Patient History and Progress

Female/44 years old, pre-menopause.

Screen detected mass lesion on left breast 7 o'clock direction.

Family history of breast cancer, two sisters.

Family history of pancreatic cancer, mother.

No other history of disease, operation, or medication.

BRCA 1 and 2 mutation: Not detected, RAD50 VUS (variant of uncertain).

9.2 Important Radiologic Findings

See Figs. 48, 49 and 50.

9.3 Courses of Treatment

Operation + Adjuvant chemotherapy (#4 cycles of doxorubicin and cyclophosphamide) + Post-operative radiation therapy + Trastuzumab.

Operation: Left breast conserving surgery (Fig. 51).

9.3.1 Pathology Report

Invasive Ductal Carcinoma
1. Size of tumor: 1.3 cm (pT1c).
2. Histologic grade: 3/3 (tubule formation: 3/3, nuclear pleomorphism: 3/3, mitotic count: 3/3, 4/HPF).
3. Intraductal component: present, intratumoral/extratumoral (30%) (nuclear grade: high, necrosis: present, architectural pattern: solid/comedo, extensive intraductal component: present).
4. Skin: no involvement of tumor.

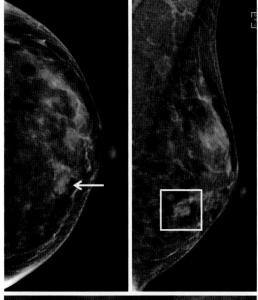
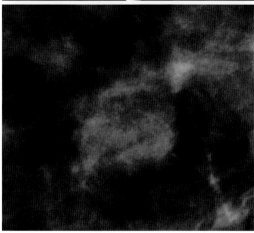

Fig. 48 Left mammography (Jan. 2021): an irregular mass at lower inner quadrant

5. Surgical margins:
   (a) superior margin: 5 mm,
   (b) inferior margin: (see Note 1),
   (c) medial margin: (see Note 2),
   (d) lateral margin: 10 mm,
   (e) deep margin: 2 mm,
   (f) superficial margin: 2 mm.

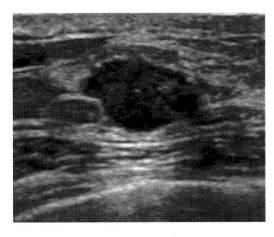

Fig. 49 Left breast US (Jan. 2021): a hypoechoic mass with microlobulated margins. US-CNB = IDC

6. Arteriovenous invasion: absent.
7. Lymphovascular invasion: present, intratumoral.
8. Tumor border: infiltrative.
9. Microcalcification: present, tumoral/non-tumoral.
10. Pathological TN category (AJCC 2017): pT1c.

Note: 1. The inferior margin of the lumpectomy specimen (slide 2) is close to ductal carcinoma in situ (3 mm) but this margin submitted for frozen diagnosis (Fro 4) is free of tumor.

2. The medial margin of the lumpectomy specimen (slide 5) is close to ductal carcinoma in

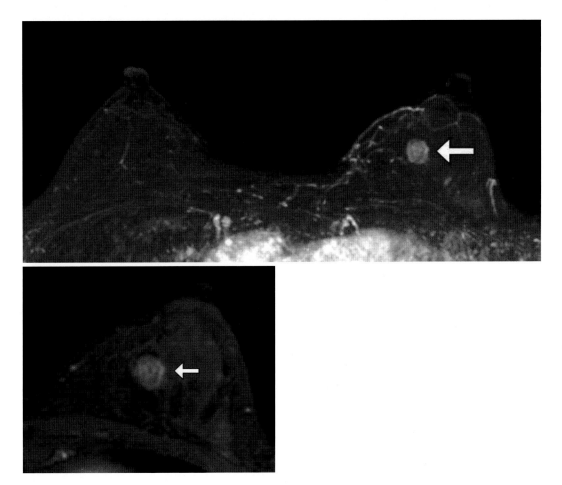

Fig. 50 Breast MRI (Jan. 2021): an irregular enhancing mass in the left breast

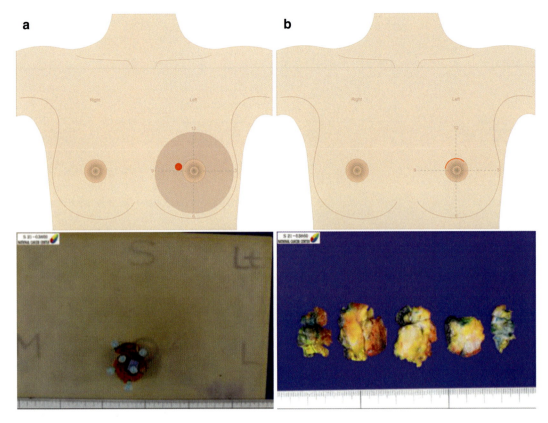

Fig. 51 (**a**) Gross pathology of lumpectomy specimen. (**b**) The margins get marked and sliced with different colors on each direction

situ (<1 mm) but this margin submitted for frozen diagnosis (Fro 4) is free of tumor.

	Result	Intensity	Positive %
Estrogen receptor	Strong (8/8)	3	>2/3
Progesterone receptor	Strong (8/8)	3	>2/3
C-erbB2	Positive (3+)		
Ki-67	Positive in 71% of tumor cells		

10 Case 10

10.1 Patient History and Progress

Female/32 years old, pre-menopause.

Self-detected skin changes and mass lesion on left breast.

Family history of breast cancer, maternal aunt. No comorbidities.

BRCA 1 and 2 mutation: Not detected, NBN and PALB2 VUS (variant of uncertain).

10.2 Important Radiologic Findings

See Figs. 52, 53, 54, 55, 56 and 57.

10.3 Courses of Treatment

Neoadjuvant chemotherapy (#6 cycles of docetaxel and carboplatin and trastuzumab and pertuzumab) + Operation + Post-operative radiation therapy + Trastuzumab emtansine + Letrozole 2.5 mg/day with goserelin.

HR(+) HER2(+) Breast Cancer

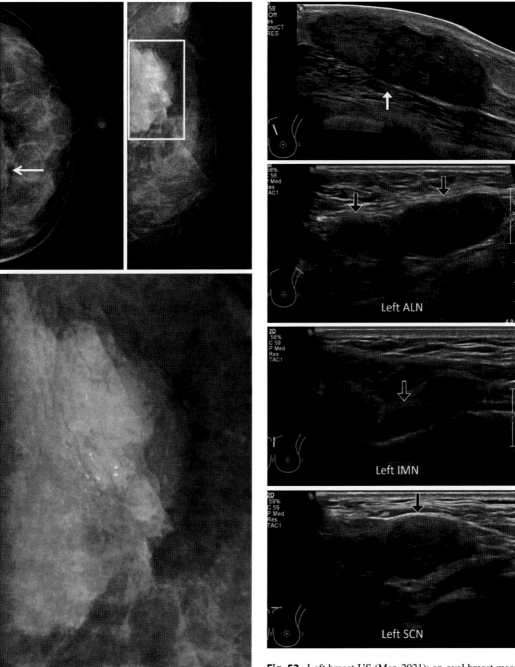

Fig. 52 Left mammography (Mar. 2021): an irregular mass with microcalcifications at upper inner quadrant

Fig. 53 Left breast US (Mar. 2021): an oval breast mass (white arrow, US-CNB = IDC) with multiple enlarged lymph nodes at ipsilateral axilla (US-CNB = metastatic ductal carcinoma), internal mammary chain, and supraclavicular area (black arrows)

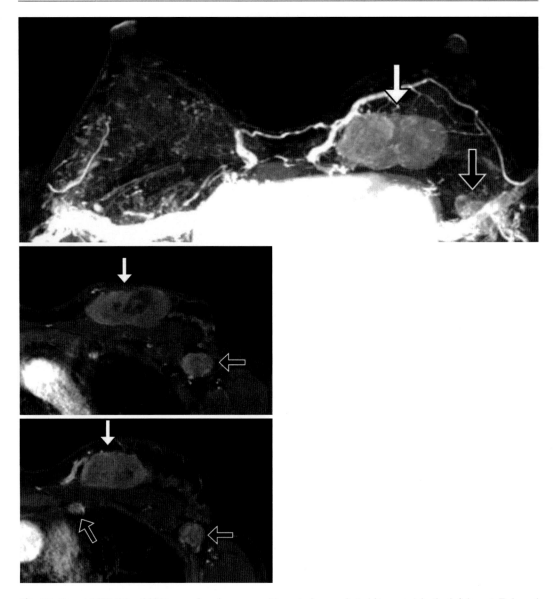

Fig. 54 Breast MRI (Mar. 2021): an enhancing mass with central necrosis (white arrow) in the left breast. Enlarged lymph nodes at the left axilla and internal mammary chain (black arrows)

Operation: Left modified radical mastectomy (Fig. 58).

10.3.1 Pathology Report

1. Invasive Ductal Carcinoma.
   (a) Post-chemotherapy status.
   (b) Size of tumor: 3.0 cm (ypT2).
   (c) Histologic grade: 2/3 (tubule formation: 3/3, nuclear pleomorphism: 3/3, mitotic count: 1/3, 3/10 HPF).
   (d) Intraductal component: present, intratumoral/extratumoral (5%) (nuclear grade: high, necrosis: present, architectural pattern: cribriform/solid/comedo, extensive intraductal component: absent).
   (e) Skin: dermal involvement of tumor.
   (f) Nipple: no involvement of tumor.
   (g) Surgical margins:
      - deep margin: (see Note 1),
      - superficial margin: (see Note 2).

Fig. 55 PET-CT shows (**a**) a hypermetabolic mass in the left breast (mSUV = 12.4) and (**b**) hypermetabolic lymph nodes in the left axilla level I–II, left internal mammary area, and (**c**) left supraclavicular fossa. (**d**) A hypermetabolic mass (white arrow) in the left breast. Hypermetabolic lymph nodes at the left axilla, internal mammary chain, and supraclavicular area (black arrows)

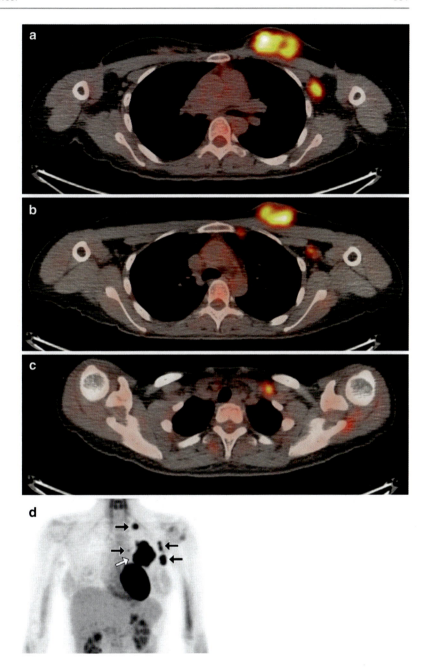

(h) Lymph nodes:
- metastasis in seven out of nine axillary lymph nodes (ypN2a) (sentinel LN: 1/3, axillary LN: 6/6),
- perinodal extension: present,
- size of metastatic carcinoma: 10 mm.

(i) Arteriovenous invasion: absent.

(j) Lymphovascular invasion: present, intratumoral/peritumoral.

(k) Tumor border: infiltrative.

(l) Microcalcification: present, tumoral/non-tumoral.

(m) Pathological TN category (AJCC 2017): ypT2N2a.

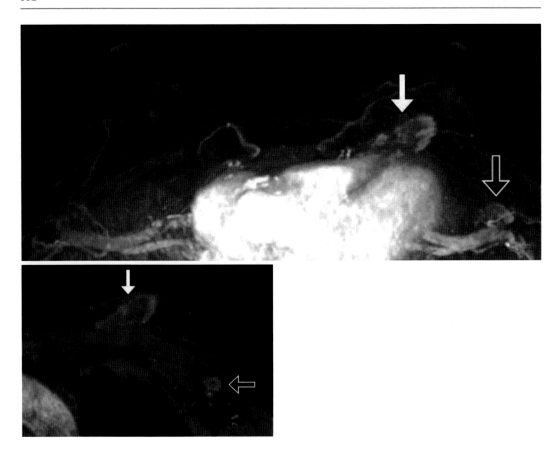

Fig. 56 Post-NAC breast MRI (July 2021): a residual left breast mass (white arrow) and axillary lymph node (black arrow) after NAC

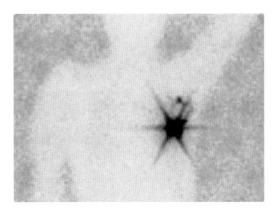

Fig. 57 Lymphoscintigraphy shows visualized sentinel lymph nodes in the left axilla

2. Fibroadenoma

Note: 1. The deep margin of the lumpectomy specimen (slides 1 and 2) is close to invasive ductal carcinoma (<1 mm) but this margin submitted for frozen diagnosis (Fro 5) is free of tumor.

2. The superficial margin of the lumpectomy specimen (slide 1) is close to invasive ductal carcinoma (<1 mm) but this margin submitted for frozen diagnosis (Fro 6) is free of tumor.

	Result	Intensity	Positive %
Estrogen receptor	Strong (8/8)	3	>2/3
Progesterone receptor	Weak (3/8)	2	<1%
C-erbB2	Positive (3+)		
Ki-67	Positive in 4% of tumor cells		

HR(+) HER2(+) Breast Cancer

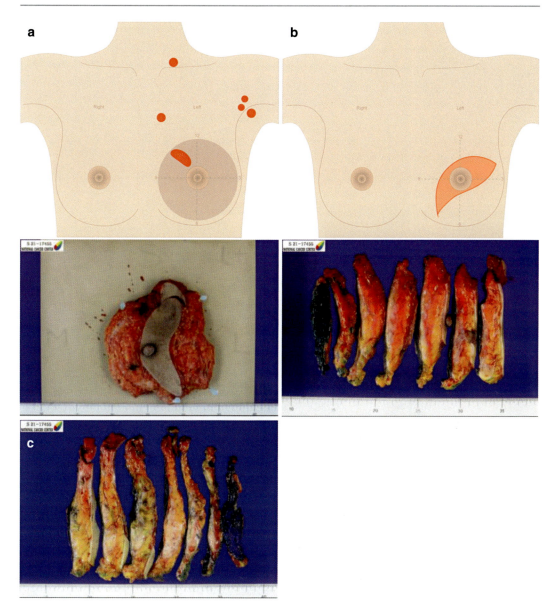

Fig. 58 (**a**) Gross pathology of mastectomy specimen. (**b**, **c**) The margins get marked and sliced with different colors on each direction

11 Case 11

11.1 Patient History and Progress

Female/60 years old, post-menopause.
Screen detected microcalcification on upper outer portion of right breast.

No family history.
Hypertension.

11.2 Important Radiologic Findings

See Figs. 59, 60, 61 and 62.

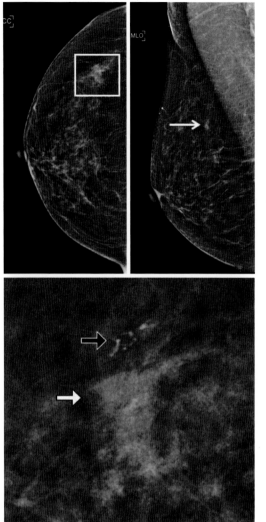

Fig. 59 Right mammography (Oct. 2020): an irregular mass (white arrow) with adjacent microcalcifications (black arrow)

11.3 Courses of Treatment

Operation + Adjuvant chemotherapy (#4 cycles of doxorubicin and cyclophosphamide) + Post-operative radiation therapy + Trastuzumab + Letrozole 2.5 mg/day.

Operation: Right breast conserving surgery (first operation), sentinel lymph node biopsy (second operation) (Fig. 63).

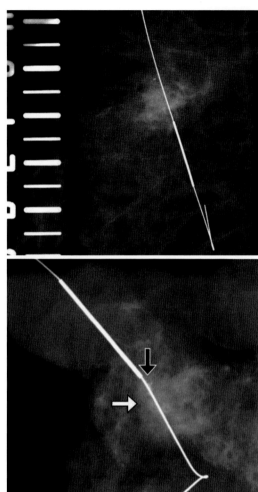

Fig. 60 MG-guided needle localization and excision (Jan. 2021): retrieval of the microcalcifications (black arrow) and mass (white arrow) in the surgical specimen

11.3.1 Pathology Report

1. Invasive Ductal Carcinoma.
   (a) Size of tumor: 1.1 cm (pT1c).
   (b) Histologic grade: 2/3 (tubule formation: 3/3, nuclear pleomorphism: 2/3, mitotic count: 1/3, 2/10HPF).
   (c) Intraductal component: present, intratumoral (20%) (nuclear grade: low, necrosis: absent, architectural pattern: cribriform, extensive intraductal component: absent).

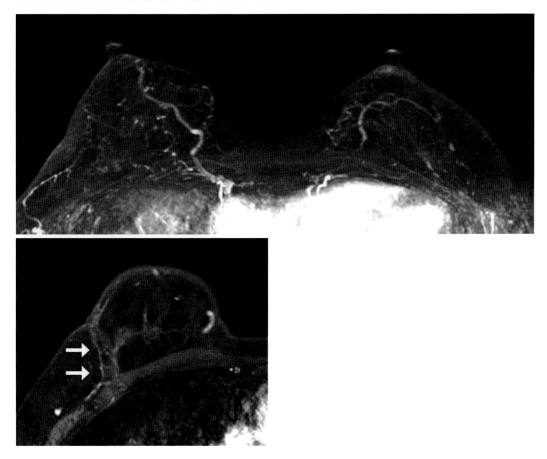

Fig. 61 Breast MRI (Feb. 2021): post-operative change (white arrows) without residual enhancing lesion in the right breast

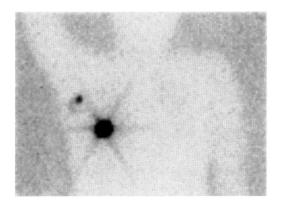

Fig. 62 Lymphoscintigraphy shows visualized sentinel lymph nodes in the right axilla

(d) Surgical margins:
- superior margin: 30 mm,
- inferior margin: 2 mm from invasive ductal carcinoma (slide 5),
- medial margin: 15 mm,
- lateral margin: 10 mm,
- deep margin: 2 mm,
- superficial margin: 10 mm.

(e) Arteriovenous invasion: absent.
(f) Lymphovascular invasion: absent.
(g) Tumor border: infiltrative.
(h) Microcalcification: present, non-tumoral.
(i) Pathological TN category (AJCC 2017): pT1cNx.

2. Intraductal papilloma

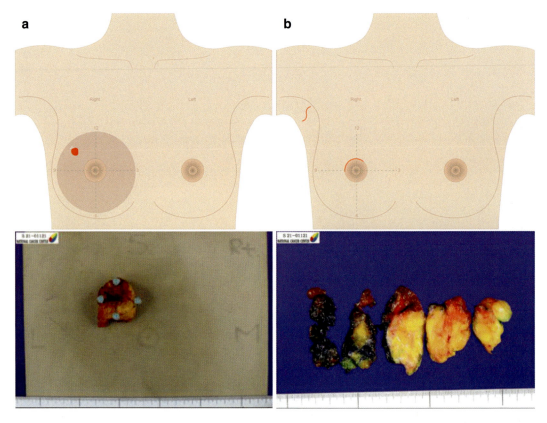

Fig. 63 (**a**) Gross pathology of lumpectomy specimen. (**b**) The margins get marked and sliced with different colors on each direction

Lymph node, right sentinel, excision: No metastasis in five axillary lymph nodes (pN0(sn)) (right sentinel LN: 0/5).

1. Post-excision status.

	Result	Intensity	Positive %
Estrogen receptor	Strong (8/8)	3	>2/3
Progesterone receptor	Weak (4/8)	2	1–10%
C-erbB2	Positive (3+)		
Ki-67	Positive in 17% of tumor cells		

12 Case 12

12.1 Patient History and Progress

Female/63 years old, post-menopause.

Screen detected mass lesion on left breast 10 o'clock direction.

No family history.

s/p Idiopathic thrombocytopenic purpura (2020).

12.2 Important Radiologic Findings

See Figs. 64, 65, 66, 67 and 68.

HR(+) HER2(+) Breast Cancer

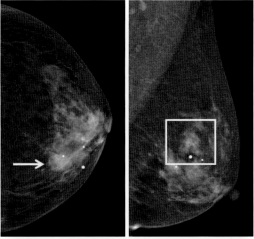

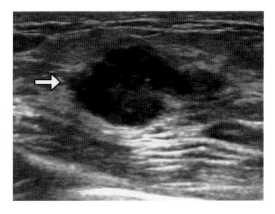

Fig. 65 Left breast US (Oct. 2020): an irregular hypoechoic mass. US-CNB = IDC

12.3.1 Pathology Report

Invasive Ductal Carcinoma
1. Post-chemotherapy status.
2. Size of tumor: 0.3 cm (ypT1a).
3. Histologic grade: 3/3 (tubule formation: 3/3, nuclear pleomorphism: 3/3, mitotic count: 2/3, 11/10HPF).
4. Intraductal component: present, intratumoral/extratumoral (50%) (nuclear grade: high, necrosis: absent, architectural pattern: micropapillary, extensive intraductal component: present).
5. Skin: no involvement of tumor.
6. Surgical margins:
   (a) superior margin: 10 mm,
   (b) inferior margin: (see Note 1),
   (c) medial margin: (see Note 2),
   (d) lateral margin: 20 mm,
   (e) deep margin: 2 mm,
   (f) superficial margin: 2 mm.
7. Lymph nodes: no metastasis in one axillary lymph node (ypN0(sn)) (sentinel LN: 0/1).
8. Arteriovenous invasion: absent.
9. Lymphovascular invasion: absent.
10. Tumor border: infiltrative.
11. Microcalcification: present, tumoral/non-tumoral.
12. Pathological TN category (AJCC 2017): ypT1aN0(sn).

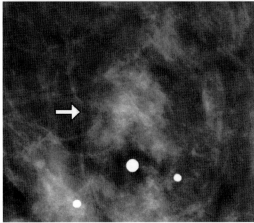

Fig. 64 Left mammography (Sep. 2020): an irregular mass at upper inner quadrant

12.3 Courses of Treatment

Neoadjuvant chemotherapy (#1 cycle of docetaxel and carboplatin and trastuzumab and pertuzumab followed by #5 cycles of docetaxel and carboplatin) + Operation + Adjuvant chemotherapy (doxorubicin and cyclophosphamide) + Post-operative radiation therapy + Letrozole 2.5 mg/day.

Operation: Left breast conserving surgery, sentinel lymph node biopsy (Fig. 69).

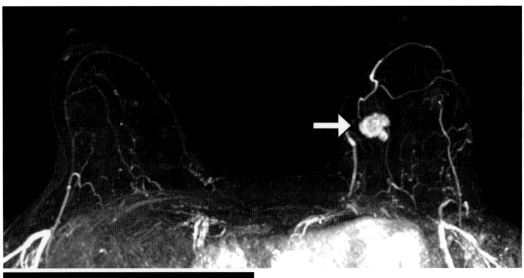
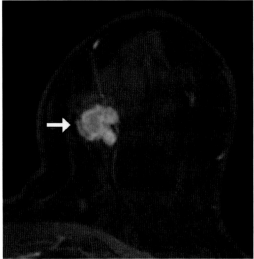

Fig. 66 Breast MRI (Oct. 2020): an irregular enhancing mass in the left breast

Note: 1. The inferior margin of the lumpectomy specimen (slide A3) is close to ductal carcinoma in situ (2 mm) but this margin submitted for frozen diagnosis (Fro 2) is free of tumor.

2. The medial margin of the lumpectomy specimen (slide 1) is close to ductal carcinoma in situ (<1 mm) but this margin submitted for frozen diagnosis (Fro 3) is free of tumor.

	Result	Intensity	Positive %
Estrogen receptor	Strong (8/8)	3	>2/3
Progesterone receptor	Weak (3/8)	1	1–10%
C-erbB2	Negative (1+)		
	Equivocal (2+) in core needle biopsy		
Ki-67	Positive in 4% of tumor cells		
SISH	Positive		

HR(+) HER2(+) Breast Cancer

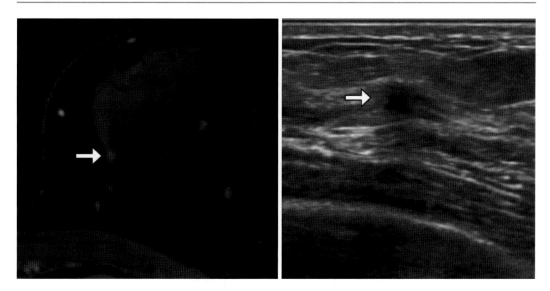

Fig. 67 Post-NAC breast MRI and US (Mar. 2021): decreased size of the tumor after NAC

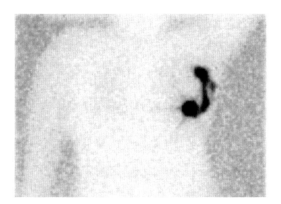

Fig. 68 Lymphoscintigraphy shows visualized sentinel lymph nodes in the left axilla

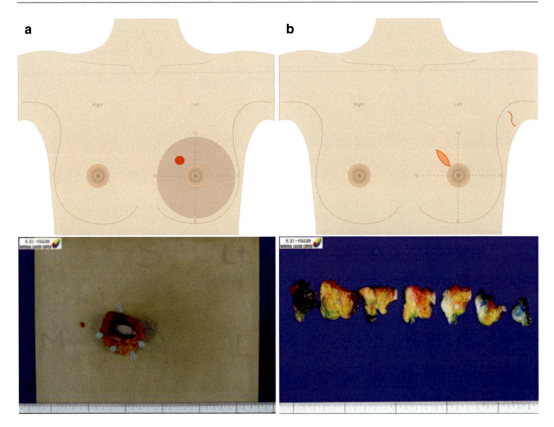

Fig. 69 (**a**) Gross pathology of lumpectomy specimen. (**b**) The margins get marked and sliced with different colors on each direction

13 Case 13

13.1 Patient History and Progress

Female/53 years old, post-menopause.
  Screen detected mass lesion on left breast 1:30 o'clock direction.
  No family history.
  Hypertension, arrhythmia, s/p myomectomy.

13.2 Important Radiologic Findings

See Figs. 70, 71 and 72.

13.3 Courses of Treatment

Operation + Adjuvant chemotherapy (#4 cycles of docetaxel and cyclophosphamide) + Post-operative radiation therapy + Trastuzumab + Letrozole 2.5 mg/day.
  Operation: Left breast conserving surgery, sentinel lymph node biopsy (Fig. 73).

13.3.1 Pathology Report

Invasive Ductal Carcinoma
1. Size of tumor: 2.1 cm (pT2).
2. Histologic grade: 2/3 (tubule formation: 3/3, nuclear pleomorphism: 2/3, mitotic count: 1/3, 15/10 HPF).

HR(+) HER2(+) Breast Cancer

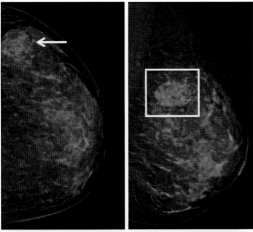

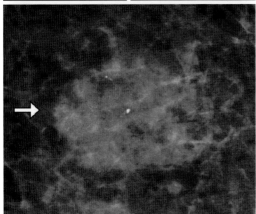

Fig. 70 Left mammography (Feb. 2021): an irregular mass with microcalcifications at upper outer quadrant

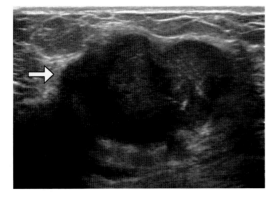

Fig. 71 Left breast US (Mar. 2021): an irregular hypoechoic mass. US-CNB = IDC

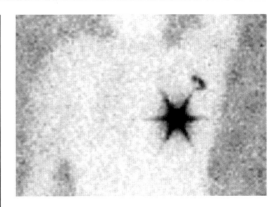

Fig. 72 Lymphoscintigraphy shows visualized sentinel lymph nodes in the left axilla

3. Intraductal component: present, intratumoral/extratumoral (10%) (nuclear grade: low, necrosis: present, architectural pattern: solid/comedo, extensive intraductal component: absent).
4. Skin: no involvement of tumor.
5. Surgical margins:
   (a) superior margin: 10 mm,
   (b) inferior margin: 10 mm,
   (c) medial margin: 5 mm,
   (d) lateral margin: 5 mm,
   (e) deep margin: 2 mm,
   (f) superficial margin: 2 mm.
6. Lymph nodes: no metastasis in one axillary lymph node (pN0(sn)) (sentinel LN: 0/1).
7. Arteriovenous invasion: absent.
8. Lymphovascular invasion: present, intratumoral.
9. Tumor border: infiltrative.
10. Microcalcification: present, tumoral/non-tumoral.
11. Pathological TN category (AJCC 2017): pT2N0(sn).

	Result	Intensity	Positive %
Estrogen receptor	Strong (8/8)	3	>2/3
Progesterone receptor	Strong (7/8)	3	1/3–2/3
C-erbB2	Positive (3+)		
Ki-67	Positive in 42% of tumor cells		

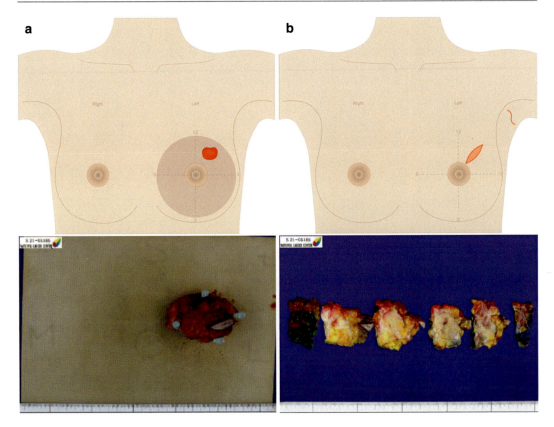

Fig. 73 (**a**) Gross pathology of lumpectomy specimen. (**b**) The margins get marked and sliced with different colors on each direction

14 Case 14

14.1 Patient History and Progress

Female/51 years old, peri-menopause.
Screen detected mass lesion on portion of lower of right breast.
Family history of breast cancer, sister.
Hypothyroidism (taking on synthroid).
BRCA 1 and 2 mutation: Not detected.

14.2 Important Radiologic Findings

See Figs. 74, 75 and 76.

14.3 Courses of Treatment

Operation + Adjuvant chemotherapy (#4 cycles of doxorubicin and cyclophosphamide followed by #4 cycles of docetaxel and trastuzumab) + Post-operative radiation therapy + Trastuzumab + Tamoxifen 20 mg/day.
Operation: Right breast conserving surgery, sentinel lymph node biopsy (Fig. 77).

14.3.1 Pathology Report

Invasive Ductal Carcinoma
1. Size of tumor: 1.5 cm (pT1c(m)).
2. Histologic grade: 2/3 (tubule formation: 2/3, nuclear pleomorphism: 3/3, mitotic count: 2/3, 11/10 HPF).

HR(+) HER2(+) Breast Cancer

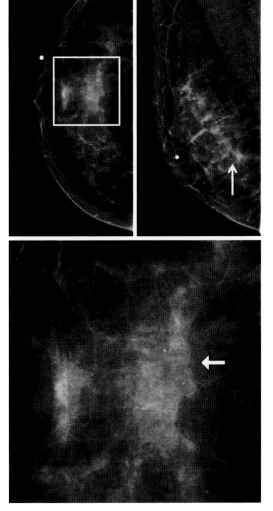

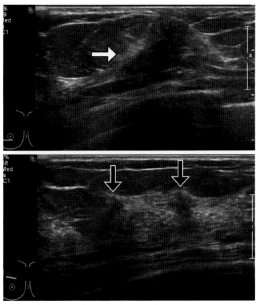

Fig. 75 Right breast US (Mar. 2021): an irregular enhancing mass at 7 o'clock direction (white arrow, US-CNB = IDC). Two isoechoic masses with non-parallel orientation at 12 o'clock direction (black arrows, US-CNB = IDC)

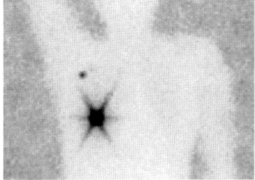

Fig. 74 Right mammography (Mar. 2021): an irregular mass with microcalcifications at lower outer quadrant

Fig. 76 Lymphoscintigraphy shows visualized sentinel lymph nodes in the right axilla

3. Intraductal component: present, intratumoral/extratumoral (50%) (nuclear grade: high, necrosis: present, architectural pattern: cribriform/solid/comedo, extensive intraductal component: present).
4. Skin: no involvement of tumor.
5. Surgical margins:
   (a) superior margin: 10 mm,
   (b) inferior margin: 10 mm,
   (c) medial margin: 10 mm,
   (d) lateral margin: 5 mm,
   (e) deep margin: 2 mm,
   (f) superficial margin: 2 mm.
6. Lymph nodes:
   (a) metastasis in one out of one axillary lymph node (pN1mi(sn)) (sentinel LN: 1/1),
   (b) perinodal extension: present,
   (c) size of metastatic carcinoma: 2 mm.
7. Arteriovenous invasion: absent.

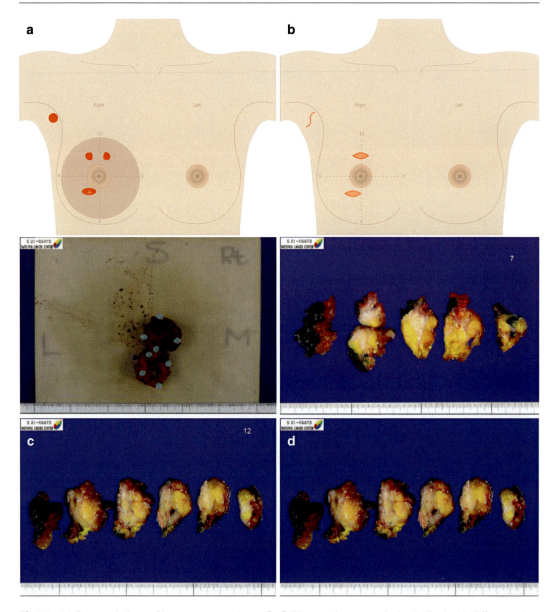

Fig. 77 (**a**) Gross pathology of lumpectomy specimen. (**b–d**) The margins get marked and sliced with different colors on each direction

8. Lymphovascular invasion: present, intratumoral.
9. Tumor border: infiltrative.
10. Microcalcification: present, tumoral/non-tumoral.
11. Pathological TN category (AJCC 2017): pT1c(m)N1mi(sn).

Invasive Ductal Carcinoma
1. Size of tumor: 0.6, 0.5 and 0.5 cm.
2. Histologic grade: 2/3 (tubule formation: 2/3, nuclear pleomorphism: 2/3, mitotic count: 2/3, 11/10 HPF).
3. Intraductal component: absent.
4. Skin: no involvement of tumor.

5. Surgical margins:
   (a) superior margin: 10 mm,
   (b) inferior margin: 10 mm,
   (c) medial margin: 5 mm,
   (d) lateral margin: 5 mm,
   (e) deep margin: 2 mm,
   (f) superficial margin: 2 mm.
6. Arteriovenous invasion: absent.
7. Lymphovascular invasion: absent.
8. Tumor border: infiltrative.
9. Microcalcification: present, tumoral.

	Result	Intensity	Positive %
Estrogen receptor	IDC—strong (8/8)	3	>2/3
	In situ—negative (2/8)	1	<1%
Progesterone receptor	IDC—strong (8/8)	3	>2/3
	In situ—negative (0/8)	0	0
C-erbB2	Positive (3+)		
Ki-67	Positive in 17% of tumor cells		

15 Case 15

15.1 Patient History and Progress

Female/42 years old, pre-menopause.

Self-detected palpable mass lesion on right breast 6 o'clock direction.

Family history of breast cancer, maternal aunt. No comorbidities.

BRCA 1 and 2 mutation: Not detected.

15.2 Important Radiologic Findings

See Figs. 78, 79, 80 and 81.

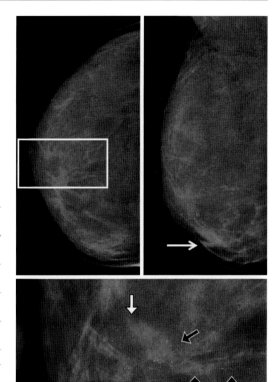

Fig. 78 Right mammography (Mar. 2021): linear distributed microcalcifications (black arrows) with an asymmetry (white arrow)

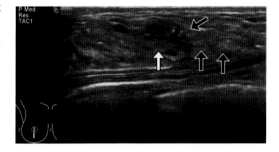

Fig. 79 Right breast US (Mar. 2021): an irregular hypoechoic mass (white arrow) with microcalcifications (black arrow). US-CNB = IDC

15.3 Courses of Treatment

Operation + Adjuvant chemotherapy (#4 cycles of doxorubicin and cyclophosphamide) + Post-operative radiation therapy + Trastuzumab + Tamoxifen 20 mg/day.

Operation: Right breast conserving surgery, sentinel lymph node biopsy (Fig. 82).

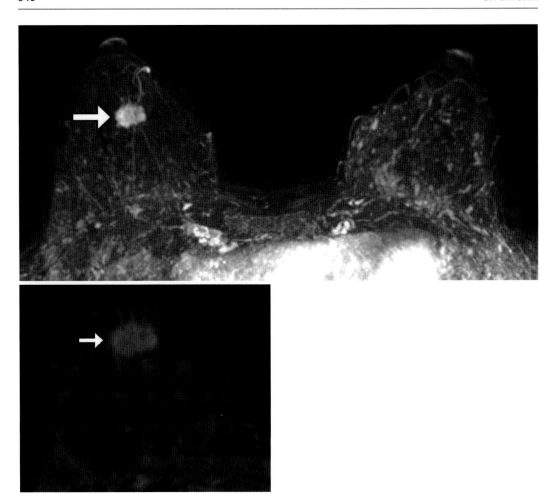

Fig. 80 Breast MRI (Mar. 2021): an irregular enhancing mass in the right breast

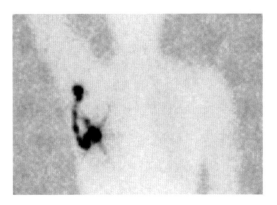

Fig. 81 Lymphoscintigraphy shows visualized sentinel lymph nodes in the right axilla

15.3.1 Pathology Report

1. Invasive Ductal Carcinoma with apocrine differentiation.
   (a) Size of tumor: 1.3 cm (pT1c).
   (b) Histologic grade: 2/3 (tubule formation: 3/3, nuclear pleomorphism: 2/3, mitotic count: 1/3, 5/10 HPF).
   (c) Intraductal component: present, intratumoral/extratumoral (15%) (nuclear grade: low, necrosis: absent, architectural pattern: solid, extensive intraductal component: absent).
   (d) Skin: no involvement of tumor.

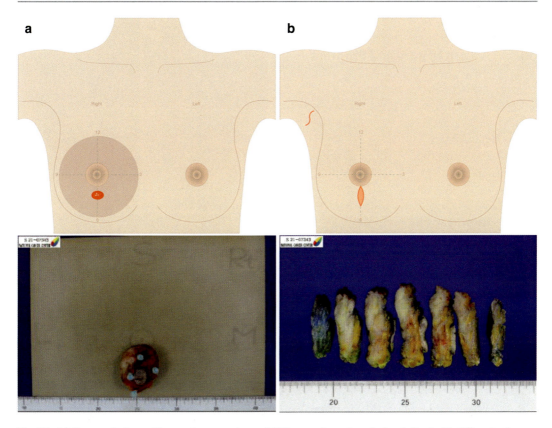

Fig. 82 (**a**) Gross pathology of lumpectomy specimen. (**b**) The margins get marked and sliced with different colors on each direction

(e) Surgical margins:
- nipple margin: positive for ductal carcinoma in situ (Fro 1),
- superior margin: 10 mm,
- inferior margin: 15 mm,
- medial margin: 20 mm,
- lateral margin: (see note),
- deep margin: 5 mm,
- superficial margin: <1 mm from invasive ductal carcinoma (slide 2).

(f) Lymph nodes: no metastasis in one axillary lymph node (pN0(sn)) (sentinel LN: 0/1).
(g) Arteriovenous invasion: absent.
(h) Lymphovascular invasion: absent.
(i) Tumor border: infiltrative.
(j) Microcalcification: present, tumoral/non-tumoral.
(k) Pathological TN category (AJCC 2017): pT1cN0(sn).

2. Fibroadenoma
3. Capillary hemangioma

Note: 1. The lateral margin of the lumpectomy specimen (slide 13) is close to ductal carcinoma in situ (3 mm) but this margin submitted for frozen diagnosis (Fro 5) is free of tumor.

	Result	Intensity	Positive %
Estrogen receptor	Strong (7/8)	2	>2/3
Progesterone receptor	Strong (7/8)	2	>2/3
C-erbB2	Positive (3+)		
Ki-67	Positive in 12% of tumor cells		

16 Case 16

16.1 Patient History and Progress

Female/54 years old, peri-menopause.

Self-detected palpable mass lesion on right breast 6 o'clock direction.

No family history.

Diabetes mellitus, S/P hysterectomy, agoraphobia.

16.2 Important Radiologic Findings

See Figs. 83, 84, 85 and 86.

16.3 Courses of Treatment

Operation + Adjuvant chemotherapy (#4 cycles of docetaxel and cyclophosphamide) + Post-operative radiation therapy + Trastuzumab + Letrozole 2.5 mg/day.

Operation: Right breast conserving surgery, sentinel lymph node biopsy (Fig. 87).

16.3.1 Pathology Report
1. Invasive Ductal Carcinoma.
    (a) Size of tumor: 1.1 cm (pT1c).
    (b) Histologic grade: 3/3 (tubule formation: 3/3, nuclear pleomorphism: 3/3, mitotic count: 2/3, 10/10 HPF).
    (c) Intraductal component: present, extratumoral (30%) (nuclear grade: high, necrosis: present, architectural pattern: papillary/cribriform, extensive intraductal component: present).
    (d) Skin: no involvement of tumor.
    (e) Surgical margins:
        - superior margin: (see note),
        - inferior margin: 15 mm,

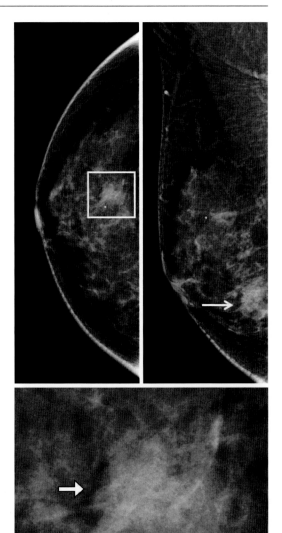

Fig. 83 Right mammography (Mar. 2021): an irregular mass at lower outer quadrant

- medial margin: 6 mm,
- lateral margin: 10 mm,
- deep margin: 3 mm,
- superficial margin: 11 mm.

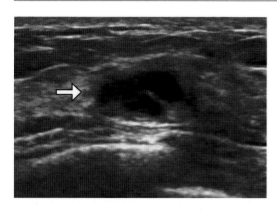

Fig. 84 Right breast US (Apr. 2021): an irregular hypoechoic mass. US-CNB = IDC

(f) Lymph nodes: no metastasis in two axillary lymph nodes (pN0(sn)) (sentinel LN: 0/2).
(g) Arteriovenous invasion: absent.
(h) Lymphovascular invasion: absent.
(i) Tumor border: infiltrative.
(j) Microcalcification: present, tumoral.
(k) Pathological TN category (AJCC 2017): pT1cN0(sn).

2. Intraductal papilloma with usual ductal hyperplasia.

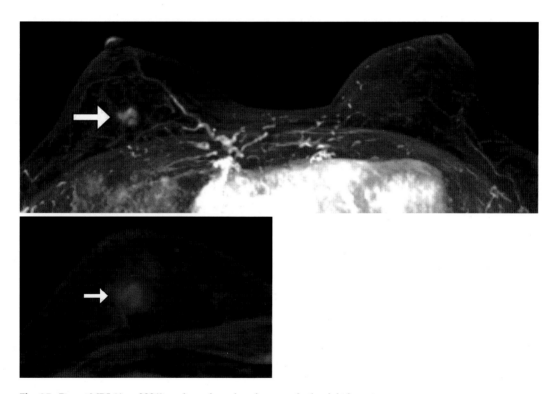

Fig. 85 Breast MRI (Apr. 2021): an irregular enhancing mass in the right breast

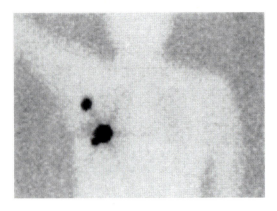

Fig. 86 Lymphoscintigraphy shows visualized sentinel lymph nodes in the right axilla

Note: 1. The superior margin of the lumpectomy specimen (slide 3) is close to ductal carcinoma in situ (2 mm) but this margin submitted for frozen diagnosis (Fro 3) is free of tumor.

	Result	Intensity	Positive %
Estrogen receptor	Strong (7/8)	2	>2/3
Progesterone receptor	Strong (7/8)	2	>2/3
C-erbB2	Positive (3+)		
Ki-67	Positive in 10% of tumor cells		

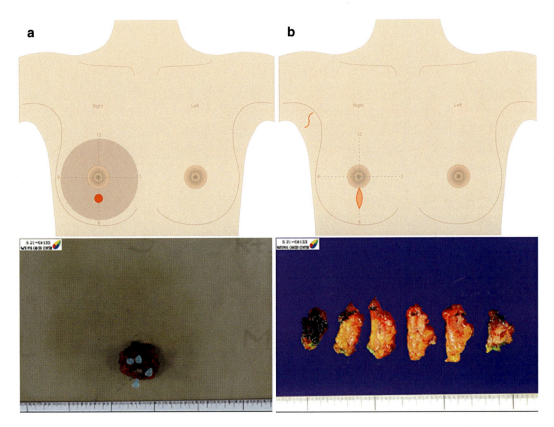

Fig. 87 (a) Gross pathology of lumpectomy specimen. (b) The margins get marked and sliced with different colors on each direction

17 Case 17

17.1 Patient History and Progress

Female/38 years old, post-menopause.
Self-detected palpable mass lesion on left breast 1 o'clock direction.
Family history of prostate cancer, maternal father.
S/P salpingo-oophorectomy (2022).
BRCA 2 mutation carrier.

17.2 Important Radiologic Findings

See Figs. 88, 89, 90 and 91.

17.3 Courses of Treatment

Operation + Adjuvant chemotherapy (#4 cycles of doxorubicin and cyclophosphamide) + Trastuzumab + Tamoxifen 20 mg/day.

Operation: Left nipple–areolar complex sparing mastectomy with immediate implant reconstruction, sentinel lymph node biopsy, Right prophylactic nipple–areolar complex sparing mastectomy with immediate implant reconstruction (Figs. 92, 93 and 94).

17.3.1 Pathology Report
[Right].

1. Ductal carcinoma in situ.
   (a) Size of tumor: 0.7 cm (pTis).
   (b) Nuclear grade: low.
   (c) Necrosis: present.
   (d) Architectural pattern: solid/comedo.
   (e) Surgical margins: (see note).
   (f) Lymph nodes: not submitted (pNx).
   (g) Microcalcification: absent.
   (h) Pathological TN category (AJCC 2017): pTisNx.
2. Fibrocystic change.

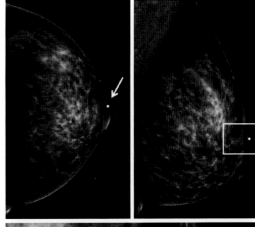

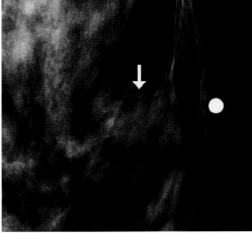

Fig. 88 Left mammography (Apr. 2021): a focal asymmetry with microcalcifications at upper outer quadrant

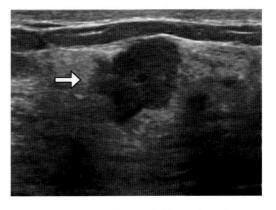

Fig. 89 Left breast US (Apr. 2021): an irregular mass with angular margins. US-CNB = IDC

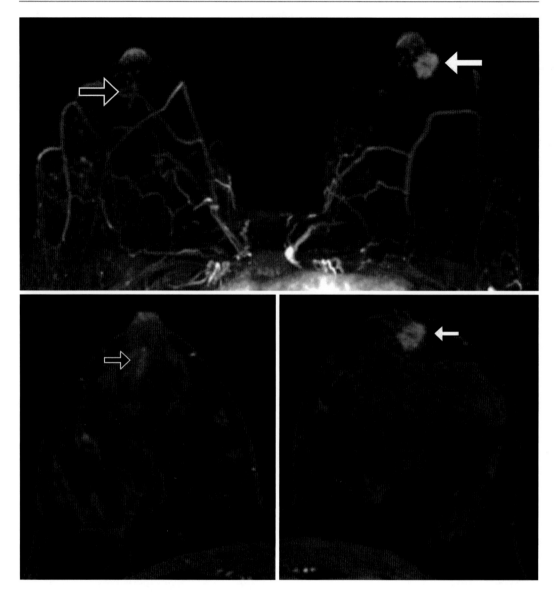

Fig. 90 Breast MRI (Apr. 2021): an irregular enhancing mass in the left breast (white arrow). Linear non-mass enhancement in the right breast (black arrow)

Note: 1. The nearest resection margin of the excision specimen (slides A1 and A2) is close to ductal carcinoma in situ (<1 mm) but this margin submitted for frozen diagnosis (Fro 13) is free of tumor.

[Left].

1. Invasive Ductal Carcinoma.
    (a) Size of tumor: 1.4 cm (pT1c).
    (b) Histologic grade: 2/3 (tubule formation: 3/3, nuclear pleomorphism: 2/3, mitotic count: 1/3, 4/10 HPF).
    (c) Intraductal component: present, intratumoral/extratumoral (5%) (nuclear grade: low, necrosis: absent, architectural pattern: cribriform, extensive intraductal component: absent).
    (d) Skin: no involvement of tumor.

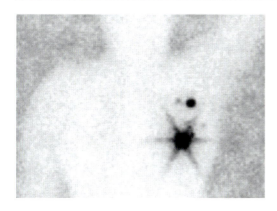

Fig. 91 Lymphoscintigraphy shows visualized sentinel lymph nodes in the left axilla

(e) Surgical margins:
- nipple margin: positive for ductal carcinoma in situ (Fro 3) (see note),
- deep margin: 27 mm,
- superficial margin: <1 mm from invasive ductal carcinoma (slide 2).

(f) Lymph nodes: no metastasis in three axillary lymph nodes (pN0(sn)) (sentinel LN: 0/3).

(g) Arteriovenous invasion: absent.

(h) Lymphovascular invasion: absent.

(i) Tumor border: infiltrative.

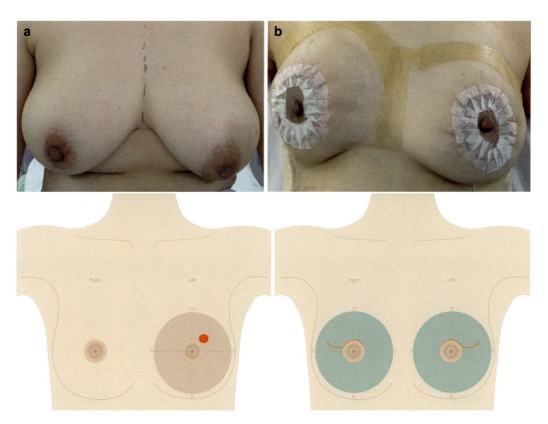

Fig. 92 (**a**) Preoperative and (**b**) immediate post-operative appearance

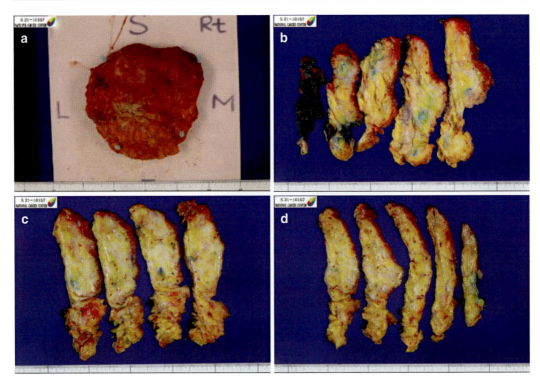

Fig. 93 (**a**) Gross pathology of right mastectomy specimen. (**b–d**) The margins get marked and sliced with different colors on each direction

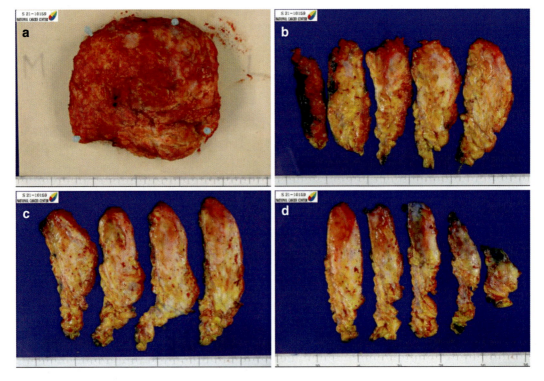

Fig. 94 (**a**) Gross pathology of left mastectomy specimen. (**b–d**) The margins get marked and sliced with different colors on each direction

HR(+) HER2(+) Breast Cancer 355

(j) Microcalcification: present, tumoral.
(k) Pathological TN category (AJCC 2017): pT1cN0(sn).
2. Fibroadenoma.

Note: 1. Ductal carcinoma in situ is present only in the permanent section of Fro 3.

	Result	Intensity	Positive %
Estrogen receptor	Strong (8/8)	3	>2/3
Progesterone receptor	Strong (7/8)	3	1/3–2/3
C-erbB2	Equivocal (2+)		
Ki-67	Positive in 19% of tumor cells		
SISH	Positive		

18 Case 18

18.1 Patient History and Progress

Female/38 years old, pre-menopause.
 Self-detected palpable mass lesion on portion of outer half of left breast.
 No family history.
 Lumbar spine disc.
 BRCA 1 and 2 mutation: Not examination.

18.2 Important Radiologic Findings

See Figs. 95, 96, 97 and 98.

18.3 Courses of Treatment

Operation + Adjuvant chemotherapy (#4 cycles of doxorubicin and cyclophosphamide followed by #4 cycles of docetaxel and trastuzumab) + Post-operative radiation therapy + Trastuzumab + Letrozole 2.5 mg/day with goserelin.

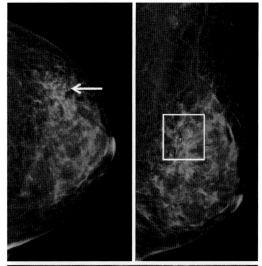

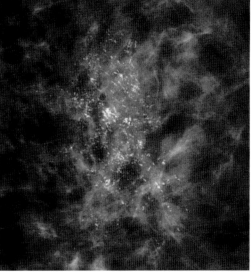

Fig. 95 Left mammography (Apr. 2021): regional fine-linear microcalcifications with architectural distortion at outer breast

Operation: Left breast conserving surgery, sentinel lymph node biopsy (Fig. 99).

18.3.1 Pathology Report

Invasive Ductal Carcinoma
1. Size of tumor: up to 3.0 cm, multifocal (pT2(Paget)).

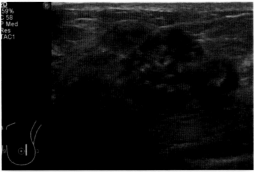
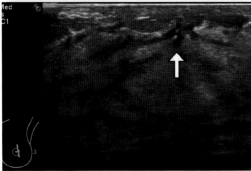
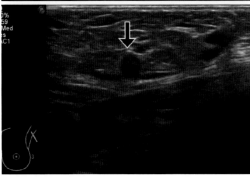

Fig. 96 Left breast US (Apr. 2021): an irregular hypoechoic mass with microcalcifications (US-CNB = IDC). Microcalcifications in subareolar ducts (white arrow). An axillary lymph node with loss of fatty hilum (black arrow)

2. Histologic grade: 3/3 (tubule formation: 3/3, nuclear pleomorphism: 3/3, mitotic count: 3/3, 23/10 HPF).
3. Intraductal component: present, intratumoral/extratumoral (20%) (nuclear grade: high, necrosis: present, architectural pattern: papillary/solid/comedo, extensive intraductal component: absent).
4. Nipple: Paget's disease.
5. Skin: no involvement of tumor.
6. Surgical margins:
   (a) superior margin: 12 mm,
   (b) inferior margin: (see Note 1),
   (c) medial margin: 15 mm,
   (d) lateral margin: 8 mm,
   (e) deep margin: <1 mm from ductal carcinoma in situ (slide 3),
   (f) superficial margin: <2 mm from invasive ductal carcinoma (slide 13).
7. Lymph nodes:
   (a) metastasis in three out of four axillary lymph nodes (pN1a(sn)) (see Note 2) (sentinel LN: 3/4),
   (b) perinodal extension: present,
   (c) size of metastatic carcinoma: 4 mm.
8. Arteriovenous invasion: absent.
9. Lymphovascular invasion: present, peritumoral.
10. Tumor border: infiltrative.
11. Microcalcification: present, tumoral/non-tumoral.
12. Pathological TN category (AJCC 2017): pT2(Paget)N1a(sn).

Note: 1. The inferior margin of the lumpectomy specimen (slide 3) is close to ductal carcinoma in situ (<1 mm) but this margin submitted for frozen diagnosis (Fro 8 and 9) is free of tumor.
2. A few isolated tumor cells are present only in the permanent section of Fro 5 for immunohistochemical staining.

	Result	Intensity	Positive %
Estrogen receptor	Strong (8/8)	3	>2/3
Progesterone receptor	Strong (8/8)	3	>2/3
C-erbB2	Positive (3+)		
Ki-67	Positive in 77% of tumor cells		

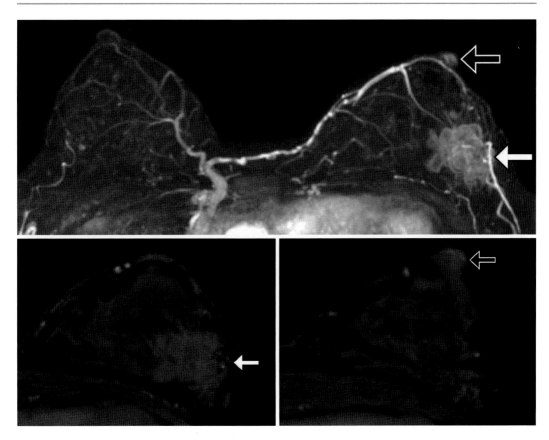

Fig. 97 Breast MRI (Apr. 2021): an irregular enhancing mass in the left breast (white arrow). Mild enhancement of the left nipple (black arrow)

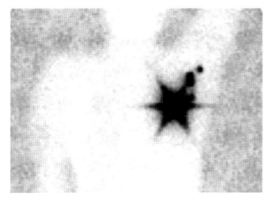

Fig. 98 Lymphoscintigraphy shows visualized sentinel lymph nodes in the left axilla

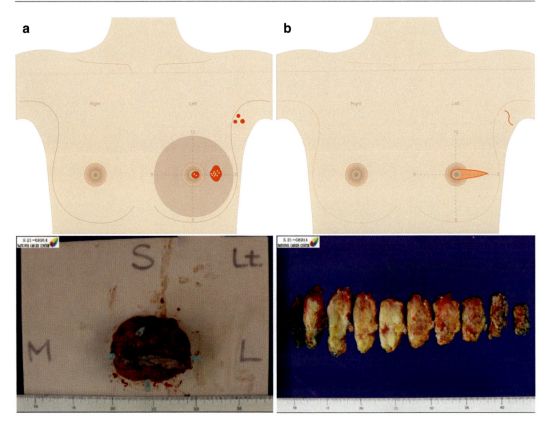

Fig. 99 (**a**) Gross pathology of lumpectomy specimen. (**b**) The margins get marked and sliced with different colors on each direction

19 Case 19

19.1 Patient History and Progress

Female/71 years old, post-menopause.

Self-detected palpable mass lesion on left breast 11 o'clock direction.

No family history.

Hypertension, dyslipidemia, s/p appendectomy.

19.2 Important Radiologic Findings

See Figs. 100, 101, 102, 103 and 104.

19.3 Courses of Treatment

Neoadjuvant chemotherapy (#6 cycles of docetaxel and carboplatin and trastuzumab and pertuzumab) + Operation + Post-operative radiation therapy + Trastuzumab + Letrozole 2.5 mg/day.

Operation: Left breast conserving surgery, sentinel lymph node biopsy (Fig. 105).

19.3.1 Pathology Report

Invasive Ductal Carcinoma
1. Post-chemotherapy status.
2. Size of tumor: 1.5 cm (ypT1c).

HR(+) HER2(+) Breast Cancer

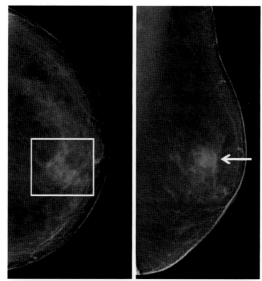

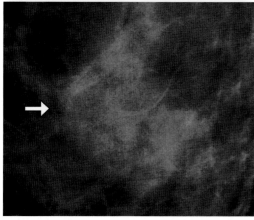

Fig. 100 Left mammography (Nov. 2020): an irregular mass at upper inner quadrant

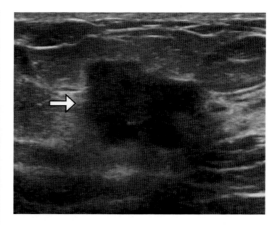

Fig. 101 Left breast US (Nov. 2020): an irregular hypoechoic mass. US-CNB = IDC

(a) superior margin: 20 mm,
(b) inferior margin: 20 mm,
(c) medial margin: 25 mm,
(d) lateral margin: 10 mm,
(e) deep margin: 13 mm,
(f) superficial margin: 18 mm.

7. Lymph nodes: no metastasis in one axillary lymph node (ypN0(sn)) (sentinel LN: 0/0, sentinel LN #2: 0/1).
8. Arteriovenous invasion: absent.
9. Lymphovascular invasion: absent.
10. Tumor border: infiltrative.
11. Microcalcification: present, non-tumoral.
12. Pathological TN category (AJCC 2017): ypT1cN0(sn).

3. Histologic grade: 3/3 (tubule formation: 3/3, nuclear pleomorphism: 3/3, mitotic count: 2/3, 10/10 HPF).
4. Intraductal component: absent.
5. Skin: no involvement of tumor.
6. Surgical margins:

	Result	Intensity	Positive %
Estrogen receptor	Intermediate (6/8)	2	1/3–2/3
Progesterone receptor	Negative (2/8)	1	<1%
C-erbB2	Positive (3+)		
Ki-67	Positive in 3% of tumor cells		

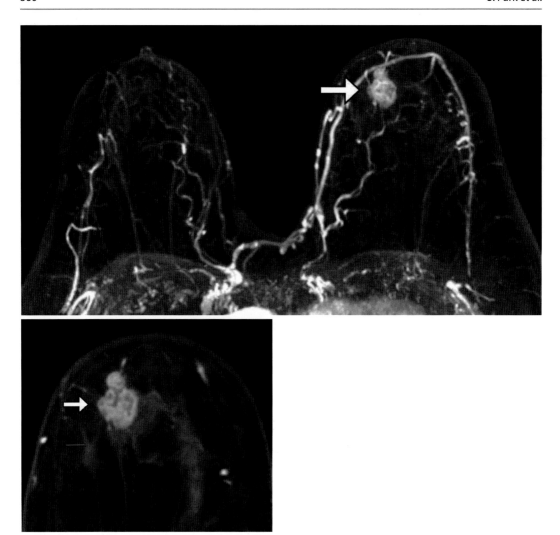

Fig. 102 Breast MRI (Nov. 2020): an irregular enhancing mass in the left breast

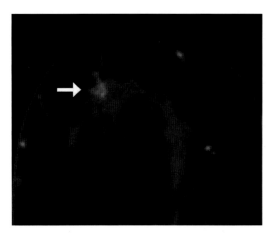

Fig. 103 Post-NAC breast MRI (Apr. 2021): decreased size of the tumor after NAC

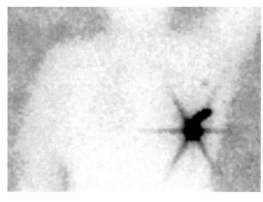

Fig. 104 Lymphoscintigraphy shows visualized sentinel lymph nodes in the left axilla

HR(+) HER2(+) Breast Cancer 361

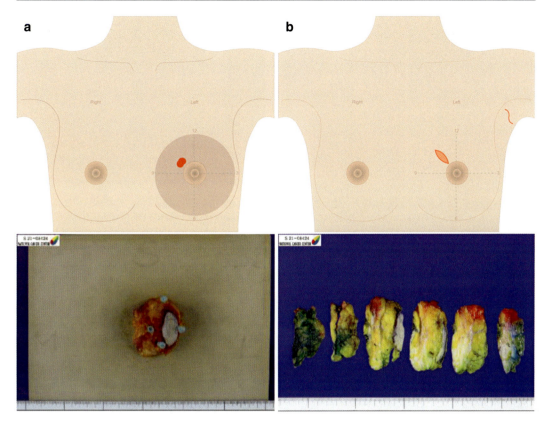

Fig. 105 (**a**) Gross pathology of lumpectomy specimen. (**b**) The margins get marked and sliced with different colors on each direction

20 Case 20

20.1 Patient History and Progress

Female/75 years old, post-menopause.
Screen detected mass lesion on right breast 8 o'clock direction.
No family history.
Asthma (follow-up).

20.2 Important Radiologic Findings

See Figs. 106, 107, 108 and 109.

20.3 Courses of Treatment

Operation + Adjuvant chemotherapy (#4 cycles of doxorubicin and cyclophosphamide followed by #11 cycles of weekly paclitaxel) + Post-operative radiation therapy + Trastuzumab + Letrozole 2.5 mg/day.
Operation: Right breast conserving surgery, sentinel lymph node biopsy (Fig. 110).

20.3.1 Pathology Report

Invasive Ductal Carcinoma
1. Post-mammotome excision status.
2. Size of tumor: 2.1 cm (pT2).

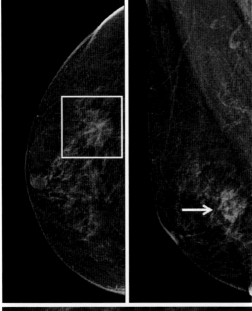

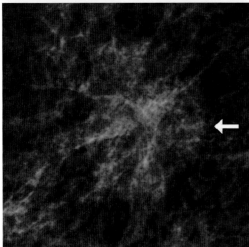

Fig. 106 Right mammography (Mar. 2021): an irregular mass at lower outer quadrant

3. Histologic grade: 2/3 (tubule formation: 3/3, nuclear pleomorphism: 2/3, mitotic count: 2/3, 10/10 HPF).

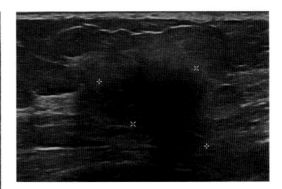

Fig. 107 Right breast US (2021-03): an irregular hypoechoic mass. Outside US-VABE = IDC

4. Intraductal component: absent.
5. Skin: no involvement of tumor.
6. Surgical margins:
    (a) superior margin: 5 mm,
    (b) inferior margin: 6 mm,
    (c) medial margin: 5 mm,
    (d) lateral margin: 5 mm,
    (e) deep margin: 4 mm,
    (f) superficial margin: 6 mm.
7. Lymph nodes: no metastasis in one axillary lymph node (pN0(sn)) (sentinel LN: 0/1).
8. Arteriovenous invasion: absent.
9. Lymphovascular invasion: absent.
10. Tumor border: infiltrative.
11. Microcalcification: present, tumoral.
12. Pathological TN category (AJCC 2017): pT2N0(sn).

	Result	Intensity	Positive %
Estrogen receptor	Strong (8/8)	3	>2/3
Progesterone receptor	Negative (0/8)	0	0
C-erbB2	Positive (3+)		
Ki-67	Positive in 15% of tumor cells		

HR(+) HER2(+) Breast Cancer

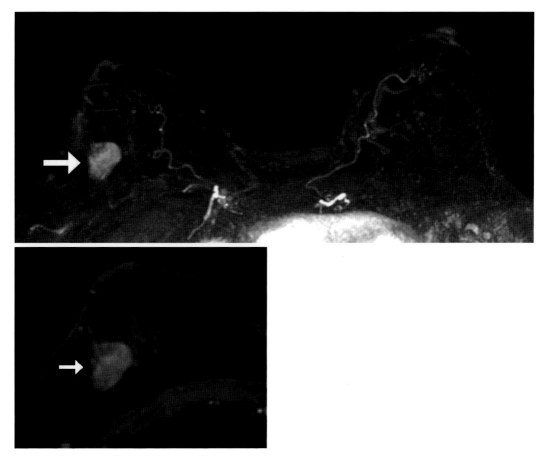

Fig. 108 Breast MRI (Apr. 2021): an enhancing mass with irregular margins in the right breast

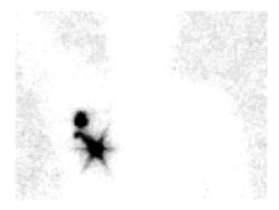

Fig. 109 Lymphoscintigraphy shows visualized sentinel lymph nodes in the right axilla

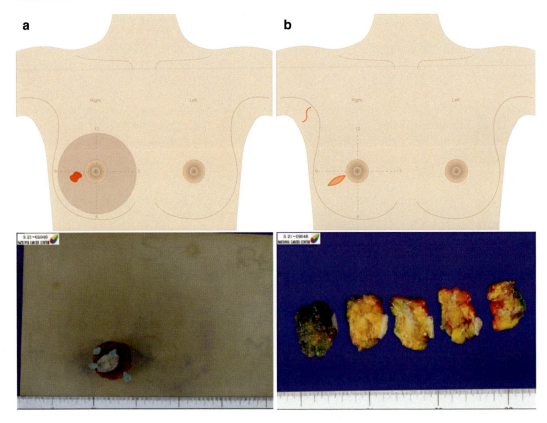

Fig. 110 (**a**) Gross pathology of lumpectomy specimen. (**b**) The margins get marked and sliced with different colors on each direction

21 Case 21

21.1 Patient History and Progress

Female/69 years old, post-menopause.
　Screen detected mass lesion on right breast 6 o'clock direction.
　Family history of breast cancer, paternal aunt, cousin (paternal).
　No comorbidities.
　BRCA 1 and 2 mutation: Not detected.

21.2 Important Radiologic Findings

See Figs. 111, 112, 113, 114, 115 and 116.

21.3 Courses of Treatment

Neoadjuvant chemotherapy (#6 cycles of docetaxel and carboplatin and trastuzumab and pertuzumab) + Operation + Postoperative radiation therapy + Letrozole 2.5 mg/day.
　Operation: Right breast conserving surgery, sentinel lymph node biopsy (Fig. 117).

21.3.1 Pathology Report

Invasive Ductal Carcinoma
1. Post-chemotherapy status.
2. Size of tumor: 1.1 cm (ypT1c).
3. Histologic grade: 2/3 (tubule formation: 3/3, nuclear pleomorphism: 2/3, mitotic count: 1/3, 1/10 HPF).

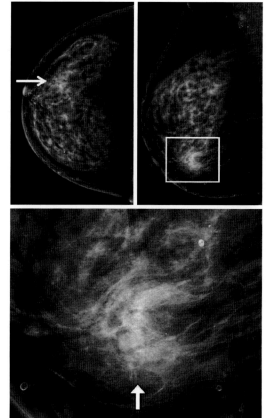

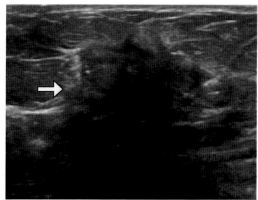

Fig. 112 Right breast US (May 2021): an irregular hypoechoic mass. US-CNB = IDC

Fig. 111 Right mammography (May 2021): an irregular mass at lower outer quadrant

4. Intraductal component: present, intratumoral/extratumoral (20%) (nuclear grade: low, necrosis: absent, architectural pattern: micropapillary/cribriform, extensive intraductal component: absent).
5. Skin: no involvement of tumor.
6. Surgical margins:
   (a) superior margin: 25 mm,
   (b) inferior margin: 50 mm,
   (c) medial margin: 10 mm,
   (d) lateral margin: 20 mm,
   (e) deep margin: 15 mm,
   (f) superficial margin: 10 mm.
7. Lymph nodes: no metastasis in one axillary lymph node (ypN0(sn)) (sentinel LN: 0/1).
8. Arteriovenous invasion: absent.
9. Lymphovascular invasion: present, intratumoral/peritumoral.
10. Tumor border: infiltrative.
11. Microcalcification: present, tumoral/non-tumoral.
12. Pathological TN category (AJCC 2017): ypT1cN0(sn).

	Result	Intensity	Positive %
Estrogen receptor	Strong (8/8)	3	>2/3
Progesterone receptor	Weak (4/8)	2	1–10%
C-erbB2	Equivocal (2+)		
Ki-67	Positive in 1% of tumor cells		
SISH	Positive		

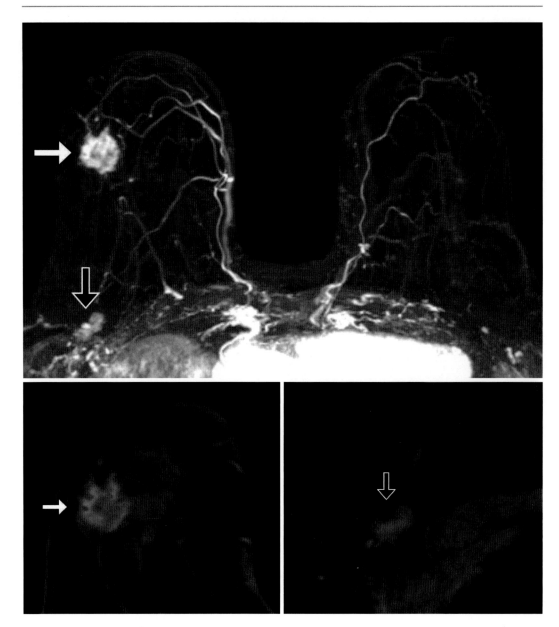

Fig. 113 Breast MRI (May 2021): an irregular enhancing mass in the right breast (white arrow). An enlarged lymph node at the right axilla (black arrow)

HR(+) HER2(+) Breast Cancer

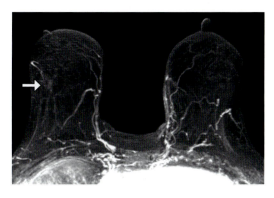

Fig. 114 Post-NAC breast MRI (Oct. 2021): decreased size of the tumor after NAC

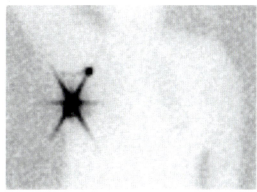

Fig. 116 Lymphoscintigraphy shows visualized sentinel lymph nodes in the right axilla

Fig. 115 PET-CT shows (**a**) focal hypermetabolic mass in the subareolar area of the right breast (mSUV = 4.3) and (**b**) mild hypermetabolic lymph node in the right axilla level I (mSUV = 0.9)

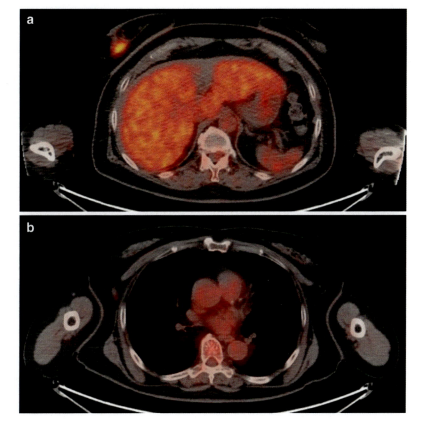

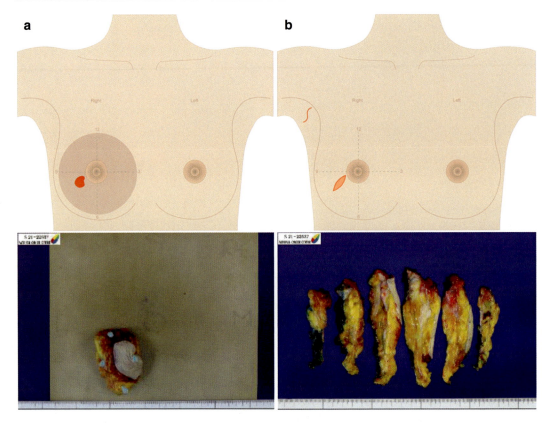

Fig. 117 (**a**) Gross pathology of lumpectomy specimen. (**b**) The margins get marked and sliced with different colors on each direction

22　Case 22

22.1　Patient History and Progress

Female/54 years old, post-menopause.
　Self-detected nipple retraction on left breast.
　No family history.
　Hepatitis B carrier.

22.2　Important Radiologic Findings

See Figs. 118, 119, 120, 121, 122, 123 and 124.

22.3　Courses of Treatment

Neoadjuvant chemotherapy (#6 cycles of docetaxel and carboplatin and trastuzumab and pertuzumab) + Operation + Trastuzumab + Letrozole 2.5 mg/day.
　Operation: Left breast conserving surgery, sentinel lymph node biopsy (Fig. 125).

22.3.1　Pathology Report

Invasive Ductal Carcinoma
1. Post-chemotherapy status.
2. Size of tumor: 0.5 cm (ypT1a).

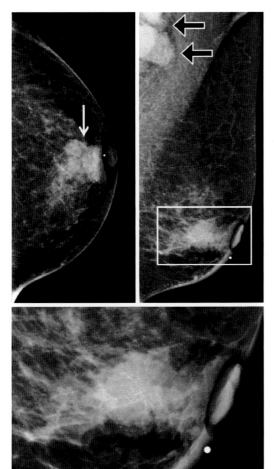
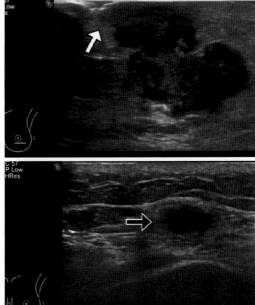

Fig. 118 Left mammography (Apr. 2021): an irregular subareolar mass with nipple retraction. Multiple enlarged lymph nodes at the axilla (black arrows)

Fig. 119 Left breast US (May 2021): an irregular subareolar mass with nipple invasion (white arrow, US-CNB = IDC). Another irregular hypoechoic mass at 6 o'clock direction (black arrow)

3. Histologic grade: 2/3 (tubule formation: 3/3, nuclear pleomorphism: 2/3, mitotic count: 1/3, <1/10HPF).
4. Intraductal component: absent.
5. Surgical margins:
   (a) superior margin: 10 mm,
   (b) inferior margin: (see Note 1),
   (c) medial margin: 5 mm,
   (d) lateral margin: 5 mm,
   (e) deep margin: <1 mm from invasive ductal carcinoma (slide 1),
   (f) superficial margin: 1 mm from invasive ductal carcinoma (slide 3).
6. Lymph nodes:
   (a) metastasis in two out of three axillary lymph nodes (ypN1mi(sn)) (see note) (sentinel LN: 1/1, axillary LN: 1/2),
   (b) perinodal extension: absent,
   (c) size of metastatic carcinoma: 0.3 mm.
7. Arteriovenous invasion: absent.
8. Lymphovascular invasion: absent.
9. Tumor border: infiltrative.
10. Microcalcification: present, non-tumoral.
11. Pathological TN category (AJCC 2017): ypT1aN1mi(sn).

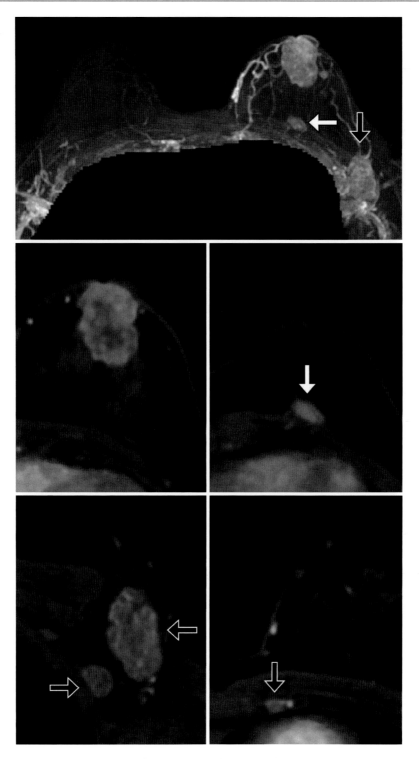

Fig. 120 Breast MRI (May 2021): an irregular enhancing mass with nipple invasion in the left breast. A satellite mass or enlarged intramammary lymph node at 6 o'clock direction (white arrow). Multiple enlarged lymph nodes at the left axilla and internal mammary chains (black arrows)

HR(+) HER2(+) Breast Cancer

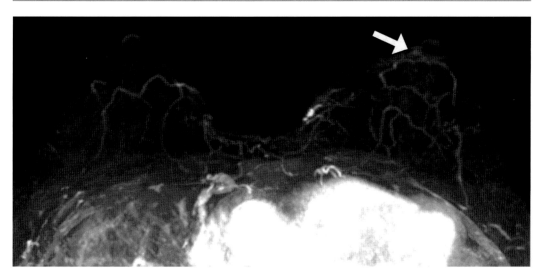

Fig. 121 Post-NAC breast MRI (Sep. 2021): residual enhancing focus after NAC

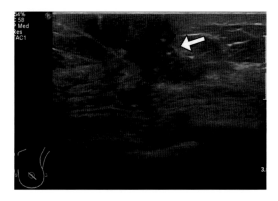

Fig. 122 Post-NAC left breast US (Oct. 2021): decreased size of the tumor after NAC

Note: 1. The inferior margin of the lumpectomy specimen (slide 3) is close to invasive ductal carcinoma (<1 mm) but this margin submitted for frozen diagnosis (Fro 5) is free of tumor.

2. Micrometastasis is present only in the permanent section of Fro 1.

	Result	Intensity	Positive %
Estrogen receptor	Strong (8/8)	3	>2/3
Progesterone receptor	Negative (0/8)	0	0
C-erbB2	Equivocal (2+)		
Ki-67	Positive in <1% of tumor cells		
SISH	Positive		

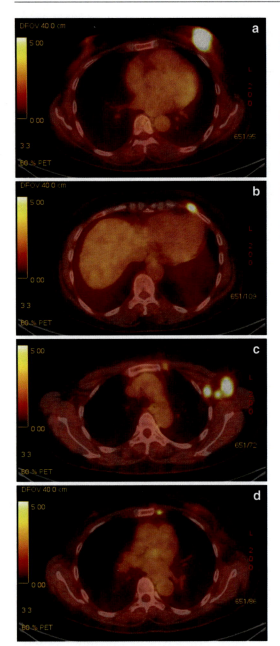

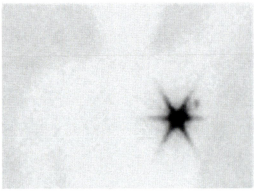

Fig. 124 Lymphoscintigraphy shows visualized sentinel lymph nodes in the left axilla

Fig. 123 PET-CT shows (**a**) a hypermetabolic mass in subareolar area of the left breast, (**b**) a hypermetabolic nodule in the left lower inner breast near the chest wall, and (**c**) multiple hypermetabolic lymph nodes in the left axilla level I–II and (**d**) left internal mammary area

HR(+) HER2(+) Breast Cancer

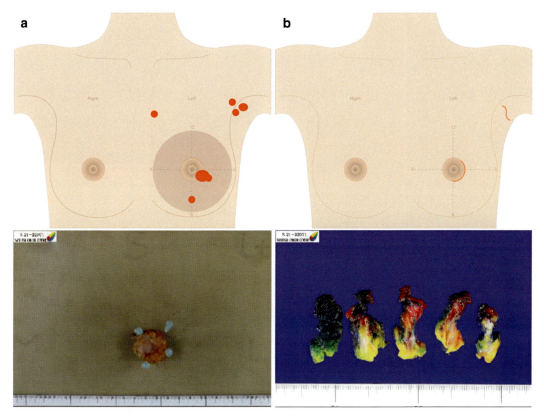

Fig. 125 (**a**) Gross pathology of lumpectomy specimen. (**b**) The margins get marked and sliced with different colors on each direction

23 Case 23

23.1 Patient History and Progress

Female/46 years old, pre-menopause.

Self-detected palpable mass lesion on both breast.

Family history of breast cancer, sister.

Hypertension, S/P varicose veins operation.

BRCA 1 and 2 mutation: Not detected (BRCAPRO mutation probability 0.118).

23.2 Important Radiologic Findings

See Figs. 126, 127, 128, 129, 130 and 131.

23.3 Courses of Treatment

Neoadjuvant chemotherapy (#6 cycles of docetaxel and carboplatin and trastuzumab and pertuzumab) + Operation + Post-

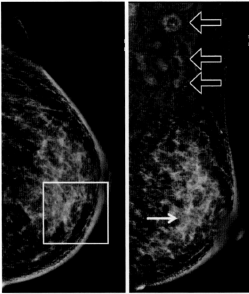

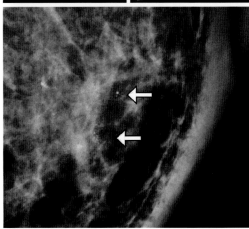

Fig. 126 Left mammography (Apr. 2021): a focal asymmetry with microcalcifications at inner center (white arrows). Diffuse edema and skin thickening of the left breast. Multiple enlarged lymph nodes at the left axilla (black arrows)

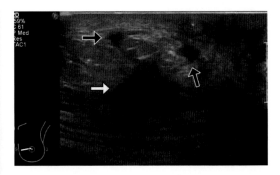

Fig. 127 Left breast US (May 2021): an irregular hypoechoic mass (white arrow) with adjacent smaller masses (black arrows). US-CNB = IDC

operative radiation therapy + Trastuzumab + Tamoxifen 20 mg/day.

Operation: Left nipple–areolar complex sparing mastectomy with immediate implant reconstruction, axillary lymph node dissection (Figs. 132 and 133).

23.3.1 Pathology Report

1. No residual tumor with stromal degeneration.
   (a) Post-chemotherapy status.
   (b) Lymph nodes: no metastasis in six axillary lymph nodes (ypN0) (axillary LN: 0/6).
2. Atypical ductal hyperplasia, focal.
3. Intraductal papilloma.
4. Fibroadenoma.

	Result	Intensity	Positive %
Estrogen receptor	Weak (4/8)	2	1–10%
Progesterone receptor	Strong (8/8)	3	>2/3
C-erbB2	Positive (3+)		
Ki-67	Positive in 30% of tumor cells		

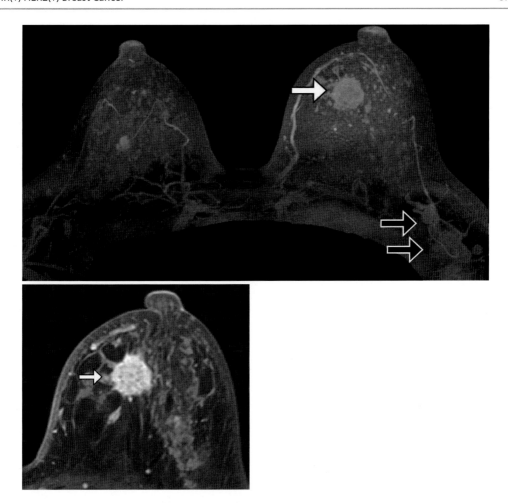

Fig. 128 Breast MRI (May 2021): an irregular enhancing mass (white arrow) with diffuse edema of the left breast. Multiple enlarged lymph nodes at the left axilla (black arrows)

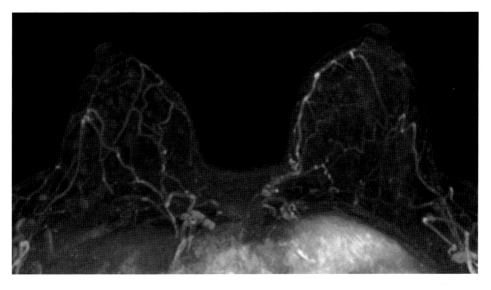

Fig. 129 Post-NAC breast MRI (Oct. 2021): no residual enhancing lesion in the left breast after NAC

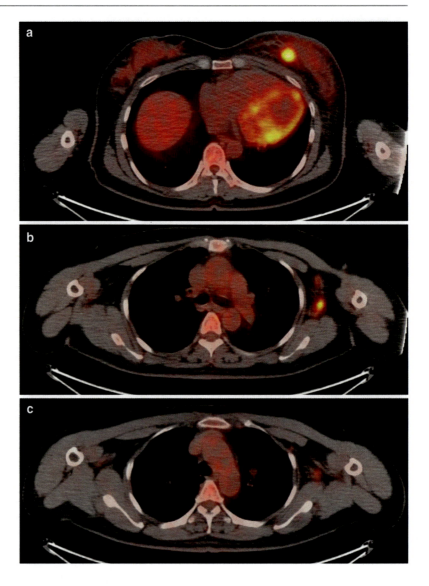

Fig. 130 PET-CT shows (**a**) a hypermetabolic mass in the left lower inner breast (mSUV = 7.7) and (**b**) multiple hypermetabolic lymph nodes in the left axilla level I–III and (**c**) left internal mammary area

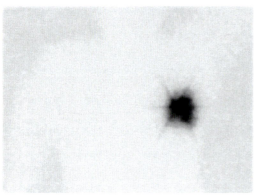

Fig. 131 Lymphoscintigraphy did not show the visualized sentinel lymph node in the left axilla

HR(+) HER2(+) Breast Cancer

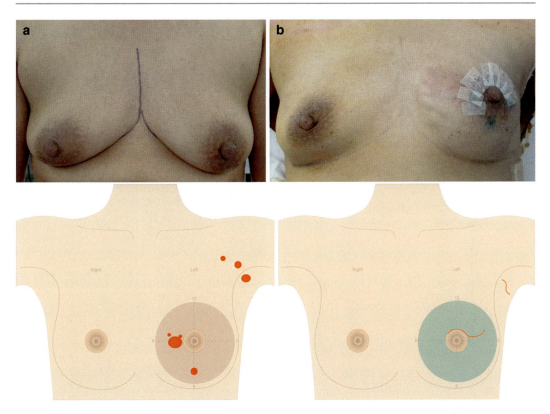

Fig. 132 (**a**) Preoperative and (**b**) immediate post-operative appearance

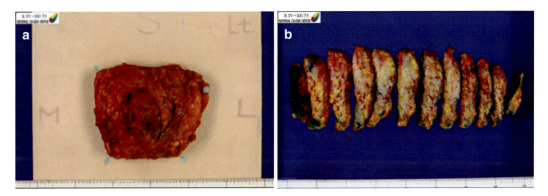

Fig. 133 (**a**) Gross pathology of mastectomy specimen. (**b**) The margins get marked and sliced with different colors on each direction

24 Case 24

24.1 Patient History and Progress

Female/41 years old, pre-menopause.
Self-detected palpable mass lesion and nipple discharge on right breast.
No family history.
S/P appendectomy, s/p hepatitis A.

24.2 Important Radiologic Findings

See Figs. 134, 135, 136, 137, 138 and 139.

24.3 Courses of Treatment

Neoadjuvant chemotherapy (#6 cycles of docetaxel and carboplatin and trastuzumab and pertuzumab) + Operation + Postoperative radiation therapy + Trastuzumab + Tamoxifen 20 mg/day.

Operation: Right breast conserving surgery, sentinel lymph node biopsy (Fig. 140).

24.3.1 Pathology Report

Ductal Carcinoma In Situ
1. Post-chemotherapy status.
2. Size of tumor: 0.2 cm (ypTis).
3. Nuclear grade: low.
4. Necrosis: absent.
5. Architectural pattern: solid.
6. Surgical margins:
    (a) superior margin: 5 mm,
    (b) inferior margin: 5 mm,
    (c) medial margin: 15 mm,
    (d) lateral margin: 10 mm,
    (e) deep margin: 5 mm,
    (f) superficial margin: 5 mm.
7. Lymph nodes: no metastasis in two axillary lymph nodes (ypN0(sn)) (sentinel LN: 0/2).
8. Microcalcification: present, tumoral/non-tumoral.
9. Pathological TN category (AJCC 2017): ypTisN0(sn).

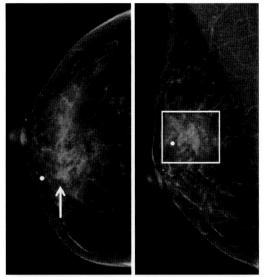

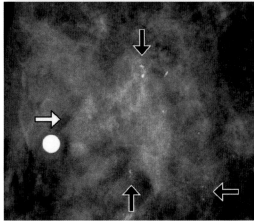

Fig. 134 Right mammography (May 2021): an irregular mass (white arrow) with microcalcifications (black arrows) at upper inner quadrant

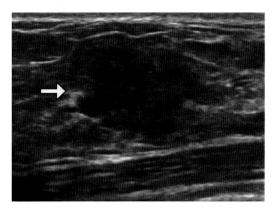

Fig. 135 Right breast US (May 2021): an irregular hypoechoic mass. US-CNB = IDC

HR(+) HER2(+) Breast Cancer

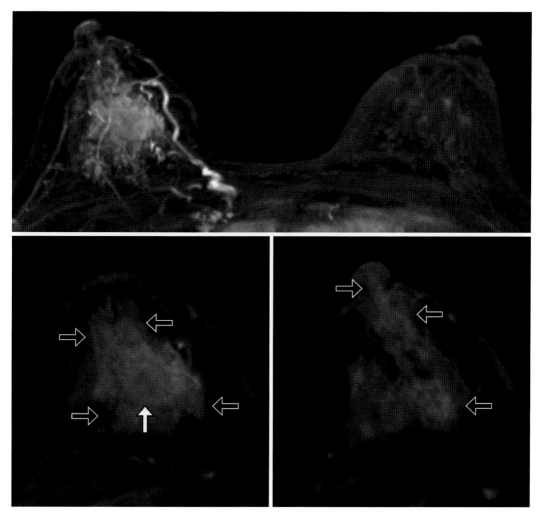

Fig. 136 Breast MRI (May 2021): an irregular enhancing mass (white arrow) with segmental non-mass enhancement involving the nipple (black arrows)

	Result	Intensity	Positive %
Estrogen receptor	Negative (0/8)	0	0
	Strong (8/8) in core needle biopsy	3	>2/3
Progesterone receptor	Negative (0/8)	0	0
	Intermediate (6/8) in core needle biopsy	3	10%-1/3
C-erbB2	Positive (3+)		
Ki-67	Not informative due to low cellularity		

Fig. 137 PET-CT shows (**a**) a hypermetabolic mass in the right breast (mSUV = 13.7) and (**b**) small lymph nodes without significant hypermetabolism in the right axilla

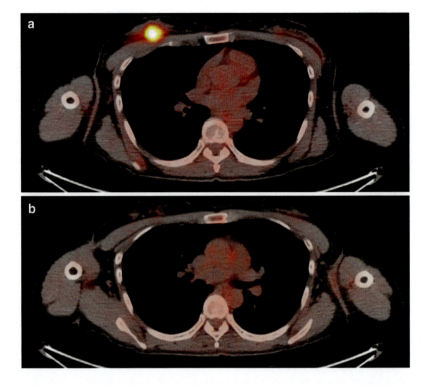

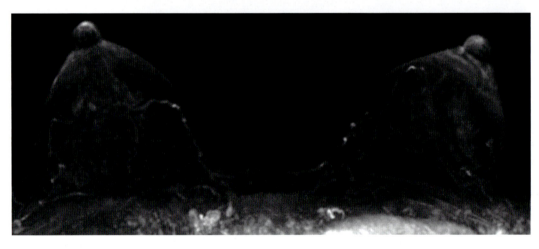

Fig. 138 Post-NAC breast MRI (Oct. 2021): nearly disappeared enhancing lesions after NAC

HR(+) HER2(+) Breast Cancer

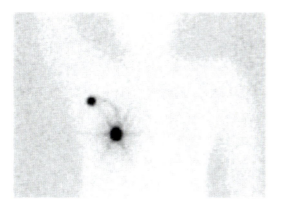

Fig. 139 Lymphoscintigraphy shows visualized sentinel lymph nodes in the right axilla

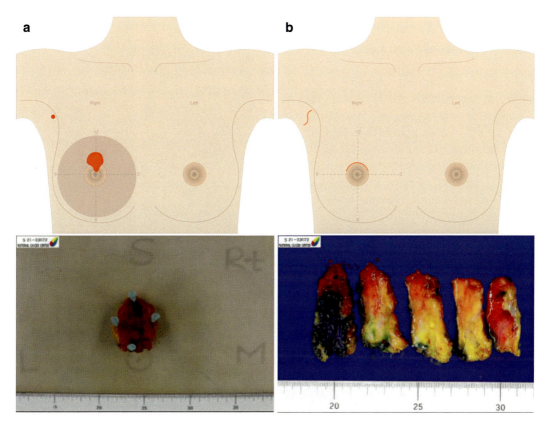

Fig. 140 (**a**) Gross pathology of lumpectomy specimen. (**b**) The margins get marked and sliced with different colors on each direction

25 Case 25

25.1 Patient History and Progress

Female/62 years old, post-menopause.

Screen detected mass lesion on right breast 5 o'clock direction and left breast subareolar area.

No family history.

Hypertension, dyslipidemia.

25.2 Important Radiologic Findings

See Figs. 141, 142, 143 and 144.

25.3 Courses of Treatment

Operation + Adjuvant chemotherapy (#4 cycles of doxorubicin and cyclophosphamide followed by #4 cycles of docetaxel and trastuzumab) + Post-operative radiation therapy + Trastuzumab + Letrozole 2.5 mg/day.

Operation: Right breast conserving surgery, sentinel lymph node biopsy, left breast conserving surgery, sentinel lymph node biopsy (Figs. 145 and 146).

25.3.1 Pathology Report
[Right].

1. Invasive Ductal Carcinoma
   (a) Size of tumor: 1.2 cm (pT1c).
   (b) Histologic grade: 2/3 (tubule formation: 2/3, nuclear pleomorphism: 2/3, mitotic count: 3/3, 15/10 HPF).
   (c) Intraductal component: present, extratumoral (30%) (nuclear grade: low, necrosis: present, architectural pattern: cribriform/solid/comedo, extensive intraductal component: absent).
   (d) Skin: no involvement of tumor.
   (e) Surgical margins:
      - superior margin: 8 mm,
      - inferior margin: 15 mm,
      - medial margin: 15 mm,
      - lateral margin: 15 mm,
      - deep margin: 2 mm,
      - superficial margin: 10 mm.
   (f) Lymph nodes: no metastasis in one axillary lymph node (pN0(sn)) (sentinel LN: 0/1).
   (g) Arteriovenous invasion: absent.
   (h) Lymphovascular invasion: present, peritumoral.

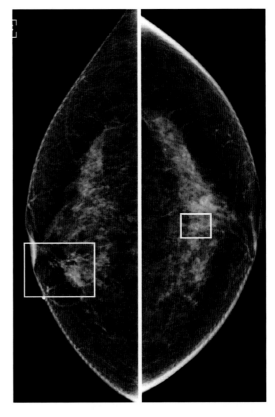

Fig. 141 Both mammography (Apr. 2021): an irregular mass with fine-linear microcalcifications at lower inner quadrant of the right breast (white arrows). Grouped fine-pleomorphic microcalcifications with asymmetry at subareolar area of the left breast (black arrow)

HR(+) HER2(+) Breast Cancer

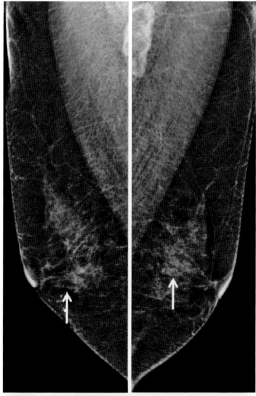

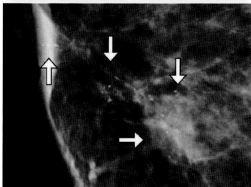

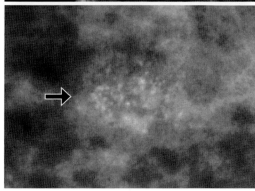

Fig. 6.141 (continued)

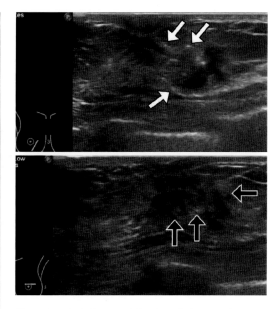

Fig. 142 Both breasts US (Apr. 2021): an irregular hypoechoic mass with microcalcifications in the right breast (white arrows). An irregular hypoechoic mass with microcalcifications in the left breast (black arrows). Both US-CNB = IDC

   (i) Tumor border: infiltrative.
   (j) Microcalcification: present, tumoral.
   (k) Pathological TN category (AJCC 2017): pT1cN0(sn).
2. Intraductal papilloma with (1) usual ductal hyperplasia, (2) microcalcification.

	Result	Intensity	Positive %
Estrogen receptor	Strong (8/8)	3	>2/3
Progesterone receptor	Strong (8/8)	3	>2/3
C-erbB2	Positive (3+)		
Ki-67	Positive in 26% of tumor cells		

[Left].

Invasive ductal carcinoma with micropapillary pattern.
1. Size of tumor: 1.1 cm (pT1c).
2. Histologic grade: 2/3 (tubule formation: 2/3, nuclear pleomorphism: 2/3, mitotic count: 2/3, 6/10 HPF).
3. Intraductal component: present, extratumoral (26%) (nuclear grade: low, necrosis: absent,

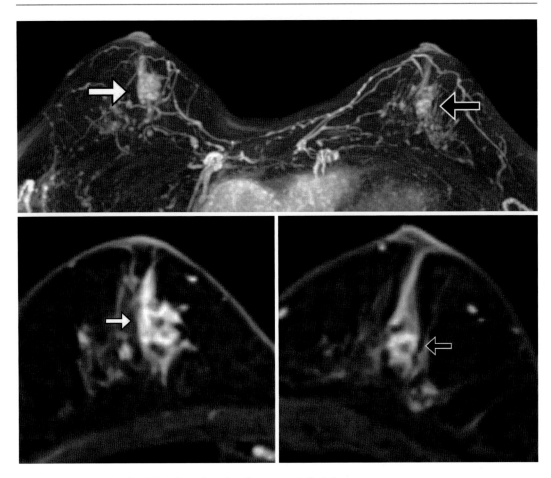

Fig. 143 Breast MRI (Mar. 2021): irregular enhancing masses in both breasts

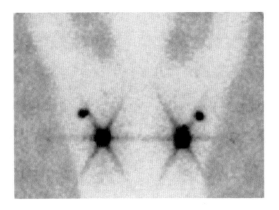

Fig. 144 Lymphoscintigraphy shows visualized sentinel lymph nodes in both axilla

architectural pattern: micropapillary/cribriform, extensive intraductal component: absent).
4. Surgical margins:
   (a) superior margin: 16 mm,
   (b) inferior margin: (see note),
   (c) medial margin: 20 mm,
   (d) lateral margin: (see note),
   (e) deep margin: 2 mm,
   (f) superficial margin: <1 mm from invasive ductal carcinoma (slides 2 and 3).
5. Lymph nodes:
   (a) metastasis in one out of seven axillary lymph nodes (pN1a) (sentinel LN: 1/3, non-sentinel LN: 0/4),

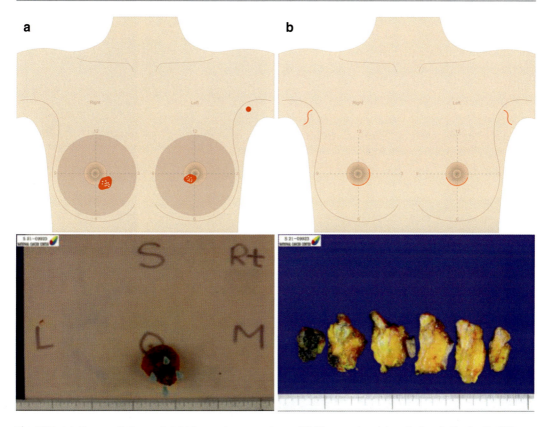

Fig. 145 (**a**) Gross pathology of right lumpectomy specimen. (**b**) The margins get marked and sliced with different colors on each direction

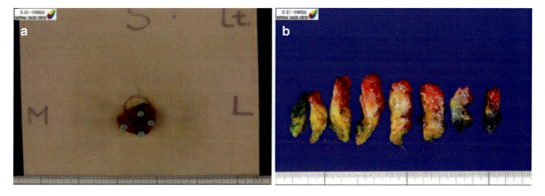

Fig. 146 (**a**) Gross pathology of left lumpectomy specimen. (**b**) The margins get marked and sliced with different colors on each direction

- (b) perinodal extension: absent,
- (c) size of metastatic carcinoma: 6 mm.
6. Arteriovenous invasion: absent.
7. Lymphovascular invasion: absent.
8. Tumor border: infiltrative.
9. Microcalcification: present, tumoral.
10. Pathological TN category (AJCC 2017): pT1cN1a.

Note: 1. The inferior margin of the lumpectomy specimen (slides 2 and 3) is close to invasive ductal carcinoma (<1 mm) but this margin submitted for frozen diagnosis (Fro 3) is free of tumor.

2. The lateral margin of the lumpectomy specimen (slide 8) is close to ductal carcinoma in situ (<1 mm) but this margin submitted for frozen diagnosis (Fro 5) is free of tumor.

	Result	Intensity	Positive %
Estrogen receptor	Strong (8/8)	3	>2/3
Progesterone receptor	Strong (8/8)	3	>2/3
C-erbB2	Equivocal (2+)		
Ki-67	Positive in 19% of tumor cells		
SISH	Negative		

26 Case 26

26.1 Patient History and Progress

Female/61 years old, post-menopause.

Self-detected palpable mass lesion on right breast 11 o'clock direction.

No family history.

S/P Tuberculosis, diabetes mellitus, dyslipidemia.

26.2 Important Radiologic Findings

See Figs. 147, 148, 149, 150, 151 and 152.

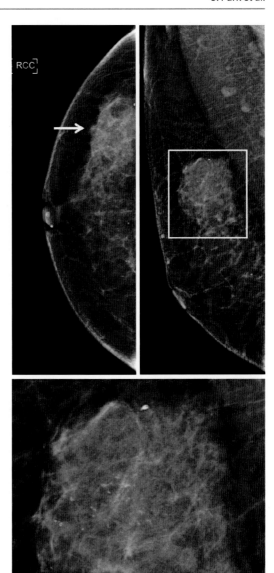

Fig. 147 Right mammography (May 2021): an irregular mass with fine-linear microcalcifications at upper outer quadrant

HR(+) HER2(+) Breast Cancer

26.3 Courses of Treatment

Neoadjuvant chemotherapy (#6 cycles of docetaxel and carboplatin and trastuzumab and pertuzumab) + Operation + Postoperative radiation therapy + Trastuzumab + Letrozole 2.5 mg/day.

Operation: Right nipple–areolar complex sparing mastectomy with immediate implant reconstruction, sentinel lymph node biopsy (Figs. 153 and 154).

26.3.1 Pathology Report

Invasive Ductal Carcinoma
1. Post-chemotherapy status.
2. Size of tumor: 2.3 cm (ypT2).

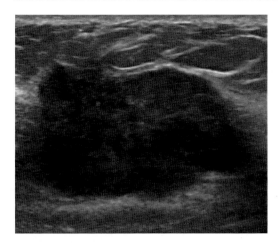

Fig. 148 Right breast US (May 2021): an irregular hypoechoic mass with microcalcifications. US-CNB = IDC

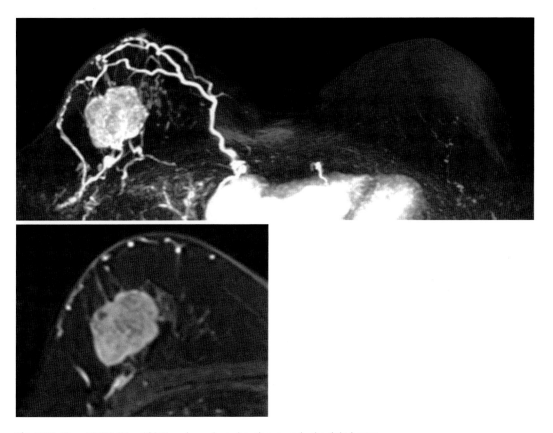

Fig. 149 Breast MRI (May 2021): an irregular enhancing mass in the right breast

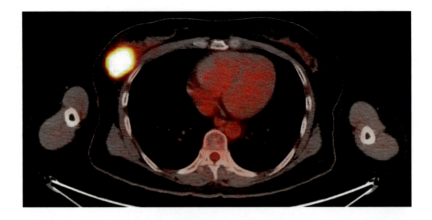

Fig. 150 PET-CT shows a hypermetabolic mass in the right upper outer breast (mSUV = 14.3)

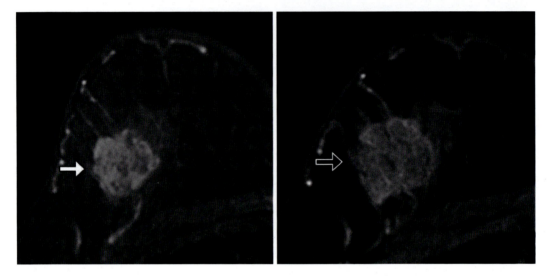

Fig. 151 Breast MRI during and after NAC (Aug. 2021, Oct. 2021): size of the tumor had decreased (white arrow) and then increased again (black arrow)

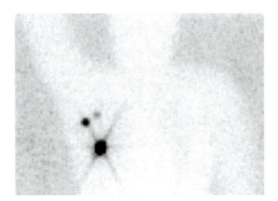

Fig. 152 Lymphoscintigraphy shows visualized sentinel lymph nodes in the right axilla

3. Histologic grade: 3/3 (tubule formation: 3/3, nuclear pleomorphism: 3/3, mitotic count: 3/3, 25/10 HPF).
4. Intraductal component: present, intratumoral/extratumoral (50%) (nuclear grade: high, necrosis: present, architectural pattern: solid/comedo, extensive intraductal component: present).
5. Surgical margins:
   (a) deep margin: <1 mm from ductal carcinoma in situ (slides 1 and 2),
   (b) superficial margin: <1 mm from ductal carcinoma in situ (slide 3).

HR(+) HER2(+) Breast Cancer

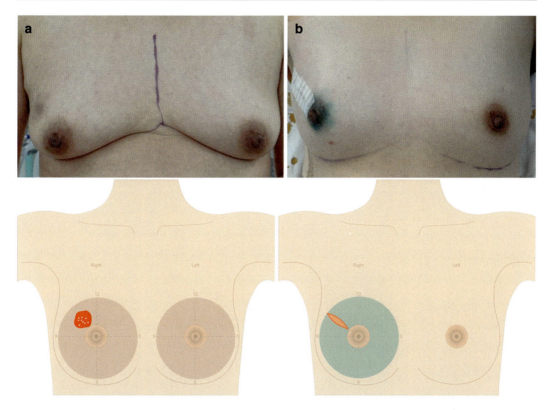

Fig. 153 (**a**) Preoperative and (**b**) immediate post-operative appearance

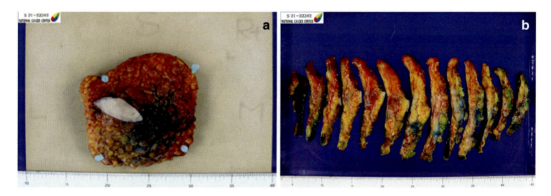

Fig. 154 (**a**) Gross pathology of mastectomy specimen. (**b**) The margins get marked and sliced with different colors on each direction

6. Lymph nodes: no metastasis in three axillary lymph nodes (ypN0(sn)) (sentinel LN: 0/3).
7. Arteriovenous invasion: absent.
8. Lymphovascular invasion: absent.
9. Tumor border: infiltrative.
10. Microcalcification: present, tumoral.
11. Pathological TN category (AJCC 2017): ypT2N0(sn).

	Result	Intensity	Positive %
Estrogen receptor	Weak (4/8)	2	1–10%
Progesterone receptor	Negative (0/8)	0	0
C-erbB2	Positive (3+)		
Ki-67	Positive in 46% of tumor cells		

27 Case 27

27.1 Patient History and Progress

Female/52 years old, peri-menopause.

Self-detected palpable mass lesion on left breast 11 o'clock direction.

Family history of breast cancer, cousin (maternal).

s/p Ovarian cyst excision.

BRCA 1 and 2 mutation: Not detected, NBN VUS (variant of uncertain).

27.2 Important Radiologic Findings

See Figs. 155, 156, 157, 158 and 159.

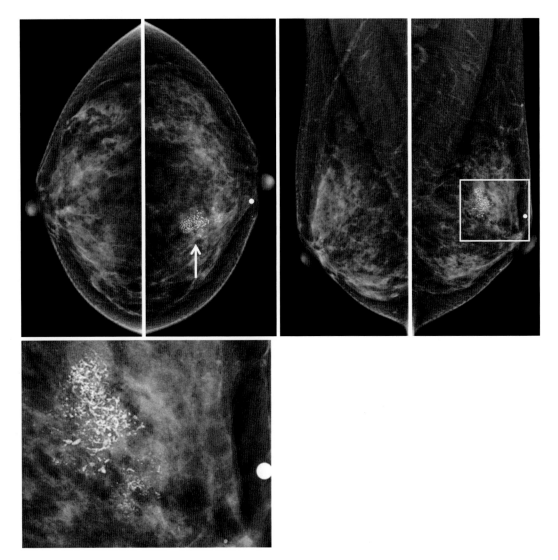

Fig. 155 Both mammography (June 2021): segmental fine-linear microcalcifications at upper inner quadrant of the left breast. Negative finding in the right breast

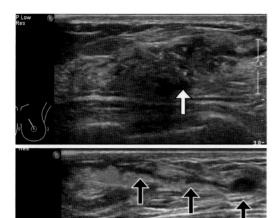

Fig. 156 Both breast US (June 2021): an irregular hypoechoic mass with microcalcifications at upper inner quadrant of the left breast (white arrow, US-CNB = IDC). An oval hypoechoic mass with associated ductal dilatation at 6 o'clock direction of the right breast (black arrows, US-CNB = DCIS)

27.3 Courses of Treatment

Neoadjuvant chemotherapy (#6 cycles of docetaxel and carboplatin and trastuzumab and pertuzumab) + Operation + Postoperative radiation therapy + Trastuzumab + Tamoxifen 20 mg/day.

Operation: Left breast conserving surgery, sentinel lymph node biopsy, Right breast conserving surgery (Figs. 160 and 161).

27.3.1 Pathology Report
[Right].

1. Ductal carcinoma in situ involving sclerosing adenosis.
   (a) Post-chemotherapy status.
   (b) Size of tumor: 0.3 cm (ypTis).
   (c) Nuclear grade: low.
   (d) Necrosis: absent.
   (e) Architectural pattern: cribriform/solid.
   (f) Skin: no involvement of tumor.
   (g) Surgical margins:
      - superior margin: 10 mm,
      - inferior margin: 20 mm,
      - medial margin: 5 mm,
      - lateral margin: 15 mm,
      - deep margin: 5 mm,
      - superficial margin: 5 mm.
   (h) Microcalcification: present, non-tumoral.
   (i) Pathological TN category (AJCC 2017): ypTis.
2. Fibroadenoma.

	Result	Intensity	Positive %
Estrogen receptor	Strong (8/8)	3	>2/3
Progesterone receptor	Intermediate (5/8)	2	10%-1/3
C-erbB2	Negative (0)		
Ki-67	Positive in <1% of tumor cells		

[Left].

Invasive ductal carcinoma, histologic grade 2 with extensive intraductal component

1. No residual tumor with (1) necrotic detritus, (2) foamy histiocytic collection.
   (a) Post-chemotherapy status
   (b) Lymph nodes: no metastasis in one axillary lymph node (ypN0(sn)) (sentinel LN: 0/1)
   (c) Microcalcification: present, non-tumoral
2. Sclerosing adenosis with microcalcification.

	Result	Intensity	Positive %
Estrogen receptor	Strong (7/8)	3	1/3–2/3
Progesterone receptor	Weak (3/8)	1	1–10%
C-erbB2	Positive (3+)		
Ki-67	Positive in 32% of tumor cells		

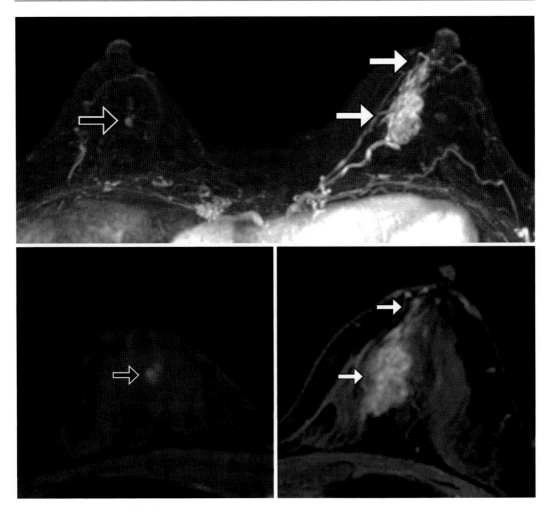

Fig. 157 Breast MRI (June 2021): an irregular enhancing mass with linear non-mass enhancement in the left breast (white arrows). An oval enhancing mass in the right breast (black arrow)

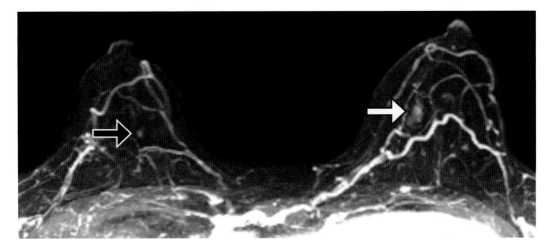

Fig. 158 Post-NAC breast MRI (June 2021): decreased size of the tumors in both breasts after NAC

HR(+) HER2(+) Breast Cancer

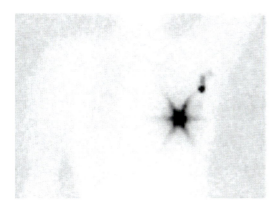

Fig. 159 Lymphoscintigraphy shows visualized sentinel lymph nodes in the left axilla

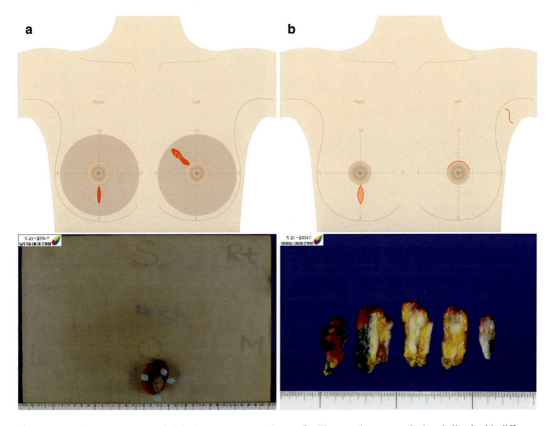

Fig. 160 (**a**) Gross pathology of right lumpectomy specimen. (**b**) The margins get marked and sliced with different colors on each direction

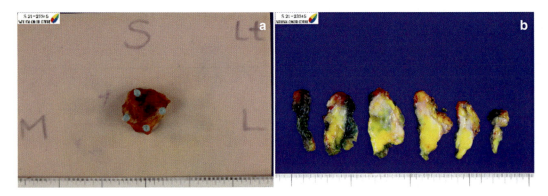

Fig. 161 (a) Gross pathology of left lumpectomy specimen. (b) The margins get marked and sliced with different colors on each direction

28 Case 28

28.1 Patient History and Progress

Female/47 years old, pre-menopause.

Self-detected palpable mass lesion on right breast 6 o'clock direction.

No family history.

Hepatitis B carrier.

28.2 Important Radiologic Findings

See Figs. 162, 163, 164 and 165.

28.3 Courses of Treatment

Operation + Adjuvant chemotherapy (#3 cycles of doxorubicin and cyclophosphamide) + Post-operative radiation therapy + Trastuzumab + Tamoxifen 20 mg/day.

Operation: Right breast conserving surgery, sentinel lymph node biopsy (Fig. 166).

28.3.1 Pathology Report
1. Invasive Ductal Carcinoma.
    (a) Size of invasive component: 1.6 cm (pT1c).
    (b) Size of intraductal component: 3.0 cm.

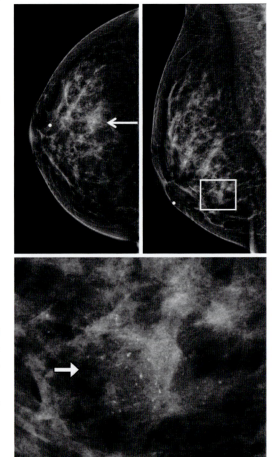

Fig. 162 Right mammography (May 2021): a focal asymmetry with fine pleomorphic microcalcifications at lower outer quadrant

HR(+) HER2(+) Breast Cancer

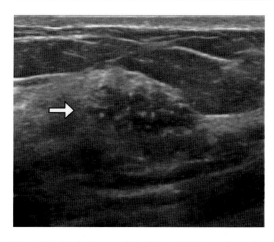

Fig. 163 Right breast US (May 2021): an irregular hypoechoic mass with microcalcifications. US-CNB = IDC

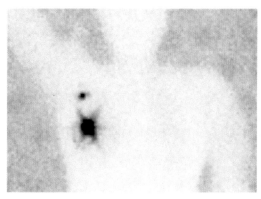

Fig. 165 Lymphoscintigraphy shows visualized sentinel lymph nodes in the right axilla

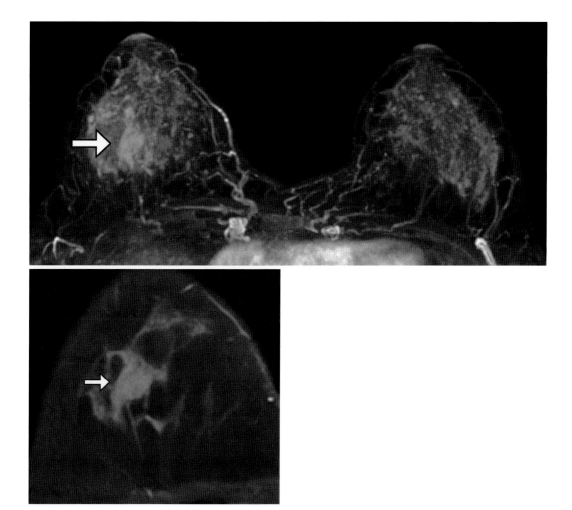

Fig. 164 Breast MRI (May 2021): an irregular enhancing mass with adjacent non-mass enhancement in the right breast

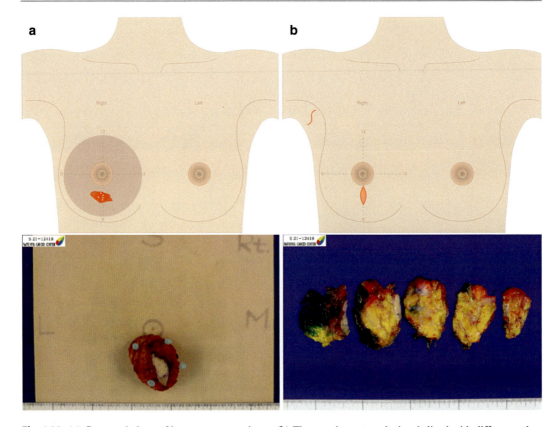

Fig. 166 (**a**) Gross pathology of lumpectomy specimen. (**b**) The margins get marked and sliced with different colors on each direction

(c) Histologic grade: 3/3 (tubule formation: 3/3, nuclear pleomorphism: 3/3, mitotic count: 3/3, 3/HPF).
(d) Intraductal component: present, intratumoral/extratumoral (50%) (nuclear grade: high, necrosis: present, architectural pattern: solid/comedo, extensive intraductal component: present).
(e) Skin: no involvement of tumor.
(f) Surgical margins:
  - superior margin: 10 mm,
  - inferior margin: 10 mm,
  - medial margin: 5 mm,
  - lateral margin: 5 mm,
  - deep margin: 2 mm,
  - superficial margin: 2 mm.
(g) Lymph nodes: no metastasis in two axillary lymph nodes (pN0(sn)) (sentinel LN: 0/2).
(h) Arteriovenous invasion: absent.
(i) Lymphovascular invasion: present, intratumoral.
(j) Tumor border: infiltrative.
(k) Microcalcification: present, tumoral/non-tumoral.
(l) Pathological TN category (AJCC 2017): pT1cN0(sn).

2. Intraductal papilloma with usual ductal hyperplasia.

	Result	Intensity	Positive %
Estrogen receptor	Strong (8/8)	3	>2/3
Progesterone receptor	Strong (8/8)	3	>2/3
C-erbB2	Equivocal (2+)		
Ki-67	Positive in 44% of tumor cells		
SISH	Positive		

29 Case 29

29.1 Patient History and Progress

Female/80 years old, post-menopause.

Self-detected mass lesion on right breast 8 o'clock direction.

No family history.

Hypertension, dyslipidemia, s/p tympanoplasty.

29.2 Important Radiologic Findings

See Figs. 167, 168, 169 and 170.

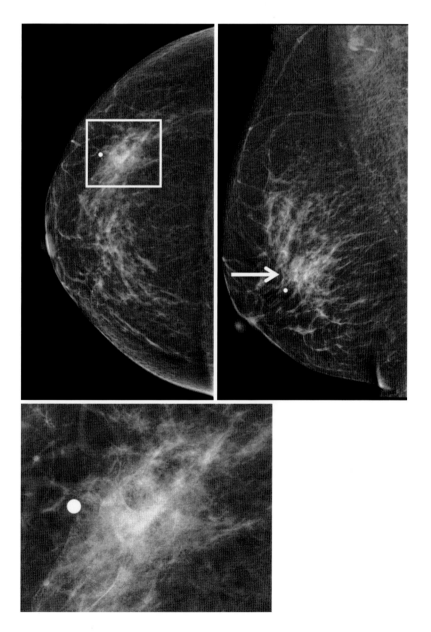

Fig. 167 Right mammography (May 2021): an irregular mass at lower outer quadrant

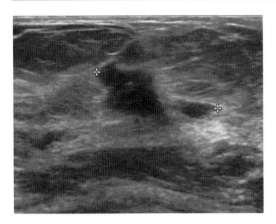

Fig. 168 Right breast US (June 2021): an irregular hypoechoic mass with angular margins. US-CNB = IDC

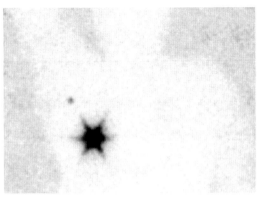

Fig. 170 Lymphoscintigraphy shows visualized sentinel lymph nodes in the right axilla

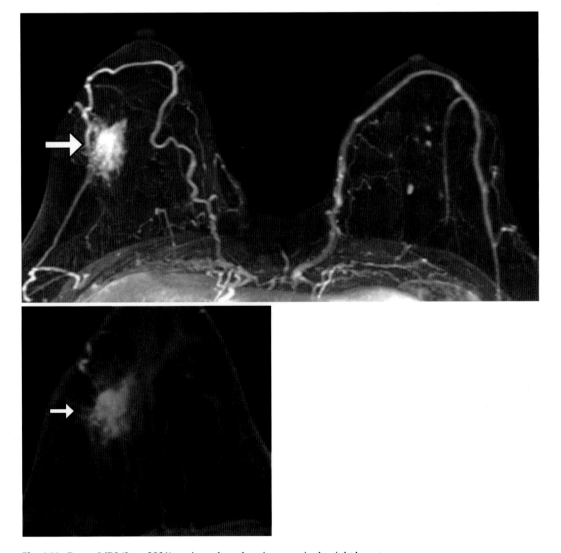

Fig. 169 Breast MRI (June 2021): an irregular enhancing mass in the right breast

29.3 Courses of Treatment

Operation + Adjuvant chemotherapy (#4 cycles of docetaxel and cyclophosphamide and trastuzumab) + Post-operative radiation therapy + Trastuzumab + Letrozole 2.5 mg/day.

Operation: Right breast conserving surgery, sentinel lymph node biopsy (Fig. 171).

29.3.1 Pathology Report

Invasive Ductal Carcinoma

1. Size of tumor: 2.1 cm (pT2).
2. Histologic grade: 2/3 (tubule formation: 3/3, nuclear pleomorphism: 2/3, mitotic count: 2/3, 11/10 HPF).
3. Intraductal component: present, intratumoral/extratumoral (5%) (nuclear grade: low, necrosis: absent, architectural pattern: papillary/cribriform/solid, extensive intraductal component: absent).
4. Skin: no involvement of tumor.
5. Surgical margins:
   (a) superior margin: 10 mm,
   (b) inferior margin: 10 mm,
   (c) medial margin: 10 mm,
   (d) lateral margin: 4 mm,
   (e) deep margin: 2 mm,
   (f) superficial margin: <1 mm from invasive ductal carcinoma (slide 4).
6. Lymph nodes: no metastasis in three axillary lymph nodes (pN0(sn)) (sentinel LN: 0/3).

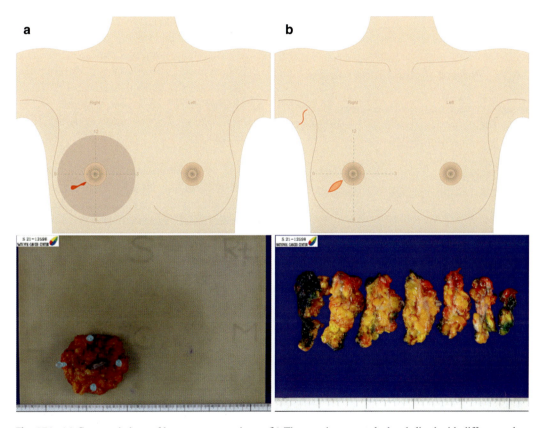

Fig. 171 (**a**) Gross pathology of lumpectomy specimen. (**b**) The margins get marked and sliced with different colors on each direction

7. Arteriovenous invasion: absent.
8. Lymphovascular invasion: present, intratumoral.
9. Tumor border: infiltrative.
10. Microcalcification: present, tumoral/non-tumoral.
11. Pathological TN category (AJCC 2017): pT2N0(sn).

	Result	Intensity	Positive %
Estrogen receptor	Strong (8/8)	3	>2/3
Progesterone receptor	Strong (7/8)	3	1/3–2/3
C-erbB2	Positive (3+)		
Ki-67	Positive in 28% of tumor cells		

30 Case 30

30.1 Patient History and Progress

Female/31 years old, pre-menopause.

Self-detected palpable mass lesion on outer inner portion of right breast.

No family history.

No comorbidities.

BRCA 1 and 2 mutation: Not detected.

30.2 Important Radiologic Findings

See Figs. 172, 173, 174, 175, 176, 177 and 178.

30.2.1 Courses of Treatment

Neoadjuvant chemotherapy (#6 cycles of docetaxel and carboplatin and trastuzumab and pertuzumab) + Operation + Postoperative radiation therapy.

Operation: Right breast conserving surgery, sentinel lymph node biopsy (Fig. 179).

30.2.2 Pathology Report

Ductal Carcinoma In Situ
1. Post-chemotherapy status.
2. Size of tumor: 2.0 cm (ypTis).
3. Nuclear grade: high.
4. Necrosis: present.
5. Architectural pattern: papillary/micropapillary/cribriform/solid/comedo.
6. Surgical margins:
   (a) superior margin: 8 mm,
   (b) inferior margin: 7 mm,
   (c) medial margin: 15 mm,
   (d) lateral margin: (see note),
   (e) deep margin: 3 mm,
   (f) superficial margin: 7 mm.
7. Lymph nodes: no metastasis in three axillary lymph nodes (ypN0(sn)) (sentinel LN: 0/3).
8. Microcalcification: present, tumoral.
9. Pathological TN category (AJCC 2017): ypTisN0(sn).

Note: 1. The lateral margin of the lumpectomy specimen (slide 4) is close to ductal carcinoma in situ (3 mm) but this margin submitted for frozen diagnosis (Fro 4) is free of tumor.

	Result	Intensity	Positive %
Estrogen receptor	Strong (7/8)	3	1/3–2/3
Progesterone receptor	Intermediate (5/8)	2	10%-1/3
C-erbB2	Positive (3+)		
Ki-67	Positive in 9% of tumor cells		

HR(+) HER2(+) Breast Cancer

Fig. 172 Right mammography (May 2021): a focal asymmetry at upper inner quadrant

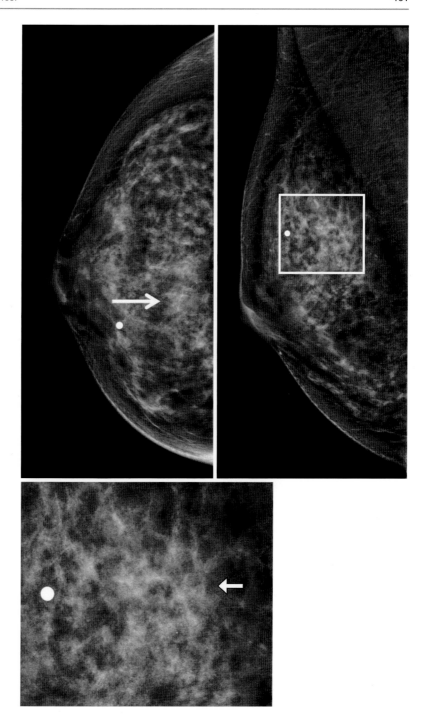

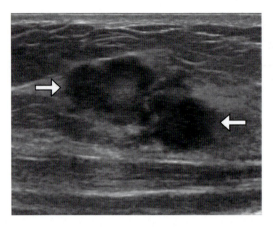

Fig. 173 Right breast US (May 2021): an irregular hypoechoic mass. US-CNB = IDC

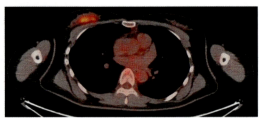

Fig. 175 PET-CT shows a hypermetabolic mass in the right breast (mSUV = 4.7)

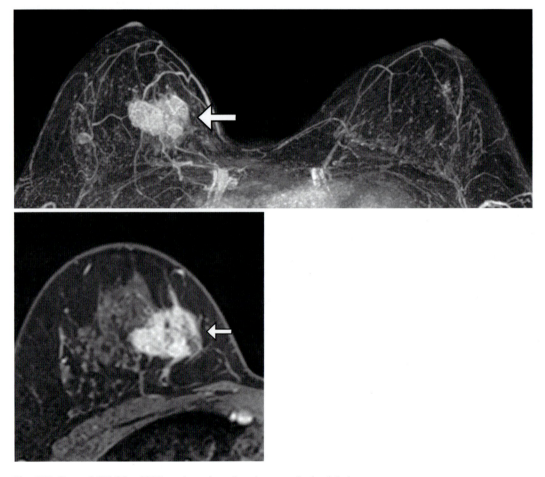

Fig. 174 Breast MRI (May 2021): an irregular enhancing mass in the right breast

HR(+) HER2(+) Breast Cancer

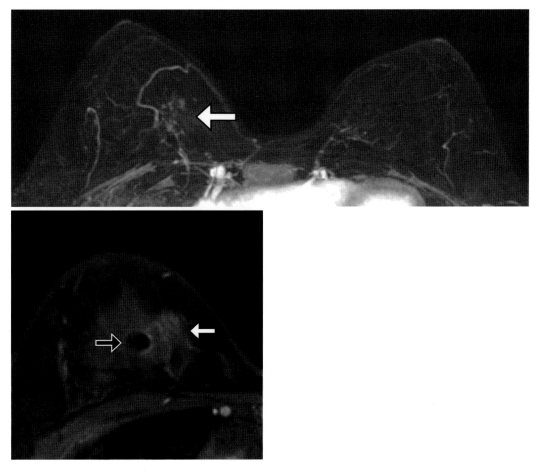

Fig. 176 Post-NAC breast MRI (Sep. 2021): residual focal non-mass enhancement (white arrow) with signal void due to an inserted marker (black arrow)

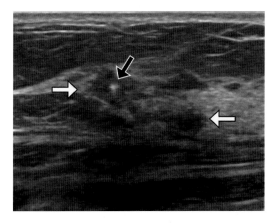

Fig. 177 Post-NAC breast US (Oct. 2021): decreased size of the tumor (white arrows) with an inserted marker (black arrow)

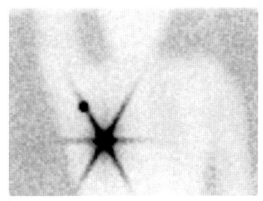

Fig. 178 Lymphoscintigraphy shows visualized sentinel lymph nodes in the right axilla

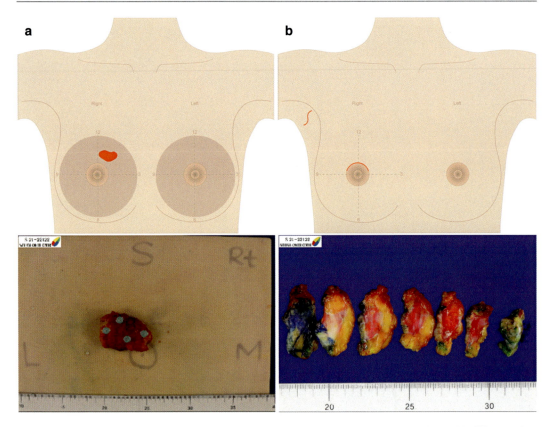

Fig. 179 (**a**) Gross pathology of lumpectomy specimen. (**b**) The margins get marked and sliced with different colors on each direction

31   Case 31

31.1   Patient History and Progress

Female/69 years old, post-menopause.
  Self-detected nipple retraction on left breast.
  No family history.
  Hypertension.

31.2   Important Radiologic Findings

See Figs. 180, 181, 182 and 183.

31.3   Courses of Treatment

Operation + Adjuvant chemotherapy (#4 cycles of doxorubicin and cyclophosphamide followed by #4 cycles of docetaxel and trastuzumab) + Post-operative radiation therapy + Trastuzumab + Letrozole 2.5 mg/day.
  Operation: Left breast conserving surgery, axillary lymph node dissection (Fig. 184).

31.3.1   Pathology Report
Invasive Ductal Carcinoma
1. Size of tumor: 1.7 cm (pT1c).

HR(+) HER2(+) Breast Cancer

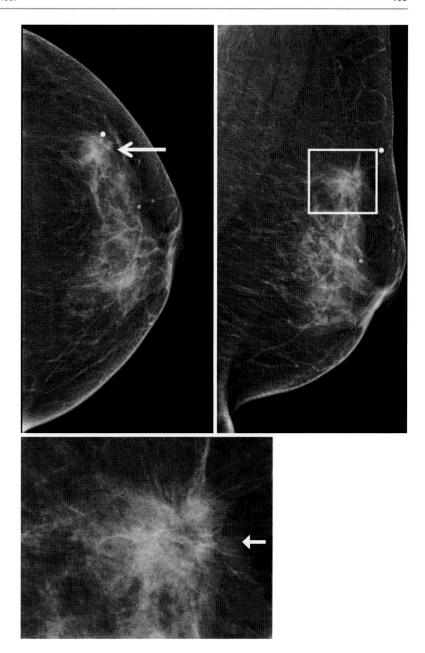

Fig. 180 Left mammography (June 2021): an irregular mass with spiculated margins at upper outer quadrant

2. Histologic grade: 2/3 (tubule formation: 2/3, nuclear pleomorphism: 3/3, mitotic count: 2/3, 11/10 HPF).
3. Intraductal component: present, intratumoral/extratumoral (20%) (nuclear grade: high, necrosis: present, architectural pattern: micropapillary/comedo, extensive intraductal component: absent).
4. Skin: no involvement of tumor.
5. Surgical margins:
    (a) superior margin: 10 mm,
    (b) inferior margin: 15 mm,
    (c) medial margin: 15 mm,
    (d) lateral margin: 10 mm,
    (e) deep margin: 2 mm,
    (f) superficial margin: 2 mm.

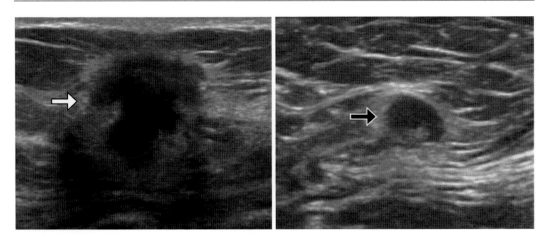

Fig. 181 Left breast US (June 2021): an irregular hypoechoic mass with non-parallel orientation (white arrow, US-CNB = IDC). A lymph node with eccentric cortical thickening at the left axilla (black arrow)

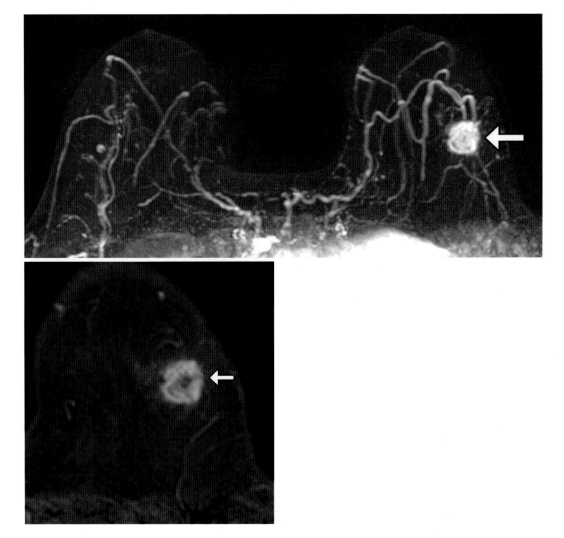

Fig. 182 Breast MRI (June 2021): an irregular rim-enhancing mass in the left breast

HR(+) HER2(+) Breast Cancer

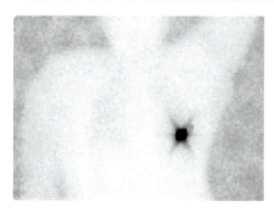

Fig. 183 Lymphoscintigraphy did not show visualized sentinel lymph nodes in the left axilla

6. Lymph nodes:
   (a) metastasis in one out of two axillary lymph nodes (pN1a(sn)) (sentinel LN: 1/1, axillary LN: 0/1),
   (b) perinodal extension: present,
   (c) size of metastatic carcinoma: 8 mm.
7. Arteriovenous invasion: absent.
8. Lymphovascular invasion: present, intratumoral.
9. Tumor border: infiltrative.
10. Microcalcification: present, tumoral/non-tumoral.
11. Pathological TN category (AJCC 2017): pT1cN1a(sn).

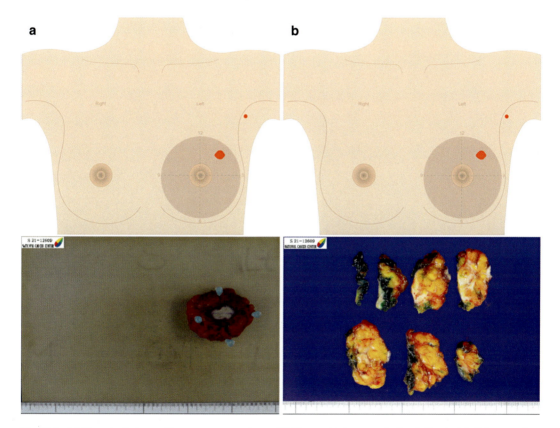

Fig. 184 (**a**) Gross pathology of lumpectomy specimen. (**b**) The margins get marked and sliced with different colors on each direction

	Result	Intensity	Positive %
Estrogen receptor	Strong (8/8)	3	>2/3
Progesterone receptor	Strong (7/8)	3	1/3–2/3
C-erbB2	Positive (3+)		
Ki-67	Positive in 19% of tumor cells		

32 Case 32

32.1 Patient History and Progress

Female/74 years old, post-menopause.
  Self-detected mass lesion on left axillary.
  No family history.
  S/P Tuberculosis, asthma.

32.2 Important Radiologic Findings

See Figs. 185, 186, 187, 188 and 189.

32.3 Courses of Treatment

Neoadjuvant chemotherapy (#3 cycles of docetaxel and trastuzumab and pertuzumab) + Operation + Post-operative radiation therapy + Trastuzumab emtansine + Letrozole 2.5 mg/day.
  Operation: Left axillary lymph node dissection.

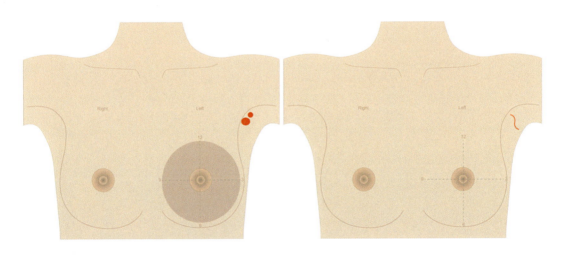

32.3.1 Pathology Report

Metastatic Ductal Carcinoma
1. Post-chemotherapy status.
2. metastasis in 7 out of 20 axillary lymph nodes (axillary LN: 7/20).
3. perinodal extension: present.
4. size of metastatic carcinoma: 40 mm.

	Result	Intensity	Positive %
Estrogen receptor	Intermediate (5/8)	2	10%-1/3
Progesterone receptor	Negative (2/8)	1	<1%
C-erbB2	Positive (3+)		
Ki-67	Positive in 48% of tumor cells		

HR(+) HER2(+) Breast Cancer

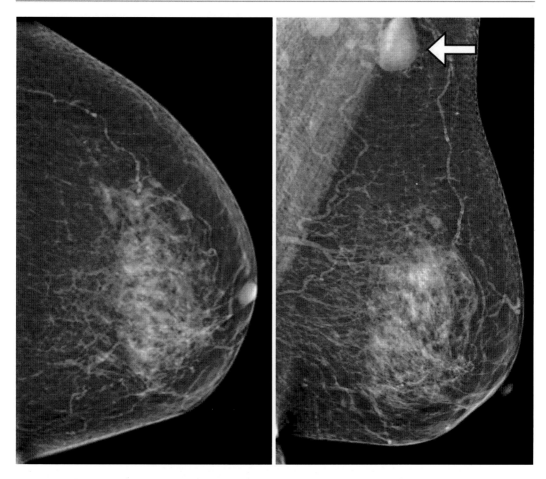

Fig. 185 Left mammography (Feb. 2021): enlarged lymph nodes at the axilla. Negative finding in the breast

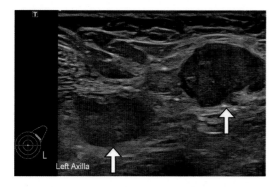

Fig. 186 Left breast US (Mar. 2021): enlarged lymph nodes at the axilla. US-CNB = Metastatic ductal carcinoma

Fig. 187 Breast MRI (Mar. 2021): enlarged lymph nodes at the axilla. No abnormal finding in both breasts

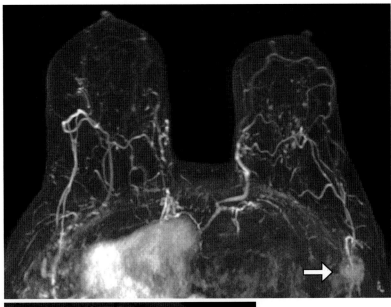

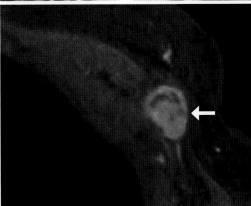

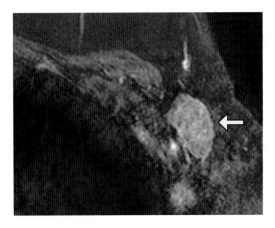

Fig. 188 Post-NAC breast MRI (May 2021): slightly increased number and size of the multiple enlarged lymph nodes at the left axilla (partly shown)

HR(+) HER2(+) Breast Cancer

Fig. 189 Breast MRI for routine surveillance (May 2022): no abnormal finding in both breasts and axillae

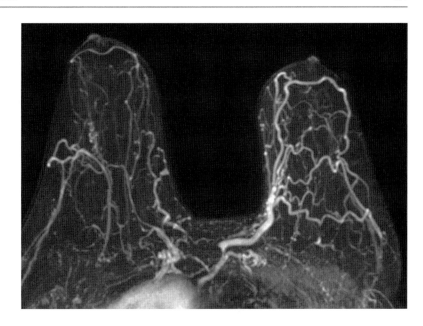

33 Case 33

33.1 Patient History and Progress

Female/50 years old, pre-menopause.

Self-detected palpable mass lesion on left breast.

No family history.

No comorbidities.

33.2 Important Radiologic Findings

See Figs. 190, 191, 192 and 193.

33.3 Courses of Treatment

Neoadjuvant chemotherapy (#6 cycles of docetaxel and carboplatin and trastuzumab and pertuzumab) + Operation + Postoperative radiation therapy + Trastuzumab + Tamoxifen 20 mg/day.

Operation: Left breast conserving surgery, sentinel lymph node biopsy (Fig. 194).

33.3.1 Pathology Report

Invasive ductal carcinoma, histologic grade 2.

No residual tumor with stromal degeneration.

1. Post-chemotherapy status.
2. Lymph nodes: no metastasis in four axillary lymph nodes (ypN0(sn)) (sentinel LN: 0/4).

	Result	Intensity	Positive %
Estrogen receptor	Strong (8/8)	3	>2/3
Progesterone receptor	Weak (3/8)	1	1–10%
C-erbB2	Equivocal (2+)		
Ki-67	Positive in 46% of tumor cells		
SISH	Positive		

Fig. 190 Left mammography (Jan. 2021): a focal asymmetry with microcalcifications at the subareolar area (white arrow). Enlarged lymph nodes at the axilla (black arrow)

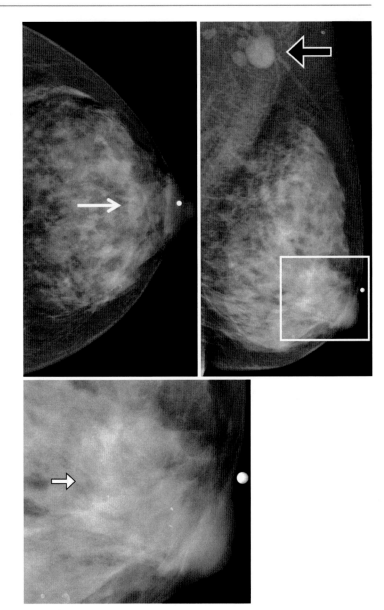

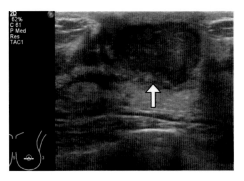

Fig. 191 Left breast US (Jan. 2021): an irregular hypoechoic mass with microcalcifications. US-CNB = IDC

HR(+) HER2(+) Breast Cancer

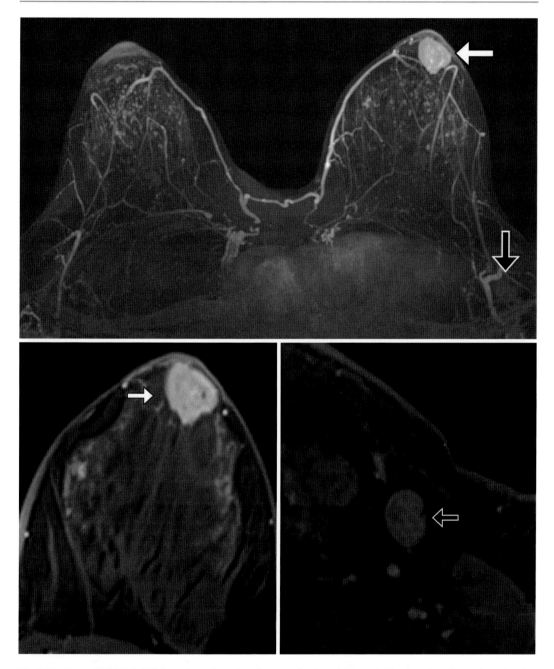

Fig. 192 Breast MRI (Jan. 2021): an irregular enhancing mass in the left breast (white arrow). Enlarged lymph nodes at the left axilla (black arrow)

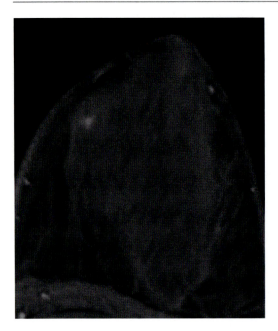

Fig. 193 Post-NAC breast MRI (Apr. 2021): no residual enhancing lesion at the tumor bed after NAC

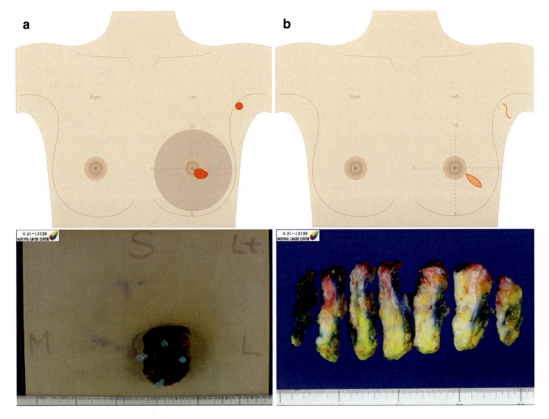

Fig. 194 (a) Gross pathology of lumpectomy specimen. (b) The margins get marked and sliced with different colors on each direction

34 Case 34

34.1 Patient History and Progress

Female/55 years old, post-menopause.
Self-detected palpable mass lesion on right breast 9 o'clock direction.
No family history.
No comorbidities.

34.2 Important Radiologic Findings

See Figs. 195, 196, 197, 198, 199 and 200.

34.3 Courses of Treatment

Neoadjuvant chemotherapy (#6 cycles of docetaxel and carboplatin and trastuzumab and pertuzumab) + Operation + Post-operative radiation therapy + Trastuzumab and Pertuzumab + Letrozole 2.5 mg/day.

Operation: Right breast conserving surgery, sentinel lymph node biopsy (Fig. 201).

34.3.1 Pathology Report
Invasive ductal carcinoma, histologic grade 2.
No residual tumor with stromal degeneration

1. Post-chemotherapy status.
2. Lymph nodes: no metastasis in three axillary lymph nodes (pN0(sn)) (sentinel LN: 0/3).

	Result	Intensity	Positive %
Estrogen receptor	Intermediate (6/8)	3	10%-1/3
Progesterone receptor	Negative (0/8)	0	0
C-erbB2	Positive (3+)		
Ki-67	Positive in 61% of tumor cells		

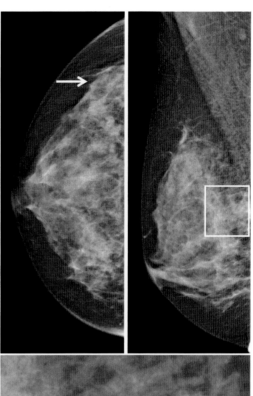

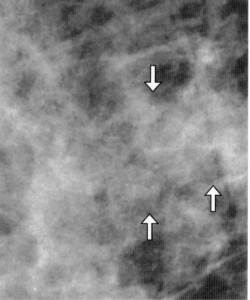

Fig. 195 Right mammography (Dec. 2020): a focal asymmetry with microcalcifications at outer center

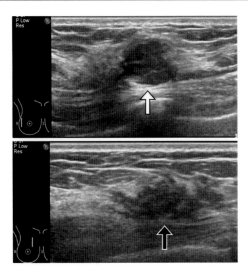

Fig. 196 Right breast US (Jan. 2021): an irregular hypoechoic mass with microcalcifications at 9 o'clock direction (white arrow, US-CNB = IDC). Another irregular mass at 1 o'clock direction (black arrow)

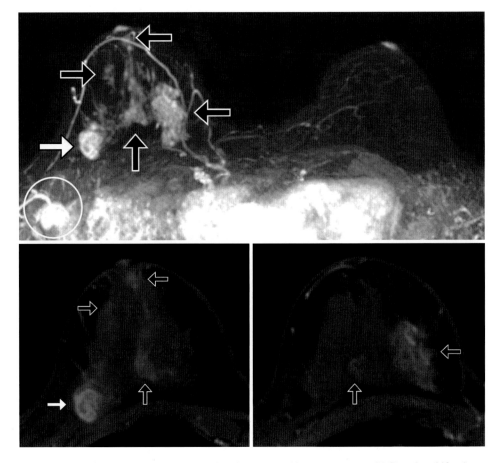

Fig. 197 Breast MRI (Jan. 2021): an irregular enhancing mass (white arrow, proven IDC) and multifocal non-mass enhancement (black arrows) in the right breast. Enlarged lymph node at the right axilla (circle)

HR(+) HER2(+) Breast Cancer 417

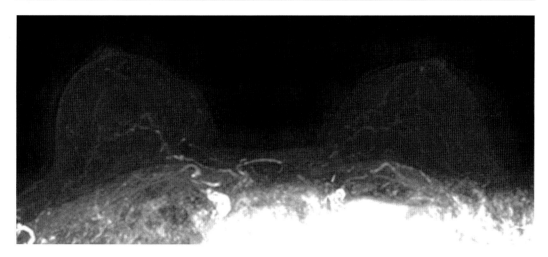

Fig. 198 Post-NAC breast MRI (June 2021): no residual enhancing lesion after NAC

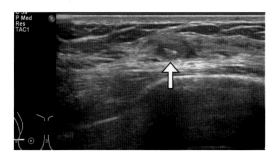

Fig. 199 Post-NAC right breast US (June 2021): an inserted marker with surrounding isoechoic change at the tumor bed

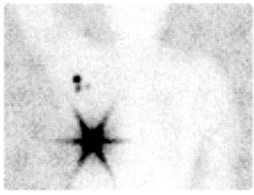

Fig. 200 Lymphoscintigraphy shows visualized sentinel lymph nodes in the right axilla

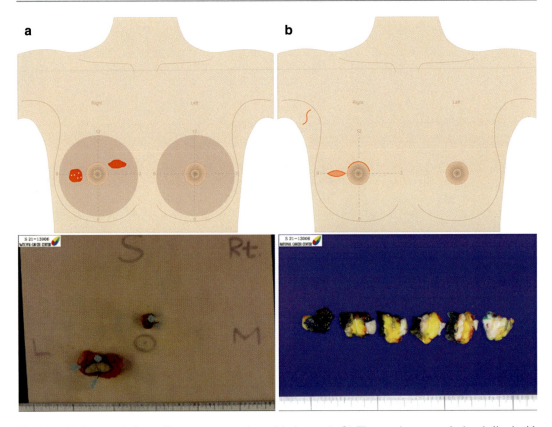

Fig. 201 (**a**) Gross pathology of lumpectomy specimen (black arrow). (**b**) The margins get marked and sliced with different colors on each direction

35 Case 35

35.1 Patient History and Progress

Female/39 years old, pre-menopause.
 Self-detected skin change and palpable mass lesion on right breast 9:30 o'clock direction.
 No family history.
 No comorbidities.
 BRCA 1 and 2 mutation: Not detected.

35.2 Important Radiologic Findings

See Figs. 202, 203, 204, 205, 206, 207 and 208.

35.3 Courses of Treatment

Neoadjuvant chemotherapy (#6 cycles of docetaxel and carboplatin and trastuzumab

Fig. 202 Right mammography (Jan. 2021): an irregular mass with fine pleomorphic microcalcifications at upper outer quadrant

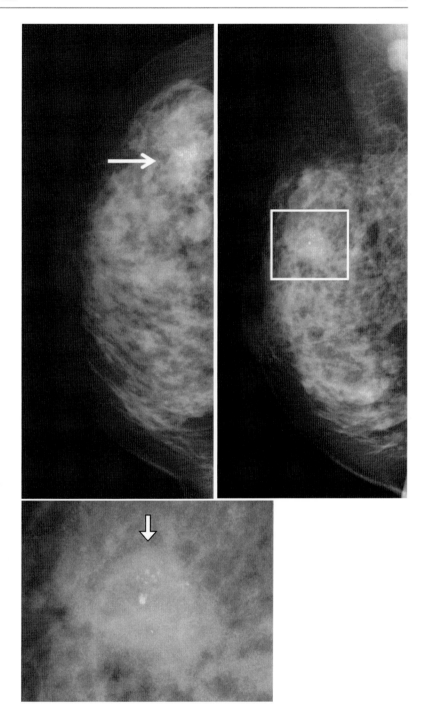

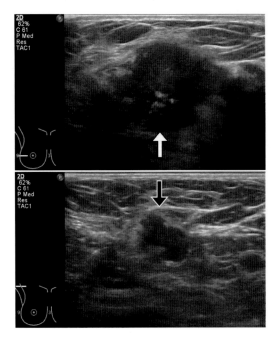

Fig. 203 Right breast US (Jan. 2021): an irregular hypoechoic mass with microcalcifications in the right breast (white arrow, US-CNB = IDC). An enlarged lymph node at the right axilla (black arrow)

and pertuzumab) + Operation + Postoperative radiation therapy + Trastuzumab + Tamoxifen 20 mg/day.

Operation: Right nipple–areolar complex sparing mastectomy with immediate implant reconstruction, axillary lymph node dissection (Figs. 209 and 210).

35.3.1 Pathology Report

Invasive ductal carcinoma, histologic grade 3.

No residual tumor with stromal degeneration.

1. Post-chemotherapy status.
2. Lymph nodes: no metastasis in seven axillary lymph nodes (ypN0) (axillary LN (Fro 4): 0/4, axillary LN: 0/3).

	Result	Intensity	Positive %
Estrogen receptor	Intermediate (5/8)	2	10%-1/3
Progesterone receptor	Intermediate (6/8)	2	10%-1/3
C-erbB2	Positive (3+)		
Ki-67	Positive in 49% of tumor cells		

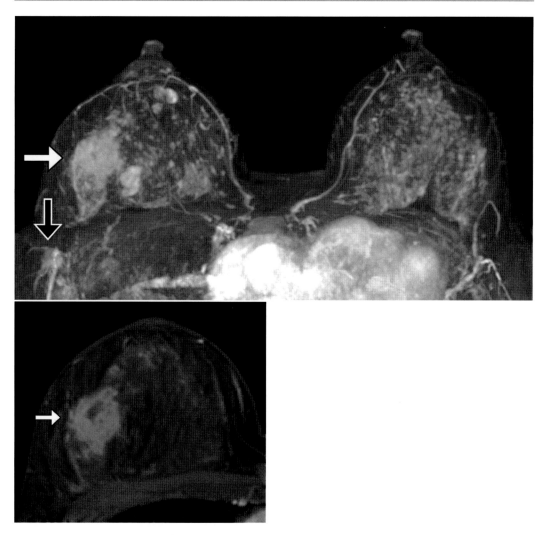

Fig. 204 Breast MRI (Jan. 2021): an irregular enhancing mass in the right breast (white arrow). Enlarged lymph node at the right axilla (black arrow)

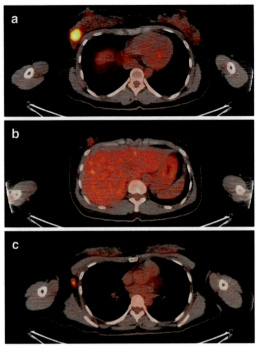

Fig. 205 PET-CT shows (**a**) a hypermetabolic mass in the right outer breast (mSUV = 8.5), (**b**) another hypermetabolic nodule in the right lower breast (mSUV = 2.1), and (**c**) hypermetabolic lymph nodes in the right axilla level I–II (mSUV = 4.6)

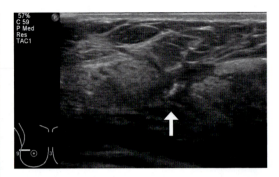

Fig. 207 Post-NAC right breast US (June 2021): decreased size of the tumor after NAC

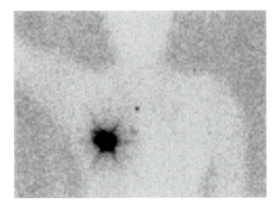

Fig. 208 Lymphoscintigraphy shows faintly visualized sentinel lymph nodes in the right axilla

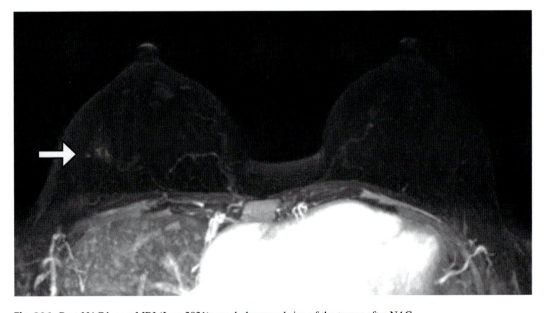

Fig. 206 Post-NAC breast MRI (June 2021): much decreased size of the tumor after NAC

HR(+) HER2(+) Breast Cancer   423

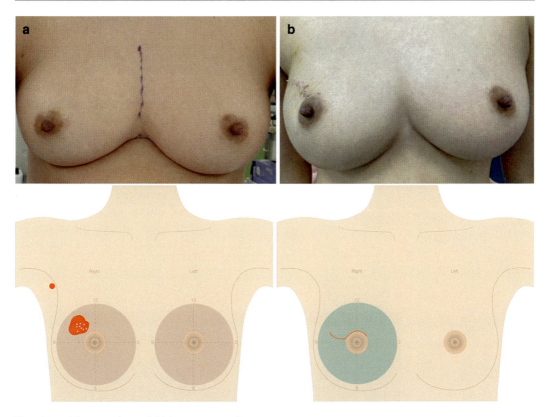

Fig. 209 (**a**) Preoperative and (**b**) late post-operative appearance

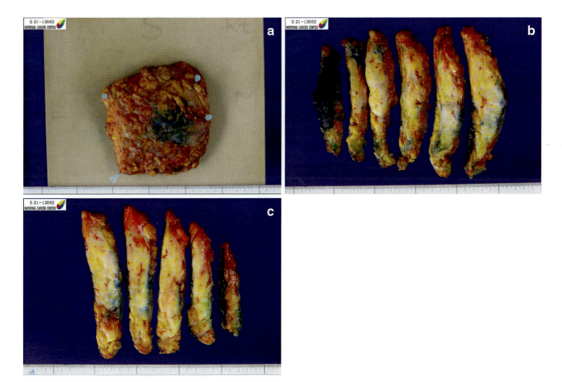

Fig. 210 (**a**) Gross pathology of mastectomy specimen. (**b**, **c**) The margins get marked and sliced with different colors on each direction

36 Case 36

36.1 Patient History and Progress

Female/42 years old, pre-menopause.

Self-detected palpable mass lesion on left breast 5:30 o'clock direction.

No family history.

S/P Right pneumonectomy (lung cancer).

BRCA 1 and 2 mutation: Not examination.

36.2 Important Radiologic Findings

See Figs. 211, 212, 213 and 214

36.3 Courses of Treatment

Operation + Adjuvant chemotherapy (#4 cycles of docetaxel and cyclophosphamide and trastuzumab) + Post-operative radiation therapy + Trastuzumab + Tamoxifen 20 mg/day.

Operation: Left breast conserving surgery, sentinel lymph node biopsy (Fig. 215).

36.3.1 Pathology Report

Invasive Ductal Carcinoma

1. Size of tumor: 1.5 cm (pT1c).
2. Histologic grade: 3/3 (tubule formation: 3/3, nuclear pleomorphism: 3/3, mitotic count: 3/3, 5/HPF).

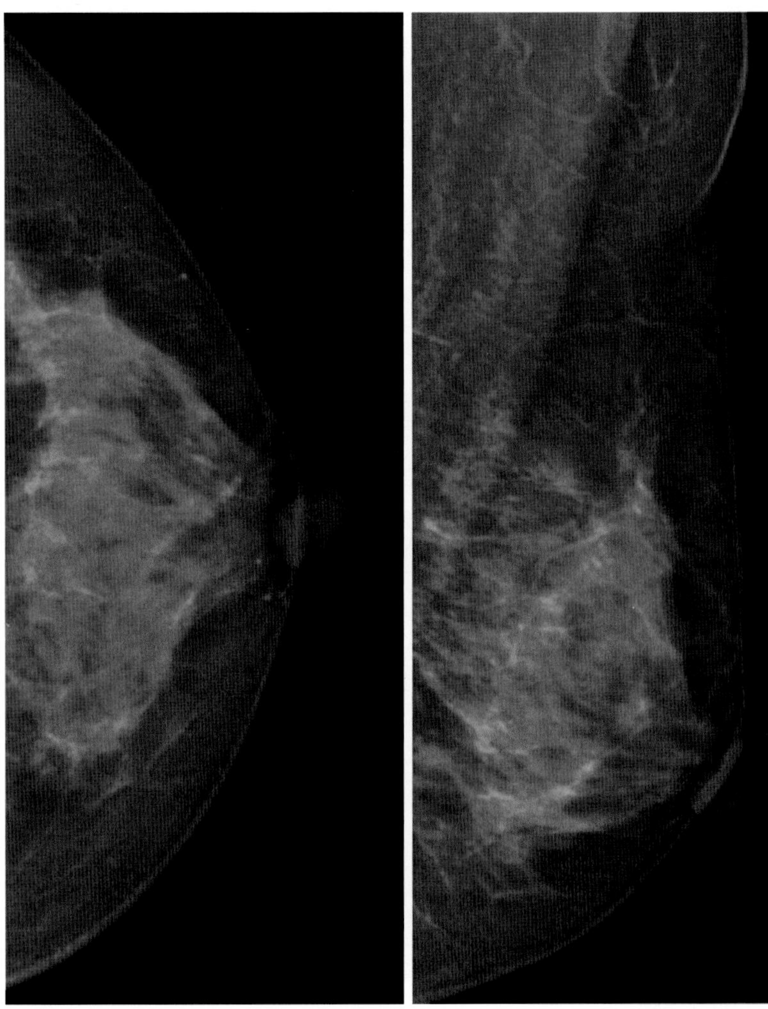

Fig. 211 Left mammography (May 2021): negative finding

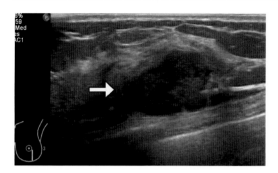

Fig. 212 Left breast US (June 2021): a circumscribed hypoechoic mass at 5 o'clock direction. US-CNB = IDC

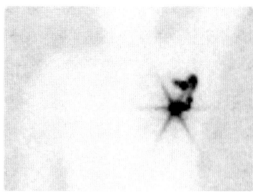

Fig. 214 Lymphoscintigraphy shows visualized sentinel lymph nodes in the left axilla

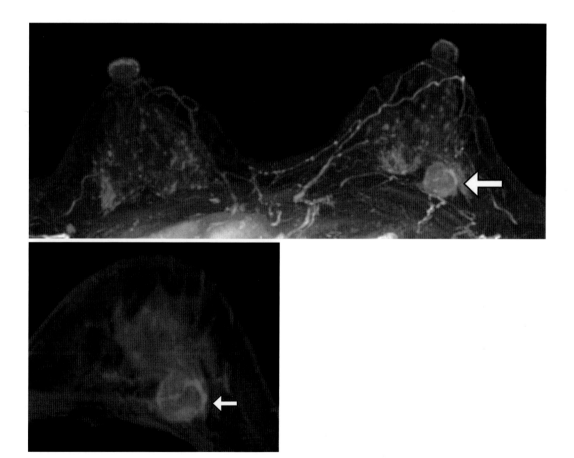

Fig. 213 Breast MRI (June 2021): a circumscribed enhancing mass in the left breast

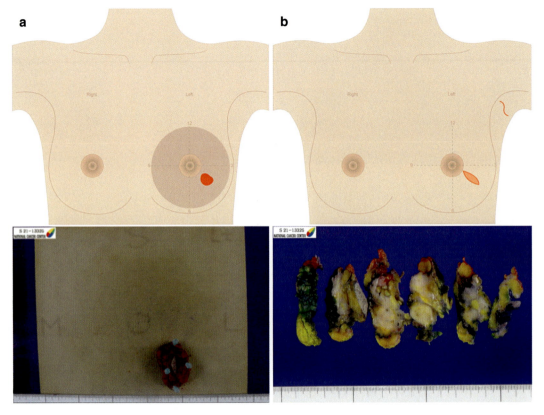

Fig. 215 (**a**) Gross pathology of lumpectomy specimen. (**b**) The margins get marked and sliced with different colors on each direction

3. Intraductal component: present, intratumoral/extratumoral (5%) (nuclear grade: high, necrosis: absent, architectural pattern: solid, extensive intraductal component: absent).
4. Skin: no involvement of tumor.
5. Surgical margins:
   (a) superior margin: 10 mm,
   (b) inferior margin: 10 mm,
   (c) medial margin: 5 mm,
   (d) lateral margin: 5 mm,
   (e) deep margin: <1 mm from invasive ductal carcinoma (slide 2),
   (f) superficial margin: 2 mm.
6. Lymph nodes: no metastasis in two axillary lymph nodes (pN0(sn)) (sentinel LN: 0/2).
7. Arteriovenous invasion: absent.
8. Lymphovascular invasion: absent.
9. Tumor border: infiltrative.
10. Microcalcification: present, tumoral/non-tumoral.
11. Pathological TN category (AJCC 2017): pT1cN0(sn).

	Result	Intensity	Positive %
Estrogen receptor	Negative (0/8)	0	0
Progesterone receptor	Weak (3/8)	2	<1%
C-erbB2	Equivocal (2+)		
Ki-67	Positive in 54% of tumor cells		
SISH	Tumor heterogeneity		

HR(−) HER2(+) Breast Cancer

Youngmi Kwon, Yunju Kim, Bo Hwa Choi,
Ji Young You, Ran Song, Jeayeon Woo,
and Soojin Park

1 Case 1

1.1 Patient History and Progress

Female/59 years old, post-menopause.

Y. Kwon
Department of Radiology, Center for Breast Cancer,
National Cancer Center, Goyang, Gyeonggi,
Republic of Korea
e-mail: ymk@ncc.re.kr

Y. Kim
Department of Pathology, National Cancer Center,
Goyang, Gyeonggi, Republic of Korea
e-mail: radkyj@ncc.re.kr

B. H. Choi
Division of Diagnostic Radiology,
Center for Breast Cancer, National Cancer Center,
Goyang, Gyeonggi, Republic of Korea
e-mail: iawy82@ncc.re.kr

J. Y. You
Division of Breast and Endocrine,
Department of General Surgery,
Korea University Medical Center, Seoul,
Republic of Korea
e-mail: joliejean@korea.ac.kr

R. Song · J. Woo
Division of Surgery, Center for Breast Cancer,
National Cancer Center, Goyang, Gyeonggi, Republic
of Korea
e-mail: thdfks37@ncc.re.kr; jaeyeon1205@ncc.re.kr

S. Park (✉)
Department of Surgery, Wonkwang University
Sanbon Hospital, Gunpo, Gyeonggi,
Republic of Korea
e-mail: amiamo.com@gmail.com

Self-detected mass lesion on right breast 12
o'clock direction.
No family history.
S/P Tuberculosis.

1.2 Important Radiologic Findings

See Figs. 1, 2, 3 and 4.

© The Author(s), under exclusive license to Springer Nature Singapore Pte Ltd. 2023
E. S. Lee (ed.), *A Practical Guide to Breast Cancer Treatment*,
https://doi.org/10.1007/978-981-19-9044-1_7

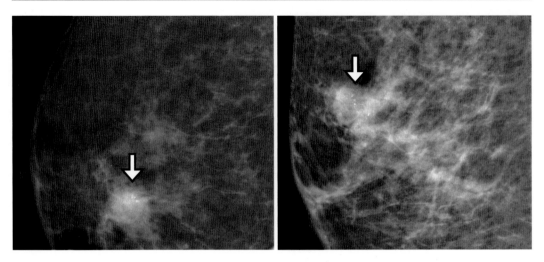

Fig. 1 Magnification CC/ML (July 2020): indistinct irregular hyperdense mass with fine pleomorphic microcalcifications at the 12 o'clock direction of right breast

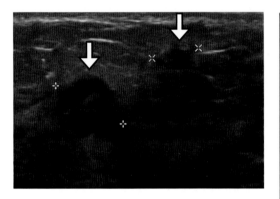

Fig. 2 Breast US (July 2020): two irregular hypoechoic masses with spiculated margin at the 12 o'clock direction of right breast

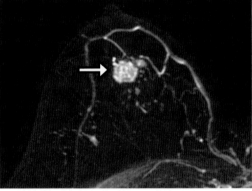

Fig. 3 Breast MRI (July 2020): irregular enhancing mass at the 12 o'clock direction of right breast

Fig. 4 PET-CT shows (**a**) hypermetabolic nodule in right upper breast (mSUV = 5.5) and (**b**) prominent right axillary LN with hypermetabolism (mSUV = 3.1)

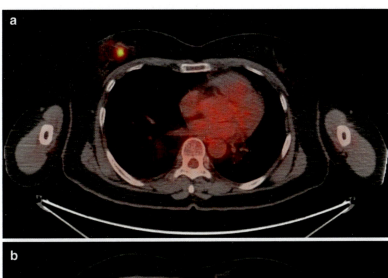
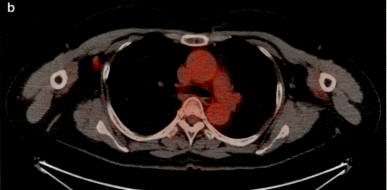

1.3 After Neoadjuvant Chemotherapy

See Figs. 5, 6 and 7.

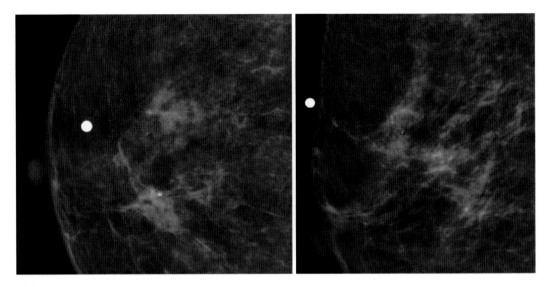

Fig. 5 Magnification (Dec. 2020): mammography after treatment demonstrates residual mass and fine pleomorphic microcalcifications that are decreased in the longest diameter (marked by BB marker)

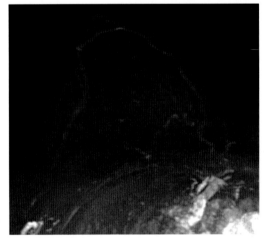

Fig. 6 Breast MRI (Dec. 2020): MRI after treatment shows complete resolution of enhancement in the right breast

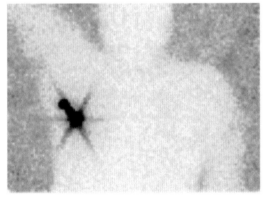

Fig. 7 Lymphoscintigraphy shows visualized sentinel lymph nodes in the right axilla

1.4 Courses of Treatment

Neoadjuvant chemotherapy (#6 cycles of docetaxel and carboplatin and trastuzumab and pertuzumab) + Operation + Post-operative radiation therapy + Trastuzumab.

	Result	Intensity	Positive %
Estrogen receptor	Negative (0/8)	0	0
Progesterone receptor	Negative (0/8)	0	0
C-erbB2	Positive (3+)		
Ki-67	Positive in 42% of tumor cells		

1.4.1 Operation

Right breast conserving surgery, sentinel lymph node biopsy (Fig. 8).

1.4.2 Pathology Report

No residual tumor with stromal fibrosis.
1. Post-chemotherapy status.
2. Lymph nodes: no metastasis in six axillary lymph nodes (ypN0) (sentinel LN: 0/1, non-sentinel LN: 0/5).

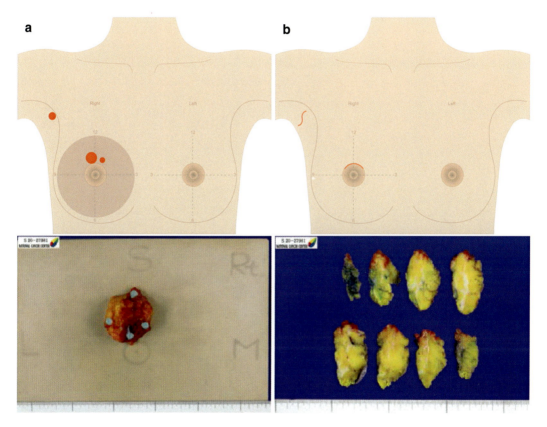

Fig. 8 (**a**) Gross pathology of lumpectomy specimen. (**b**) The margins get marked and sliced with different colors on each direction

2 Case 2

2.1 Patient History and Progress

Female/68 years old, post-menopause.
A self-detected skin change and nipple retraction on left breast.

No family history.
Hypothyroidism.

2.2 Important Radiologic Findings

See Figs. 9, 10, 11 and 12.

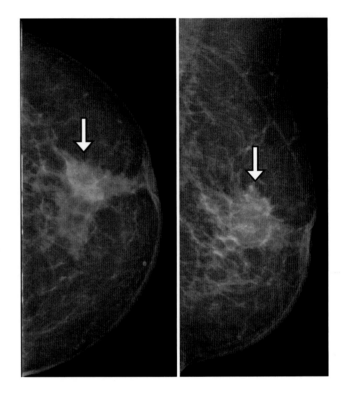

Fig. 9 Mammography (July 2020): irregular hyperdense mass in left subareolar area

HR(−) HER2(+) Breast Cancer

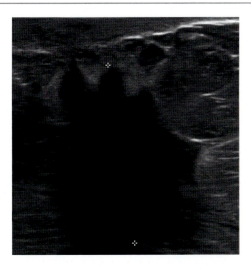

Fig. 10 Breast US (July 2020): irregular hypoechoic mass with echogenic halo in the left subareolar area

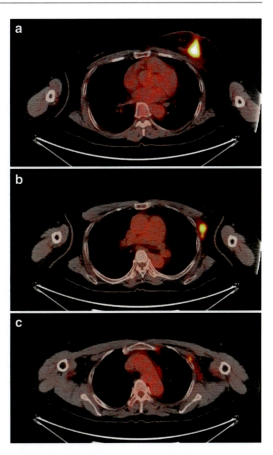

Fig. 12 PET-CT shows (**a**) hypermetabolic mass in Lt breast subareolar area (mSUV = 11.5), (**b**) hypermetabolic LNs in left axilla, level I–II (mSUV = 8.3), and (**c**) mild hypermetabolic nodule in left internal mammary area (mSUV = 2.1)

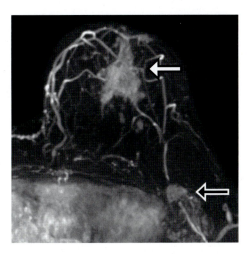

Fig. 11 Breast MRI (July 2020): irregular enhancing mass (white arrow) with small satellite nodules in left subareolar breast. Enlarged heterogeneously enhancing lymph node in the left axilla (black arrow)

2.3 After Neoadjuvant Chemotherapy

See Figs. 13, 14, 15 and 16.

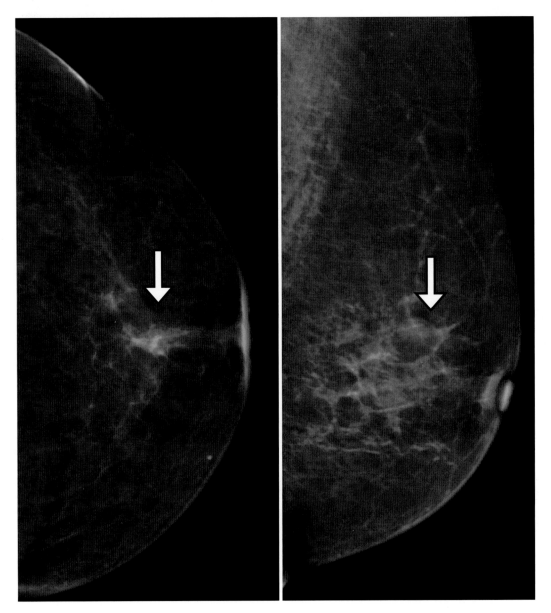

Fig. 13 Mammography (Dec.2020): mammography after treatment demonstrates residual mass that is decreased in the longest diameter

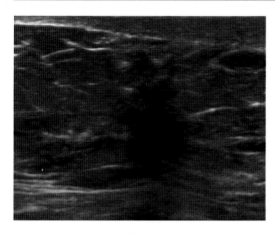

Fig. 14 Breast US (Dec. 2020): US after treatment demonstrates residual hypoechoic mass that is decreased in the longest diameter

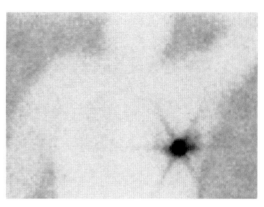

Fig. 16 Lymphoscintigraphy shows faintly visualized sentinel lymph node in left axilla

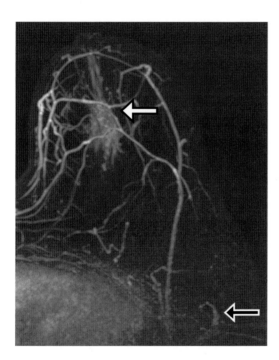

Fig. 15 Breast MRI (Dec. 2020): MRI after treatment demonstrates residual non-mass enhancement (white arrow) that is decreased in the longest diameter and in the degree of enhancement and a normal-appearing axillary lymph node (black arrow)

2.4 Courses of Treatment

Neoadjuvant chemotherapy (#2 cycles of docetaxel and carboplatin and trastuzumab and pertuzumab + #4 cycles of docetaxel and trastuzumab and pertuzumab) + Operation + Postoperative radiation therapy + Trastuzumab emtansine.

2.4.1 Operation
Left breast conserving surgery, sentinel lymph node biopsy (Fig. 17).

2.4.2 Pathology Report

Invasive Ductal Carcinoma
1. Post-chemotherapy status.
2. Size of invasive component: 0.6 cm, multifocal (pT1b).
3. Size of intraductal component: 3.0 cm.
4. Histologic grade: 2/3 (tubule formation: 3/3, nuclear pleomorphism: 2/3, mitotic count: 2/3, 10/10HPF).
5. Intraductal component: present, extratumoral (80%) (nuclear grade: high, necrosis: present, architectural pattern: solid/comedo, extensive intraductal component: present).
6. Skin: no involvement of tumor.
7. Surgical margins:
    (a) subareolar margin: positive for ductal carcinoma in situ (Fro 6),
    (b) superior margin: 10 mm,
    (c) inferior margin: positive for ductal carcinoma in situ (Fro 3) (see note),
    (d) medial margin: 5 mm,
    (e) lateral margin: (see note),
    (f) deep margin: (see note),
    (g) superficial margin: <1 mm from ductal carcinoma in situ (slide 7).

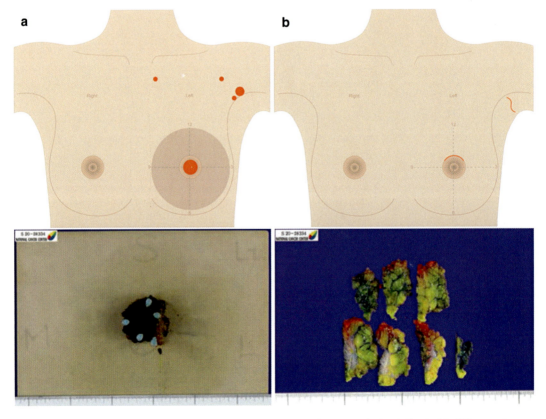

Fig. 17 (**a**) Gross pathology of lumpectomy specimen. (**b**) The margins get marked and sliced with different colors on each direction

8. Lymph nodes: no metastasis in two axillary lymph nodes (ypN0(sn)) (sentinel LN: 0/2).
9. Arteriovenous invasion: absent.
10. Lymphovascular invasion: absent.
11. Tumor border: infiltrative.
12. Microcalcification: present, non-tumoral.
13. Pathological TN category (AJCC 2017): ypT1bN0(sn).

	Result	Intensity	Positive %
Estrogen receptor	Negative (0/8)	0	0
Progesterone receptor	Negative (0/8)	0	0
C-erbB2	Positive (3+)		
Ki-67	Positive in 79% of tumor cells		

3 Case 3

3.1 Patient History and Progress

Female/61 years old, post-menopause.
Self-detected nipple retraction on right breast.
Family history of breast cancer, cousin (maternal).
No comorbidities.
BRCA 1 and 2 mutation: Not detected.

3.2 Important Radiologic Findings

See Figs. 18, 19, 20 and 21.

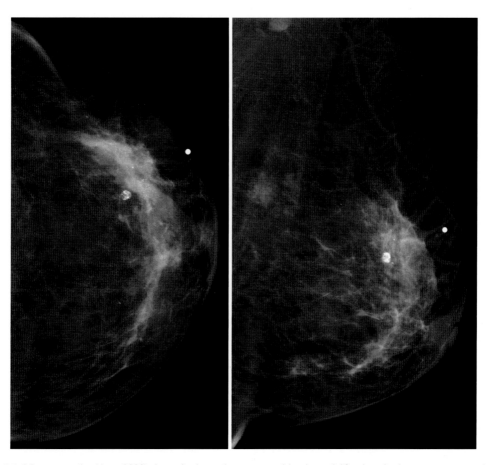

Fig. 18 Mammography (Aug. 2020): irregular hyperdense mass with microcalcifications in the upper outer quadrant of left breast (marked by BB marker)

Fig. 19 Breast US (Aug. 2020): irregular hypoechoic mass with microcalcifications at the 2 o'clock direction of left breast

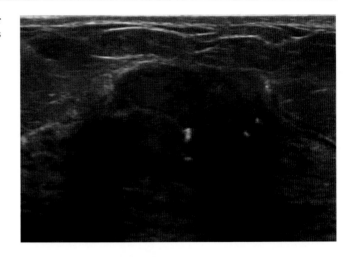

Fig. 20 Breast MRI (Aug. 2020): irregular enhancing mass (white arrow) with small satellite nodules at the 2 o'clock direction of left breast. Multiple enlarged heterogeneously enhancing lymph node in the left axilla (black arrow)

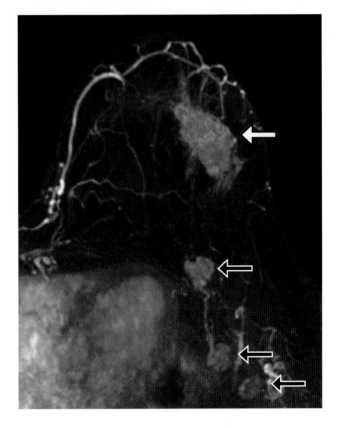

Fig. 21 PET-CT shows (**a**) hypermetabolic mass in the left upper outer breast (mSUV = 11.7), (**b**) enlarged hypermetabolic LNs in the left axilla level I–II (mSUV = 5.9), (**c**) hypermetabolic nodule in the left pectoralis muscle (mSUV = 4.9), and (**d**) focal hypermetabolic osteolytic lesion in L5 (mSUV = 5.0)

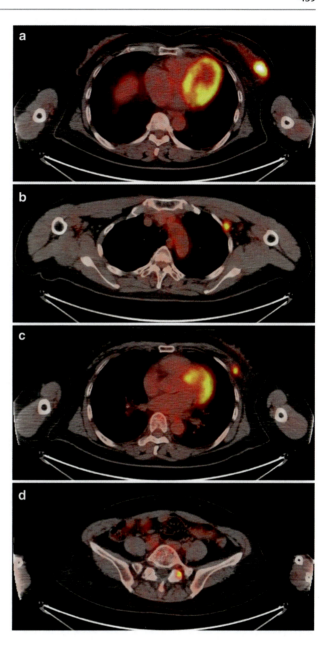

3.3 After Neoadjuvant Chemotherapy

See Figs. 22, 23, 24 and 25.

Fig. 22 Mammography (Dec. 2020): mammography after treatment demonstrates residual mass and microcalcifications that are decreased in the longest diameter

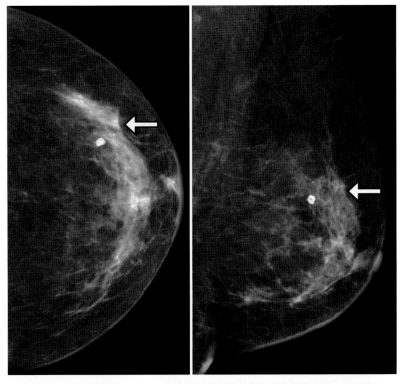

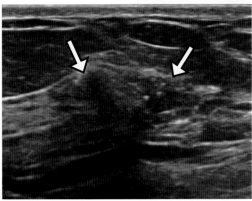

Fig. 23 Breast US (Dec. 2020): US after treatment demonstrates residual hypoechoic mass with microcalcifications that are decreased in the longest diameter

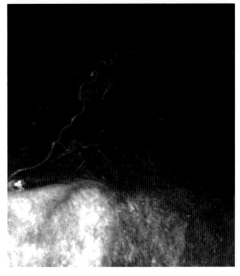

Fig. 24 Breast MRI (Dec. 2020): MRI after treatment shows complete resolution of enhancement in the left breast and enlarged lymph nodes in left axilla

3.4 Courses of Treatment

Palliative chemotherapy (#7 cycles of docetaxel and trastuzumab and pertuzumab) + Operation + Post-operative radiation therapy + Palliative trastuzumab and pertuzumab.

3.4.1 Operation
Left breast conserving surgery, axillary lymph node sampling (Fig. 26).

3.4.2 Pathology Report

Ductal Carcinoma In Situ
1. Post-chemotherapy status.
2. Size of tumor: 0.2 cm (ypTis).
3. Nuclear grade: high.
4. Necrosis: absent.
5. Architectural pattern: solid.
6. Skin: no involvement of tumor.
7. Surgical margins:
   (a) superior margin: 12 mm,
   (b) inferior margin: (see note),
   (c) medial margin: 10 mm,
   (d) lateral margin: 20 mm,
   (e) deep margin: 10 mm,
   (f) superficial margin: 12 mm.
8. Lymph nodes: no metastasis in four axillary lymph nodes (ypN0(sn)) (sentinel LN: 0/4).
9. Arteriovenous invasion: absent.
10. Lymphovascular invasion: absent.
11. Tumor border: pushing.
12. Microcalcification: present, tumoral/non-tumoral.
13. Pathological TN category (AJCC 2017): ypTisN0(sn).

	Result	Intensity	Positive %
Estrogen receptor	Negative (0/8)	0	0
Progesterone receptor	Negative (0/8)	0	0
C-erbB2	Positive (3+)		
Ki-67	Positive in 14% of tumor cells		

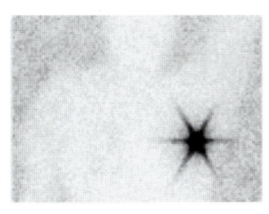

Fig. 25 Lymphoscintigraphy shows non-visualized sentinel lymph node in left axilla

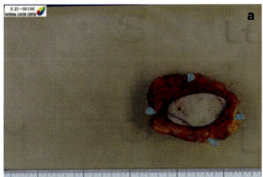
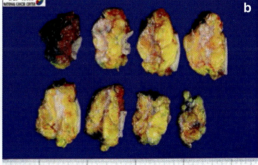

Fig. 26 (a) Gross pathology of lumpectomy specimen. (b) The margins get marked and sliced with different colors on each direction

4 Case 4

4.1 Patient History and Progress

Female/58 years old, post-menopause.

Self-detected mass lesion on left breast 3:30 o'clock direction.

No family history.
No comorbidities.

4.2 Important Radiologic Findings

See Figs. 27, 28, 29 and 30.

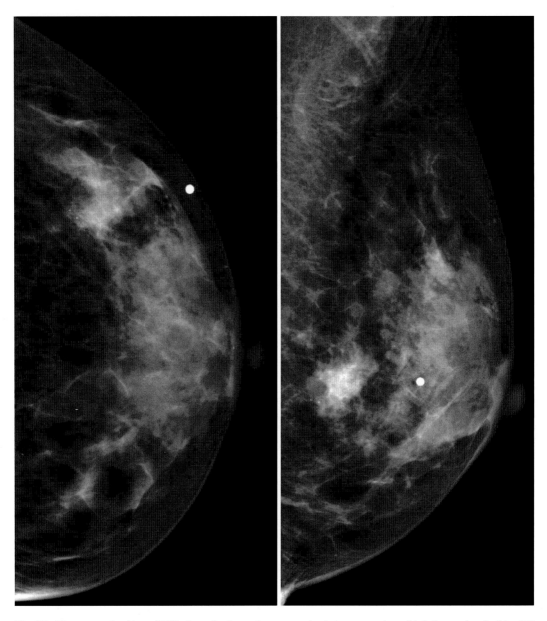

Fig. 27 Mammography (Aug. 2020): irregular hyperdense mass in the outer portion of left breast (marked by BB marker)

HR(−) HER2(+) Breast Cancer

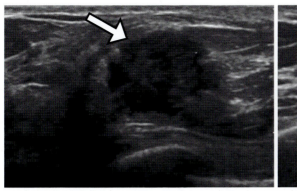

Fig. 28 Breast US (Aug. 2020): irregular hypoechoic mass (white arrow) at the 3 o'clock direction of left breast. Round hypoechoic mass (black arrow) at the 6 o'clock direction of left breast, biopsy proven metastatic intramammary LN

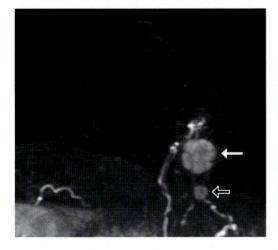

Fig. 29 Breast MRI (Aug. 2020): irregular enhancing mass (white arrow) at the 3 o'clock direction of left breast. Enlarged intramammary lymph node at the 6 o'clock direction of left breast (black arrow)

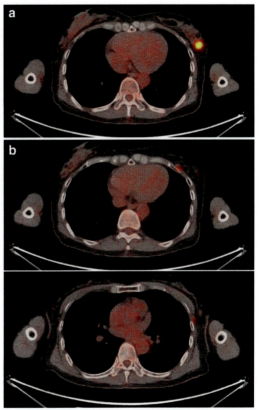

Fig. 30 PET-CT shows (**a**) hypermetabolic mass in LOQ of left breast (mSUV = 7.5), (**b**) small soft tissue lesions in left chest wall, medial side of mass (mSUV = 3.7) and superior aspect (2.2) (mSUV = 2.2)

4.3 After Neoadjuvant Chemotherapy

See Figs. 31, 32, 33 and 34.

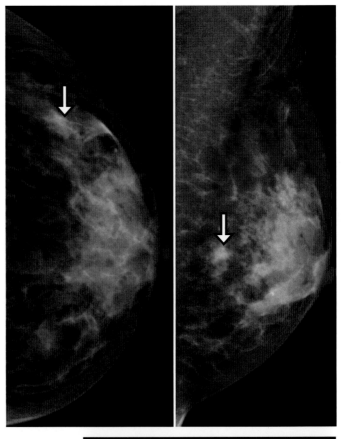

Fig. 31 Mammography (Jan. 2021): mammography after treatment demonstrates residual mass that is decreased in the longest diameter

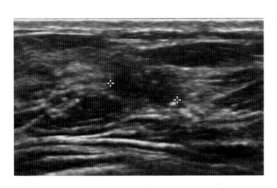

Fig. 32 Breast US (Jan. 2021): US after treatment demonstrates residual hypoechoic mass that is decreased in the longest diameter. Disappearance of enlarged intramammary lymph node at the 6 o'clock direction of left breast

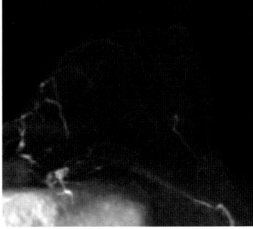

Fig. 33 Breast MRI (Jan. 2021): MRI after treatment shows complete resolution of enhancement in the left breast and disappearance of enlarged intramammary lymph node

Fig. 34 Lymphoscintigraphy shows visualized sentinel lymph nodes in the left axilla

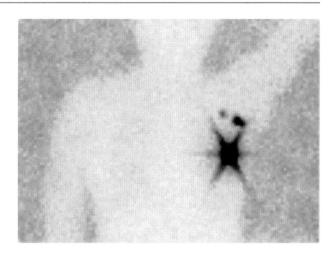

4.4 Courses of Treatment

Neoadjuvant chemotherapy (#6 cycles of docetaxel and carboplatin and trastuzumab and pertuzumab) + Operation + Post-operative radiation therapy.

4.4.1 Operation

Left breast conserving surgery, sentinel lymph node biopsy (Fig. 35).

4.4.2 Pathology Report
1. No residual tumor with stromal fibrosis.
    (a) Post-chemotherapy status.
    (b) Lymph nodes: no metastasis in nine axillary lymph nodes (ypN0) (sentinel LN: 0/4, non-sentinel LN: 0/5).
2. Fibroadenomatous change.
    Note: Histologic mapping has been done.

	Result	Intensity	Positive %
Estrogen receptor	Negative (0/8)	0	0
Progesterone receptor	Negative (0/8)	0	0
C-erbB2	Positive (3+)		
Ki-67	Positive in 35% of tumor cells		

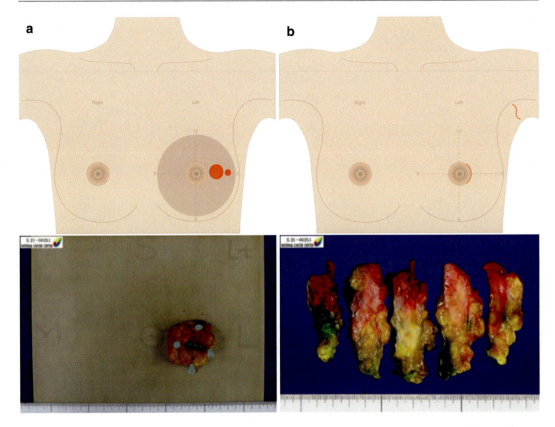

Fig. 35 (**a**) Gross pathology of lumpectomy specimen. (**b**) The margins get marked and sliced with different colors on each direction

5 Case 5

5.1 Patient History and Progress

Female/58 years old, post-menopause.

Screen detected mass lesion on upper inner portion of left breast 8 o'clock.

No family history.

S/P myomectomy, dyslipidemia.

5.2 Important Radiologic Findings

See Figs. 36, 37, 38 and 39.

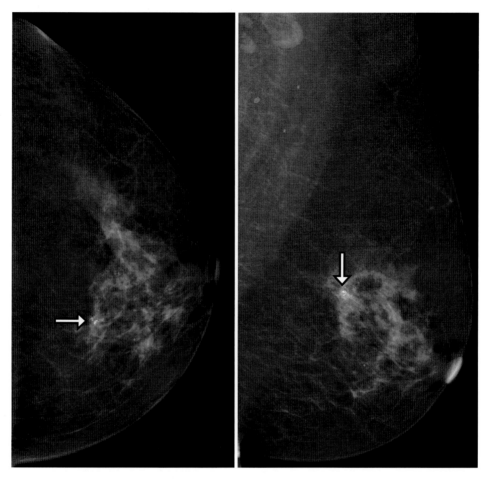

Fig. 36 Mammography (Nov. 2020): regional fine pleomorphic microcalcifications in the upper inner quadrant of left breast

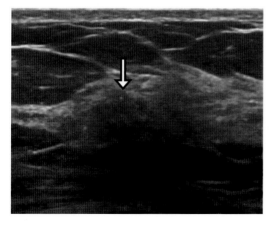

Fig. 37 Breast US (Nov. 2020): indistinct hypoechoic mass with microcalcifications at the 11 o'clock direction of left breast

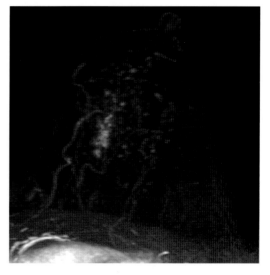

Fig. 38 Breast MRI (Nov. 2020): segmental heterogeneous non-mass enhancement at the 11 o'clock direction of left breast

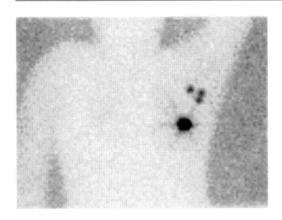

Fig. 39 Lymphoscintigraphy shows visualized sentinel lymph nodes in the left axilla

5.3 Courses of Treatment

Operation + Post-operative radiation therapy.

5.3.1 Operation
Left breast conserving surgery, sentinel lymph node biopsy (Fig. 40).

5.3.2 Pathology Report
1. Invasive ductal carcinoma.
   (a) Size of invasive component: 0.2 cm (pT1a).
   (b) Size of intraductal component: 2.0 cm.
   (c) Histologic grade: 3/3 (tubule formation: 3/3, nuclear pleomorphism: 3/3, mitotic count: 2/3, 10/10HPF).
   (d) Intraductal component: present, intratumoral/extratumoral (99%) (nuclear grade: high, necrosis: present, architectural pattern: cribriform/solid/comedo, extensive intraductal component: present).
   (e) Skin: no involvement of tumor.
   (f) Surgical margins:
   - superior margin: 10 mm,
   - inferior margin: 40 mm,
   - medial margin: 15 mm,
   - lateral margin: 15 mm,
   - deep margin: 2 mm,
   - superficial margin: 30 mm.
   (g) Lymph nodes: no metastasis in four axillary lymph nodes (pN0(sn)) (sentinel LN: 0/4).
   (h) Arteriovenous invasion: absent.
   (i) Lymphovascular invasion: absent.
   (j) Tumor border: infiltrative.
   (k) Microcalcification: present, tumoral/non-tumoral.
   (l) Pathological TN category (AJCC 2017): pT1aN0(sn).
2. Intraductal papilloma.
3. Mucocele-like lesion.

	Result	Intensity	Positive %
Estrogen receptor	Negative (0/8)	0	0
Progesterone receptor	Negative (0/8)	0	0
C-erbB2	Positive (3+)		
Ki-67	Positive in 28% of tumor cells		

HR(−) HER2(+) Breast Cancer

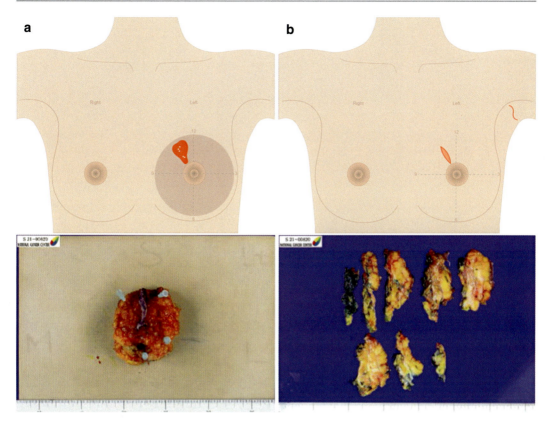

Fig. 40 (**a**) Gross pathology of lumpectomy specimen. (**b**) The margins get marked and sliced with different colors on each direction

6 Case 6

6.1 Patient History and Progress

Female/66 years old, post-menopause.

Self-detected nipple retraction on left breast.

Family history of breast cancer, cousin (maternal).

S/P cholecystectomy, hypertension, dyslipidemia.

BRCA 1 and 2 mutation: Not detected.

6.2 Important Radiologic Findings

See Figs. 41, 42 and 43.

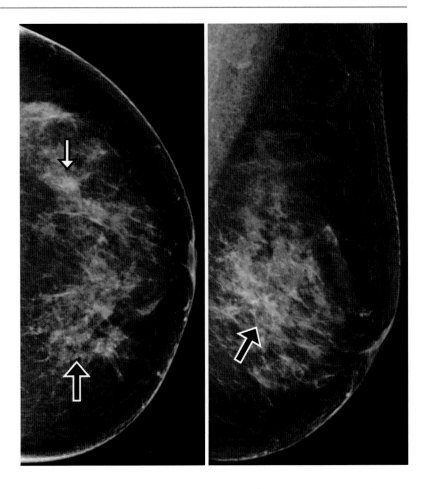

Fig. 41 Mammography (Aug. 2020): asymmetry (white arrow) in the outer portion of left breast. Segmental fine linear or fine-linear branching microcalcifications (black arrows) in left upper inner breast

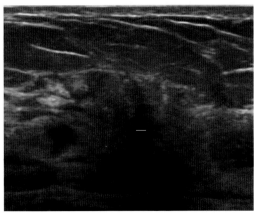

Fig. 42 Breast US (Aug. 2020): irregular hypoechoic mass with indistinct margin at the 3 o'clock direction of left breast

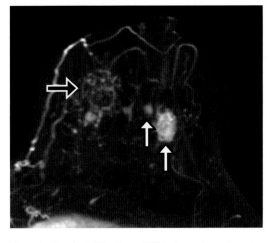

Fig. 43 Breast MRI (Aug. 2020): irregular enhancing masses (white arrows) in the left center breast. Regional heterogeneous non-mass enhancement (black arrow) at the corresponding area of the microcalcifications on mammography

6.3 After Neoadjuvant Chemotherapy

See Figs. 44, 45 and 46.

Fig. 44 Mammography: mammography after treatment demonstrates residual mass is decreased in the longest diameter and no change in extent of microcalcifications in left upper inner breast

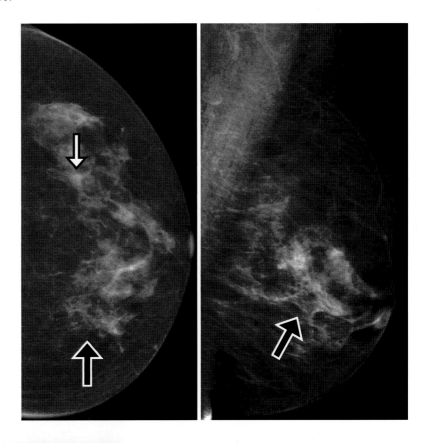

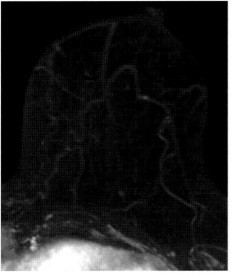

Fig. 45 Breast MRI: MRI after treatment shows complete resolution of enhancement in the left breast

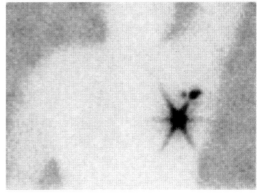

Fig. 46 Lymphoscintigraphy shows visualized sentinel lymph nodes in the left axilla

6.4 Courses of Treatment

Neoadjuvant chemotherapy (#1 cycle of docetaxel and carboplatin and #6 cycles of trastuzumab and pertuzumab) + Operation + Postoperative radiation therapy + Trastuzumab + Letrozole 2.5 mg.

6.4.1 Operation
Left modified radical mastectomy, sentinel lymph node biopsy (Fig. 47).

6.4.2 Pathology Report
1. No residual tumor with stromal degeneration.
    (a) Post-chemotherapy status.

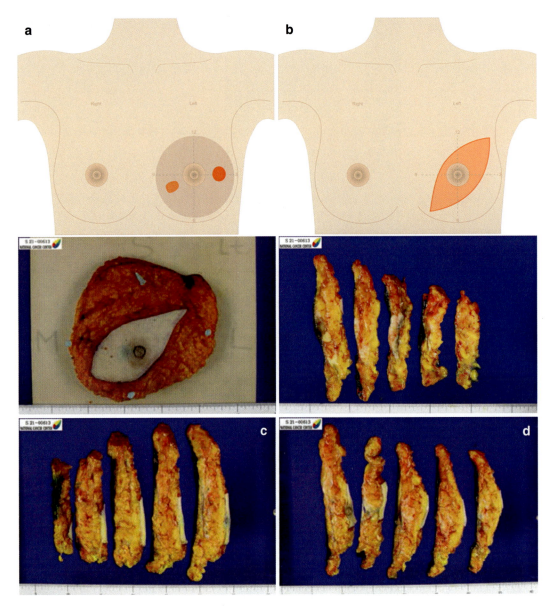

Fig. 47 (**a**) Gross pathology of mastectomy specimen. (**b–d**) The margins get marked and sliced with different colors on each direction

(b) Lymph nodes: no metastasis in ten axillary lymph nodes (ypN0) (sentinel LN: 0/3, axillary LN: 0/7).
2. Atypical ductal hyperplasia, focal with microcalcification.

	Result	Intensity	Positive %
Estrogen receptor	Negative (0/8)	0	0
Progesterone receptor	Negative (0/8)	2	0
C-erbB2	Positive (3+)		
Ki-67	Positive in 22% of tumor cells		

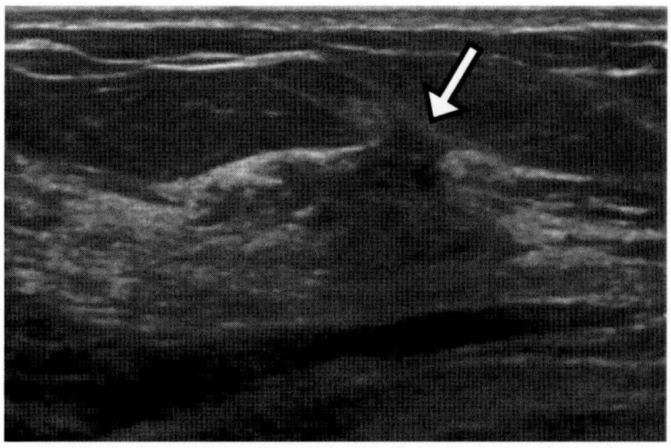

7 Case 7

7.1 Patient History and Progress

Female/58 years old, post-menopause.
Screen detected mass lesion on upper outer portion of left breast.
No family history.
S/P Nodules of vocal cord, operation.

7.2 Important Radiologic Findings

See Figs. 48 and 49.

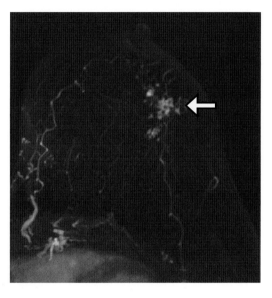

Fig. 48 Breast US: spiculated irregular heterogeneous echoic mass at the 2 o'clock direction of left breast

Fig. 49 Breast MRI: segmental heterogenous non-mass enhancement at the corresponding area of the mass on US

7.3 After Neoadjuvant Chemotherapy

See Figs. 50, 51 and 52.

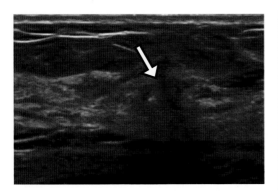

Fig. 50 Breast US (June 2021): US after treatment demonstrates residual hypoechoic mass that is decreased in the longest diameter

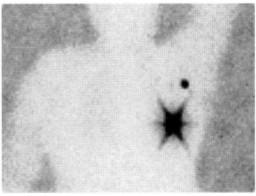

Fig. 52 Lymphoscintigraphy shows visualized sentinel lymph nodes in the left axilla

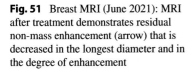

Fig. 51 Breast MRI (June 2021): MRI after treatment demonstrates residual non-mass enhancement (arrow) that is decreased in the longest diameter and in the degree of enhancement

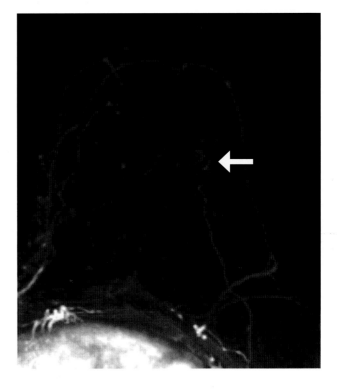

7.4 Courses of Treatment

Neoadjuvant chemotherapy (#6 cycles of docetaxel and carboplatin and trastuzumab and pertuzumab) + Operation + Post-operative radiation therapy.

7.4.1 Operation
Left breast conserving surgery, sentinel lymph node biopsy (Fig. 53).

7.4.2 Pathology Report
No residual tumor with stromal degeneration.

1. Post-chemotherapy status.
2. Lymph nodes: no metastasis in two axillary lymph nodes (ypN0(sn)) (sentinel LN: 0/2, non-sentinel LN: 0/0).

	Result	Intensity	Positive %
Estrogen receptor	Negative (2/8)	1	<1%
Progesterone receptor	Negative (2/8)	1	<1%
C-erbB2	Positive (3+)		
Ki-67	Positive in 16% of tumor cells		

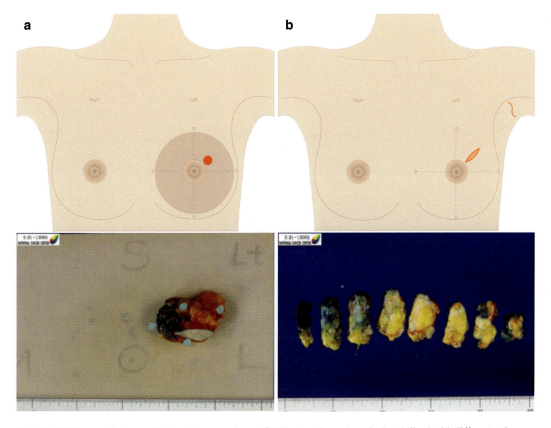

Fig. 53 (**a**) Gross pathology of lumpectomy specimen. (**b**) The margins get marked and sliced with different colors on each direction

8 Case 8

8.1 Patient History and Progress

Female/53 years old, peri-menopause.

Screen detected microcalcification on right breast 1 and 10 o'clock direction.

No family history.

No comorbidities.

8.2 Important Radiologic Findings

See Figs. 54, 55, 56 and 57.

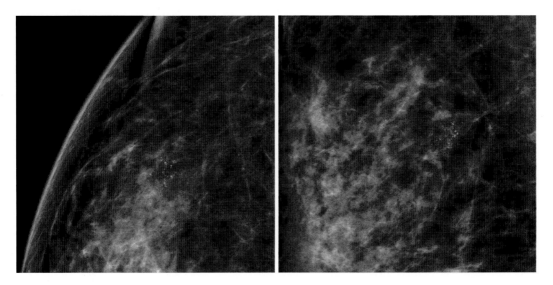

Fig. 54 Magnification CC/ML: segmental fine pleomorphic microcalcifications in right upper outer quadrant

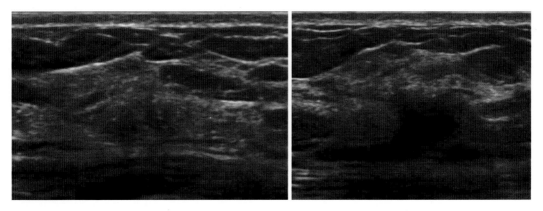

Fig. 55 Breast US: echogenic foci, suggesting microcalcifications at the 10 o'clock direction of right breast. Irregular hypoechoic mass at the 1 o'clock direction of right breast

HR(−) HER2(+) Breast Cancer

Fig. 56 PET-CT shows hypermetabolic lesions in Rt. breast (mSUV = 2.5)

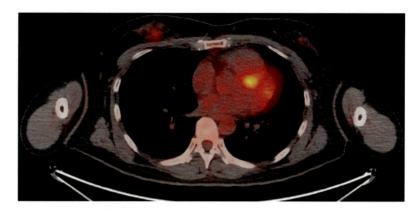

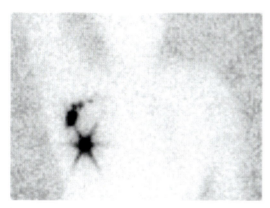

Fig. 57 Lymphoscintigraphy shows visualized sentinel lymph nodes in the right axilla

8.3 Courses of Treatment

Operation + Adjuvant chemotherapy (#4 cycles of Doxorubicin and Cyclophosphamide) + Operation + Trastuzumab.

8.3.1 Operation

Right nipple–areolar complex sparing mastectomy + implant reconstruction, sentinel lymph node biopsy left mastopexy, both accessory breast excision (Figs. 58 and 59).

8.3.2 Pathology Report

Invasive Ductal Carcinoma
1. Size of invasive component: 1.1 cm (pT1c).
2. Size of intraductal component: 3.0 cm.
3. Histologic grade: 3/3 (tubule formation: 3/3, nuclear pleomorphism: 3/3, mitotic count: 3/3, 5/HPF).
4. Intraductal component: present, intratumoral/extratumoral (60%) (nuclear grade: high, necrosis: present, architectural pattern: solid/comedo, extensive intraductal component: present).
5. Skin: no involvement of tumor.
6. Surgical margins:
   (a) deep margin: 2 mm,
   (b) superficial margin: 2 mm.
7. Lymph nodes: no metastasis in four axillary lymph nodes (pN0(sn)) (sentinel LN: 0/1, axillary LN: 0/3).
8. Arteriovenous invasion: absent.
9. Lymphovascular invasion: present, intratumoral.
10. Tumor border: infiltrative.
11. Microcalcification: present, tumoral/non-tumoral.
12. Pathological TN category (AJCC 2017): pT1cN0(sn).

Breast, right "accessary," excision:
Mammary ducts and lobules in fibroadipose tissue, suggestive of accessory breast.

	Result	Intensity	Positive %
Estrogen receptor	Negative (0/8)	0	0
Progesterone receptor	Negative (0/8)	0	0
C-erbB2	Positive (3+)		
Ki-67	Positive in 23% of tumor cells		

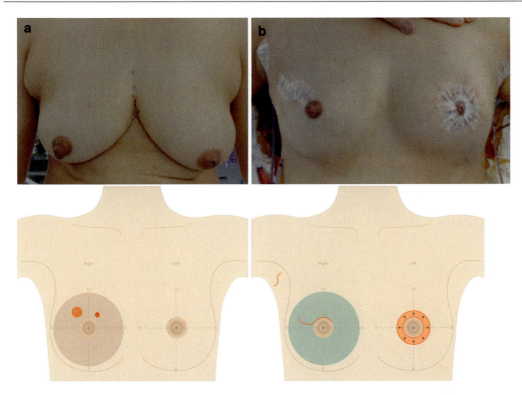

Fig. 58 (**a**) Preoperative and (**b**) immediate post-operative appearance

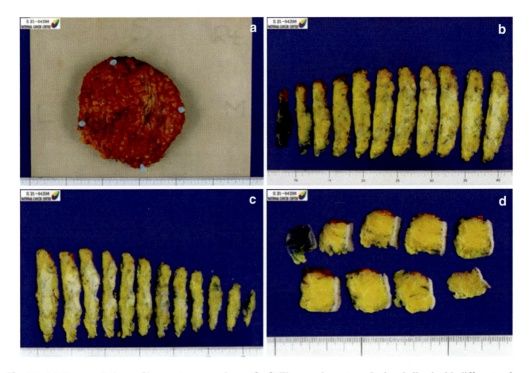

Fig. 59 (**a**) Gross pathology of lumpectomy specimen. (**b–d**) The margins get marked and sliced with different colors on each direction

9 Case 9

9.1 Patient History and Progress

Female/51 years old, pre-menopause.
Screen detected mass lesion on left breast 2 o'clock direction.
No family history.
Hypothyroidism.

9.2 Important Radiologic Findings

See Figs. 60, 61, 62 and 63.

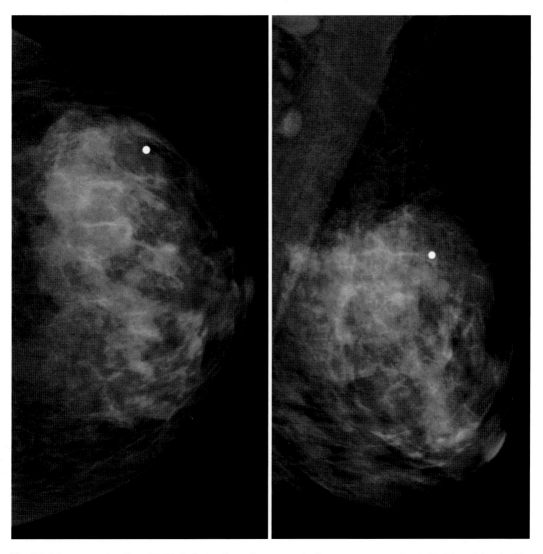

Fig. 60 Mammography (Sept. 2020): indistinct hyperdense mass in the upper outer quadrant of left breast (marked by BB marker). Several enlarged lymph nodes in Lt. Axilla

Fig. 61 Breast US (Sept. 2020): irregular hypoechoic mass at the 2 o'clock direction of left breast

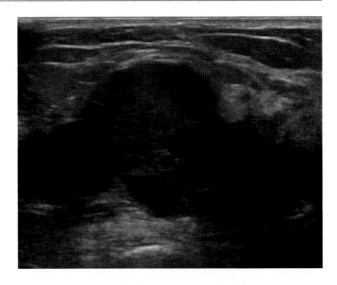

Fig. 62 Breast MRI (Sept. 2020): irregular heterogeneous enhancing mass at the 2 o'clock direction of left breast

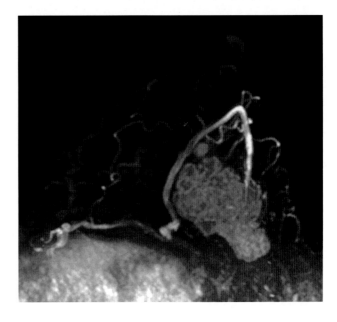

Fig. 63 PET-CT shows (**a**) hypermetabolic mass in the left upper outer breast (mSUV = 23.1) with satellite nodules and (**b**) hypermetabolic LNs in the left axilla level I–II (mSUV = ~10.5)

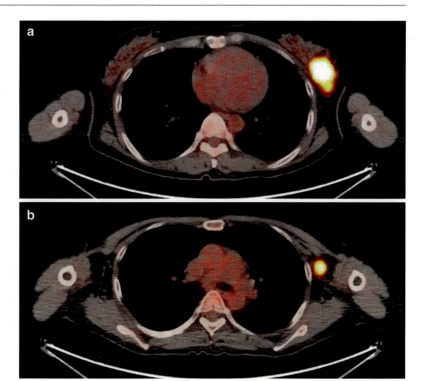

9.3 After Neoadjuvant Chemotherapy

See Figs. 64, 65, 66 and 67.

Fig. 64 Mammography (Jan. 2021): mammography after treatment demonstrates residual mass that is decreased in the longest diameter. Decrease in size of enlarged lymph nodes in left axilla

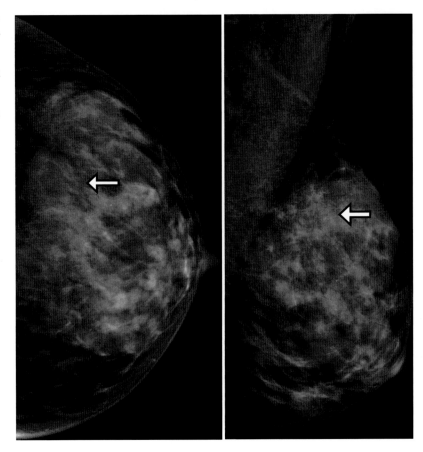

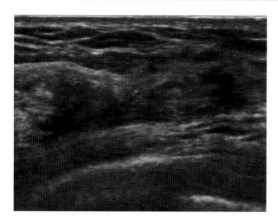

Fig. 65 Breast US (Jan. 2021): US after treatment demonstrates residual hypoechoic mass that is decreased in the longest diameter

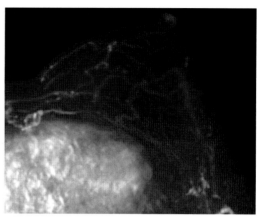

Fig. 66 Breast MRI (Jan. 2021): MRI after treatment shows complete resolution of enhancement in the left breast

Fig. 67 Lymphoscintigraphy shows visualized sentinel lymph nodes in the left axilla

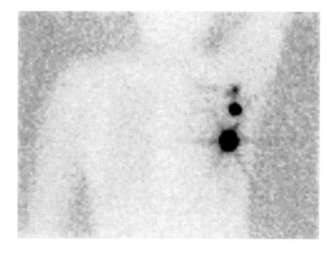

9.4 Courses of Treatment

Neoadjuvant chemotherapy (#2 cycles of docetaxel and carboplatin and trastuzumab and pertuzumab after followed #4 cycles of docetaxel and trastuzumab and pertuzumab) + Operation + Post-operative radiation therapy + Trastuzumab and pertuzumab.

9.4.1 Operation
Left breast conserving surgery, sentinel lymph node biopsy (Fig. 68).

9.4.2 Pathology Report
1. No residual tumor with stromal fibrosis.
   (a) Post-chemotherapy status.
   (b) Lymph nodes: no metastasis in eight axillary lymph nodes (ypN0) (sentinel LN: 0/8).
2. Atypical ductal hyperplasia with microcalcification.

	Result	Intensity	Positive %
Estrogen receptor	Negative (1/8)	1	<1%
Progesterone receptor	Negative (2/8)	1	<1%
C-erbB2	Positive (3+)		
Ki-67	Positive in 79% of tumor cells		

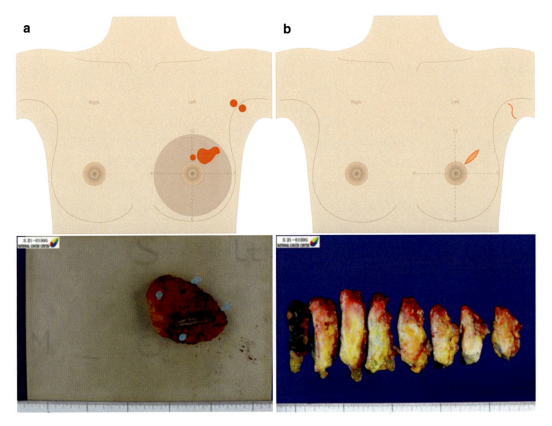

Fig. 68 (**a**) Gross pathology of lumpectomy specimen. (**b**) The margins get marked and sliced with different colors on each direction

10 Case 10

10.1 Patient History and Progress

Female/36 years old, pre-menopause.

Self-detected palpable mass lesion on left breast 9 o'clock direction.

Family history of breast cancer, aunt (paternal).

S/P Tuberculosis, s/p salpingectomy.

BRCA 1 and 2 mutation: Not detected, ATM VUS (variant of uncertain).

10.2 Important Radiologic Findings

See Figs. 69, 70, 71 and 72.

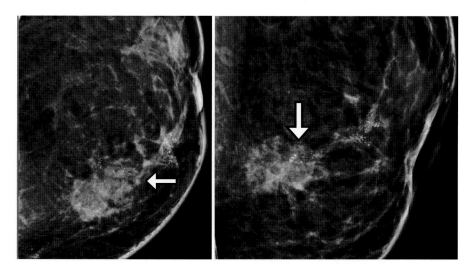

Fig. 69 Magnification CC/ML (Feb. 2021): irregular hyperdense masses with fine pleomorphic microcalcifications in left mid-inner breast mass with microcalcifications at the 9 o'clock direction of left breast

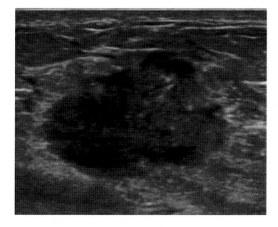

Fig. 70 Breast US (Feb. 2021): irregular hypoechoic mass with microcalcifications at the 9 o'clock direction of left breast

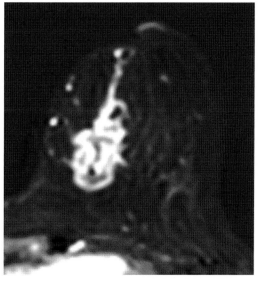

Fig. 71 Breast MRI (Feb. 2021): irregular enhancing mass at the 9 o'clock direction of left breast

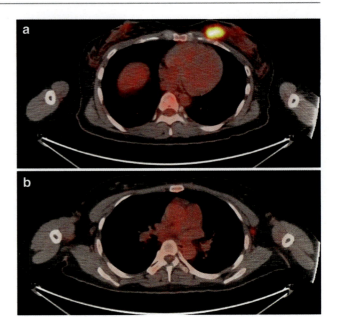

Fig. 72 PET-CT shows (**a**) hypermetabolic mass in left breast 9′ (mSUV = 10.5) and (**b**) hypermetabolic LN in left axilla, level I–II (mSUV = 2.6)

HR(−) HER2(+) Breast Cancer   467

10.3 After Neoadjuvant Chemotherapy

See Figs. 73, 74, 75 and 76.

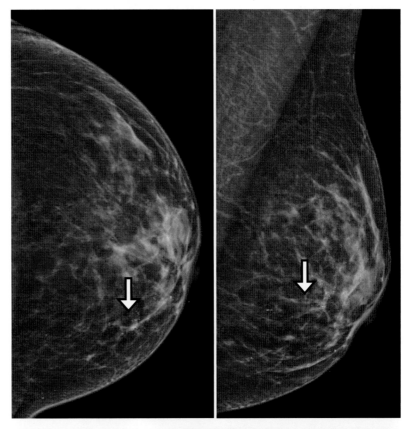

Fig. 73 Mammography (July 2021): mammography after treatment demonstrates residual fine pleomorphic microcalcifications

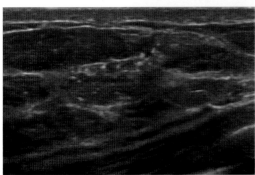

Fig. 74 Breast US (July 2021): US after treatment demonstrates residual microcalcifications

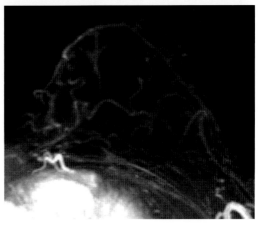

Fig. 75 Breast MRI (July 2021): MRI after treatment demonstrates residual non-mass enhancement (white arrow) that is decreased in the longest diameter and in the degree of enhancement

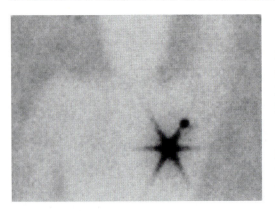

Fig. 76 Lymphoscintigraphy shows visualized sentinel lymph nodes in the left axilla

10.4 Courses of Treatment

Neoadjuvant chemotherapy (#6 cycles of docetaxel and carboplatin and trastuzumab and pertuzumab) + Operation + Trastuzumab and pertuzumab.

10.4.1 Operation

Left nipple–areolar complex sparing mastectomy with implant reconstruction, axillary lymph node sampling (Fig. 77).

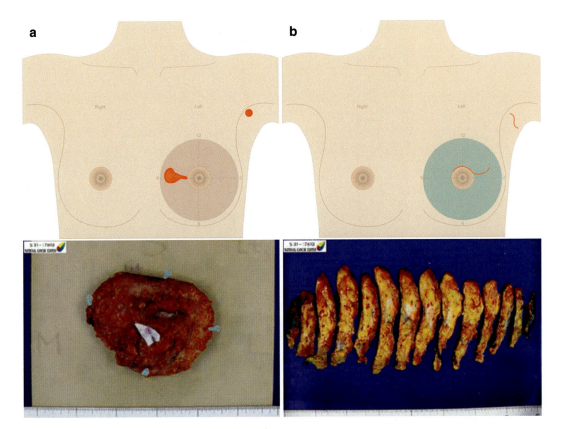

Fig. 77 (**a**) Gross pathology of nipple–areolar complex sparing mastectomy specimen. (**b**) The margins get marked and sliced with different colors on each direction

10.4.2 Pathology Report

No residual tumor with stromal degeneration.
1. Post-chemotherapy status.
2. Lymph nodes: no metastasis in six axillary lymph nodes (ypN0(sn)) (sentinel LN: 0/1, non-sentinel LN: 0/5).

	Result	Intensity	Positive %
Estrogen receptor	Negative (2/8)	1	<1%
Progesterone receptor	Negative (2/8)	1	<1%
C-erbB2	Positive (3+)		
Ki-67	Positive in 33% of tumor cells		

11 Case 11

11.1 Patient History and Progress

Female/56 years old, post-menopause.
Self-detected palpable mass lesion on right breast.
No family history.
Diabetes mellitus, hepatitis C virus carrier.

11.2 Important Radiologic Findings

See Figs. 78, 79, 80 and 81.

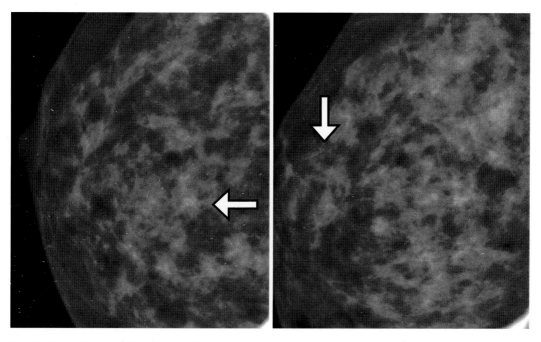

Fig. 78 Magnification CC/ML (June 2020): segmental fine pleomorphic microcalcifications in the upper inner quadrant of right breast

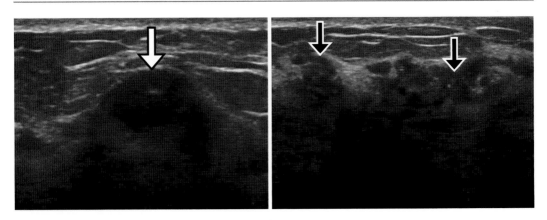

Fig. 79 Breast US (June 2020): irregular hypoechoic mass (white arrow) at the 1 o'clock direction of right breast. Associated microcalcifications (black arrow) at the 12 o'clock direction of right breast

Fig. 80 Breast MRI (June 2020): segmental heterogeneous non-mass enhancement in the upper inner quadrant of right breast

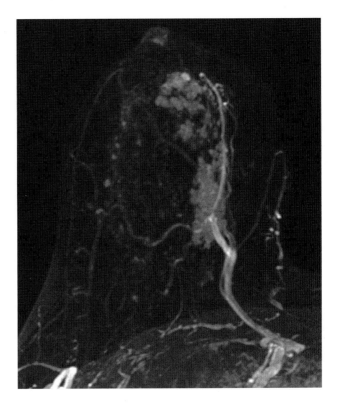

Fig. 81 PET-CT shows (**a**) hypermetabolic mass in the right upper breast (mSUV = 6.2) with mild hypermetabolic satellite nodules and (**b**) mild hypermetabolic LNs in the right axilla level I (mSUV = 1.3)

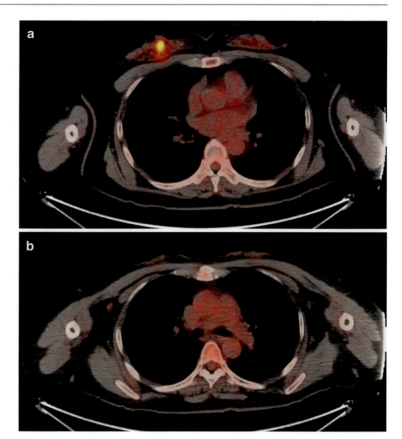

11.3 After Neoadjuvant Chemotherapy

See Figs. 82, 83, 84 and 85.

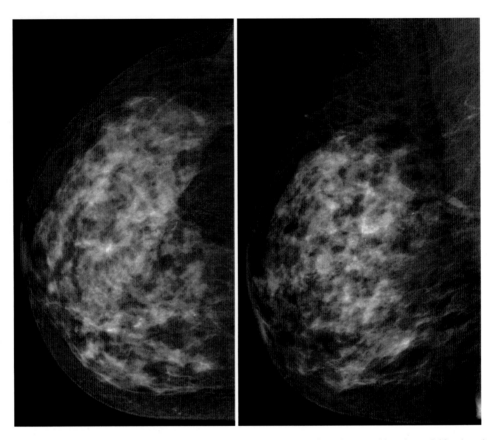

Fig. 82 Mammography (Dec. 2020): no significant change of segmental fine pleomorphic microcalcifications in the upper inner quadrant of right breast

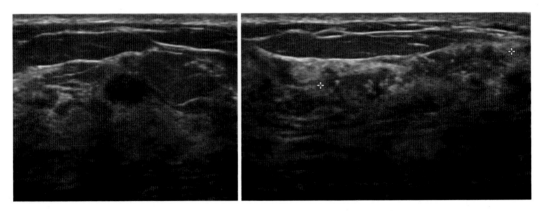

Fig. 83 Breast US (Dec. 2020): US after treatment demonstrates residual hypoechoic mass and microcalcifications that are decreased in the extent of the lesions

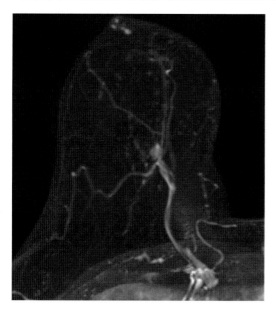

Fig. 84 Breast MRI (Dec. 2020): MRI after treatment demonstrates residual non-mass enhancement (white arrow) that is decreased in the longest diameter and in the degree of enhancement

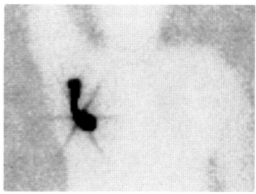

Fig. 85 Lymphoscintigraphy shows visualized sentinel lymph nodes in the right axilla

11.4 Courses of Treatment

Neoadjuvant chemotherapy (#4 cycles of doxorubicin and cyclophosphamide + #4 cycles of docetaxel and trastuzumab) + Operation + Postoperative radiation therapy + Trastuzumab.

11.4.1 Operation

Right modified radical mastectomy, axillary lymph node sampling (Fig. 86).

11.4.2 Pathology Report

Invasive Ductal Carcinoma
1. Post-chemotherapy status.
2. Size of tumor: 1.5 cm (ypT1c).
3. Histologic grade: 3/3 (tubule formation: 3/3, nuclear pleomorphism: 3/3, mitotic count: 3/3, 5/HPF).
4. Intraductal component: present, intratumoral/extratumoral (40%) (nuclear grade: high, necrosis: present, architectural pattern: solid/comedo, extensive intraductal component: present).
5. Skin and nipple: no involvement of tumor.
6. Surgical margins:
    (a) deep margin: 2 mm,
    (b) superficial margin: 2 mm.
7. Lymph nodes: no metastasis in six axillary lymph nodes (ypN0) (sentinel LN: 0/3, non-sentinel LN: 0/3).
8. Arteriovenous invasion: absent.
9. Lymphovascular invasion: present, intratumoral.
10. Tumor border: infiltrative.
11. Microcalcification: present, tumoral/non-tumoral.
12. Pathological TN category (AJCC 2017): ypT1cN0.

	Result	Intensity	Positive %
Estrogen receptor	Negative (0/8)	0	0
Progesterone receptor	Negative (0/8)	0	0
C-erbB2	Positive (3+)		
Ki-67	Positive in 77% of tumor cells		

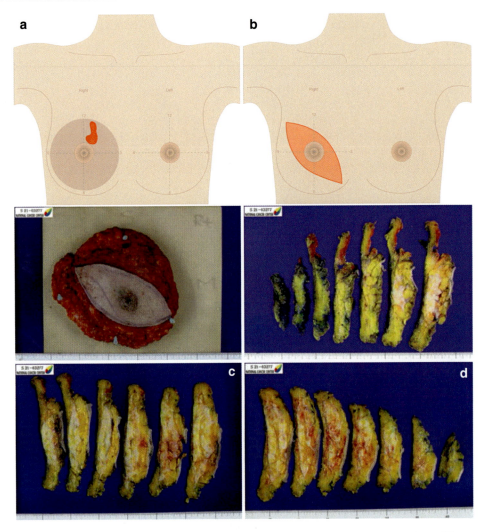

Fig. 86 (**a**) Gross pathology of mastectomy specimen. (**b–d**) The margins get marked and sliced with different colors on each direction

12　Case 12

12.1　Patient History and Progress

Female/66 years old, post-menopause.

Self-detected palpable mass lesion on left breast.

No family history.

Hypertension, thyroidectomy (hyperthyroidism), s/p salpingectomy.

12.2　Important Radiologic Findings

See Fig. 87, 88, 89 and 90.

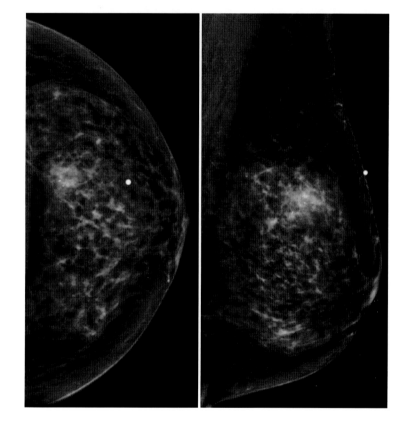

Fig. 87 Mammography: irregular hyperdense mass with microcalcifications in the upper outer quadrant of left breast (marked by BB marker)

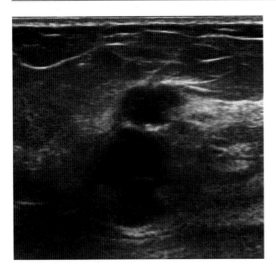

Fig. 88 Breast US: two irregular hypoechoic masses at the 2 o'clock direction of left breast

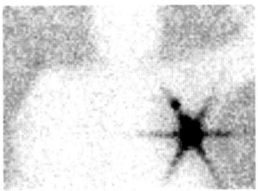

Fig. 90 Lymphoscintigraphy shows visualized sentinel lymph nodes in the left axilla

12.3 Courses of Treatment

Operation + Adjuvant chemotherapy (#4 cycles of docetaxel and cyclophosphamide) + Postoperative radiation therapy + Trastuzumab.

12.3.1 Operation
Left breast conserving surgery, sentinel lymph node biopsy (Fig. 91).

12.3.2 Pathology Report

Invasive Ductal Carcinoma with medullary pattern
1. Size of tumor: 2.9 cm (pT2).
2. Histologic grade: 3/3 (tubule formation: 3/3, nuclear pleomorphism: 3/3, mitotic count: 3/3, 5/HPF).
3. Intraductal component: present, intratumoral/extratumoral (30%) (nuclear grade: high, necrosis: present, architectural pattern:

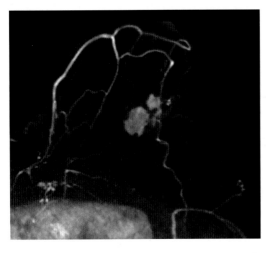

Fig. 89 Breast MRI: two irregular enhancing masses in the upper portion of left breast

HR(−) HER2(+) Breast Cancer

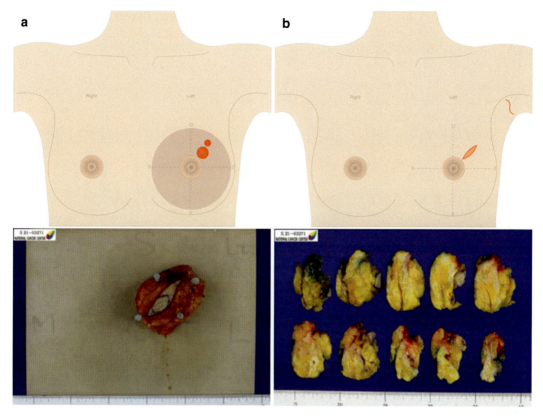

Fig. 91 (a) Gross pathology of lumpectomy specimen. (b) The margins get marked and sliced with different colors on each direction

solid/comedo, extensive intraductal component: present).
4. Skin: no involvement of tumor.
5. Surgical margins:
    (a) superior margin: 10 mm,
    (b) inferior margin: 5 mm,
    (c) medial margin: 20 mm,
    (d) lateral margin: 15 mm,
    (e) deep margin: 2 mm,
    (f) superficial margin: 2 mm.
6. Lymph nodes: no metastasis in four axillary lymph nodes (pN0(sn)) (sentinel LN (frozen): 0/4, sentinel LN (A): 0/0, non-sentinel LN: 0/0).
7. Arteriovenous invasion: absent.
8. Lymphovascular invasion: present, intratumoral.
9. Tumor border: infiltrative.
10. Microcalcification: present, tumoral/non-tumoral.
11. Pathological TN category (AJCC 2017): pT2N0(sn).

	Result	Intensity	Positive %
Estrogen receptor	Negative (0/8)	0	0
Progesterone receptor	Negative (0/8)	0	0
C-erbB2	Positive (3+)		
Ki-67	Positive in 52% of tumor cells		

13 Case 13

13.1 Patient History and Progress

Female/44 years old, pre-menopause.

Self-detected palpable mass lesion on left breast 11 o'clock direction.

No family history.

No comorbidities.

13.2 Important Radiologic Findings

See Figs. 92, 93 and 94.

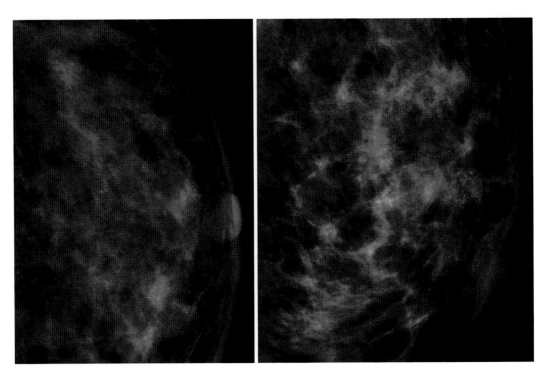

Fig. 92 Magnification (Oct. 2020): irregular hyperdense masses with associated fine pleomorphic microcalcifications in the upper portion of left breast and thickening of left nipple–areolar complex

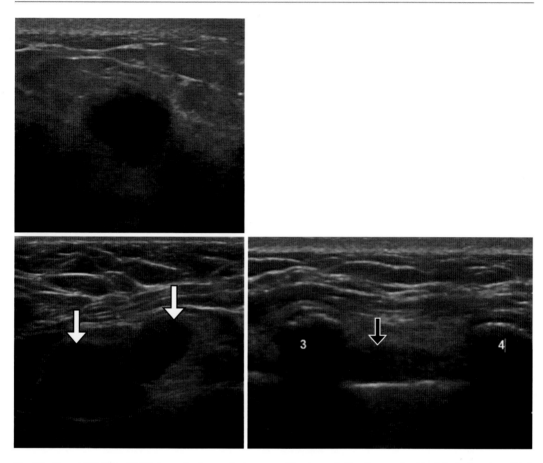

Fig. 93 Breast US (Oct. 2020): irregular hypoechoic mass with microcalcifications at the 11 o'clock direction of left breast. Enlarged lymph nodes in left axilla (white arrows) and left third intercostal space, parasternal area (black arrow)

Fig. 94 Breast MRI (Oct. 2020): multicentric irregular enhancing masses and heterogeneous non-mass enhancement in the upper portion of left breast. Enhancing lesion (black arrow) in left nipple

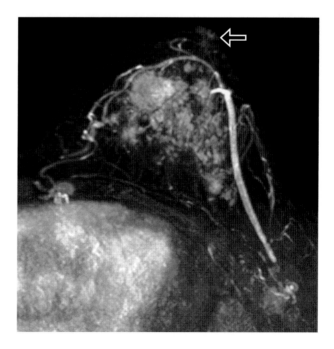

13.3 After Neoadjuvant Chemotherapy

See Figs. 95, 96, 97 and 98.

13.4 Courses of Treatment

Neoadjuvant chemotherapy (#6 cycles of docetaxel and carboplatin and trastuzumab and pertuzumab) + Operation + Post-operative radiation therapy + Trastuzumab emtansine.

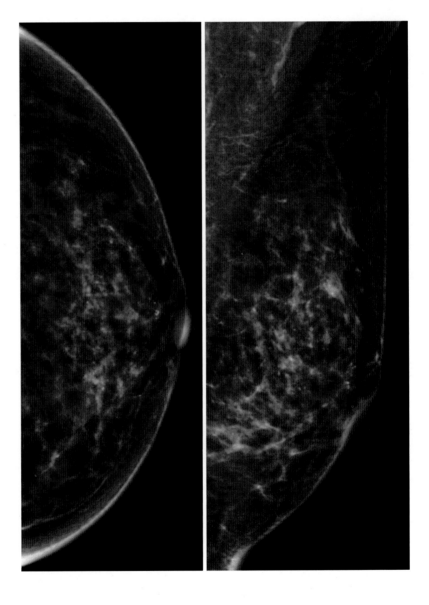

Fig. 95 Mammography (Feb. 2021): no significant change of segmental fine pleomorphic microcalcifications in the upper portion of left breast

Fig. 96 Breast US (Feb. 2021): US after treatment demonstrates residual hypoechoic mass that is decreased in the longest diameter. Decrease in size of previous enlarged LNs of left axilla and left third intercostal space

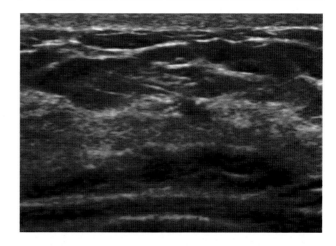

Fig. 97 Breast MR (Feb. 2021): MRI after treatment demonstrates residual non-mass enhancement (white arrow) that is decreased in the longest diameter and in the degree of enhancement

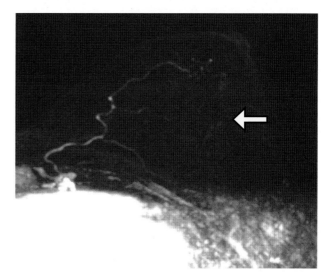

Fig. 98 Lymphoscintigraphy shows visualized sentinel lymph node in left axilla and left internal mammary area

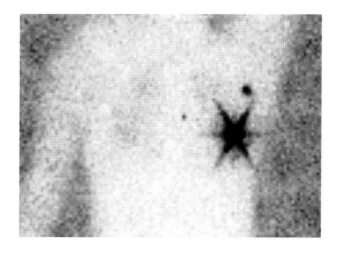

13.4.1 Operation

Left modified radical mastectomy, axillary lymph node sampling (Fig. 99).

13.4.2 Pathology Report

Invasive Ductal Carcinoma with apocrine differentiation

1. Post-chemotherapy status.
2. Size of tumor: 0.3 cm (ypT1a).
3. Histologic grade: 3/3 (tubule formation: 3/3, nuclear pleomorphism: 3/3, mitotic count: 3/3, 4/HPF).
4. Intraductal component: present, intratumoral/extratumoral (30%) (nuclear grade: high, necrosis: present, architectural pattern: cribriform/solid, extensive intraductal component: present).

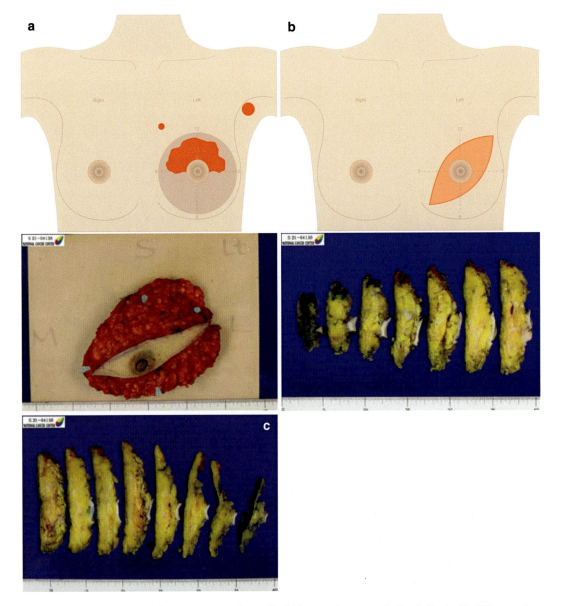

Fig. 99 (**a**) Gross pathology of mastectomy specimen. (**b, c**) The margins get marked and sliced with different colors on each direction

5. Skin and nipple: no involvement of tumor.
6. Surgical margins:
   (a) deep margin: 2 mm,
   (b) superficial margin: 2 mm.
7. Lymph nodes: no metastasis in six axillary lymph nodes (ypN0) (sentinel LN: 0/3, non-sentinel LN: 0/3).
8. Arteriovenous invasion: absent.
9. Lymphovascular invasion: present, intratumoral.
10. Tumor border: infiltrative.
11. Microcalcification: present, tumoral/non-tumoral.
12. Pathological TN category (AJCC 2017): ypT1aN0.

	Result	Intensity	Positive %
Estrogen receptor	Negative (0/8)	0	0
Progesterone receptor	Negative (0/8)	0	0
C-erbB2	Positive (3+)		

	Result	Intensity	Positive %
Ki-67	Positive in 4% of tumor cells		

14   Case 14

14.1   Patient History and Progress

Female/74 years old, post-menopause.

Screen detected mass lesion on right breast 12 o'clock direction.

No family history.

S/P retroperitoneum, excision (paraganglioma).

14.2   Important Radiologic Findings

See Figs. 100, 101, 102 and 103.

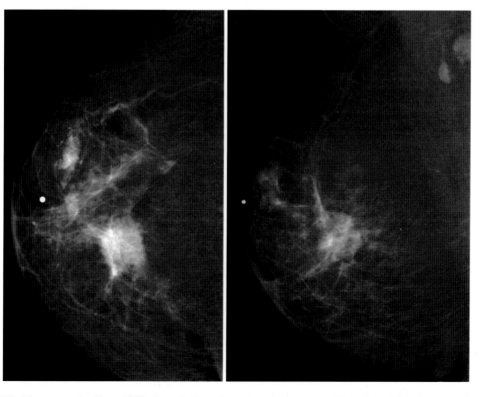

Fig. 100 Mammography (Sept. 2020): irregular hyperdense mass in the upper mid portion of right breast (marked by BB marker). Enlarged lymph nodes in right axilla

Fig. 101 Breast US (Sept. 2020): irregular hypoechoic mass at the 12 o'clock direction of right breast

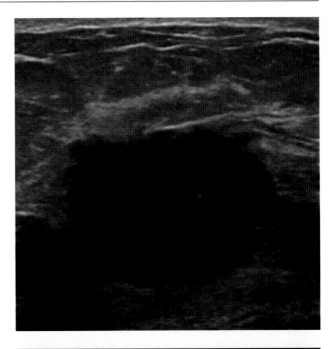

Fig. 102 Breast MRI (Sept. 2020): irregular enhancing mass at the 12 o'clock direction of right breast. Enlarged lymph nodes in right axilla

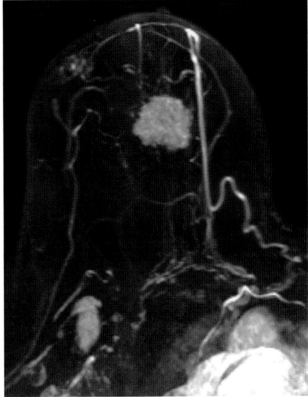

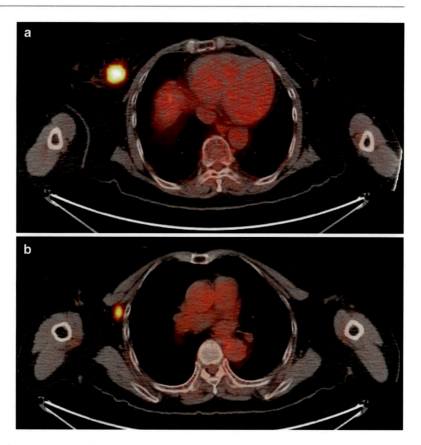

Fig. 103 PET-CT shows (**a**) hypermetabolic mass in the right upper breast (mSUV = 10.3) and (**b**) enlarged hypermetabolic LNs in the right axilla level I–II (mSUV = 5.5)

14.3 After Neoadjuvant Chemotherapy

See Figs. 104, 105, 106 and 107.

14.4 Courses of Treatment

Neoadjuvant chemotherapy (#3 cycles of docetaxel and trastuzumab and pertuzumab after followed #3 cycles of trastuzumab and pertuzumab #4) + Operation + Post-operative radiation therapy + Trastuzumab emtansine.

14.4.1 Operation

Right breast conserving surgery, axillary lymph node dissection (level II) (Fig. 108).

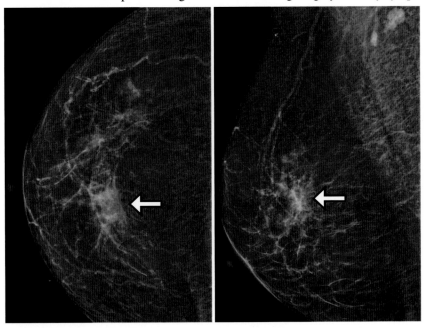

Fig. 104 Mammography (Mar. 2021): mammography after treatment demonstrates residual mass that is decreased in the longest diameter. Decreased size of lymph nodes, Rt. Axilla

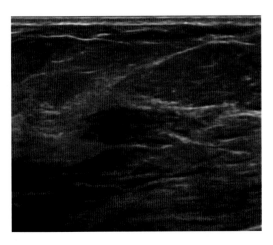

Fig. 105 Breast US (Mar. 2021): US after treatment demonstrates residual hypoechoic mass that is decreased in the longest diameter

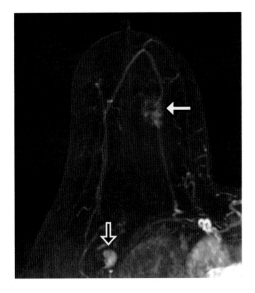

Fig. 106 Breast MRI (Dec. 2020): MRI after treatment demonstrates residual enhancing mass (white arrow) that is decreased in the longest diameter and in the degree of enhancement Decrease in size of suspicious lymph nodes (black arrow) in right axilla

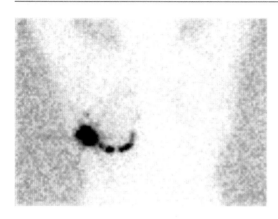

Fig. 107 Lymphoscintigraphy shows visualized sentinel lymph nodes in the right axilla

14.4.2 Pathology Report

Microinvasive Ductal Carcinoma

1. Size of invasive component: <0.1 cm (pT1mi).
2. Size of intraductal component: 2.5 cm.
3. Histologic grade: 3/3 (tubule formation: 3/3, nuclear pleomorphism: 3/3, mitotic count: 3/3, 4/HPF).
4. Intraductal component: present, intratumoral/extratumoral (99%) (nuclear grade: high, necrosis: present, architectural pattern: cribriform/solid/comedo, extensive intraductal component: present).
5. Skin: no involvement of tumor.
6. Surgical margins:
   (a) superior margin: (see Note 1),
   (b) inferior margin: (see Note 2),
   (c) medial margin: positive for ductal carcinoma in situ (Fro 3) (see Note 3),
   (d) lateral margin: 10 mm,
   (e) deep margin: <1 mm from ductal carcinoma in situ (slide 8),
   (f) superficial margin: 2 mm.
7. Lymph nodes:
   (a) metastasis in four out of nine axillary lymph nodes (pN2a),
   (b) perinodal extension: present,
   (c) size of metastatic carcinoma: 19 mm.
8. Arteriovenous invasion: absent.
9. Lymphovascular invasion: present, intratumoral.
10. Tumor border: infiltrative.
11. Microcalcification: present, tumoral/non-tumoral.
12. Pathological TN category (AJCC 2017): pT1miN2a.

Note: 1. The superior margin of the lumpectomy specimen (slide 1) is close to ductal carcinoma in situ (<1 mm) but this margin submitted for frozen diagnosis (Fro 1) is free of tumor.

2. The inferior margin of the lumpectomy specimen (slide 5) is close to ductal carcinoma in situ (2 mm) but this margin submitted for frozen diagnosis (Fro 2) is free of tumor.

3. Ductal carcinoma in situ is present only in the permanent section of Fro 3.

	Result	Intensity	Positive %
Estrogen receptor	Negative (2/8)	1	<1%
Progesterone receptor	Negative (0/8)	0	0
C-erbB2	Positive (3+)		
Ki-67	Positive in 41% of tumor cells		

15 Case 15

15.1 Patient History and Progress

Female/61 years old, post-menopause.

Self-detected palpable mass lesion on right breast 12 o'clock direction.

No family history.

Hypertension.

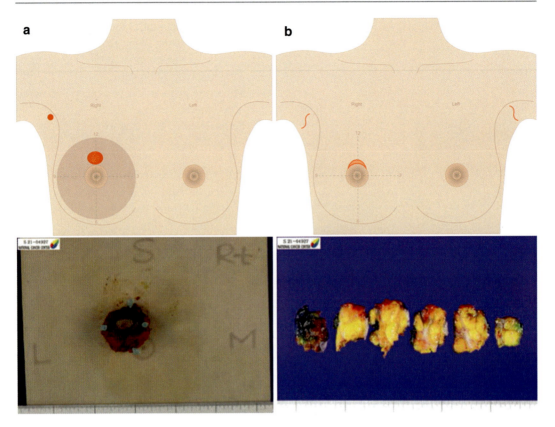

Fig. 108 (**a**) Gross pathology of lumpectomy specimen. (**b**) The margins get marked and sliced with different colors on each direction

15.2 Important Radiologic Findings

See Figs. 109, 110, 111 and 112.

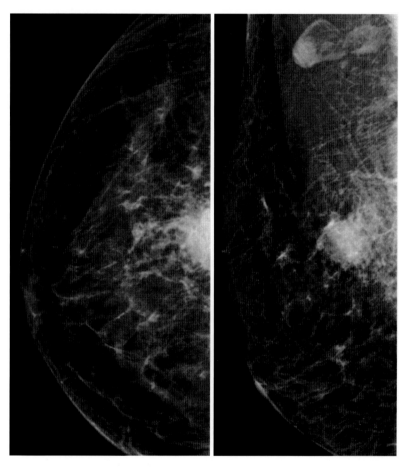

Fig. 109 Mammography (Mar. 2021): irregular hyperdense mass in the upper mid portion of right breast. Enlarged lymph nodes in right axilla

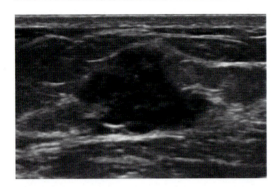

Fig. 110 Breast US (Mar. 2021): irregular hypoechoic mass at the 12 o'clock direction of right breast

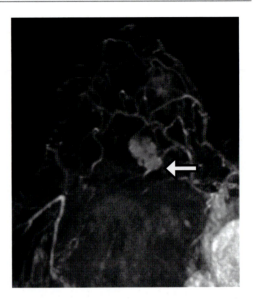

Fig. 111 Breast MRI (Mar. 2021): irregular enhancing mass at the 12 o'clock direction of right breast

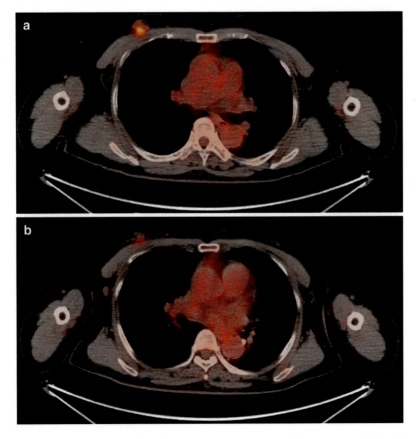

Fig. 112 PET-CT shows (**a**) hypermetabolic lesion in right breast, upper inner quadrant (mSUV = 4.1) and (**b**) mild hypermetabolic lymph node in right axilla level I area (mSUV = 1.1)

15.3 After Neoadjuvant Chemotherapy

See Figs. 113, 114 and 115.

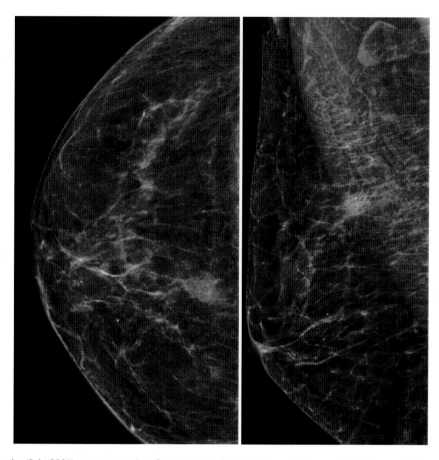

Fig. 113 Mammography (July 2021): mammography after treatment demonstrates residual mass that is decreased in the longest diameter. Decreased size of lymph nodes, Rt. Axilla

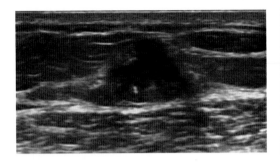

Fig. 114 Breast MRI (July 2021): MRI after treatment demonstrates residual enhancing mass that is decreased in the longest diameter

15.4 Courses of Treatment

Neoadjuvant chemotherapy (#6 cycles of docetaxel and carboplatin and trastuzumab and pertuzumab) + Operation + Post-operative radiation therapy + Trastuzumab.

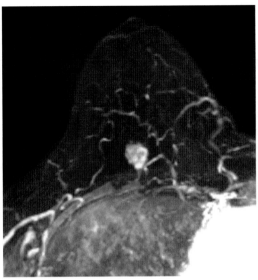

Fig. 115 Breast US (July 2021): US after treatment demonstrates residual hypoechoic mass that is decreased in the longest diameter

15.4.1 Operation

Right breast conserving surgery, sentinel lymph node biopsy (Fig. 116).

15.4.2 Pathology Report

Invasive Ductal Carcinoma
1. Post-chemotherapy status.
2. Size of tumor: 1.9 cm (ypT1c).
3. Histologic grade: 3/3 (tubule formation: 3/3, nuclear pleomorphism: 3/3, mitotic count: 2/3, 12/10HPF).
4. Intraductal component: absent.
5. Skin: no involvement of tumor.
6. Surgical margins:
    (a) superior margin: 30 mm,
    (b) inferior margin: 55 mm,
    (c) medial margin: 20 mm,
    (d) lateral margin: 15 mm,
    (e) deep margin: 1 mm from invasive ductal carcinoma (slide 2),
    (f) superficial margin: 10 mm.
7. Lymph nodes:
    (a) metastasis in two out of seven axillary lymph nodes (ypN1a) (sentinel LN: 1/2, axillary LN: 1/5),
    (b) perinodal extension: absent,
    (c) size of metastatic carcinoma: 5 mm.
8. Arteriovenous invasion: absent.
9. Lymphovascular invasion: present, intratumoral/peritumoral.
10. Tumor border: infiltrative.
11. Microcalcification: present, non-tumoral.
12. Pathological TN category (AJCC 2017): ypT1cN1a.

	Result	Intensity	Positive %
Estrogen receptor	Negative (0/8)	0	0
Progesterone receptor	Negative (0/8)	0	0
C-erbB2	Positive (3+)		
Ki-67	Positive in 25% of tumor cells		

HR(−) HER2(+) Breast Cancer

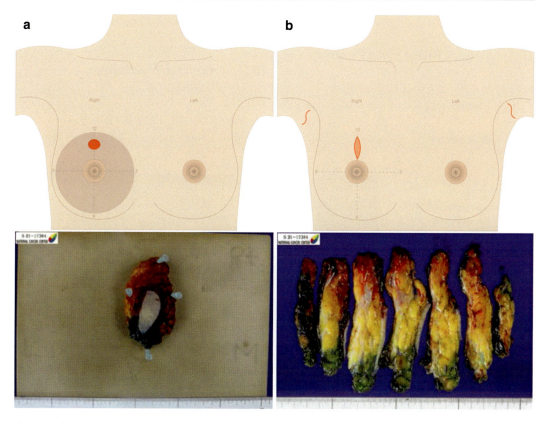

Fig. 116 (**a**) Gross pathology of lumpectomy specimen. (**b**) The margins get marked and sliced with different colors on each direction

16 Case 16

16.1 Patient History and Progress

Female/57 years old, post-menopause.

Self-detected palpable mass lesion on left breast.

No family history.

Hypothyroidism (taking on synthroid).

16.2 Important Radiologic Findings

See Figs. 117, 118, 119 and 120.

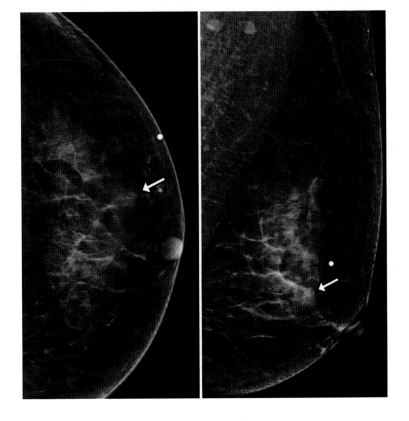

Fig. 117 Mammography (Feb. 2021): irregular isodense mass with obscured margin in the mid-outer portion of left breast

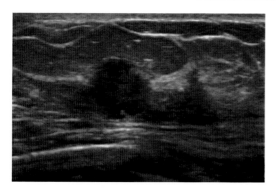

Fig. 118 Breast US (Feb. 2021): irregular hypoechoic mass at the 3 o'clock direction of left breast

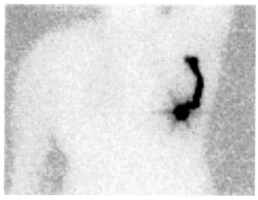

Fig. 120 Lymphoscintigraphy shows visualized sentinel lymph nodes in the left axilla

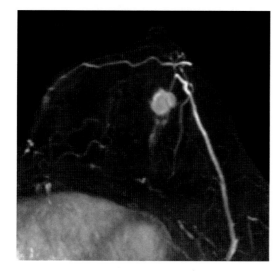

Fig. 119 Breast MRI (Feb. 2021): irregular enhancing mass with associated segmental non-mass enhancement at the 3 o'clock direction of left breast

16.3 Courses of Treatment

Operation + adjuvant chemotherapy (#4 cycles of docetaxel and cyclophosphamide) + Postoperative radiation therapy + Trastuzumab.

16.3.1 Operation

Left breast conserving surgery, sentinel lymph node biopsy (Fig. 121).

16.3.2 Pathology Report

Invasive Ductal Carcinoma
1. Size of tumor: 1.5 cm (pT1c).
2. Histologic grade: 3/3 (tubule formation: 3/3, nuclear pleomorphism: 3/3, mitotic count: 3/3, 4/HPF).

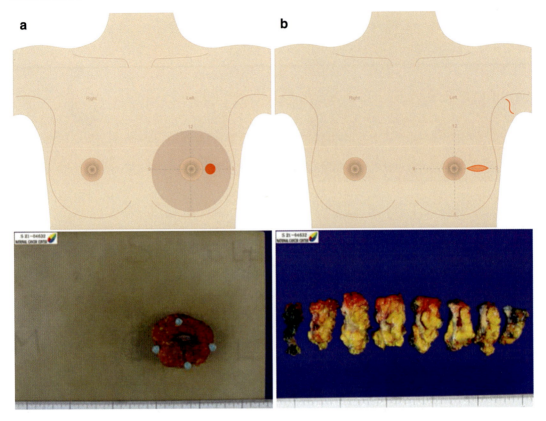

Fig. 121 (**a**) Gross pathology of lumpectomy specimen. (**b**) The margins get marked and sliced with different colors on each direction

3. Intraductal component: present, intratumoral/extratumoral (30%) (nuclear grade: high, necrosis: present, architectural pattern: cribriform/solid/comedo, extensive intraductal component: present).
4. Skin: no involvement of tumor.
5. Surgical margins:
   (a) superior margin: 10 mm,
   (b) inferior margin: 10 mm,
   (c) medial margin: (see note),
   (d) lateral margin: 10 mm,
   (e) deep margin: 2 mm,
   (f) superficial margin: 2 mm.
6. Lymph nodes: no metastasis in three axillary lymph nodes (pN0(sn)) (sentinel LN: 0/1, non-sentinel LN: 0/2).
7. Arteriovenous invasion: absent.
8. Lymphovascular invasion: present, intratumoral.
9. Tumor border: infiltrative.
10. Microcalcification: present, tumoral/non-tumoral.
11. Pathological TN category (AJCC 2017): pT1cN0(sn).

	Result	Intensity	Positive %
Estrogen receptor	Negative (0/8)	0	0
Progesterone receptor	Negative (0/8)	0	0
C-erbB2	Positive (3+)		
Ki-67	Positive in 64% of tumor cells		

17 Case 17

17.1 Patient History and Progress

Female/41 years old, pre-menopause.

Self-detected palpable mass lesion on left breast.

Family history of breast cancer, aunt (maternal).

S/P Lumbar spine disc operation.

BRCA 1 and 2 mutation: Not detected, MUTYH VUS (variant of uncertain).

17.2 Important Radiologic Findings

See Figs. 122, 123, 124 and 125.

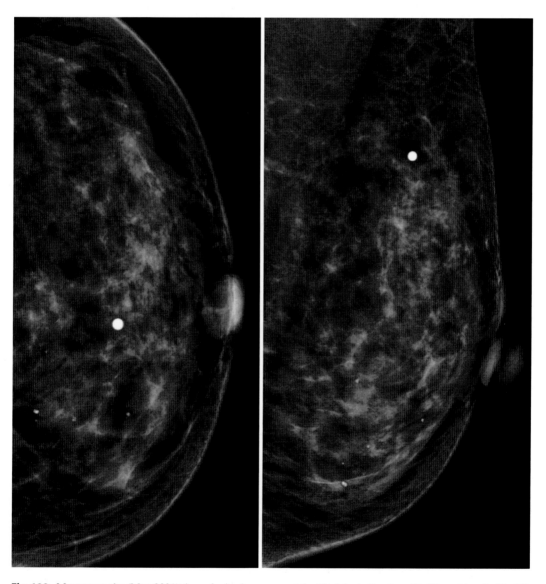

Fig. 122 Mammography (Mar. 2021): irregular isodense mass at the 12 o'clock direction of left breast (marked by BB marker)

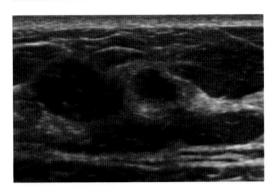

Fig. 123 Breast US (Mar. 2021): irregular masses at the 12 o'clock direction of left breast

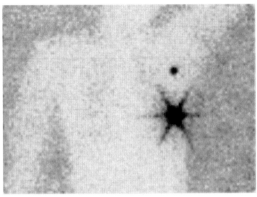

Fig. 125 Lymphoscintigraphy shows visualized sentinel lymph nodes in the left axilla

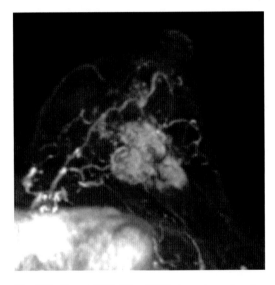

Fig. 124 Breast MRI (Mar. 2021): irregular enhancing masses with associated non-mass enhancement in the upper portion of left breast

17.3 Courses of Treatment

Operation + Adjuvant chemotherapy (#4 cycles of doxorubicin and cyclophosphamide + #4 cycles of docetaxel and trastuzumab) + Postoperative radiation therapy + Trastuzumab.

17.3.1 Operation

Left breast conserving surgery, axillary lymph node dissection (Fig. 126).

17.3.2 Pathology Report

Invasive Ductal Carcinoma
1. Size of tumor: 1.8 and 1.5 cm (pT1c(2)).
2. Histologic grade: 3/3 (tubule formation: 3/3, nuclear pleomorphism: 3/3, mitotic count: 3/3, 3/HPF).

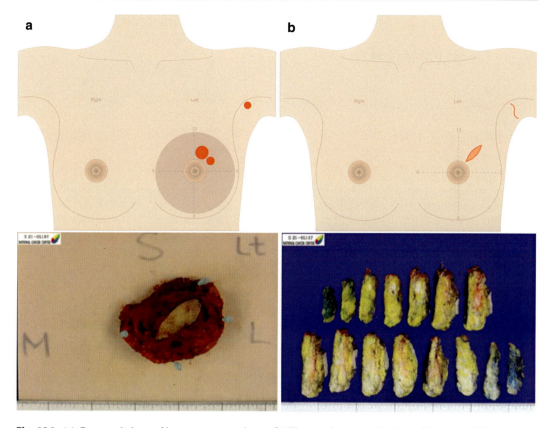

Fig. 126 (**a**) Gross pathology of lumpectomy specimen. (**b**) The margins get marked and sliced with different colors on each direction

3. Intraductal component: present, intratumoral/extratumoral (50%) (nuclear grade: high, necrosis: present, architectural pattern: solid/comedo, extensive intraductal component: present).
4. Skin: no involvement of tumor.
5. Surgical margins:
   (a) superior margin: (see note),
   (b) inferior margin: 10 mm,
   (c) medial margin: 5 mm,
   (d) lateral margin: 30 mm,
   (e) deep margin: 2 mm,
   (f) superficial margin: 2 mm.
6. Lymph nodes:
   (a) metastasis in one out of three axillary lymph nodes (pN1a(sn)) (sentinel LN: 1/2, axillary LN: 0/1),
   (b) perinodal extension: present,
   (c) size of metastatic carcinoma: 9 mm.
7. Arteriovenous invasion: absent.
8. Lymphovascular invasion: present, intratumoral.
9. Tumor border: infiltrative.
10. Microcalcification: present, tumoral/non-tumoral.
11. Pathological TN category (AJCC 2017): pT1c(2)N1a(sn).

	Result	Intensity	Positive %
Estrogen receptor	Negative (0/8)	0	0
Progesterone receptor	Negative (0/8)	0	0
C-erbB2	Positive (3+)		
Ki-67	Positive in 20% of tumor cells		

18 Case 18

18.1 Patient History and Progress

Female/61 years old, post-menopause.

Self-detected bloody discharge on nipple of left breast.

No family history.

S/p hysterectomy.

18.2 Important Radiologic Findings

See Figs. 127, 128, 129 and 130.

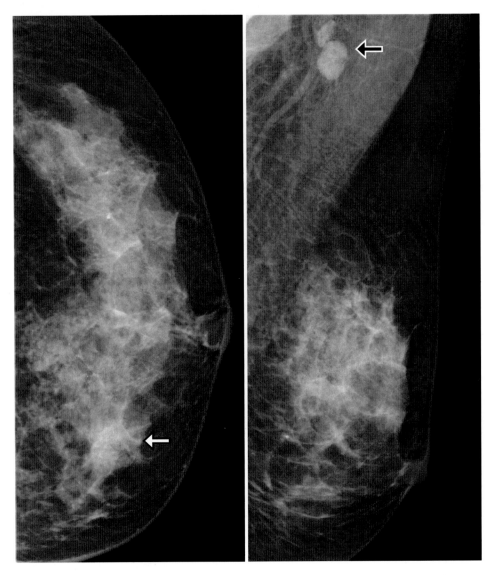

Fig. 127 Mammography (Mar. 2021): irregular hyperdense mass in the inner portion of left breast (white arrow). The mass is almost invisible on the mediolateral oblique view. Enlarged lymph nodes in left axilla (black arrow)

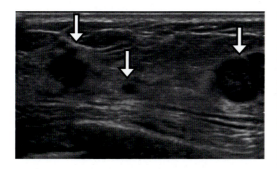

Fig. 128 Breast US (Mar. 2021): multiple irregular masses in the upper portion of left breast

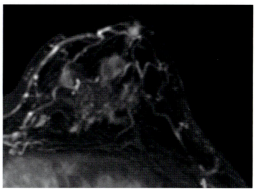

Fig. 129 Breast MRI (Mar. 2021): irregular masses with associated regional non-mass enhancement in the upper portion of left breast

Fig. 130 PET-CT shows (**a**) hypermetabolic uptake in the known left breast cancer and (**b**) hypermetabolic enlarged LN at left axillary level I

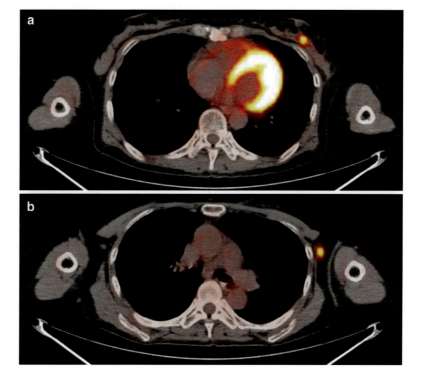

18.3 After Neoadjuvant Chemotherapy

See Figs. 131, 132, 133 and 134.

18.4 Courses of Treatment

Neoadjuvant chemotherapy (#6 cycles of docetaxel and carboplatin and trastuzumab and pertuzumab) + Operation + Post-operative radiation therapy + Trastuzumab.

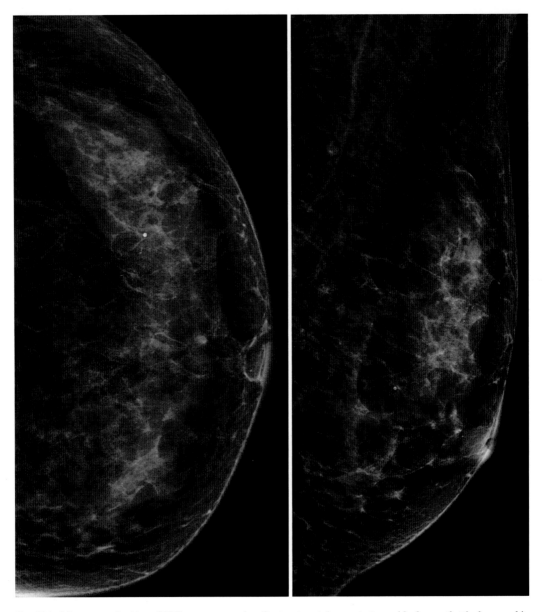

Fig. 131 Mammography (Aug. 2021): mammography after treatment demonstrates residual mass that is decreased in the longest diameter. Decrease in size of lymph nodes in left axilla

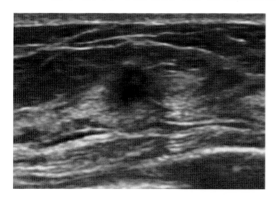

Fig. 132 Breast US (Aug. 2021): US after treatment demonstrates residual hypoechoic mass that is decreased in the longest diameter

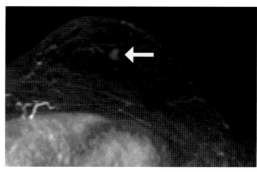

Fig. 133 Breast MRI (Aug. 2021): MRI after treatment demonstrates residual irregular mass (white arrow) that is decreased in the longest diameter

Fig. 134 Lymphoscintigraphy shows visualized sentinel lymph nodes in the left axilla

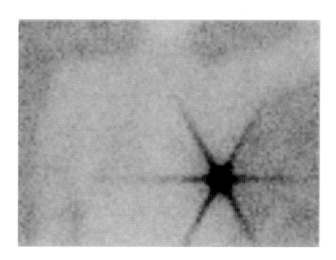

18.4.1 Operation

Left breast conserving surgery, axillary lymph node sampling (Fig. 135).

18.4.2 Pathology Report

Invasive Ductal Carcinoma
1. Post-chemotherapy status.
2. Size of tumor: 0.7 cm (ypT1b).
3. Histologic grade: 3/3 (tubule formation: 3/3, nuclear pleomorphism: 3/3, mitotic count: 3/3, 3/1HPF).
4. Intraductal component: absent.
5. Surgical margins:
   (a) superior margin: 40 mm,
   (b) inferior margin: 15 mm,
   (c) medial margin: 10 mm,
   (d) lateral margin: 15 mm,
   (e) deep margin: 5 mm,
   (f) superficial margin: 8 mm.
6. Lymph nodes: no metastasis in two axillary lymph nodes (ypN0(sn)) (sentinel LN: 0/1, axillary LN: 0/1).
7. Arteriovenous invasion: absent.
8. Lymphovascular invasion: present, intratumoral.

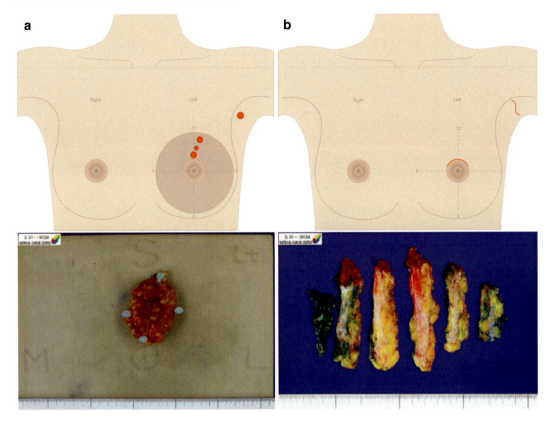

Fig. 135 (**a**) Gross pathology of lumpectomy specimen. (**b**) The margins get marked and sliced with different colors on each direction

9. Tumor border: infiltrative.
10. Microcalcification: present, non-tumoral.
11. Pathological TN category (AJCC 2017): ypT1bN0(sn).

	Result	Intensity	Positive %
Estrogen receptor	Negative (0/8)	0	0
Progesterone receptor	Negative (0/8)	0	0
C-erbB2	Positive (3+)		
Ki-67	Positive in 41% of tumor cells		

19 Case 19

19.1 Patient History and Progress

Female/52 years old, pre-menopause.

Self-detected palpable mass lesion on left breast 1 and 2 o'clock direction.

No family history.

Hepatitis B virus carrier, liver cirrhosis.

19.2 Important Radiologic Findings

See Figs. 136, 137, 138 and 139.

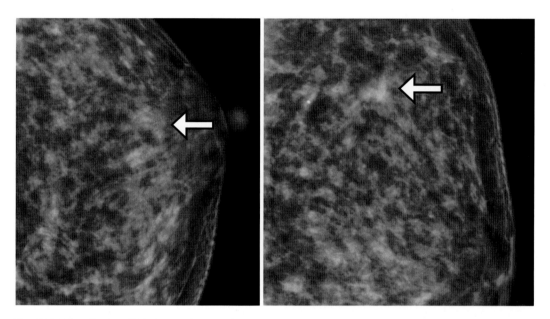

Fig. 136 Magnification CC/ML (Apr. 2021): ML Irregular mass with microcalcifications in the upper mid portion of left breast

Fig. 137 Breast US (Apr. 2021): US irregular hypoechoic mass at the 12 o'clock direction of left breast

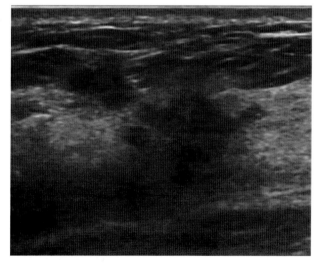

19.3 Courses of Treatment

Operation + Adjuvant chemotherapy (#4 cycles of doxorubicin and cyclophosphamide) + Postoperative radiation therapy + Trastuzumab.

19.3.1 Operation
Left breast conserving surgery, sentinel lymph node biopsy (Fig. 140).

19.3.2 Pathology Report

Invasive Ductal Carcinoma
1. Size of tumor: 2.1 cm (pT2).
2. Histologic grade: 3/3 (tubule formation: 3/3, nuclear pleomorphism: 3/3, mitotic count: 12/3, 2/10HPF).
3. Intraductal component: present, extratumoral (5%) (nuclear grade: high, necrosis: present, architectural pattern: solid/comedo, extensive intraductal component: absent).
4. Surgical margins:
    (a) superior margin: 10 mm,
    (b) inferior margin: 20 mm,
    (c) medial margin: 10 mm,
    (d) lateral margin: 10 mm,
    (e) deep margin: 2 mm,
    (f) superficial margin: 5 mm.
5. Lymph nodes: no metastasis in two axillary lymph nodes (pN0(sn)) (sentinel LN: 0/2).
6. Arteriovenous invasion: absent.
7. Lymphovascular invasion: present, peritumoral.
8. Tumor border: infiltrative.
9. Microcalcification: present, tumoral/non-tumoral.
10. Pathological TN category (AJCC 2017): pT2N0(sn).

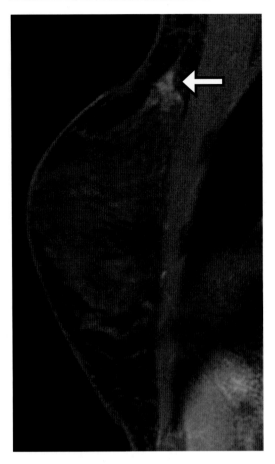

Fig. 138 Breast MRI (Apr. 2021): sagittal T1 weighted image with contrast enhancement shows irregular enhancing mass at the 12 o'clock direction of left breast

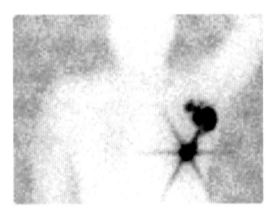

Fig. 139 Lymphoscintigraphy shows visualized sentinel lymph nodes in the left axilla

	Result	Intensity	Positive %
Estrogen receptor	Negative (0/8)	0	0
Progesterone receptor	Negative (0/8)	0	0
C-erbB2	Positive (3+)		
Ki-67	Positive in 39% of tumor cells		

HR(−) HER2(+) Breast Cancer

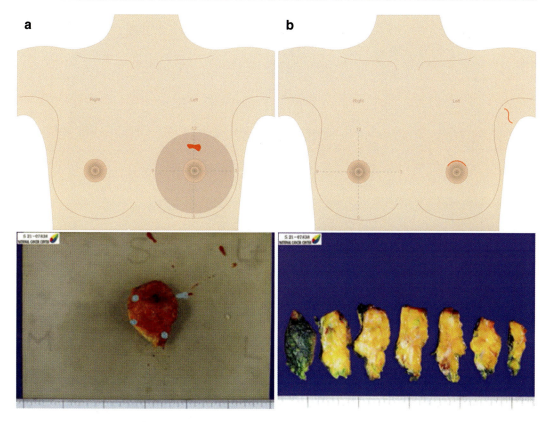

Fig. 140 (**a**) Gross pathology of lumpectomy specimen. (**b**) The margins get marked and sliced with different colors on each direction

20　Case 20

20.1　Patient History and Progress

Female/54 years old, post-menopause.

Screen detected mass lesion on left breast 11 o'clock direction.

Family history of breast cancer, aunt (paternal).

No comorbidities.
BRCA 1 and 2 mutation: Not detected.

20.2　Important Radiologic Findings

See Figs. 141, 142 and 143.

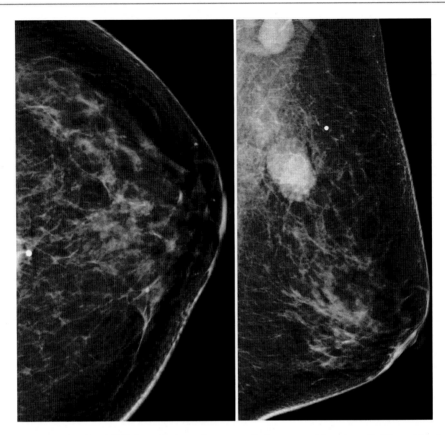

Fig. 141 Mammography (Oct. 2020): irregular hyperdense mass in the upper mid portion of left breast (marked by BB marker). Enlarged lymph node in left axilla

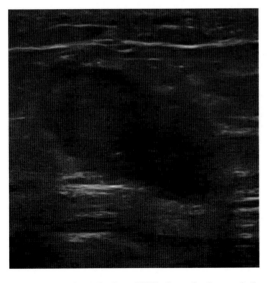

Fig. 142 Breast US (Oct. 2020): irregular hypoechoic mass at the 12 o'clock direction of left breast

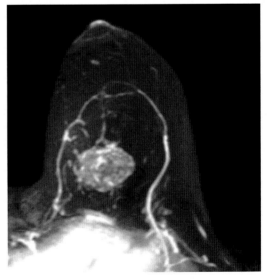

Fig. 143 Breast MRI (Oct. 2020): irregular enhancing mass at the 12 o'clock direction of left breast

20.3 After Neoadjuvant Chemotherapy

See Figs. 144, 145 and 146.

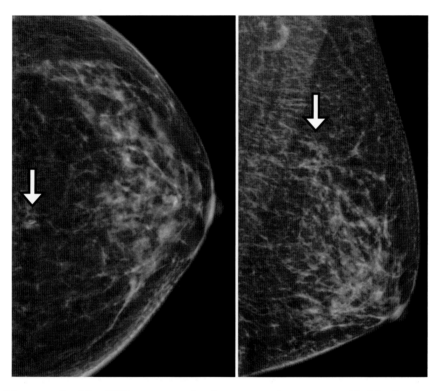

Fig. 144 Mammography (Mar. 2021): mammography after treatment demonstrates residual focal asymmetry that is decreased in the longest diameter (marked by radiopaque marker)

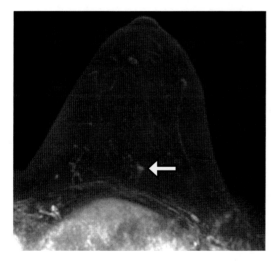

Fig. 145 Breast MRI (Mar. 2021): MRI after treatment demonstrates residual non-mass enhancement (white arrow) that is decreased in the longest diameter

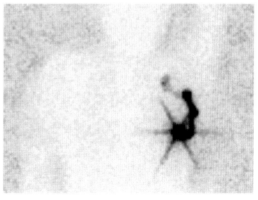

Fig. 146 Lymphoscintigraphy shows visualized sentinel lymph nodes in the left axilla

20.4 Courses of Treatment

Neoadjuvant chemotherapy (#6 cycles of docetaxel and carboplatin and trastuzumab and pertuzumab) + Operation + Post-operative radiation therapy + Trastuzumab.

20.4.1 Operation

Left breast conserving surgery, sentinel lymph node biopsy (Fig. 147).

20.4.2 Pathology Report

Invasive Ductal Carcinoma
1. Post-chemotherapy status.
2. Size of tumor: 1.1 cm (ypT1c).
3. Histologic grade: 3/3 (tubule formation: 3/3, nuclear pleomorphism: 3/3, mitotic count: 3/3, 3/HPF).
4. Intraductal component: present, intratumoral/extratumoral (10%) (nuclear grade: high, necrosis: absent, architectural pattern: solid, extensive intraductal component: absent).
5. Skin: no involvement of tumor.
6. Surgical margins:
    (a) superior margin: 10 mm,
    (b) inferior margin: 10 mm,
    (c) medial margin: 15 mm,
    (d) lateral margin: 10 mm,
    (e) deep margin: 2 mm,
    (f) superficial margin: 2 mm.
7. Lymph nodes:
    (a) metastasis in one out of two axillary lymph nodes (ypN1a(sn)) (sentinel LN: 1/2),
    (b) perinodal extension: absent,
    (c) size of metastatic carcinoma: 2.5 mm.

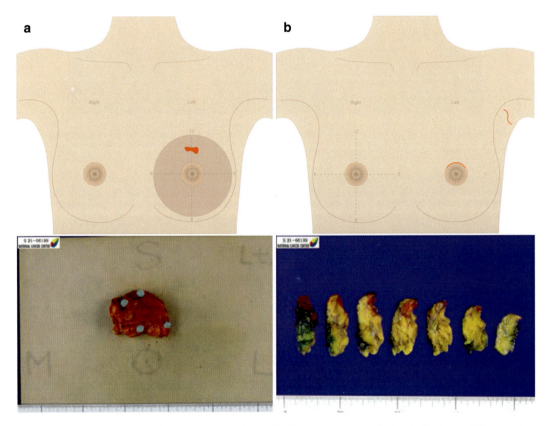

Fig. 147 (**a**) Gross pathology of lumpectomy specimen. (**b**) The margins get marked and sliced with different colors on each direction

8. Arteriovenous invasion: absent.
 9. Lymphovascular invasion: present, intratumoral.
 10. Tumor border: infiltrative.
 11. Microcalcification: present, tumoral/non-tumoral.
 12. Pathological TN category (AJCC 2017): ypT1cN1a(sn).

	Result	Intensity	Positive %
Estrogen receptor	Negative (0/8)	0	0
Progesterone receptor	Negative (0/8)	0	0
C-erbB2	Positive (3+)		
Ki-67	Positive in 45% of tumor cells		

21 Case 21

21.1 Patient History and Progress

Female/55 years old, pre-menopause.

Self-detected palpable mass lesion on right breast.

No family history.

S/P Tuberculosis.

21.2 Important Radiologic Findings

See Figs. 148, 149, 150 and 151.

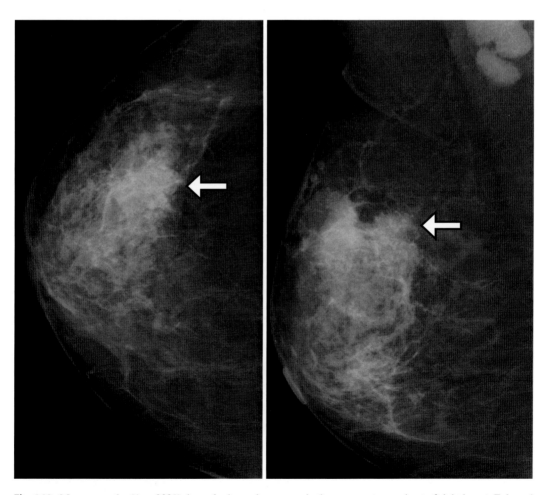

Fig. 148 Mammography (Apr. 2021): irregular hyperdense mass in the upper outer quadrant of right breast. Enlarged lymph nodes in right axilla

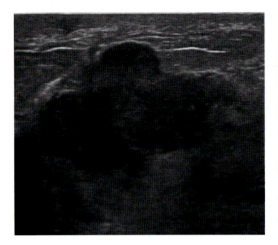

Fig. 149 Breast US (Apr. 2021): irregular hypoechoic mass at the 11 o'clock direction of right breast

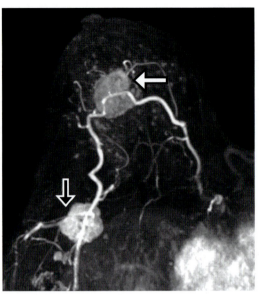

Fig. 150 Breast MRI (Apr. 2021): irregular enhancing mass (white arrow) at the 11 o'clock direction of right breast. Several enlarged lymph nodes (black arrow) in right axilla

Fig. 151 PET-CT shows (**a**) hypermetabolic mass in right breast, upper outer quadrant (mSUV = ~12.0) and (**b**) hypermetabolic lymph nodes in right axilla level I area

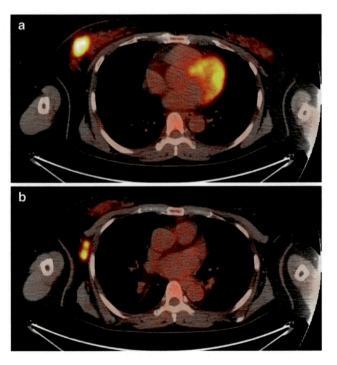

21.3 After Neoadjuvant Chemotherapy

See Figs. 152, 153, 154 and 155.

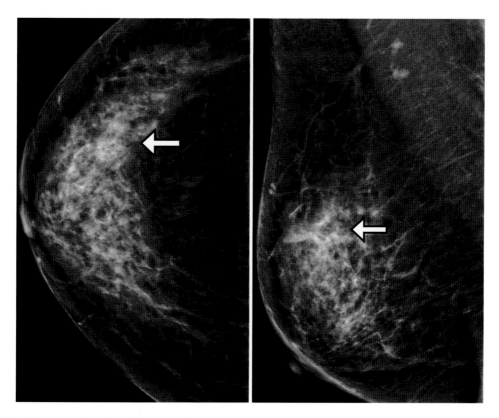

Fig. 152 Mammography (Sept. 2021): mammography after treatment demonstrates residual mass that is decreased in the longest diameter. Decrease in size of enlarged lymph nodes in right axilla

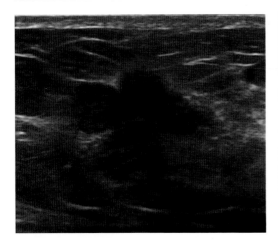

Fig. 153 Breast US (Sept. 2021): US after treatment demonstrates residual hypoechoic mass that is decreased in the longest diameter

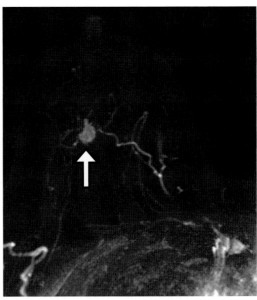

Fig. 154 Breast MRI (Sept. 2021): MRI after treatment demonstrates residual enhancing mass (white arrow) that is decreased in the longest diameter and disappearance of enlarged lymph nodes in right axilla

Fig. 155 Lymphoscintigraphy shows visualized sentinel lymph nodes in the right axilla

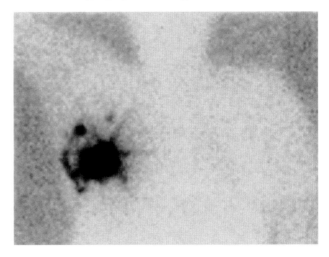

21.4 Courses of Treatment

Neoadjuvant chemotherapy (#6 cycles of docetaxel and carboplatin and trastuzumab and pertuzumab) + Operation + Post-operative radiation therapy + Trastuzumab and Pertuzumab.

21.4.1 Operation

Right breast conserving surgery, sentinel lymph node biopsy (Fig. 156).

21.4.2 Pathology Report

Invasive Ductal Carcinoma
1. Post-chemotherapy status.
2. Size of tumor: 1.0 cm (ypT1b).
3. Histologic grade: 3/3 (tubule formation: 2/3, nuclear pleomorphism: 3/3, mitotic count: 3/3, 49/10HPF).
4. Intraductal component: absent.

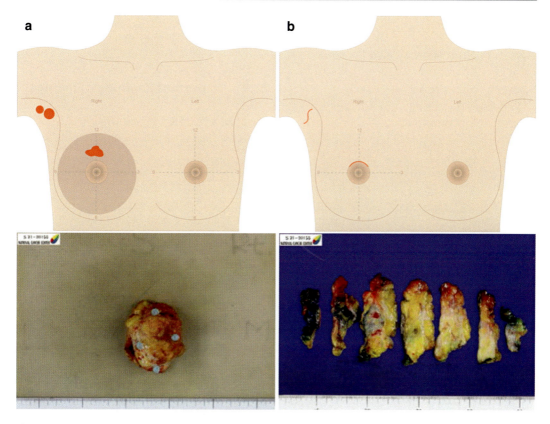

Fig. 156 (**a**) Gross pathology of lumpectomy specimen. (**b**) The margins get marked and sliced with different colors on each direction

5. Surgical margins:
   (a) superior margin: 15 mm,
   (b) inferior margin: 35 mm,
   (c) medial margin: 5 mm,
   (d) lateral margin: 15 mm,
   (e) deep margin: 10 mm,
   (f) superficial margin: 3 mm.
6. Lymph nodes: no metastasis in three axillary lymph nodes (ypN0(sn)) (sentinel LN: 0/2, axillary LN: 0/1).
7. Arteriovenous invasion: absent.
8. Lymphovascular invasion: absent.
9. Tumor border: infiltrative.
10. Microcalcification: present, non-tumoral.
11. Pathological TN category (AJCC 2017): ypT1bN0(sn).

	Result	Intensity	Positive %
Estrogen receptor	Negative (0/8)	0	0
Progesterone receptor	Negative (0/8)	0	0
C-erbB2	Positive (3+)		
Ki-67	Positive in 39% of tumor cells		

22 Case 22

22.1 Patient History and Progress

Female/53 years old, peri-menopause.
Self-detected palpable mass lesion on right breast 4 o'clock direction.

No family history.
S/P hemorrhoids operation.

22.2 Important Radiologic Findings

See Figs. 157, 158, 159 and 160.

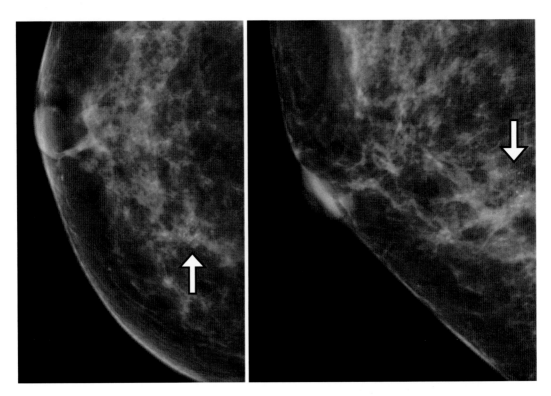

Fig. 157 Magnification (Mar. 2021): irregular mass with fine pleomorphic microcalcifications in the lower inner of right breast

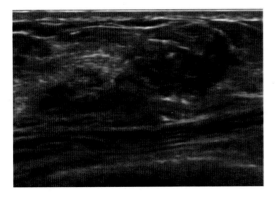

Fig. 158 Breast US (Mar. 2021): irregular hypoechoic mass with microcalcifications at the 4 o'clock direction of right breast

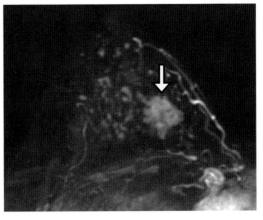

Fig. 159 Breast MRI (Mar. 2021): irregular enhancing mass at the 4 o'clock direction of right breast

HR(−) HER2(+) Breast Cancer

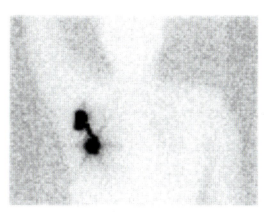

Fig. 160 Lymphoscintigraphy shows visualized sentinel lymph nodes in the right axilla

22.3 Courses of Treatment

Operation + Adjuvant chemotherapy (#4 cycles of doxorubicin and cyclophosphamide) + Postoperative radiation therapy + Trastuzumab.

22.3.1 Operation

Right breast conserving surgery, sentinel lymph node biopsy (Fig. 161).

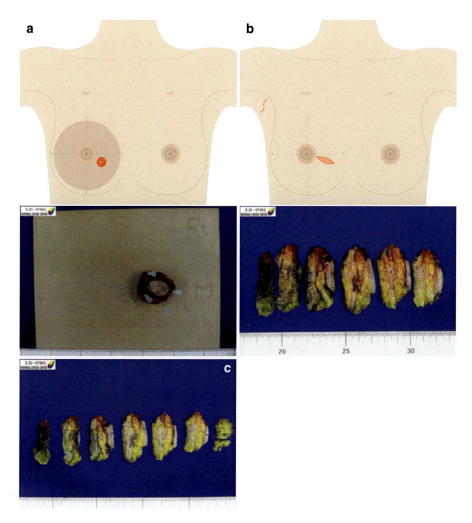

Fig. 161 (**a**) Gross pathology of lumpectomy specimen. (**b, c**) The margins get marked and sliced with different colors on each direction

22.3.2 Pathology Report

Invasive Ductal Carcinoma with apocrine differentiation and medullary pattern

1. Size of invasive component: 1.3 cm (pT1c).
2. Size of intraductal component: 3.0 cm.
3. Histologic grade: 3/3 (tubule formation: 3/3, nuclear pleomorphism: 3/3, mitotic count: 2/3, 15/10HPF).
4. Intraductal component: present, extratumoral (70%) (nuclear grade: high, necrosis: present, architectural pattern: solid/comedo, extensive intraductal component: present).
5. Skin: no involvement of tumor.
6. Surgical margins:
   (a) superior margin: 6 mm,
   (b) inferior margin: 6 mm,
   (c) medial margin: positive for ductal carcinoma in situ (Fro 4) (see note),
   (d) lateral margin: 6 mm,
   (e) deep margin: 2 mm,
   (f) superficial margin: 5 mm.
7. Lymph nodes: no metastasis in two axillary lymph nodes (pN0(sn)) (sentinel LN: 0/2).
8. Arteriovenous invasion: absent.
9. Lymphovascular invasion: absent.
10. Tumor border: infiltrative.
11. Microcalcification: present, tumoral/non-tumoral.
12. Pathological TN category (AJCC 2017): pT1cN0(sn).

Note: 1. Ductal carcinoma in situ is present only in the permanent section of Fro 4.

	Result	Intensity	Positive %
Estrogen receptor	Negative (2/8)	1	<1%
Progesterone receptor	Negative (0/8)	0	0
C-erbB2	Positive (3+)		
Ki-67	Positive in 49% of tumor cells		

23 Case 23

23.1 Patient History and Progress

Female/49 years old, pre-menopause.
Self-detected bloody discharge on nipple of right breast.
No family history.
No comorbidities.

23.2 Important Radiologic Findings

See Figs. 162, 163, 164 and 165.

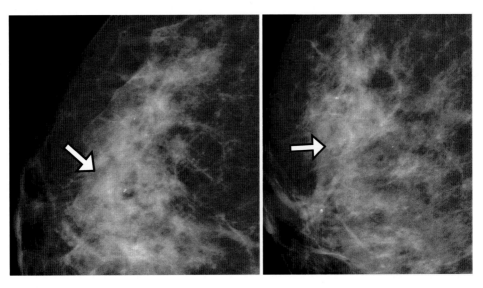

Fig. 162 Magnification (Aug. 2020): regional fine pleomorphic microcalcifications in right upper outer quadrant

HR(−) HER2(+) Breast Cancer

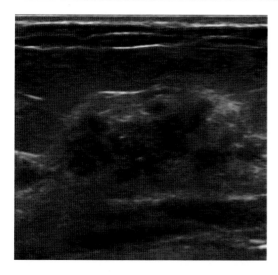

Fig. 163 Breast US (Aug. 2020): irregular hypoechoic mass with microcalcifications at the 10 o'clock direction of right breast

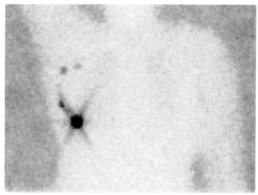

Fig. 165 Lymphoscintigraphy shows visualized sentinel lymph nodes in the right axilla

23.3.1 Operation

Right nipple–areolar complex sparing mastectomy+ implant reconstruction, sentinel lymph node biopsy (1st, Sept. 2020) (Fig. 166).

23.3.2 Pathology Report

Breast, right, nipple-sparing mastectomy:

Microinvasive Ductal Carcinoma

1. Size of invasive component: <0.1 cm (pT1mi).
2. Size of intraductal component: 6.0 cm.
3. Histologic grade: 3/3 (tubule formation: 3/3, nuclear pleomorphism: 3/3, mitotic count: 3/3, 3/10HPF).
4. Intraductal component: present, intratumoral/extratumoral (99%) (nuclear grade: high, necrosis: present, architectural pattern: micropapillary/cribriform/solid/comedo, extensive intraductal component: present).
5. Skin: no involvement of tumor.
6. Surgical margins:
   (a) deep margin: 2 mm,
   (b) superficial margin: 2 mm.
7. Lymph nodes: no metastasis in one axillary lymph node (pN0(sn)) (sentinel LN: 0/1).
8. Arteriovenous invasion: absent.
9. Lymphovascular invasion: absent.
10. Tumor border: infiltrative.

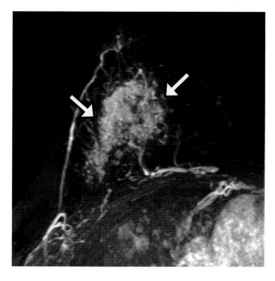

Fig. 164 Breast MRI (Aug. 2020): regional heterogeneous non-mass enhancement in the upper portion of right breast

23.3 Courses of Treatment

Operation + Operation + Adjuvant paclitaxel and trastuzumab.

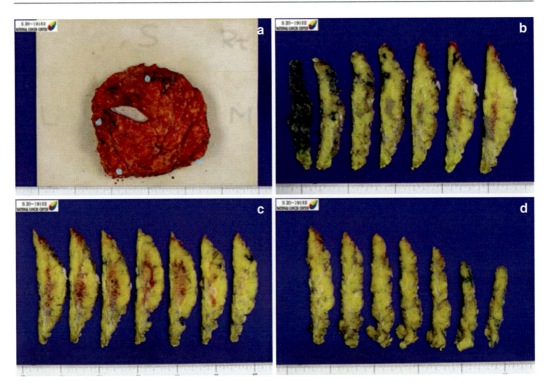

Fig. 166 (a) Gross pathology of lumpectomy specimen. (b–d) The margins get marked and sliced with different colors on each direction

11. Microcalcification: present, tumoral/non-tumoral.
12. Pathological TN category (AJCC 2017): pT1miN0(sn).

	Result	Intensity	Positive %
Estrogen receptor	Negative (0/8)	0	0
Progesterone receptor	Negative (0/8)	0	0
C-erbB2	Positive (3+)		
Ki-67	Positive in 32% of tumor cells		

23.3.3 Operation

Right nipple excision + left breast partial mastectomy with reduction mammoplasty (2nd, May 2020) (Fig. 167).

23.3.4 Pathology Report

Invasive Ductal Carcinoma
1. Post nipple-sparing mastectomy status.
2. Size of tumor: 0.7 cm (rpT1b).
3. Histologic grade: 3/3 (tubule formation: 3/3, nuclear pleomorphism: 3/3, mitotic count: 3/3, 21/10HPF).

HR(−) HER2(+) Breast Cancer

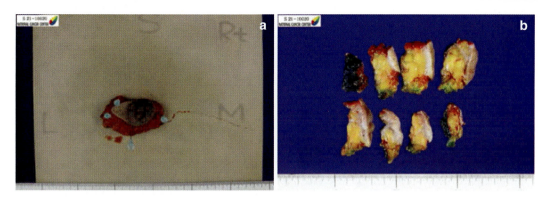

Fig. 167 (**a**) Gross pathology of lumpectomy specimen. (**b**) The margins get marked and sliced with different colors on each direction

4. Intraductal component: absent.
5. Skin and nipple: no involvement of tumor.
6. Surgical margins:
   (a) superior margin: 3 mm,
   (b) inferior margin: 21 mm,
   (c) medial margin: 25 mm,
   (d) lateral margin: 10 mm,
   (e) deep margin: 2 mm,
   (f) superficial margin: 18 mm.
7. Lymph nodes: not submitted (rpNx).
8. Arteriovenous invasion: absent.
9. Lymphovascular invasion: absent.
10. Tumor border: infiltrative.
11. Microcalcification: absent.
12. Pathological TN category (AJCC 2017): rpT1bNx.

24 Case 24

24.1 Patient History and Progress

Female/55 years old, pre-menopause.
Self-detected palpable mass lesion on left breast 10–12 o'clock direction.
No family history.
Hypertension.

24.2 Important Radiologic Findings

See Figs. 168, 169, 170 and 171.

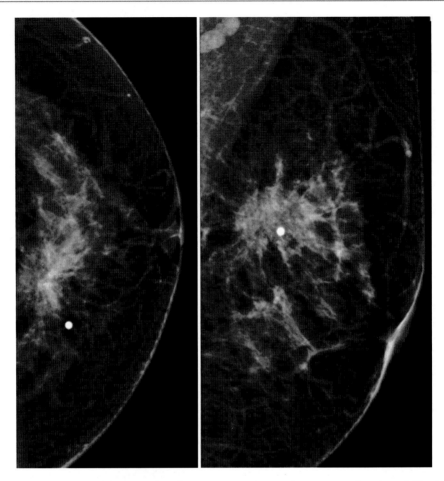

Fig. 168 Mammography (Apr. 2021): irregular hyperdense mass with fine pleomorphic microcalcifications in the upper inner quadrant of left breast (marked BB marker). Enlarged lymph nodes in left axilla

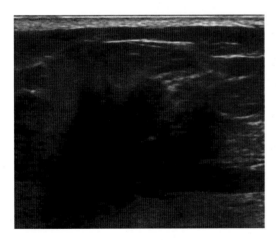

Fig. 169 Breast US (Apr. 2021): irregular hypoechoic mass with microcalcifications at the 11 o'clock direction of left breast

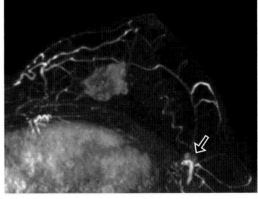

Fig. 170 Breast MRI (Apr. 2021): irregular enhancing mass at the 11 o'clock direction of left breast. Enlarged lymph node in left axilla (black arrow)

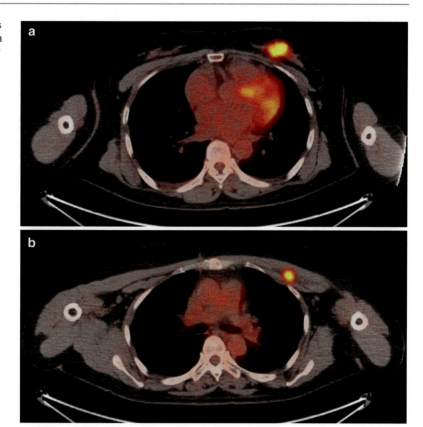

Fig. 171 PET-CT shows (**a**) hypermetabolic lesion in left breast, upper inner quadrant (mSUV = ~6.6) and (**b**) hypermetabolic lymph nodes in left SCN (2.4), left axilla level II and interpectoral area

24.3 After Neoadjuvant Chemotherapy

See Figs. 172, 173, 174 and 175.

Fig. 172 Mammography: mammography after treatment demonstrates residual mass that is decreased in the longest diameter

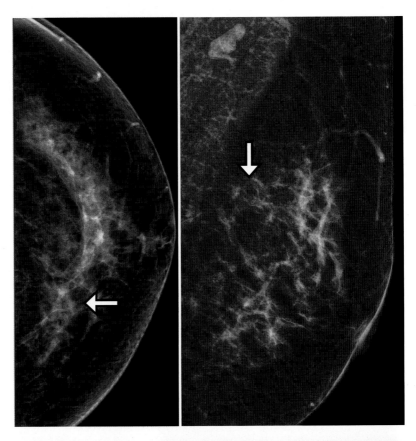

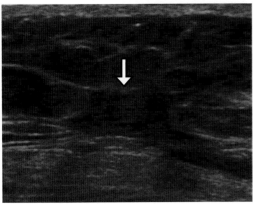

Fig. 173 Breast US: US after treatment demonstrates residual hypoechoic mass that is decreased in the longest diameter

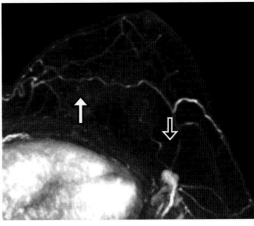

Fig. 174 Breast MRI: MRI after treatment demonstrates residual non-mass enhancement (white arrow) that is decreased in the longest diameter and in the degree of enhancement. No change of suspected metastatic lymph nodes (black arrow) in left axilla

HR(−) HER2(+) Breast Cancer

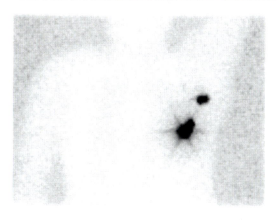

Fig. 175 Lymphoscintigraphy shows visualized sentinel lymph nodes in the left axilla

24.4 Courses of Treatment

Neoadjuvant chemotherapy (#3 cycles of docetaxel and carboplatin and trastuzumab and pertuzumab) + Operation + Post-operative radiation therapy + Trastuzumab and pertuzumab.

24.4.1 Operation
Left breast conserving surgery, sentinel lymph node biopsy (Fig. 176).

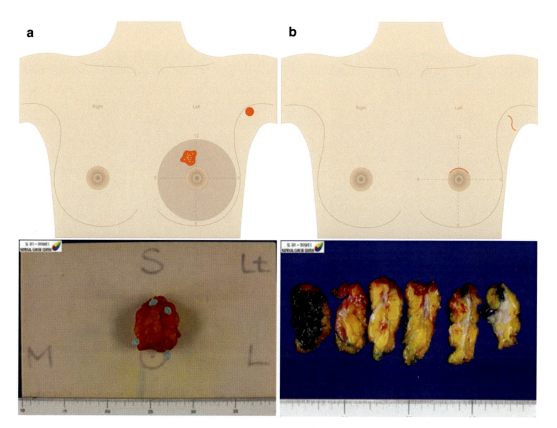

Fig. 176 (**a**) Gross pathology of lumpectomy specimen. (**b**) The margins get marked and sliced with different colors on each direction

24.4.2 Pathology Report

1. No residual tumor with stromal fibrosis.
   (a) Post-chemotherapy status.
   (b) Lymph nodes: no metastasis in two axillary lymph nodes (ypN0(sn)) (sentinel LN: 0/2).
2. Sclerosing adenosis with microcalcification.

	Result	Intensity	Positive %
Estrogen receptor	Negative (0/8)	0	0
Progesterone receptor	Negative (0/8)	0	0
C-erbB2	Positive (3+)		
Ki-67	Positive in 36% of tumor cells		

25 Case 25

25.1 Patient History and Progress

Female/82 years old, post-menopause.

Screen detected mass lesion on left breast 2:30 o'clock direction.

No family history.

S/P Left hemiplegia (due to brain hemorrhage), hypertension, S/P spinal stenosis operation, s/p Tuberculosis.

25.2 Important Radiologic Findings

See Figs. 177, 178 and 179.

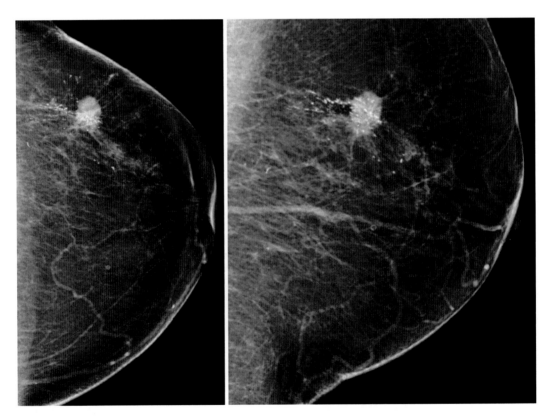

Fig. 177 Mammography (Apr. 2021): irregular hyperdense mass with fine pleomorphic microcalcifications in the upper outer quadrant of left breast

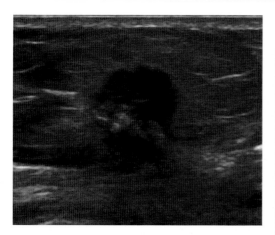

Fig. 178 Breast US (Apr. 2021): irregular hypoechoic mass with echogenic halo and microcalcifications at the 2 o'clock direction of left breast

25.3 Courses of Treatment

Operation + Post-operative radiation therapy (adjuvant chemotherapy refuse).

25.3.1 Operation

Left breast conserving surgery, sentinel lymph node biopsy (Fig. 180).

25.3.2 Pathology Report

Invasive Ductal Carcinoma
1. Size of invasive component: 2.5 cm (pT2).
2. Size of intraductal component: 4.0 cm.
3. Histologic grade: 3/3 (tubule formation: 3/3, nuclear pleomorphism: 3/3, mitotic count: 2/3, 11/10HPF).
4. Intraductal component: present, intratumoral/extratumoral (50%) (nuclear grade: high, necrosis: present, architectural pattern: cribriform/solid/comedo, extensive intraductal component: present).
5. Skin: no involvement of tumor.

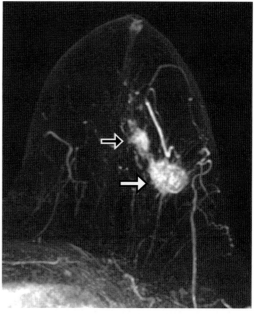

Fig. 179 Breast MRI (Apr. 2021): irregular enhancing mass (white arrow) with associated non-mass enhancement (black arrow) at the 2 o'clock direction of left breast

6. Surgical margins:
   (a) superior margin: 15 mm,
   (b) inferior margin: positive for ductal carcinoma in situ (Fro 2) (see note),
   (c) medial margin: 10 mm,
   (d) lateral margin: 20 mm,
   (e) deep margin: <2 mm from ductal carcinoma in situ (slide 11),
   (f) superficial margin: 13 mm.
7. Lymph nodes:
   (a) metastasis in two out of four axillary lymph nodes (pN1a(sn)) (sentinel LN: 2/4),
   (b) perinodal extension: present,
   (c) size of metastatic carcinoma: 8 mm.
8. Arteriovenous invasion: absent.
9. Lymphovascular invasion: present, peritumoral.

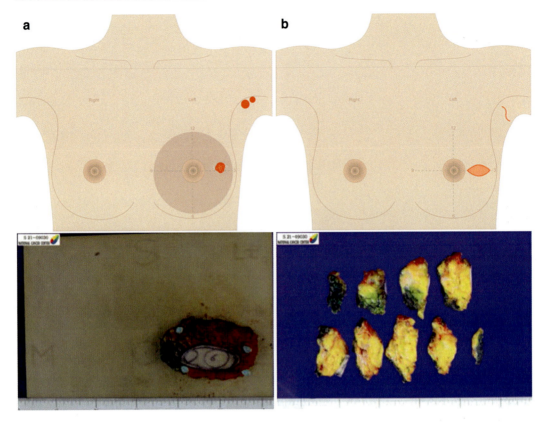

Fig. 180 (**a**) Gross pathology of lumpectomy specimen. (**b**) The margins get marked and sliced with different colors on each direction

10. Tumor border: infiltrative.
11. Microcalcification: present, tumoral/non-tumoral.
12. Pathological TN category (AJCC 2017): pT2N1a(sn).

Note: 1. Ductal carcinoma in situ is focally present only in the permanent section of Fro 2.

	Result	Intensity	Positive %
Estrogen receptor	Negative (0/8)	0	0
Progesterone receptor	Negative (0/8)	0	0
C-erbB2	Positive (3+)		
Ki-67	Positive in 52% of tumor cells		

26 Case 26

26.1 Patient History and Progress

Female/49 years old, pre-menopause.
Self-detected palpable mass lesion on right breast 1 o'clock direction.
No family history.
No comorbidities.

26.2 Important Radiologic Findings

See Figs. 181, 182 and 183.

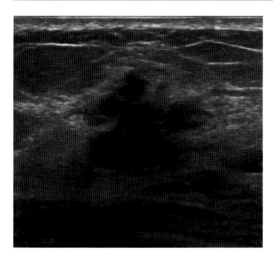

Fig. 181 Breast US (May 2021): irregular hypoechoic mass at the 2 o'clock direction of right breast

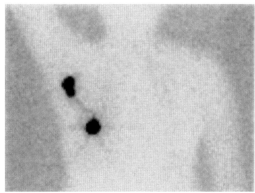

Fig. 183 Lymphoscintigraphy shows visualized sentinel lymph nodes in the right axilla

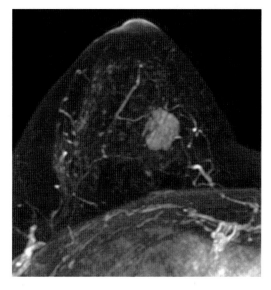

Fig. 182 Breast MRI (May 2021): irregular enhancing mass at the 2 o'clock direction of right breast

26.3 Courses of Treatment

Operation + Adjuvant chemotherapy (#4 cycles of doxorubicin + cyclophosphamide) + Postoperative radiation therapy + Trastuzumab.

26.3.1 Operation
Right breast conserving surgery, sentinel lymph node biopsy (Fig. 184).

26.3.2 Pathology Report

Invasive Ductal Carcinoma with medullary pattern
1. Size of tumor: 1.5 cm (pT1c).
2. Histologic grade: 3/3 (tubule formation: 3/3, nuclear pleomorphism: 3/3, mitotic count: 2/3, 12/10HPF).
3. Intraductal component: present, intratumoral/extratumoral (5%) (nuclear grade: high, necrosis: absent, architectural pattern: solid, extensive intraductal component: absent).

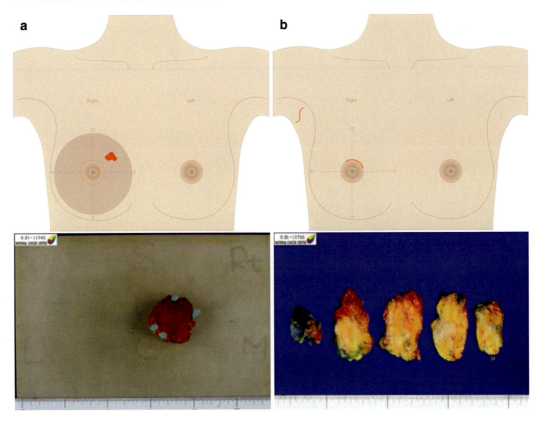

Fig. 184 (**a**) Gross pathology of lumpectomy specimen. (**b**) The margins get marked and sliced with different colors on each direction

4. Skin: no involvement of tumor.
5. Surgical margins:
   (a) superior margin: 20 mm,
   (b) inferior margin: 5 mm,
   (c) medial margin: 5 mm,
   (d) lateral margin: 5 mm,
   (e) deep margin: 2 mm,
   (f) superficial margin: 2 mm.
6. Lymph nodes: no metastasis in one axillary lymph node (pN0(sn)) (sentinel LN: 0/1).
7. Arteriovenous invasion: absent.
8. Lymphovascular invasion: present, intratumoral.
9. Tumor border: infiltrative.
10. Microcalcification: present, tumoral/non-tumoral.
11. Pathological TN category (AJCC 2017): pT1cN0(sn).

	Result	Intensity	Positive %
Estrogen receptor	Negative (0/8)	0	0
Progesterone receptor	Negative (2/8)	1	<1%
C-erbB2	Positive (3+)		
Ki-67	Positive in 23% of tumor cells		

27 Case 27

27.1 Patient History and Progress

Female/69 years old, post-menopause.
  Screen detected mass lesion on right breast 9 o'clock direction.
  Family history of breast cancer, sister.
  Hypertension, dyslipidemia.
  BRCA 1 and 2 mutation: Not examination.

27.2 Important Radiologic Findings

See Figs. 185, 186 and 187.

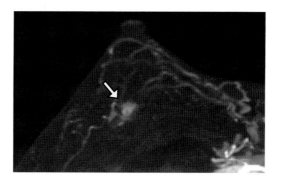

Fig. 186 Breast MRI (May 2021): irregular enhancing mass at the 9 o'clock direction of right breast

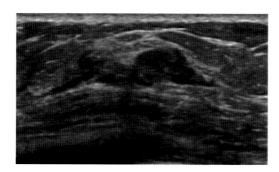

Fig. 185 Breast US (May 2021): irregular hypoechoic mass with microcalcifications at the 9 o'clock direction of right breast

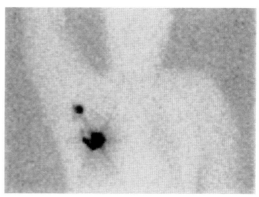

Fig. 187 Lymphoscintigraphy shows visualized sentinel lymph nodes in the right axilla

27.3 Courses of Treatment

Operation + Post-operative radiation therapy + Adjuvant paclitaxel and trastuzumab.

27.3.1 Operation
Right breast conserving surgery, sentinel lymph node biopsy (Fig. 188).

27.3.2 Pathology Report
1. Invasive ductal carcinoma with medullary pattern.
   (a) Size of tumor: 0.8 cm (pT1b).
   (b) Histologic grade: 3/3 (tubule formation: 3/3, nuclear pleomorphism: 3/3, mitotic count: 3/3, 4/HPF).
   (c) Intraductal component: present, intratumoral/extratumoral (50%) (nuclear grade: high, necrosis: absent, architectural pattern: solid, extensive intraductal component: present).
   (d) Skin: no involvement of tumor.
   (e) Surgical margins:
       - superior margin: 5 mm,
       - inferior margin: 20 mm,
       - medial margin: 5 mm,
       - lateral margin: 5 mm,
       - deep margin: 1.5 mm from ductal carcinoma in situ (slide 1),
       - superficial margin: 2 mm.
   (f) Lymph nodes: no metastasis in one axillary lymph node (pN0(sn)) (sentinel LN: 0/1).
   (g) Arteriovenous invasion: absent.
   (h) Lymphovascular invasion: present, intratumoral.

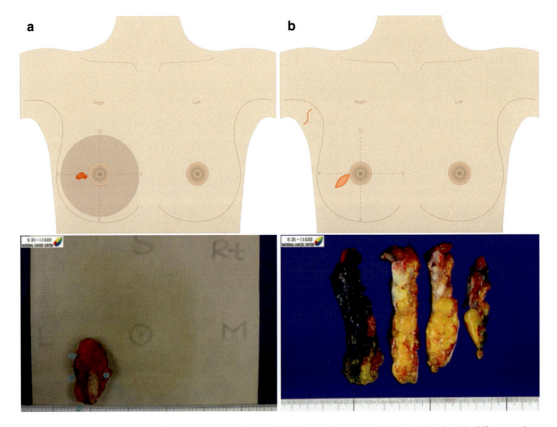

Fig. 188 (**a**) Gross pathology of lumpectomy specimen. (**b**) The margins get marked and sliced with different colors on each direction

- (i) Tumor border: infiltrative.
- (j) Microcalcification: present, tumoral/non-tumoral.
- (k) Pathological TN category (AJCC 2017): pT1bN0(sn).
2. Intraductal papilloma with usual ductal hyperplasia.

	Result	Intensity	Positive %
Estrogen receptor	Negative (0/8)	0	0
Progesterone receptor	Negative (0/8)	0	0
C-erbB2	Equivocal(2+), SISH(+)		
Ki-67	Positive in 26% of tumor cells		

28 Case 28

28.1 Patient History and Progress

Female/61 years old, post-menopause.

Screen detected mass lesion on right breast 9 o'clock direction.

No family history.

Hypertension.

28.2 Important Radiologic Findings

See Figs. 189, 190, 191 and 192.

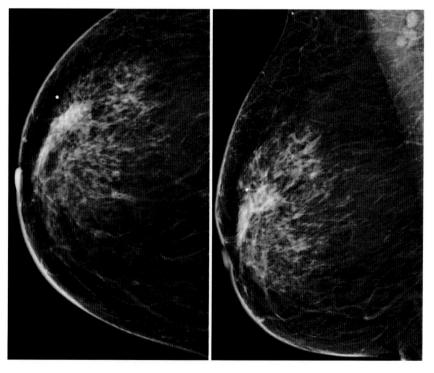

Fig. 189 Mammography (June 2021): irregular hyperdense mass in the upper outer quadrant of right breast (marked by BB marker). Enlarged lymph nodes in right axilla

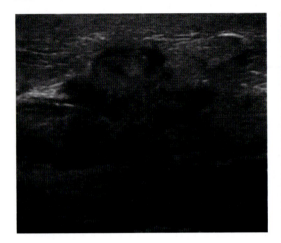

Fig. 190 Breast US (June 2021): irregular heterogeneous echoic mass at the 9 o'clock direction of right breast

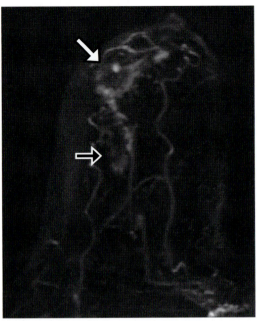

Fig. 191 Breast MRI (June 2021): irregular rim enhancing mass (white arrow) at the 9 o'clock direction of right breast. Associated non-mass enhancement (black arrow) in the outer portion of right breast

Fig. 192 PET-CT shows (**a**) a hypermetabolic breast mass, right outer (mSUV = 5.7) and (**b**) hypermetabolic LNs along right axilla, level I–III

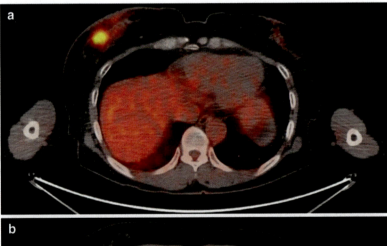

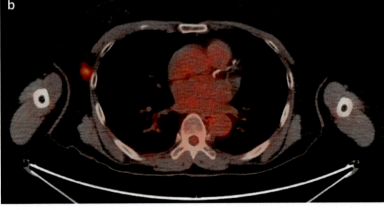

28.3 After Neoadjuvant Chemotherapy

See Figs. 193, 194 and 195.

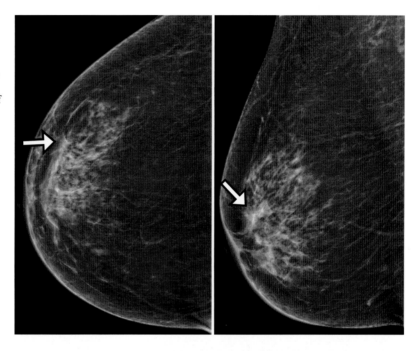

Fig. 193 Mammography (Oct. 2021): mammography after treatment demonstrates residual mass (white arrow) that is decreased in the longest diameter and no change of associated fine linear microcalcifications. Decrease in size of enlarged lymph nodes in right axilla

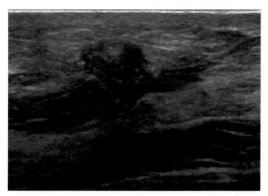

Fig. 194 Breast US (Oct. 2021): US after treatment demonstrates residual hypoechoic mass that is decreased in the longest diameter

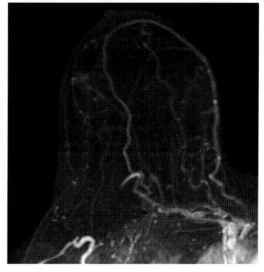

Fig. 195 Breast MRI (Oct. 2021): MRI after treatment demonstrates residual non-mass enhancement that is decreased in the longest diameter and in the degree of enhancement and decrease in size of enlarged right axillary lymph node

28.4 Courses of Treatment

Neoadjuvant chemotherapy (#6 cycles of docetaxel and carboplatin and trastuzumab and pertuzumab) + Operation + Post-operative radiation therapy + Trastuzumab and pertuzumab.

28.4.1 Operation
Right breast conserving surgery, sentinel lymph node biopsy (Fig. 196).

28.4.2 Pathology Report

Ductal Carcinoma In Situ
1. Post-chemotherapy status.
2. Size of tumor: 0.2 cm (ypTis).
3. Nuclear grade: high.
4. Necrosis: absent.
5. Architectural pattern: solid.
6. Skin: no involvement of tumor.
7. Surgical margins:
   (a) superior margin: 20 mm,
   (b) inferior margin: 10 mm,
   (c) medial margin: 30 mm,
   (d) lateral margin: 5 mm,
   (e) deep margin: 2 mm,
   (f) superficial margin: 2 mm.
8. Lymph nodes: no metastasis in three axillary lymph nodes (ypN0(sn)) (sentinel LN: 0/3).
9. Microcalcification: present, tumoral/non-tumoral.
10. Pathological TN category (AJCC 2017): ypTisN0(sn).

	Result	Intensity	Positive %
Estrogen receptor	Negative (0/8)	0	0
Progesterone receptor	Negative (0/8)	0	0
C-erbB2	Positive (3+)		
Ki-67	Positive in 38% of tumor cells		

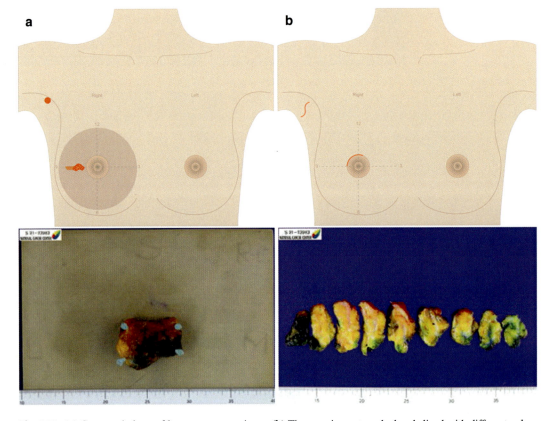

Fig. 196 (**a**) Gross pathology of lumpectomy specimen. (**b**) The margins get marked and sliced with different colors on each direction

29 Case 29

29.1 Patient History and Progress

Female/39 years old, pre-menopause.
Self-detected palpable mass lesion on upper outer portion of left breast.
No family history.
S/P Left salpingo-oophorectomy.
BRCA 1 and 2 mutation: Not detected.

29.2 Important Radiologic Findings

See Figs. 197, 198 and 199.

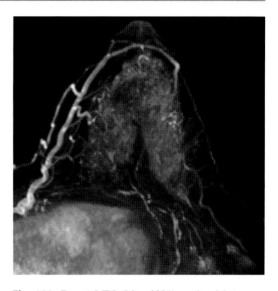

Fig. 198 Breast MRI (May 2021): regional heterogeneous non-mass enhancement in the upper portion of left breast

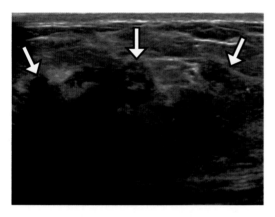

Fig. 197 Breast US (May 2021): irregular hypoechoic masses with microcalcifications in the upper portion of left breast

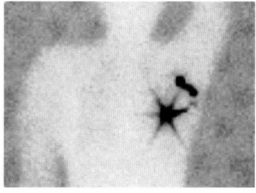

Fig. 199 Lymphoscintigraphy shows visualized sentinel lymph nodes in the right axilla

29.3 Courses of Treatment

Operation (adjuvant chemotherapy refuse).

29.3.1 Operation

Left nipple–areolar complex sparing mastectomy with implant reconstruction, sentinel lymph node biopsy (Figs. 200 and 201).

29.3.2 Pathology Report

Microinvasive Ductal Carcinoma
1. Size of invasive component: <0.1 cm (pT1mi).
2. Size of intraductal component: 5.0 cm.
3. Histologic grade: not applicable.
4. Intraductal component: present, intratumoral/extratumoral (99%) (nuclear grade: high, necrosis: present, architectural pattern: micropapillary/cribriform/comedo, extensive intraductal component: present).
5. Skin: no involvement of tumor.
6. Surgical margins: (see Note 1).
   (a) deep margin: 2 mm,
   (b) superficial margin: 2 mm.
7. Lymph nodes: no metastasis in two axillary lymph nodes (pN0(sn)) (sentinel LN: 0/2, axillary LN: 0/0).
8. Arteriovenous invasion: absent.
9. Lymphovascular invasion: absent.
10. Tumor border: infiltrative.
11. Microcalcification: present, tumoral/non-tumoral.
12. Pathological TN category (AJCC 2017): pT1miN0(sn).

Breast, left nipple, excision: Ductal carcinoma in situ (see Note 2).

Breast, left nipple margin, excision: Ductal carcinoma in situ (see Note 2).

Note: 1. The lateral border of the mastectomy specimen (slide MG8) is close to ductal carcinoma in situ (<1 mm).

2. The nipple margin separately submitted for permanent diagnosis (slides B&C) is positive for ductal carcinoma in situ but this margin submitted for frozen diagnosis (Fro 9) is free of tumor.

	Result	Intensity	Positive %
Estrogen receptor	Negative (0/8)	0	0
Progesterone receptor	Negative (0/8)	0	0
C-erbB2	Positive (3+)		
Ki-67	Positive in 29% of tumor cells		

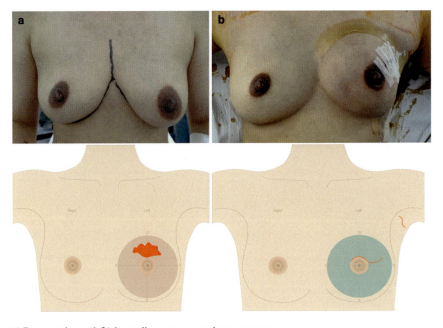

Fig. 200 (**a**) Preoperative and (**b**) immediate post-operative appearance

HR(−) HER2(+) Breast Cancer

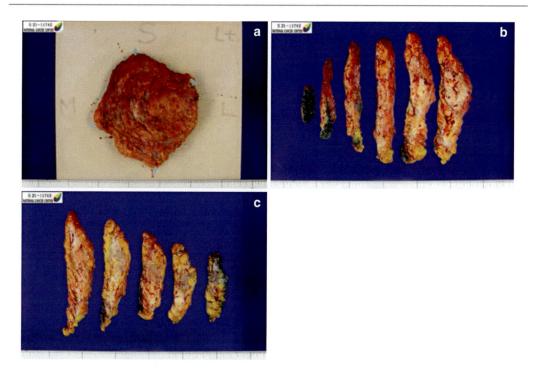

Fig. 201 (**a**) Gross pathology of mastectomy specimen. (**b**, **c**) The margins get marked and sliced with different colors on each direction

30 Case 30

30.1 Patient History and Progress

Female/41 years old, pre-menopause.

Self-detected palpable mass and nipple discharge on left breast.

No family history.
No comorbidities.
BRCA 1 and 2 mutation: Not detected.

30.2 Important Radiologic Findings

See Figs. 202, 203 and 204.

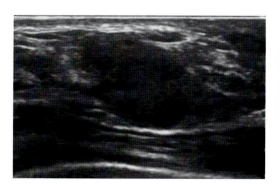

Fig. 202 Breast US (June 2021): irregular heterogeneous echoic mass at the 9 o'clock direction of left breast

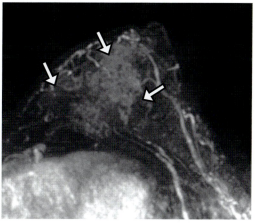

Fig. 203 Breast MRI (June 2021): regional heterogeneous non-mass enhancement in the inner portion of left breast

Fig. 204 PET-CT shows (**a**) known breast cancer with uptake, Lt 8′ (mSUV = 7.3), (**b**) another hypermetabolic lesion in left breast 9′ (mSUV = 3.6), (**c**) hypermetabolic LNs in left internal mammary area, and (**d**) hypermetabolic LNs in left axilla, level I–II

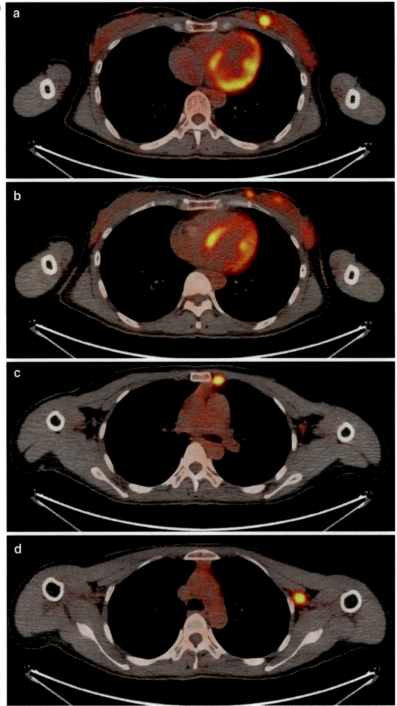

30.3 After Neoadjuvant Chemotherapy

See Figs. 205, 206 and 207.

30.4 Courses of Treatment

Neoadjuvant chemotherapy (#6 cycles of docetaxel and carboplatin and trastuzumab and pertuzumab) + Operation + Post-operative radiation therapy + Trastuzumab and pertuzumab.

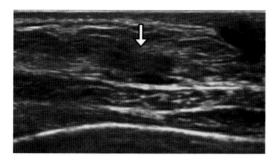

Fig. 205 Breast US (Nov. 2021): US after treatment demonstrates residual hypoechoic mass that is decreased in the longest diameter

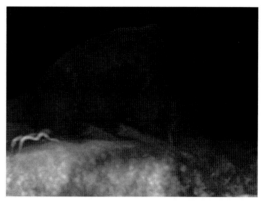

Fig. 206 Breast MRI (Nov. 2021): MRI after treatment shows complete resolution of enhancement in the left breast

Fig. 207 Lymphoscintigraphy shows visualized sentinel lymph nodes in the left axilla

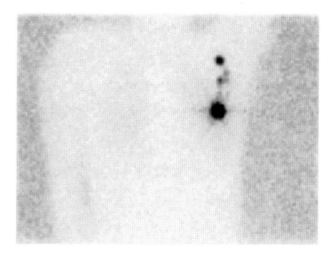

30.4.1 Operation

Left breast conserving surgery, sentinel lymph node biopsy (Fig. 208).

30.4.2 Pathology Report

Microinvasive Ductal Carcinoma
1. Post-chemotherapy status.
2. Size of tumor: <0.1 cm (ypT1mi).
3. Histologic grade: not applicable.
4. Intraductal component: absent.
5. Skin: no involvement of tumor.
6. Surgical margins:
   (a) superior margin: 10 mm,
   (b) inferior margin: (see note),
   (c) medial margin: 10 mm,
   (d) lateral margin: 10 mm,
   (e) deep margin: 2 mm,
   (f) superficial margin: 2 mm.
7. Lymph nodes: no metastasis in three axillary lymph nodes (ypN0(sn)) (sentinel LN: 0/3).
8. Arteriovenous invasion: absent.
9. Lymphovascular invasion: absent.
10. Tumor border: infiltrative.
11. Microcalcification: present, tumoral.
12. Pathological TN category (AJCC 2017): ypT1miN0(sn).

Note: 1. The inferior margin of the lumpectomy specimen (slide 5) is close to microinvasive ductal carcinoma (2 mm) but this margin submitted for frozen diagnosis (Fro 2) is free of tumor.

	Result	Intensity	Positive %
Estrogen receptor	Negative (0/8)	0	0
Progesterone receptor	Negative (0/8)	0	0
C-erbB2	Positive (3+)		
Ki-67	Positive in 19% of tumor cells		

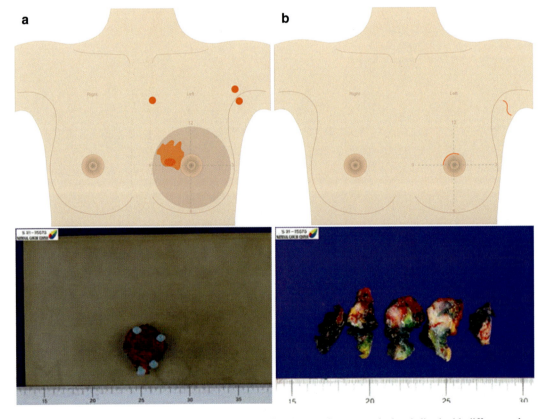

Fig. 208 (a) Gross pathology of lumpectomy specimen. (b) The margins get marked and sliced with different colors on each direction

31 Case 31

31.1 Patient History and Progress

Female/74 years old, post-menopause.

Screen detected mass lesion on left breast 1 o'clock direction.

No family history.

Hypertension.

31.2 Important Radiologic Findings

See Figs. 209, 210, 211 and 212.

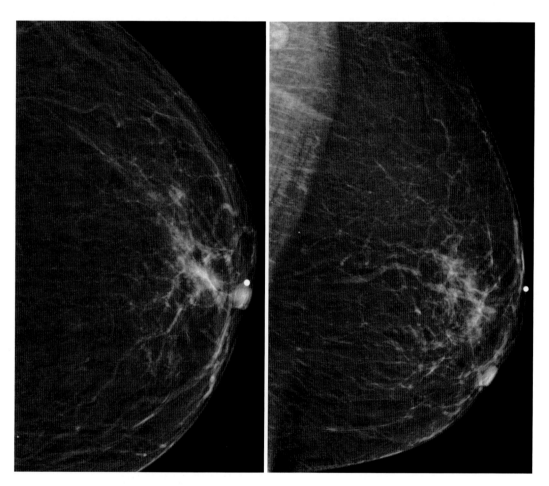

Fig. 209 Mammography (May 2021): Focal asymmetry with fine linear microcalcifications in the upper mid portion of left breast (marked by BB marker)

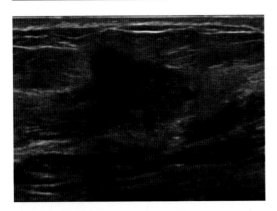

Fig. 210 Breast US (May 2021): irregular hypoechoic mass with microcalcifications at the 1 o'clock direction of left breast

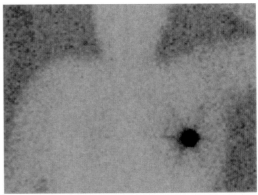

Fig. 212 Lymphoscintigraphy shows visualized sentinel lymph nodes in the left axilla

31.3 Courses of Treatment

Operation + Adjuvant chemotherapy (#4 cycles of doxorubicin and cyclophosphamide) + Postoperative radiation therapy + Trastuzumab.

31.3.1 Operation

Left breast conserving surgery, sentinel lymph node biopsy (Fig. 213).

31.3.2 Pathology Report

Invasive Ductal Carcinoma
1. Size of tumor: 2.1 cm (pT2).
2. Histologic grade: 3/3 (tubule formation: 3/3, nuclear pleomorphism: 3/3, mitotic count: 3/3, 5/HPF).
3. Intraductal component: present, intratumoral/extratumoral (50%) (nuclear grade: high, necrosis: present, architectural pattern: solid/comedo, extensive intraductal component: present).

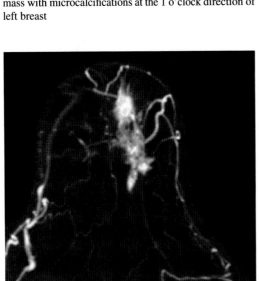

Fig. 211 Breast MRI (May 2021): irregular enhancing masses in the upper outer quadrant of left breast

HR(−) HER2(+) Breast Cancer

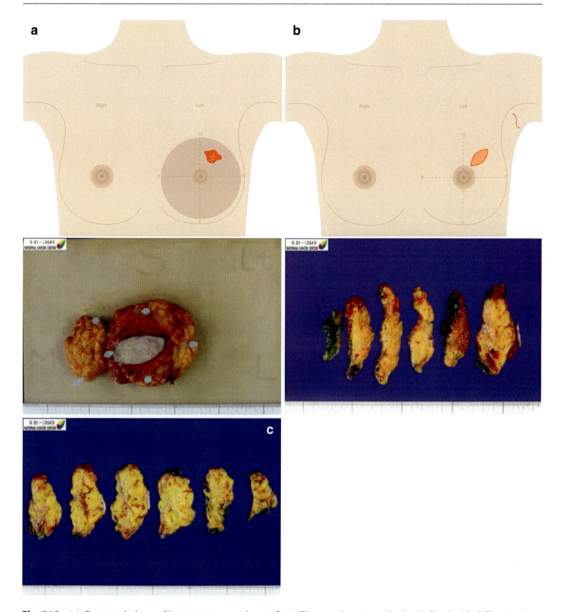

Fig. 213 (**a**) Gross pathology of lumpectomy specimen. (**b, c**) The margins get marked and sliced with different colors on each direction

4. Skin: no involvement of tumor.
5. Surgical margins:
   (a) superior margin: 10 mm,
   (b) inferior margin: 10 mm,
   (c) medial margin: 20 mm,
   (d) lateral margin: 15 mm,
   (e) deep margin: 2 mm,
   (f) superficial margin: 2 mm.
6. Lymph nodes: no metastasis in one axillary lymph node (pN0(sn)) (sentinel LN: 0/1).
7. Arteriovenous invasion: absent.
8. Lymphovascular invasion: present, intratumoral.
9. Tumor border: infiltrative.
10. Microcalcification: present, tumoral/non-tumoral.
11. Pathological TN category (AJCC 2017): pT2N0(sn).

	Result	Intensity	Positive %
Estrogen receptor	Negative (0/8)	0	0
Progesterone receptor	Negative (0/8)	0	0
C-erbB2	Positive (3+)		
Ki-67	Positive in 79% of tumor cells		

32 Case 32

32.1 Patient History and Progress

Female/55 years old, post-menopause.

Screen detected mass lesion on right breast 8 o'clock direction.

No family history.

Hypertension, thyroid nodules.

32.2 Important Radiologic Findings

See Figs. 214, 215 and 216.

32.3 After Neoadjuvant Chemotherapy

See Figs. 217, 218 and 219.

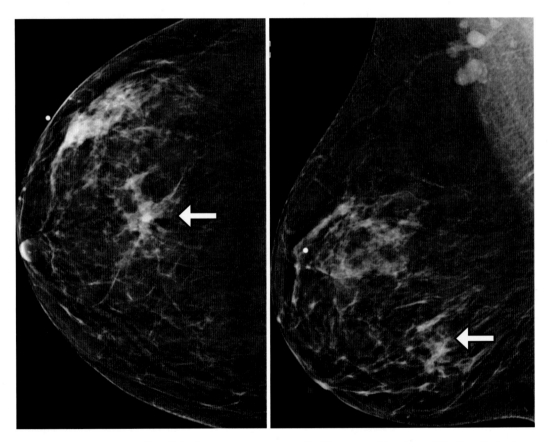

Fig. 214 Mammography (Feb. 2021): irregular hyperdense mass in the upper outer quadrant of right breast (marked BB marker). Spiculated hyperdense mass (white arrow) with pleomorphic microcalcifications in the lower outer portion of right breast. Enlarged lymph nodes in right axilla

HR(−) HER2(+) Breast Cancer

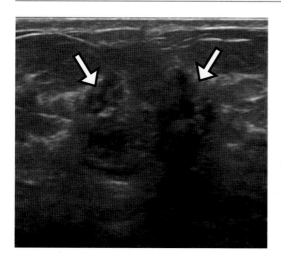

Fig. 215 Breast US (Feb. 2021): irregular heterogeneous echoic mass with microcalcifications at the 7 o'clock direction of right breast

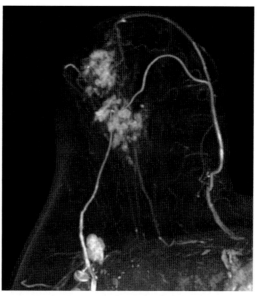

Fig. 216 Breast MRI (Feb. 2021): two irregular enhancing masses at the 9 and 7 o'clock direction of right breast. Enlarged lymph node in right axilla

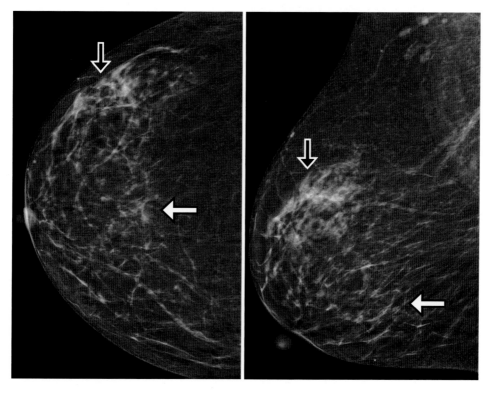

Fig. 217 Mammography (June 2021): mammography after treatment demonstrates residual masses that are decreased in the longest diameter in lower outer and upper outer portion of right breast. Decrease in size of enlarged LNs in right axilla

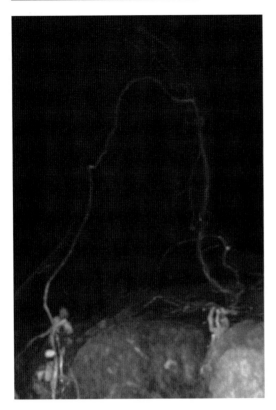

Fig. 218 Breast MRI (June 2021): MRI after treatment shows complete resolution of enhancement in the right breast and decrease in size of enlarged lymph nodes in right axilla

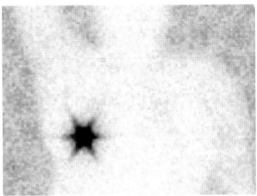

Fig. 219 Lymphoscintigraphy shows visualized sentinel lymph nodes in the right axilla

32.4 Courses of Treatment

Neoadjuvant chemotherapy (#5 cycles of docetaxel and carboplatin and trastuzumab and pertuzumab after followed #1 cycle of trastuzumab and pertuzumab) + Operation + Postoperative radiation therapy + Trastuzumab.

32.4.1 Operation
Right breast conserving surgery, sentinel lymph node biopsy (Fig. 220).

32.4.2 Pathology Report
No residual tumor with stromal degeneration.
1. Post-chemotherapy status.
2. Lymph nodes: no metastasis in three axillary lymph nodes (ypN0(sn)) (sentinel LN: 0/3).

	Result	Intensity	Positive %
Estrogen receptor	Negative (2/8)	1	<1%
Progesterone receptor	Negative (2/8)	1	<1%
C-erbB2	Positive (3+)		
Ki-67	Positive in 45% of tumor cells		

HR(−) HER2(+) Breast Cancer

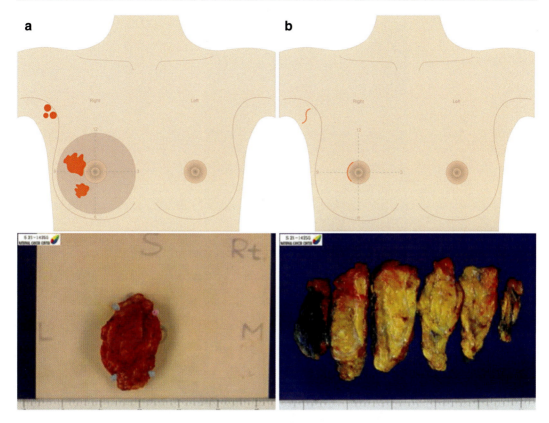

Fig. 220 (**a**) Gross pathology of lumpectomy specimen. (**b**) The margins get marked and sliced with different colors on each direction

33 Case 33

33.1 Patient History and Progress

Female/63 years old, post-menopause.

Self-detected palpable mass lesion on left breast 2 o'clock direction.

No family history.

Hypertension, chronic kidney disease, ventricular premature contraction.

33.2 Important Radiologic Findings

See Figs. 221, 222, 223 and 224.

Fig. 221 Mammography (Feb. 2021): irregular hyperdense mass in the upper outer quadrant of left breast. Enlarged lymph nodes in left axilla

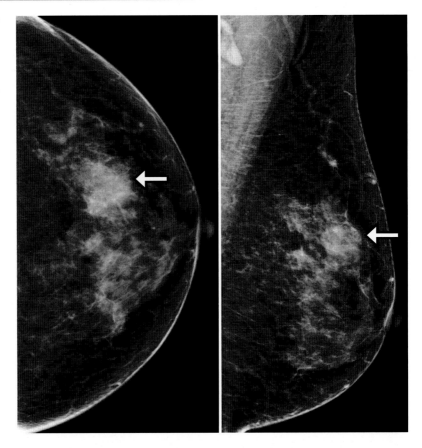

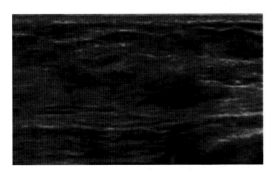

Fig. 222 Breast US (Feb. 2021): irregular hypoechoic mass at the 2 o'clock direction of left breast

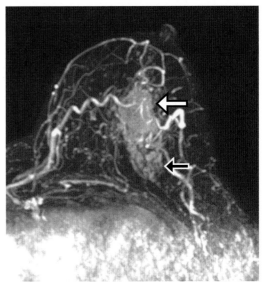

Fig. 223 Breast MRI (Feb. 2021): irregular enhancing mass (white arrow) with associated non-mass enhancement (black arrow) at the 1 o'clock direction of left breast

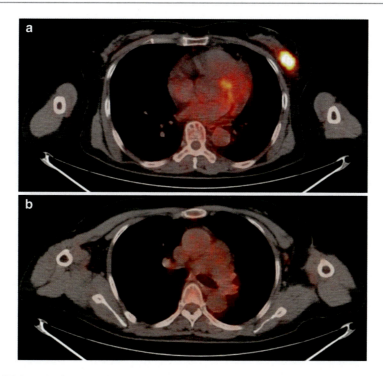

Fig. 224 PET-CT shows (**a**) hypermetabolic mass in left breast, 1′ (mSUV = 14.8) and (**b**) small left axillary LNs, level I–II (mSUV = 1.3)

33.3 After Neoadjuvant Chemotherapy

See Figs. 225, 226 and 227.

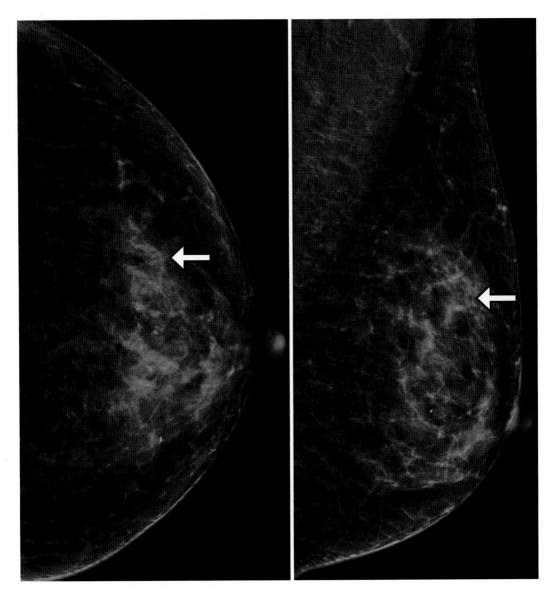

Fig. 225 Mammography (May 2021): mammography after treatment demonstrates no residual mass that is decreased in the longest diameter

Fig. 226 Breast US (May 2021): US after treatment demonstrates residual hypoechoic mass that is decreased in the longest diameter

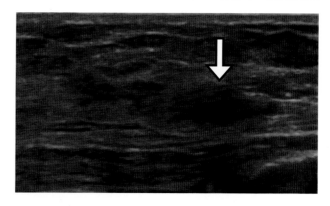

Fig. 227 Lymphoscintigraphy shows visualized sentinel lymph nodes in the left axilla

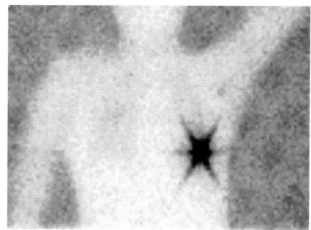

33.4 Courses of Treatment

Neoadjuvant chemotherapy (#6 cycles of docetaxel and carboplatin and trastuzumab and pertuzumab) + Operation + Post-operative radiation therapy + Trastuzumab.

33.4.1 Operation

Left breast conserving surgery, sentinel lymph node biopsy (Fig. 228).

33.4.2 Pathology Report

1. No residual tumor with foamy histiocytic collection.
   (a) Post-chemotherapy status.
   (b) Lymph nodes: no metastasis in four axillary lymph nodes (ypN0(sn)) (sentinel LN: 0/4).
   (c) Microcalcification: present, tumoral/non-tumoral.
   (d) Related slides: C21-518.

2. Intraductal papilloma.

	Result	Intensity	Positive %
Estrogen receptor	Negative (2/8)	1	<1%
Progesterone receptor	Negative (0/8)	0	0
C-erbB2	Positive (3+)		
Ki-67	Positive in 22% of tumor cells		

34 Case 34

34.1 Patient History and Progress

Female/54 years old, post-menopause.

Self-detected palpable mass lesion on left breast.

No family history.

S/P unilateral salpingo-oophorectomy, dyslipidemia.

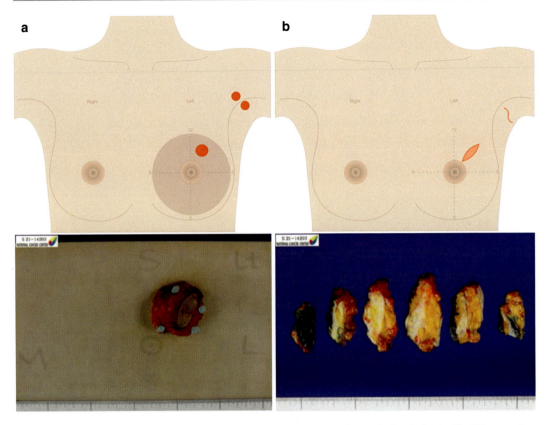

Fig. 228 (**a**) Gross pathology of lumpectomy specimen. (**b**) The margins get marked and sliced with different colors on each direction

34.2 Important Radiologic Findings

See Figs. 229, 230, 231 and 232.

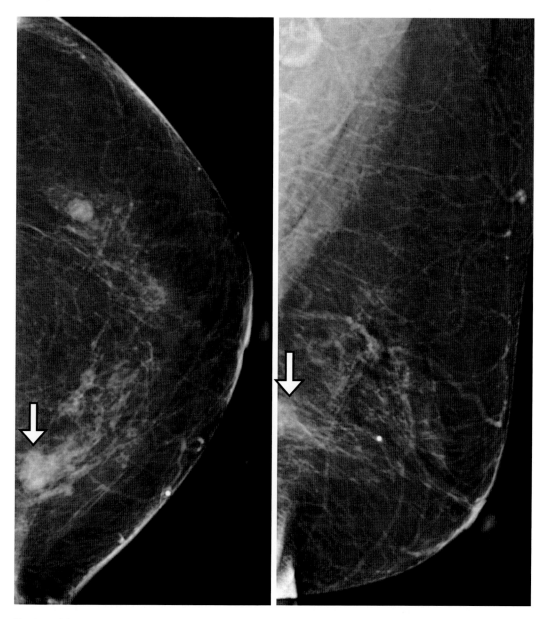

Fig. 229 Mammography (June 2021): irregular hyperdense mass in the upper inner quadrant of left breast

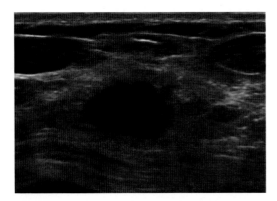

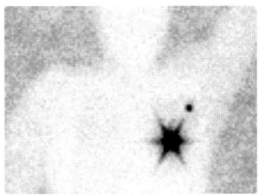

Fig. 230 Breast US (Feb. 2021): irregular hypoechoic mass with microlobulated margin at the 9 o'clock direction of left breast

Fig. 232 Lymphoscintigraphy shows visualized sentinel lymph nodes in the left axilla

34.3 Courses of Treatment

Operation + Adjuvant chemotherapy (#4 cycles of doxorubicin + cyclophosphamide) + Operation + Trastuzumab.

34.3.1 Operation

Left modified radical mastectomy, sentinel lymph node biopsy (Fig. 233).

34.3.2 Pathology Report

Invasive Ductal Carcinoma
1. Size of tumor: 1.5 cm (pT1c(Paget)).
2. Histologic grade: 3/3 (tubule formation: 3/3, nuclear pleomorphism: 3/3, mitotic count: 2/3, 11/10HPF).
3. Intraductal component: absent.
4. Nipple: Paget disease.
5. Skin: no involvement of tumor.

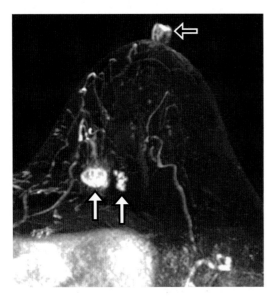

Fig. 231 Breast MRI (Feb. 2021): irregular enhancing masses (white arrow) in the inner portion of left breast. Enhancing lesion (black arrow) in left nipple

HR(−) HER2(+) Breast Cancer

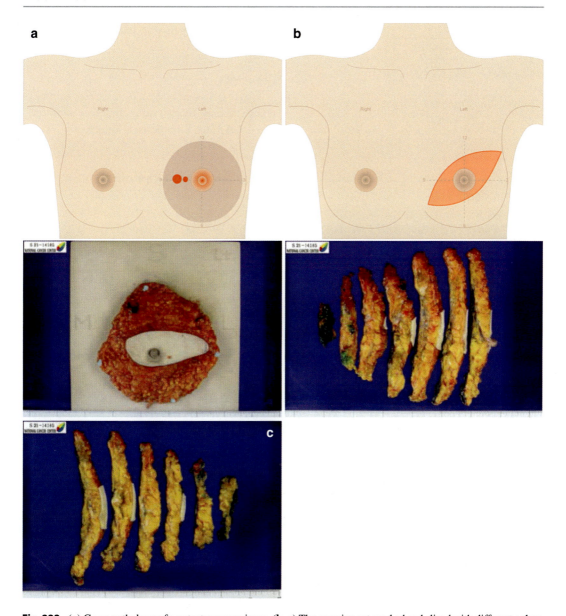

Fig. 233 (**a**) Gross pathology of mastectomy specimen. (**b**, **c**) The margins get marked and sliced with different colors on each direction

6. Surgical margins: deep margin: 2 mm.
7. Lymph nodes: no metastasis in one axillary lymph node (pN0(sn)) (sentinel LN: 0/1).
8. Arteriovenous invasion: absent.
9. Lymphovascular invasion: present, intratumoral.
10. Tumor border: infiltrative.
11. Microcalcification: present, tumoral/non-tumoral.
12. Pathological TN category (AJCC 2017): pT1c(Paget)N0(sn).

	Result	Intensity	Positive %
Estrogen receptor	Negative (2/8)	1	<1%
Progesterone receptor	Negative (0/8)	0	0
C-erbB2	Positive (3+)		
Ki-67	Positive in 25% of tumor cells		

35 Case 35

35.1 Patient History and Progress

Female/73 years old, post-menopause.

Self-detected palpable mass lesion on right breast.

Family history of breast cancer, cousin (maternal).

s/p cholecystectomy, s/p unilateral salpingo-oophorectomy, hypertension, diabetes mellitus.

BRCA 1 and 2 mutation: Not detected.

35.2 Important Radiologic Findings

See Figs. 234, 235, 236 and 237.

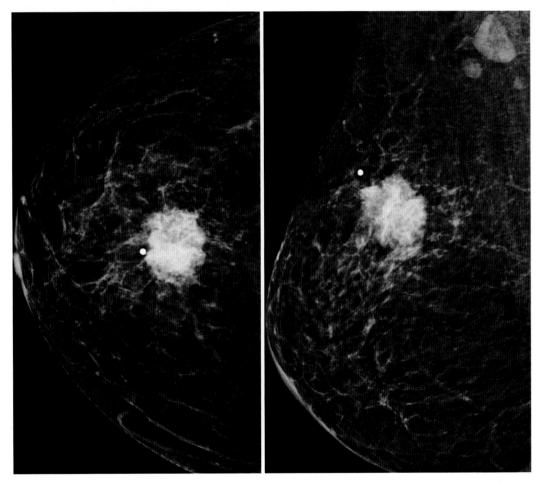

Fig. 234 Mammography (July 2021): irregular hyperdense mass in the upper mid portion of right breast (marked by BB marker). Enlarged lymph nodes in right axilla

HR(−) HER2(+) Breast Cancer

Fig. 235 Breast US (July 2021): irregular heterogeneous echoic mass with microcalcifications at the 12 o'clock direction of right breast

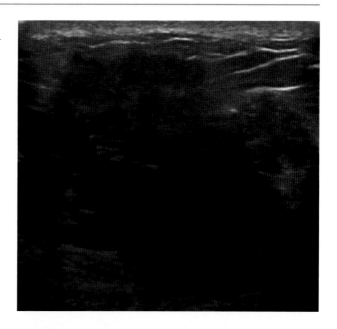

Fig. 236 Breast MRI (July 2021): irregular enhancing mass at the 12 o'clock direction of right breast. Enlarged lymph node in right axilla

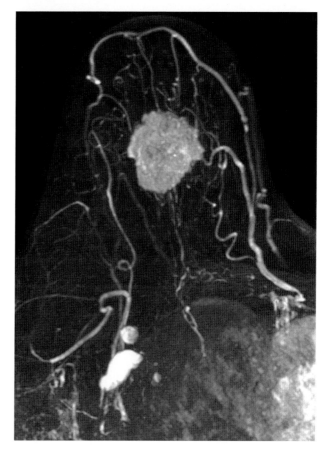

Fig. 237 PET-CT shows (**a**) a hypermetabolic mass at right breast (mSUV = 13.8) and (**b**, **c**) a few hypermetabolic lymph nodes in right axillary level I, III (mSUV = 5.5)

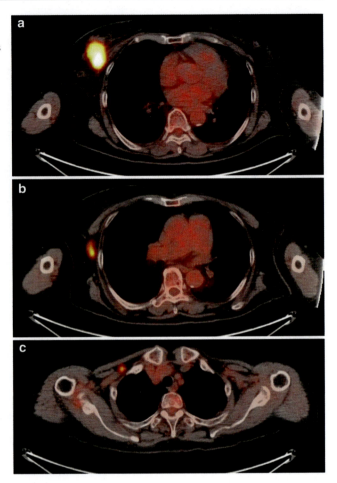

35.3 After Neoadjuvant Chemotherapy

See Figs. 238, 239, 240 and 241.

35.4 Courses of Treatment

Neoadjuvant chemotherapy (#5 cycles of docetaxel and trastuzumab and pertuzumab) + Operation + Post-operative radiation therapy + Trastuzumab and pertuzumab.

35.4.1 Operation

Right breast conserving surgery, sentinel lymph node biopsy (Fig. 242).

35.4.2 Pathology Report

Microinvasive Ductal Carcinoma
1. Post-chemotherapy status.
2. Size of invasive component: <0.1 cm (ypT1mi).
3. Size of intraductal component: 0.8 cm.
4. Histologic grade: not applicable.

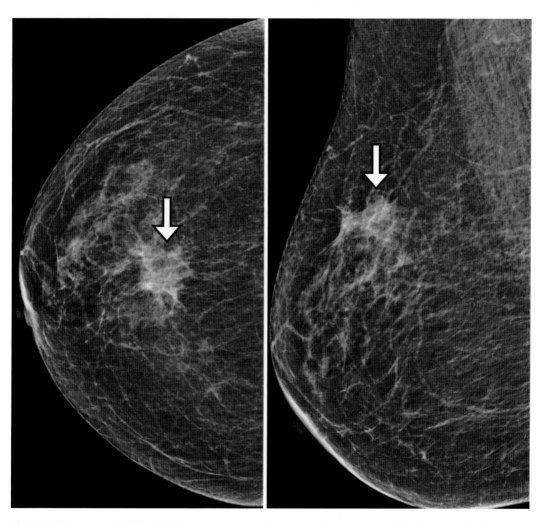

Fig. 238 Mammography (Nov. 2021): mammography after treatment demonstrates residual mass that is decreased in the longest diameter. Decrease in size of enlarged LNs in right axilla

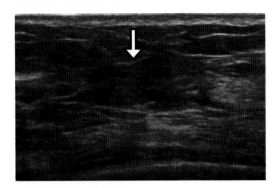

Fig. 239 Breast US (Nov. 2021): US after treatment demonstrates residual hypoechoic mass that is decreased in the longest diameter

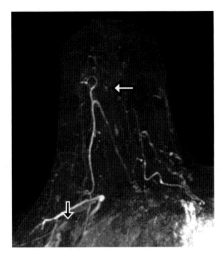

Fig. 240 Breast MRI (Nov. 2021): MRI after treatment demonstrates residual enhancing foci (white arrow) that are decreased in the longest diameter and in the degree of enhancement and a normal-appearing axillary lymph node (black arrow)

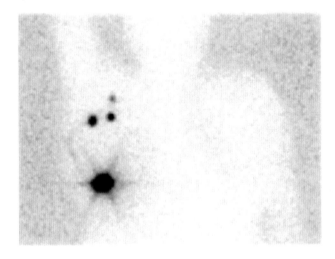

Fig. 241 Lymphoscintigraphy shows visualized sentinel lymph nodes in the right axilla

HR(−) HER2(+) Breast Cancer

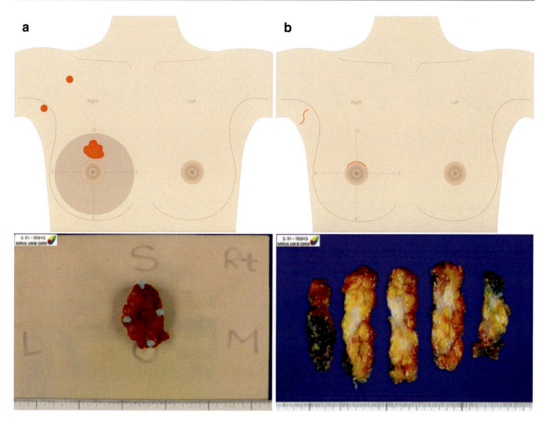

Fig. 242 (**a**) Gross pathology of mastectomy specimen. (**b**) The margins get marked and sliced with different colors on each direction

5. Intraductal component: present, intratumoral/extratumoral (99%) (nuclear grade: low, necrosis: present, architectural pattern: solid/comedo, extensive intraductal component: present).
6. Skin: no involvement of tumor.
7. Surgical margins:
   (a) superior margin: 5 mm,
   (b) inferior margin: 20 mm,
   (c) medial margin: positive for microinvasive ductal carcinoma (Fro 3) (see note),
   (d) lateral margin: 5 mm,
   (e) deep margin: 2 mm,
   (f) superficial margin: 2 mm.
8. Lymph nodes: no metastasis in three axillary lymph nodes (ypN0(sn)) (sentinel LN: 0/3).
9. Arteriovenous invasion: absent.
10. Lymphovascular invasion: absent.
11. Tumor border: infiltrative.
12. Microcalcification: present, tumoral/non-tumoral.
13. Pathological TN category (AJCC 2017): ypT1miN0(sn).

Note: 1. Microinvasive ductal carcinoma is focally present only in the permanent section of Fro 3.

	Result	Intensity	Positive %
Estrogen receptor	Negative (0/8)	0	0
Progesterone receptor	Negative (0/8)	0	0
C-erbB2	Positive (3+)		
Ki-67	Positive in 48% of tumor cells		

36 Case 36

36.1 Patient History and Progress

Female/63 years old, post-menopause.

Screen detected mass lesion on left breast 2 o'clock direction.

No family history.

Hypertension, chronic renal failure, ventricular premature contraction.

S/P cholecystectomy (due to stone).

36.2 Important Radiologic Findings

See Figs. 243 and 244.

36.3 Courses of Treatment

Neoadjuvant chemotherapy (#6 cycles of docetaxel and carboplatin and trastuzumab and pertuzumab) + Operation + Postoperative radiation therapy + Trastuzumab.

Operation: Left breast conserving surgery, sentinel lymph node biopsy (Fig. 245).

36.3.1 Pathology Report

1. No residual tumor with foamy histiocytic collection.
   (a) Post-chemotherapy status.
   (b) Lymph nodes: no metastasis in four axillary lymph nodes (ypN0(sn)) (sentinel LN: 0/4).
   (c) Microcalcification: present, tumoral/non-tumoral.
2. Intraductal papilloma.

	Result	Intensity	Positive %
Estrogen receptor	Negative (0/8)	0	0
Progesterone receptor	Negative (0/8)	0	0
C-erbB2	Positive (3+)		
Ki-67	Positive in 22% of tumor cells		

HR(−) HER2(+) Breast Cancer

Fig. 243 PET-CT shows (**a**) a hypermetabolic mass in the left breast (mSUV = 14.8), (**b**) small hypermetabolic lesions in the left upper outer breast (mSUV = 1.6), and (**c**) small lymph nodes in the left axilla level I–II (mSUV = 1.3)

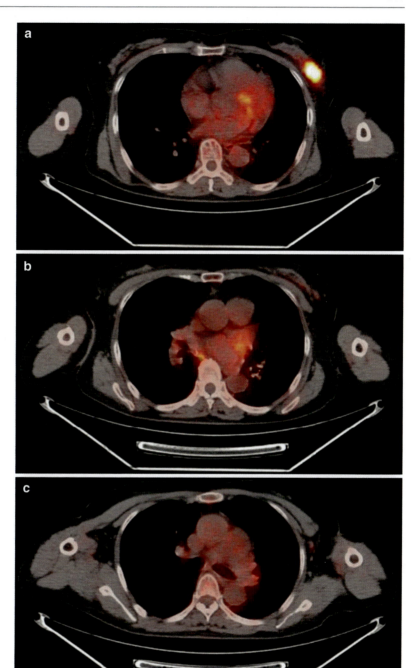

Fig. 244 Lymphoscintigraphy shows visualized sentinel lymph nodes in the left axilla

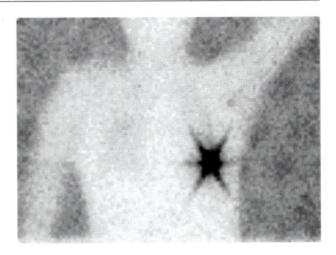

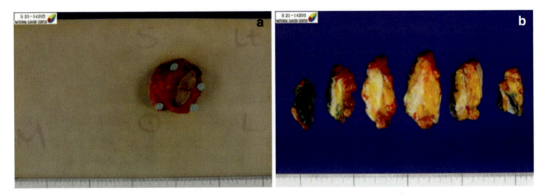

Fig. 245 (**a**) Gross pathology of lumpectomy specimen. (**b**) The margins get marked and sliced with different colors on each direction

37 Case 37

37.1 Patient History and Progress

Female/63 years old, post-menopause.
   Self-detected nipple discharge on left breast.
   No family history.
   S/P Total hysterectomy, s/p right lung lobectomy (benign), diabetes mellitus.

37.2 Important Radiologic Findings

See Figs. 246, 247 and 248.

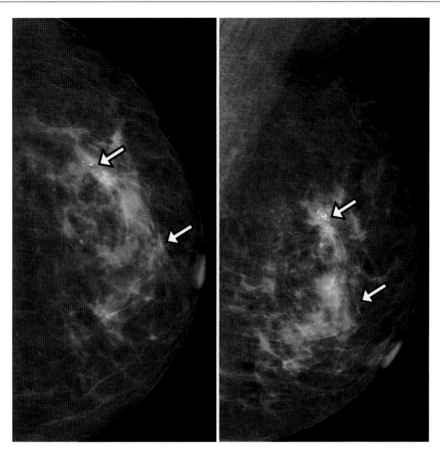

Fig. 246 Mammography: segmental fine pleomorphic microcalcifications with focal asymmetries in the upper outer quadrant of left breast, irregular hypoechoic mass with microcalcifications at the 2 o'clock direction of left breast

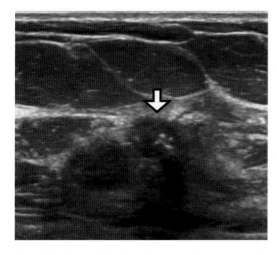

Fig. 247 Breast US: irregular hypoechoic mass with microcalcifications at the 2 o'clock direction of left breast

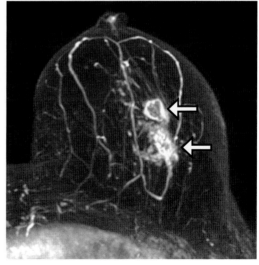

Fig. 248 Breast MRI: two irregular enhancing masses in the upper outer quadrant of left breast

37.3 After Neoadjuvant Chemotherapy

See Figs. 249, 250, 251 and 252.

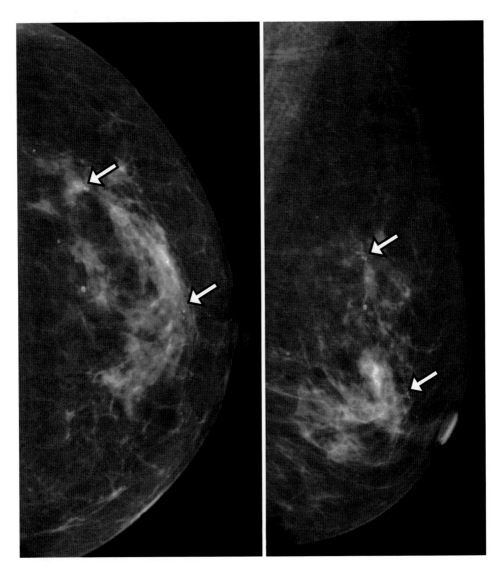

Fig. 249 Mammography (Dec. 2020): no change of segmental fine pleomorphic microcalcifications and decrease in size of focal asymmetries in the upper outer quadrant of left breast

HR(−) HER2(+) Breast Cancer

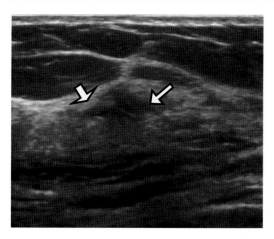

Fig. 250 Breast US (Dec. 2020): US after treatment demonstrates residual hypoechoic mass that is decreased in the longest diameter

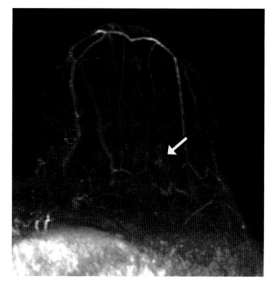

Fig. 251 Breast MRI (Dec. 2020): MRI after treatment shows residual non-mass enhancement in left breast

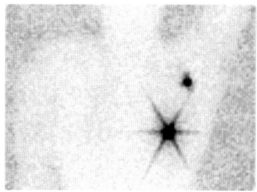

Fig. 252 Lymphoscintigraphy shows visualized sentinel lymph nodes in the left axilla

37.4 Courses of Treatment

Neoadjuvant chemotherapy (#6 cycles of docetaxel and carboplatin and trastuzumab and pertuzumab) + Operation + Postoperative radiation therapy + Trastuzumab.

Operation: Left breast conserving surgery, sentinel lymph node biopsy (Fig. 253).

37.4.1 Pathology Report

Ductal Carcinoma In Situ
1. Post-chemotherapy status.
2. Size of tumor: 0.5 cm (ypTis).
3. Nuclear grade: high.
4. Necrosis: present.
5. Architectural pattern: solid/comedo.
6. Skin: no involvement of tumor.
7. Surgical margins:
    (a) superior margin: 10 mm,
    (b) inferior margin: 10 mm,
    (c) medial margin: 30 mm,

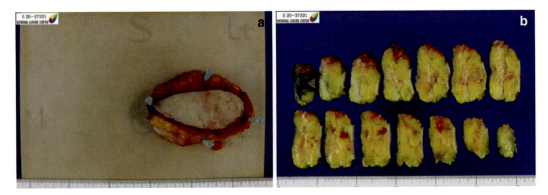

Fig. 253 (a) Gross pathology of lumpectomy specimen. (b) The margins get marked and sliced with different colors on each direction

   (d) lateral margin: 20 mm,
   (e) deep margin: 2 mm,
   (f) superficial margin: 2 mm.
8. Lymph nodes: no metastasis in two axillary lymph nodes (ypN0(sn)) (sentinel LN: 0/2).
9. Microcalcification: present, tumoral/non-tumoral.
10. Pathological TN category (AJCC 2017): ypTisN0(sn).

	Result	Intensity	Positive %
Estrogen receptor	Negative (0/8)	0	0
Progesterone receptor	Negative (0/8)	0	0
C-erbB2	Positive (3+)		
Ki-67	Positive in 39% of tumor cells		

38 Case 38

38.1 Patient History and Progress

Female/55 years old, post-menopause.

Self-detected palpable mass lesion on right breast.
Family history of breast cancer, sister.
Dyslipidemia.
BRCA 1 and 2 mutation: Not detected, MUTYH and RAD50 VUS (variant of uncertain).

38.2 Important Radiologic Findings

See Figs. 254, 255, 256 and 257.

38.3 Courses of Treatment

Operation + Adjuvant chemotherapy (#4 cycles of docetaxel and cyclophosphamide) + Post-operative radiation therapy + Trastuzumab.

Operation: Right breast conserving surgery, sentinel lymph node biopsy (Fig. 258).

HR(−) HER2(+) Breast Cancer

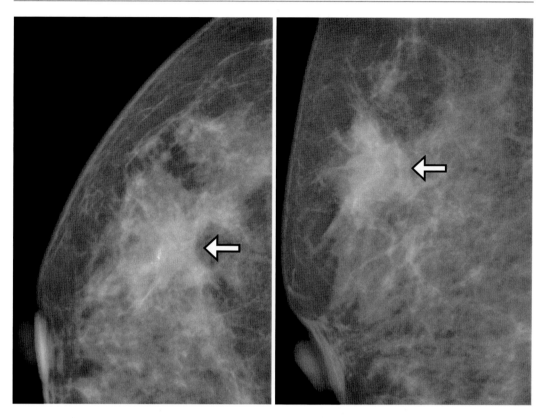

Fig. 254 Magnification (Jan. 2021): indistinct hyperdense mass with microcalcifications in right upper outer quadrant

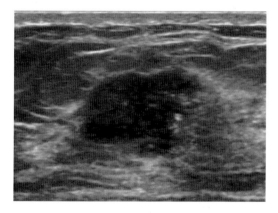

Fig. 255 Breast US (Jan. 2021): irregular hypoechoic mass with microcalcifications at the 11 o'clock direction of right breast

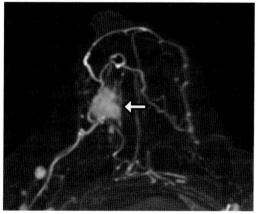

Fig. 256 Breast MRI (Jan. 2021): irregular enhancing mass at the 11 o'clock direction of right breast

Fig. 257 Lymphoscintigraphy shows visualized sentinel lymph nodes in the right axilla

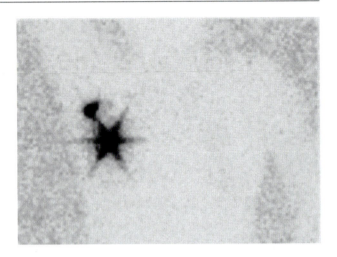

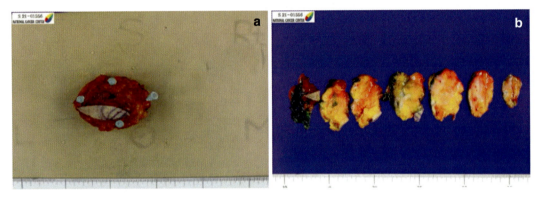

Fig. 258 (**a**) Gross pathology of lumpectomy specimen. (**b**) The margins get marked and sliced with different colors on each direction

38.3.1 Pathology Report

Invasive Ductal Carcinoma with medullary pattern
1. Size of tumor: 1.1 cm (pT1c).
2. Histologic grade: 3/3 (tubule formation: 3/3, nuclear pleomorphism: 3/3, mitotic count: 3/3, 30/10HPF).
3. Intraductal component: present, intratumoral/extratumoral (60%) (nuclear grade: high, necrosis: present, architectural pattern: cribriform/solid/comedo, extensive intraductal component: present).
4. Skin: no involvement of tumor.
5. Surgical margins:
    (a) superior margin: 10 mm,
    (b) inferior margin: 15 mm,
    (c) medial margin: 5 mm,
    (d) lateral margin: 10 mm,
    (e) deep margin: 10 mm,
    (f) superficial margin: 7 mm.

6. Lymph nodes: no metastasis in nine axillary lymph nodes (pN0) (sentinel LN: 0/4, axillary LN: 0/5).
7. Arteriovenous invasion: absent.
8. Lymphovascular invasion: absent.
9. Tumor border: infiltrative.
10. Microcalcification: present, non-tumoral.
11. Pathological TN category (AJCC 2017): pT1cN0.

	Result	Intensity	Positive %
Estrogen receptor	Negative (0/8)	0	0
Progesterone receptor	Negative (0/8)	0	0
C-erbB2	positive (3+)		
Ki-67	Positive in 59% of tumor cells		

HR(−) HER2(−) Breast Cancer

Eun Sook Lee, Chan Wha Lee, Youngmi Kwon, Jeayeon Woo, and Yunju Kim

1 Case 1

1.1 Patient History and Progress

Female/40 years old, pre-menopause.

Screen detected a mass lesion at 1 o'clock direction of the left breast.

No family history.

No comorbidities.

BRCA 1 and 2 mutation: Not detected, CHEK2 VUS (variant of uncertain).

1.2 Important Radiologic Findings

See Figs. 1, 2 and 3.

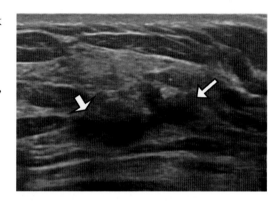

Fig. 1 Breast US (Jun. 2020): An irregular hypoechoic mass at the 2 o'clock direction of left breast

E. S. Lee
Center for Breast Cancer, National Cancer Center, Goyang, Kyonggi-do, Republic of Korea
e-mail: eslee@ncc.re.kr

C. W. Lee
Division of Diagnostic Radiology, Center for Breast Cancer, National Cancer Center, Goyang, Republic of Korea
e-mail: drlee4958@gmail.com

Y. Kwon
Department of Radiology, Center for Breast Cancer, National Cancer Center, Goyang, Republic of Korea
e-mail: ymk@ncc.re.kr

J. Woo
Division of Surgery, Center for Breast Cancer, National Cancer Center, Goyang, Republic of Korea
e-mail: jaeyeon1205@gmail.com

Y. Kim (✉)
Department of Pathology, National Cancer Center, Goyang, Gyeonggi, Republic of Korea
e-mail: radkyj@ncc.re.kr

Fig. 2 Breast MRI (Jun. 2020): An irregular enhancing mass in the upper outer quadrant of left breast

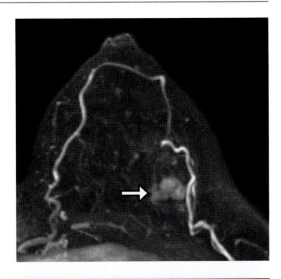

Fig. 3 PET-CT shows (**a**) a mild hypermetabolic nodule on Lt. outer breast (mSUV = 3.7), (**b**) hypermetabolic lymph node in Lt. supraclavicular area, and (**c**) hypermetabolic lymph node in Lt. axilla level I–III

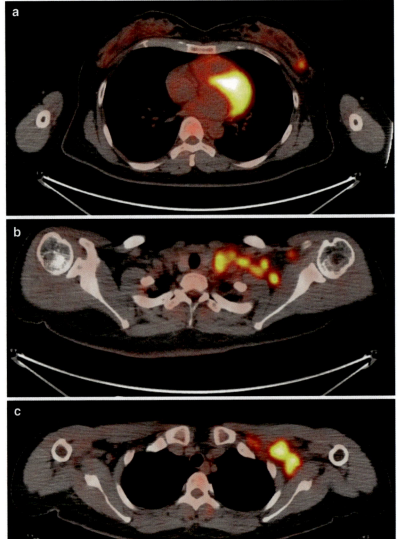

1.2.1 After Neoadjuvant Chemotherapy

See Figs. 4, 5 and 6.

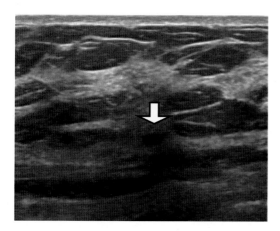

Fig. 4 Breast US (Dec. 2020): US after treatment demonstrates residual hypoechoic mass that is decreased in the longest diameter

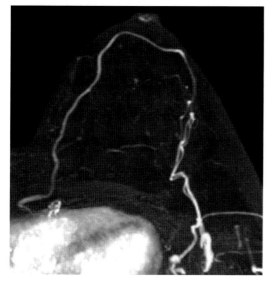

Fig. 5 Breast MRI (Dec. 2020): MRI after treatment shows complete resolution of enhancement in the left breast

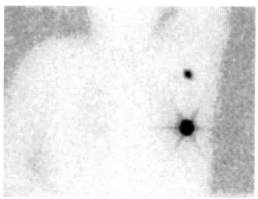

Fig. 6 Lymphoscintigraphy shows visualized sentinel lymph nodes in the left axilla

1.3 Courses of Treatment

Neoadjuvant chemotherapy (#4 cycles of doxorubicin and cyclophosphamide + #4 cycles of docetaxel) + Operation + Postoperative radiation therapy.

1.3.1 Operation

Left breast conserving surgery, sentinel lymph node biopsy (Fig. 7).

1.3.2 Pathology Report

Breast, left, lumpectomy:
1. No residual tumor with stromal degeneration.
    (a) Post-chemotherapy status.
    (b) Lymph nodes: no metastasis in four axillary lymph nodes (ypN0(sn)) (sentinel LN: 0/1, non-sentinel LN: 0/3).
2. Fibroadenomatous change.

	Result	Intensity	Positive %
Estrogen receptor	Negative (2/8)	1	<1%
Progesterone receptor	Negative (2/8)	1	<1%
C-erbB2	Negative (0)		
Ki-67	Positive in 65% of tumor cells		

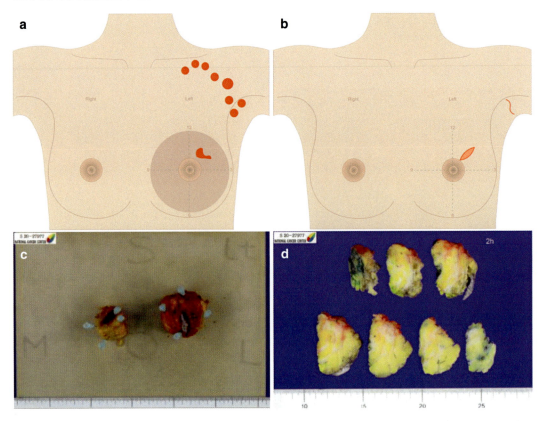

Fig. 7 (**a**) A schematic illustration of tumor location and lymph node metastasis and (**b**) breast and axillary incision lines. (**c**) Gross pathology of lumpectomy specimen. (**d**) The margins get marked and sliced with different colors on each direction

2 Case 2

2.1 Patient History and Progress

Female/49 years old, pre-menopause.

Self-detected palpable mass lesion on right breast.

No family history.
No comorbidities.

2.2 Important Radiologic Findings

See Figs. 8, 9, 10 and 11.

Fig. 8 Mammography (Apr. 2020): An irregular isodense mass in the upper portion of right breast on mediolateral oblique view. The mass is not identified on the craniocaudal view

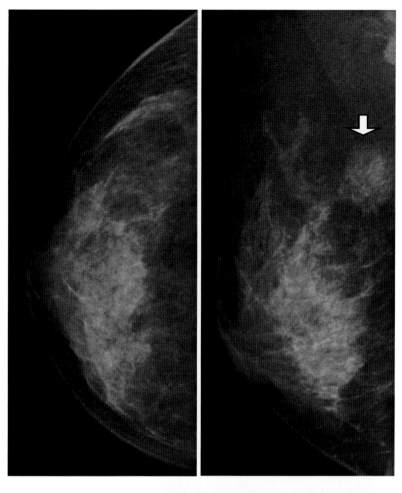

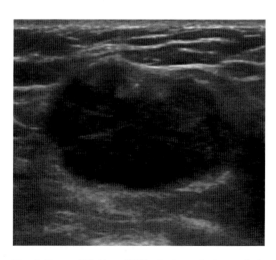

Fig. 9 Breast US (Apr. 2020): An irregular hypoechoic mass at the 10 o'clock direction of right breast

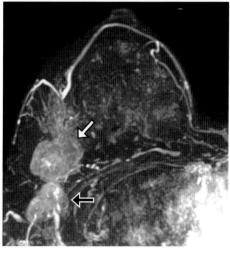

Fig. 10 Breast MRI (Apr. 2020): An irregular enhancing mass (white arrow) at the 10 o'clock direction of right breast. Multiple enlarged lymph nodes (black arrow) in right axilla

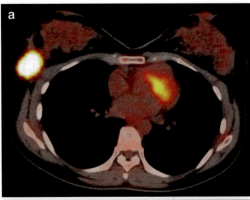

2.3.2 Pathology Report
No residual tumor with stromal fibrosis

1. Post-chemotherapy status.
2. Lymph nodes:
   (a) No metastasis in ten axillary lymph node (ypN0) (sentinel LN: 0/3, non-sentinel LN: 0/7).

	Result	Intensity	Positive %
Estrogen receptor	Negative (2/8)	1	<1%
Progesterone receptor	Negative (0/8)	0	0
C-erbB2	Equivocal (2+) SISH (−)		
Ki-67	Positive in 67% of tumor cells		

Fig. 11 PET-CT shows (**a**) an intense hypermetabolic mass in Rt. breast outer portion (mSUV = 27.9) and (**b**) multiple hypermetabolic LNs enlargement at Rt. axilla level I–II (mSUV = 14.8)

2.2.1 After Neoadjuvant Chemotherapy
See Figs. 12, 13 and 14.

2.3 Courses of Treatment

Neoadjuvant chemotherapy (#4 cycles of doxorubicin and cyclophosphamide + #4 cycles of docetaxel) + Operation + Postoperative radiation therapy.

2.3.1 Operation
Right breast conserving surgery, axillary lymph node dissection (level 1) (Fig. 15).

Fig. 12 Mammography (Dec. 2020): Invisible previous malignant lesion in the right upper breast

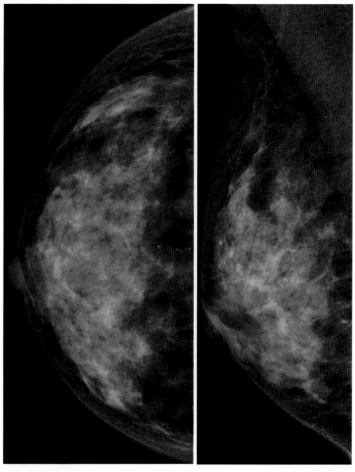

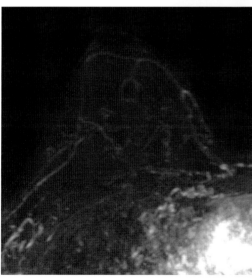

Fig. 13 Breast MRI (Dec. 2020): MRI after treatment shows complete resolution of enhancement in the right breast

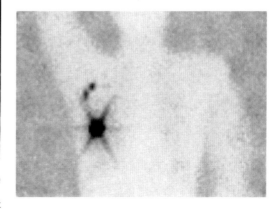

Fig. 14 Lymphoscintigraphy shows visualized sentinel lymph nodes in the right axilla

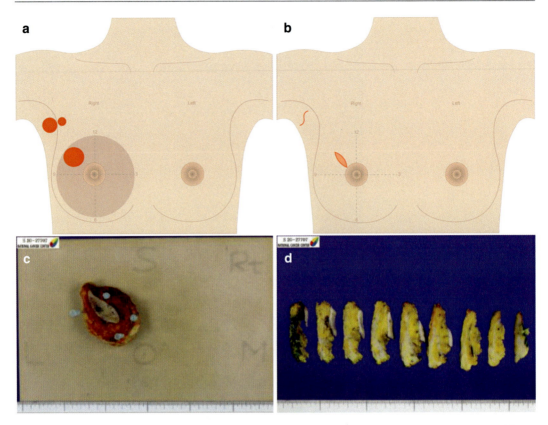

Fig. 15 (**a**) A schematic illustration of tumor location and lymph node metastasis and (**b**) breast and axillary incision lines. (**c**) Gross pathology of lumpectomy specimen. (**d**) The margins get marked and sliced with different colors on each direction

3 Case 3

3.1 Patient History and Progress

Female/41 years old, pre-menopause.

Screen detected mass lesion on left breast 3 o'clock direction.
No family history.
No comorbidities.

3.2 Important Radiologic Findings

See Figs. 16, 17, 18 and 19.

3.3 Courses of Treatment

Operation + operation, Transfer.

3.3.1 Operation

First operation: Dec. 2020 Left breast conserving surgery, sentinel lymph node biopsy (Fig. 20).

3.3.2 Pathology Report

Invasive Ductal Carcinoma
1. Size of tumor: 2.3 cm (pT2).
2. Histologic grade: 3/3 (tubule formation: 2/3, nuclear pleomorphism: 3/3, mitotic count: 3/3, 82/10HPF).
3. Intraductal component: present, extratumoral (30%) (nuclear grade: high, necrosis: present, architectural pattern: solid/comedo, extensive intraductal component: present).
4. Skin: no involvement of tumor.
5. Surgical margins:
    (a) superior margin: (see note),
    (b) inferior margin: positive for ductal carcinoma in situ (Fro 5),

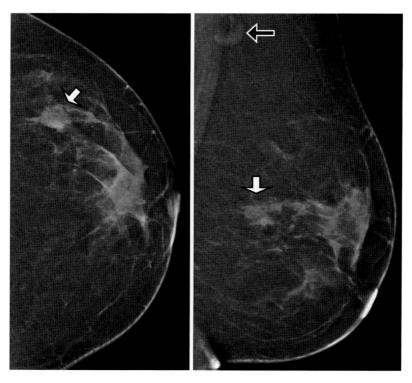

Fig. 16 Mammography (Dec. 2020): An irregular isodense mass (white arrow) at the 3 o'clock direction of the left breast. Enlarged lymph node (black arrow) in the left axilla

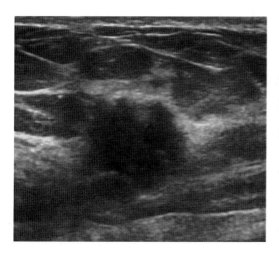

Fig. 17 Breast US (Dec. 2020): An irregular hypoechoic mass with microlobulated margins at the 3 o'clock direction of the left breast

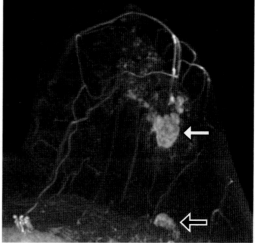

Fig. 18 Breast MRI (Dec. 2020): An irregular heterogeneous enhancing mass (white arrow) at the 3 o'clock direction of the left breast. Regional heterogeneous non-mass enhancement in the upper outer quadrant of the left breast. Enlarged lymph node (black arrow) in the left axilla

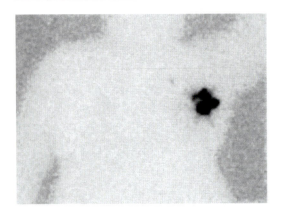

Fig. 19 Lymphoscintigraphy shows visualized sentinel lymph nodes in the left axilla

  (c) medial margin: positive for ductal carcinoma in situ (Fro 6),
  (d) lateral margin: 5 mm,
  (e) deep margin: <1 mm from ductal carcinoma in situ (slide 11),
  (f) superficial margin: 5 mm.
6. Lymph nodes: no metastasis in three axillary lymph nodes (pN0(sn)) (sentinel LN: 0/3, non-sentinel LN: 0/0).
7. Arteriovenous invasion: absent.
8. Lymphovascular invasion: present, intratumoral.

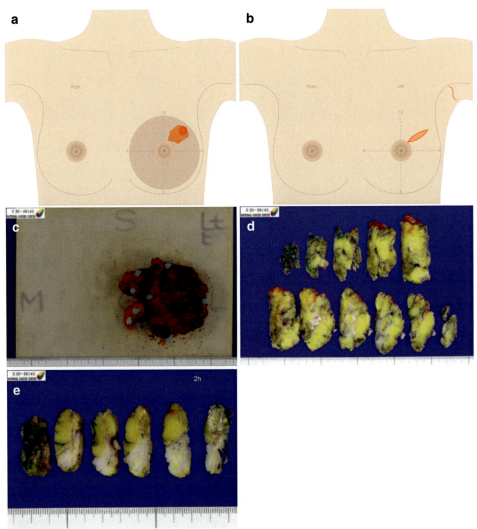

Fig. 20 (a) A schematic illustration of tumor location and (b) breast and axillary incision lines. (c) Gross pathology of lumpectomy specimen. (d) The margins get marked and sliced with different colors on each direction. (e) The margins get marked and sliced with different colors on each direction (2H)

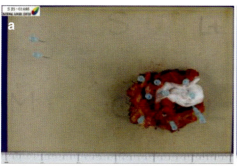
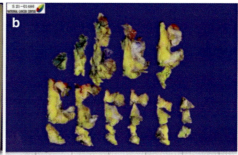

Fig. 21 (**a**) Gross pathology of lumpectomy specimen. (**b**) The margins get marked and sliced with different colors on each direction

9. Tumor border: infiltrative.
10. Microcalcification: present, tumoral.
11. Pathological TN category (AJCC 2017): pT2N0(sn).

Breast, left 2 o'clock, lumpectomy:

Invasive Ductal Carcinoma

1. Size of invasive component: 0.2 cm.
2. Size of intraductal component: 2.0 cm.
3. Histologic grade: 3/3 (tubule formation: 3/3, nuclear pleomorphism: 3/3, mitotic count: 2/3, 13/10HPF).
4. Intraductal component: present, intratumoral/extratumoral (90%) (nuclear grade: high, necrosis: present, architectural pattern: solid/comedo, extensive intraductal component: present).
5. Skin: no involvement of tumor.
6. Surgical margins:
    (a) Superior margin: 5 mm.
    (b) Inferior margin: positive for ductal carcinoma in situ (slide 21).
    (c) Medial margin: 5 mm.
    (d) Lateral margin: <1 mm from ductal carcinoma in situ (slide 22).
    (e) Deep margin: <1 mm from ductal carcinoma in situ (slide 21).
    (f) Superficial margin: 1 mm from ductal carcinoma in situ (slide 18).
7. Arteriovenous invasion: absent.
8. Lymphovascular invasion: absent.
9. Tumor border: infiltrative.
10. Microcalcification: present, non-tumoral.

Note: 1. The superior margin of the lumpectomy specimen (slide 1) is positive for ductal carcinoma in situ, but this margin submitted for frozen diagnosis (Fro 4) is free of tumor.

Second operation: Jan. 2021 superior, medial, inferior margin re-excision (Fig. 21).

	Result	Intensity	Positive %
Estrogen receptor	Negative (0/8)	0	0
Progesterone receptor	Negative (0/8)	0	0
C-erbB2	Negative (0)		
Ki-67	Positive in 53% of tumor cells		

4 Case 4

4.1 Patient History and Progress

Female/52 years old, post-menopause.
Self-detected palpable mass lesion on left breast 1–2 o'clock direction.
No family history.
Hyperthyroidism.

4.2 Important Radiologic Findings

See Figs. 22, 23, 24 and 25.

Fig. 22 Mammography (Dec. 2020): An irregular hyperdense mass in the upper outer quadrant of the left breast

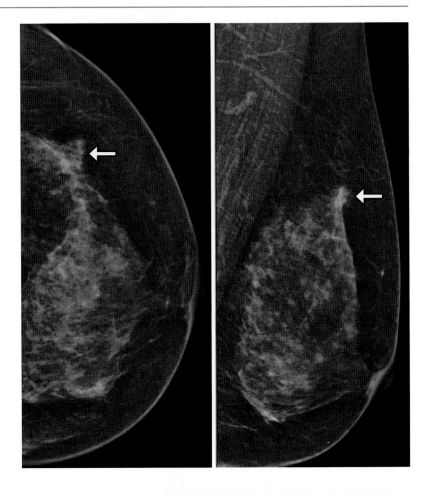

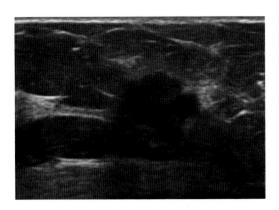

Fig. 23 Breast US (Dec. 2020): An irregular hypoechoic mass with echogenic halo at the 2 o'clock direction of the left breast

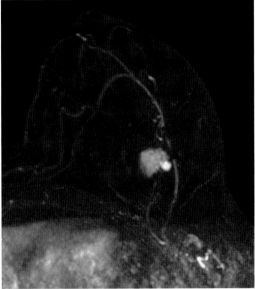

Fig. 24 Breast MRI (Dec. 2020): An irregular enhancing mass at the 2 o'clock direction of the left breast

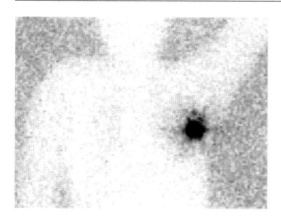

Fig. 25 Lymphoscintigraphy shows visualized sentinel lymph nodes in the left axilla

4.3 Courses of Treatment

Operation + adjuvant chemotherapy (#4 cycles of docetaxel and cyclophosphamide) + Postoperative radiation therapy.

4.3.1 Operation

Left breast conserving surgery, sentinel lymph node biopsy (Fig. 26).

4.3.2 Pathology Report

Invasive Ductal Carcinoma
1. Size of tumor: 1.5 cm (pT1c).
2. Histologic grade: 3/3 (tubule formation: 2/3, nuclear pleomorphism: 3/3, mitotic count: 3/3, 40/10HPF).
3. Intraductal component: absent.
4. Skin: no involvement of tumor.
5. Surgical margins:
    (a) Superior margin: 16 mm.
    (b) Inferior margin: 20 mm.
    (c) Medial margin: 18 mm.
    (d) Lateral margin: 26 mm.
    (e) Deep margin: 6 mm.
    (f) Superficial margin: 8 mm.
6. Lymph nodes: no metastasis in one axillary lymph node (pN0(sn)) (sentinel LN: 0/1).
7. Arteriovenous invasion: absent.
8. Lymphovascular invasion: absent.
9. Tumor border: infiltrative.
10. Microcalcification: present, non-tumoral.
11. Pathological TN category (AJCC 2017): pT1cN0(sn).

	Result	Intensity	Positive %
Estrogen receptor	Negative (0/8)	0	0
Progesterone receptor	Negative (0/8)	0	0
C-erbB2	Negative (1+)		
Ki-67	Positive in 25% of tumor cells		

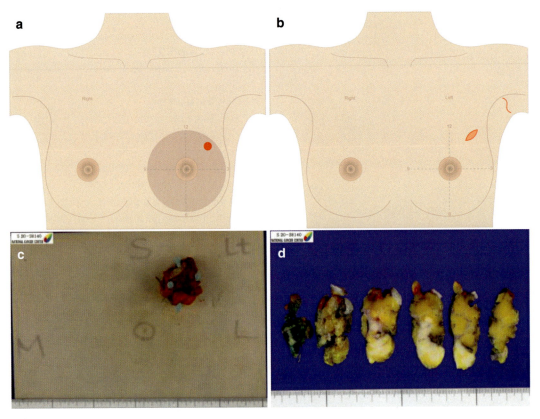

Fig. 26 (**a**) A schematic illustration of tumor location and (**b**) breast and axillary incision lines. (**c**) Gross pathology of lumpectomy specimen. (**d**) The margins get marked and sliced with different colors on each direction

5 Case 5

5.1 Patient History and Progress

Female/57 years old, post-menopause.

Screen detected a mass lesion on left breast 9 o'clock direction.

Family history of breast cancer, sister and niece.

Family history of ovarian cancer, mother.

S/P Hysterectomy, s/o bilateral salpingo-oophorectomy.

BRCA 1 mutation carrier.

5.2 Important Radiologic Findings

See Figs. 27, 28, 29 and 30.

Fig. 27 Mammography (Jun. 2020): An irregular hyperdense mass with indistinct margins (marked by BB marker) in mid inner portion of left breast. Enlarged lymph nodes (white arrow) in left axilla

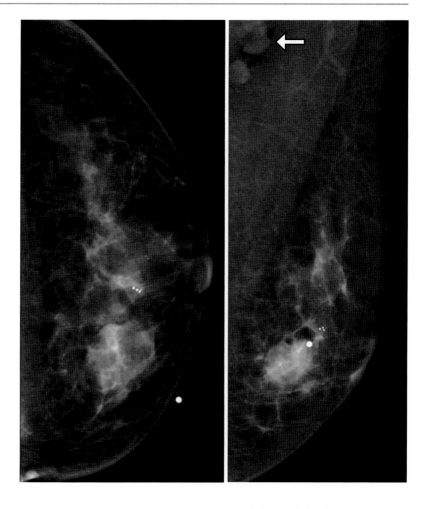

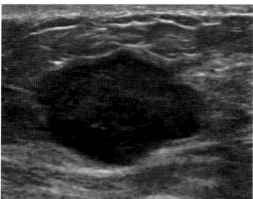

Fig. 28 Breast US (Jun. 2020): An irregular hypoechoic mass with angular margins at the 9 o'clock direction of the left breast

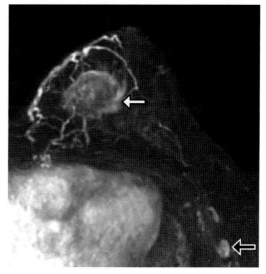

Fig. 29 Breast MRI (Jun. 2020): An irregular enhancing mass (white arrow) at the 9 o'clock direction of the left breast. Enlarged lymph node (black arrow) in the left axilla

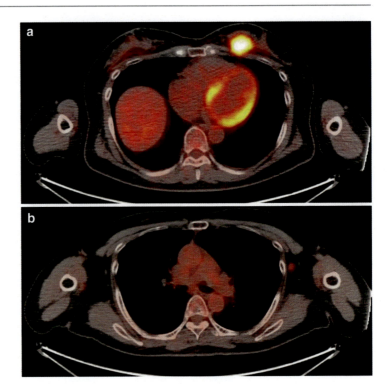

Fig. 30 PET-CT shows (**a**) Lt. breast UIQ mass with hypermetabolism (mSUV = 11.3) and (**b**) mild hypermetabolism left axillary LN (mSUV = 1.9)

5.2.1 After Neoadjuvant Chemotherapy

See Figs. 31, 32, 33 and 34.

5.3 Courses of Treatment

Neoadjuvant chemotherapy (#4 cycles of doxorubicin and cyclophosphamide + #4 cycles of docetaxel) + Operation + Postoperative radiation therapy + Adjuvant capecitabine (refuse).

5.3.1 Operation

Left breast conserving surgery, sentinel lymph node biopsy (Fig. 35).

5.3.2 Pathology Report

Invasive Ductal Carcinoma
1. Post-chemotherapy status.
2. Size of tumor: 0.3 cm (ypT1a).
3. Histologic grade: 3/3 (tubule formation: 3/3, nuclear pleomorphism: 3/3, mitotic count: 2/3, 11/10HPF).
4. Intraductal component: absent.
5. Skin: no involvement of tumor.
6. Surgical margins:
    (a) Superior margin: 13 mm.
    (b) Inferior margin: 11 mm.
    (c) Medial margin: 25 mm.
    (d) Lateral margin: 15 mm.
    (e) Deep margin: 5 mm.
    (f) Superficial margin: 6 mm.
7. Lymph nodes: no metastasis in two axillary lymph nodes (ypN0(sn)) (sentinel LN: 0/2).
8. Arteriovenous invasion: absent.
9. Lymphovascular invasion: absent.
10. Tumor border: infiltrative.
11. Microcalcification: present, non-tumoral.
12. Pathological TN category (AJCC 2017): ypT1aN0(sn).

	Result	Intensity	Positive %
Estrogen receptor	Negative (0/8)	0	0
Progesterone receptor	Negative (0/8)	0	0
C-erbB2	Negative (1+)		
Ki-67	Positive in 26% of tumor cells		

Fig. 31 Mammography (Dec. 2020): mammography after treatment demonstrates no residual mass

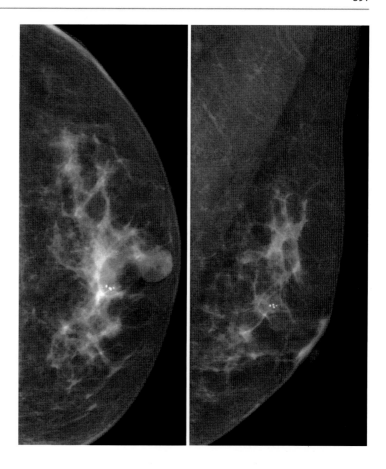

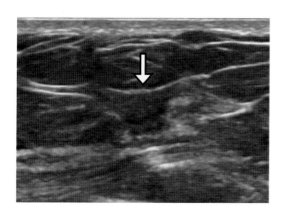

Fig. 32 Breast US (Dec. 2020): US after treatment demonstrates the residual hypoechoic mass that is decreased in the longest diameter

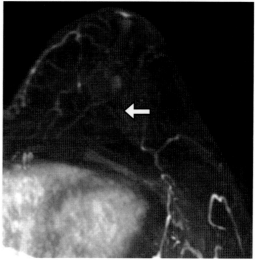

Fig. 33 Breast MRI (Dec. 2020): MRI after treatment demonstrates residual enhancing mass (white arrow) that is decreased in the longest diameter

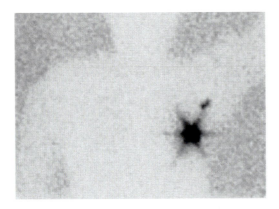

Fig. 34 Lymphoscintigraphy shows visualized sentinel lymph nodes in the left axilla

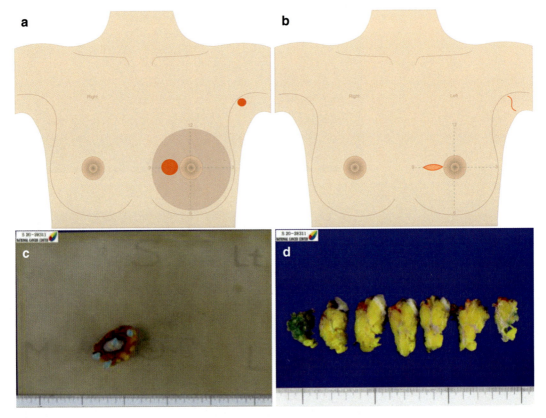

Fig. 35 (a) A schematic illustration of tumor location and lymph node metastasis and (b) breast and axillary incision lines. (c) Gross pathology of lumpectomy specimen. (d) The margins get marked and sliced with different colors on each direction

6 Case 6

6.1 Patient History and Progress

Female/49 years old, pre-menopause.

Self-detected palpable mass lesion on left breast.

No family history.

Panic disorder, lumbar spine disc.

6.2 Important Radiologic Findings

See Figs. 36, 37, 38 and 39.

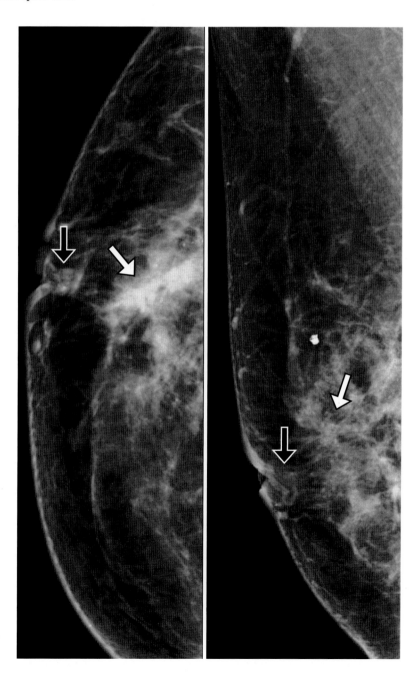

Fig. 36 Mammography (Jun. 2020): An irregular hyperdense mass with microcalcifications in the subareolar region of the right breast. Note associated nipple retraction (black arrow)

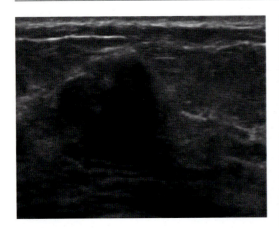

Fig. 37 Breast US (Jun. 2020): An irregular hypoechoic mass at the 9 o'clock direction of the right breast

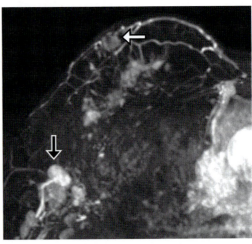

Fig. 38 Breast MRI (Jun. 2020): multicentric irregular enhancing masses in right breast. Note right nipple enhancement (white arrow), suggesting nipple invasion. Multiple enlarged lymph nodes (black arrow) in the right axilla

Fig. 39 PET-CT shows (**a**) mild hypermetabolic masses in the right whole breast (mSUV = 2.0) and (**b**) enlarged LNs with hypermetabolism in the right axilla level I (mSUV = 3.5) and II

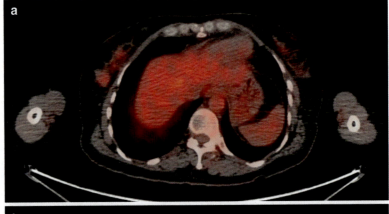

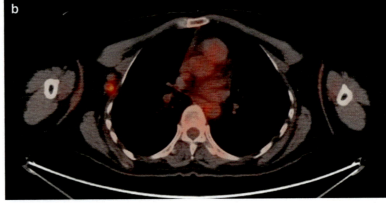

6.2.1 After Neoadjuvant Chemotherapy

See Figs. 40, 41 and 42.

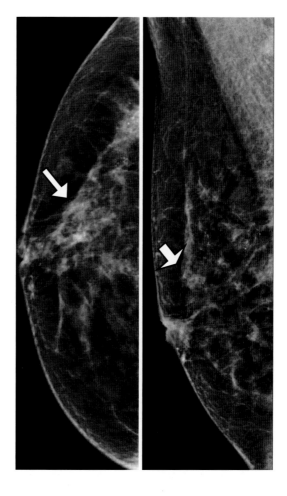

Fig. 40 Mammography (Jan. 2021): Mammography after treatment demonstrates residual mass that is decreased in the longest diameter

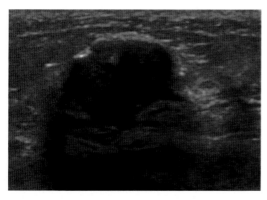

Fig. 41 Breast US (Jan. 2021): US after treatment demonstrates residual hypoechoic mass that is decreased in the longest diameter

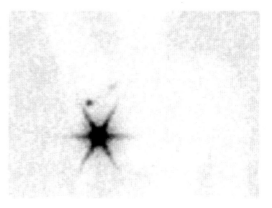

Fig. 42 Lymphoscintigraphy shows visualized sentinel lymph nodes in the right axilla

6.3 Courses of Treatment

Neoadjuvant chemotherapy (#4 cycles of doxorubicin and cyclophosphamide + #4 cycles of docetaxel) + Operation + Postoperative radiation therapy + Letrozole 2.5 mg + Adjuvant capecitabine.

6.3.1 Operation

Right modified radical mastectomy, axillary lymph node dissection (level 1) (Fig. 43).

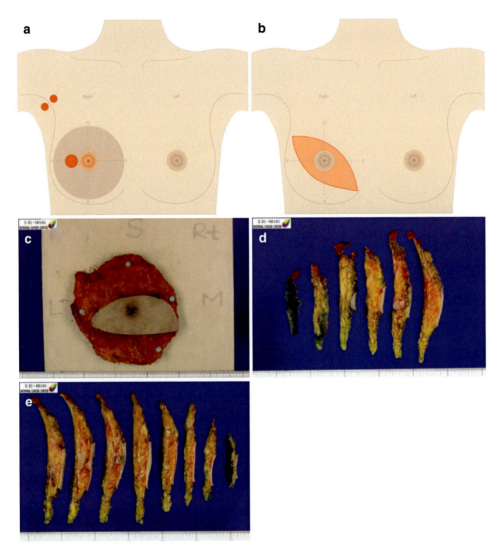

Fig. 43 (**a**) A schematic illustration of tumor location and lymph node metastasis and (**b**) incision lines on right breast. (**c**) Gross pathology of mastectomy specimen. (**d, e**) The margins get marked and sliced with different colors on each direction

6.3.2 Pathology Report

Ductal Carcinoma In Situ associated with fibroadenoma

1. Post-chemotherapy status.
2. Size of tumor: 3.0 cm and 2.2 cm (ypTis).
3. Nuclear grade: high.
4. Necrosis: present.
5. Architectural pattern: cribriform/comedo.
6. Nipple: involvement of lactiferous duct.
7. Skin: no involvement of tumor.
8. Surgical margins:
   (a) Superior margin: 80 mm.
   (b) Inferior margin: 80 mm.
   (c) Medial margin: 60 mm.
   (d) Lateral margin: 40 mm.
   (e) Deep margin: 3 mm.
   (f) Superficial margin: 10 mm.
9. Lymph nodes:
   (a) Metastasis in three out of five axillary lymph nodes (ypN1a(sn)) (axillary LN: 3/5),
   (b) Perinodal extension: present,
   (c) Size of metastatic carcinoma: 4 mm.
10. Microcalcification: present, tumoral/non-tumoral.
11. Pathological TN category (AJCC 2017): ypTisN1a(sn).

	Result	Intensity	Positive %
Estrogen receptor	Negative (2/8)	1	<1%
Progesterone receptor	Negative (2/8)	1	0
C-erbB2	Negative (1+)-metastasis Equivocal (2+)-in situ		
Ki-67	Positive in 46% of tumor cells		

7 Case 7

7.1 Patient History and Progress

Female/56 years old, post-menopause.

Self-detected palpable mass lesion on right breast.

No family history.

No comorbidities.

BRCA 1 and 2 mutation: Not detected.

7.2 Important Radiologic Findings

See Figs. 44, 45 and 46.

Fig. 44 Magnification (Jul. 2020): An irregular hyperdense mass with obscured margins in the right upper breast

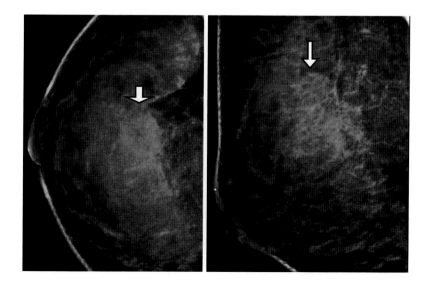

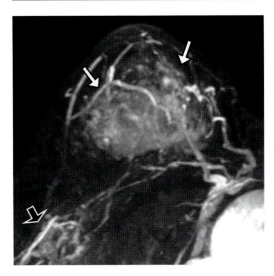

Fig. 45 Breast MRI (Jul. 2020): An irregular heterogeneous enhancing mass in the upper portion of the right breast. Enlarged lymph nodes in the right axilla

7.2.1 After Neoadjuvant Chemotherapy

See Figs. 47, 48, 49 and 50.

7.3 Courses of Treatment

Neoadjuvant chemotherapy (#4 cycles of doxorubicin and cyclophosphamide + #4 cycles of docetaxel) + Operation + Postoperative radiation therapy + Adjuvant capecitabine.

7.3.1 Operation

Right modified radical mastectomy, sentinel lymph node biopsy (Fig. 51).

7.3.2 Pathology Report

Metaplastic Carcinoma with sarcomatous differentiation

1. Post-chemotherapy status.

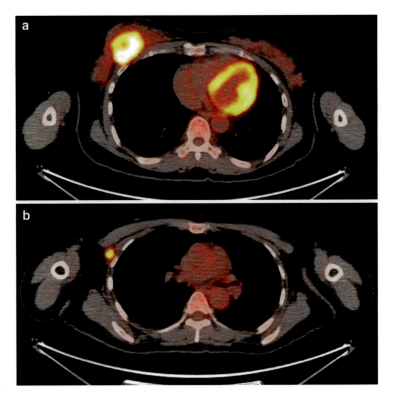

Fig. 46 PET-CT shows (**a**) hypermetabolic mass in the right upper central breast (mSUV = ~34.4), and (**b**) hypermetabolic enlarged LNs in the right axilla level I and II (mSUV = ~7.0)

Fig. 47 Mammography (Dec. 2020): Decrease in size of the irregular mass at the upper portion of the right breast

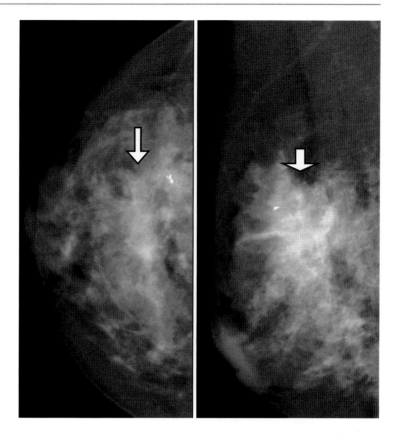

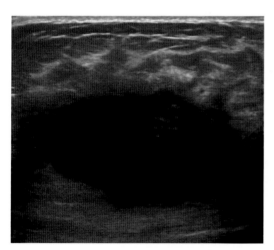

Fig. 48 Breast US (Dec. 2020): An irregular hypoechoic mass at the 12 o'clock direction of the right breast

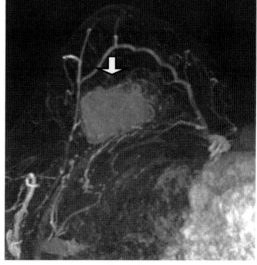

Fig. 49 Breast MRI (Dec. 2020): MRI after treatment demonstrates residual enhancing mass (white arrow) that is decreased in the longest diameter

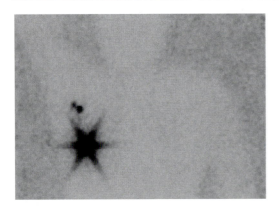

Fig. 50 Lymphoscintigraphy shows visualized sentinel lymph nodes in the right axilla

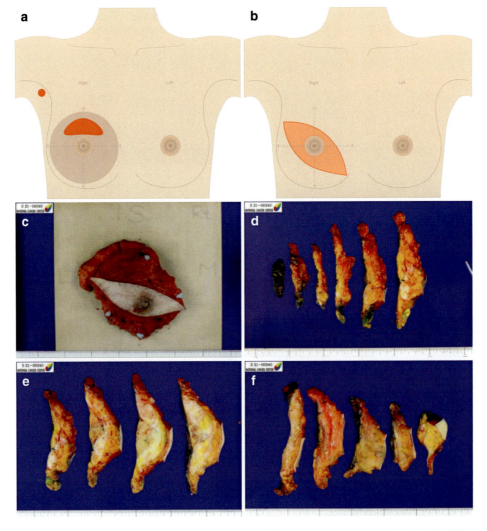

Fig. 51 (a) A schematic illustration of tumor location and lymph node metastasis and (b) incision lines on right breast. (c) Gross pathology of mastectomy specimen. (d, e, f) The margins get marked and sliced with different colors on each direction

2. Size of tumor: 4.2 cm (ypT2).
3. Histologic grade: 3/3 (tubule formation: 3/3, nuclear pleomorphism: 3/3, mitotic count: 3/3, 22/10HPF).
4. Intraductal component: present, intratumoral (<5%) (nuclear grade: high, necrosis: present, architectural pattern: comedo, extensive intraductal component: absent).
5. Skin and nipple: no involvement of tumor.
6. Surgical margins:
   (a) Deep margin: positive for metaplastic carcinoma (slides 3 and 5).
   (b) Superficial margin: 11 mm.
7. Lymph nodes: no metastasis in four axillary lymph nodes (ypN0(sn)) (sentinel LN: 0/3, non-sentinel LN: 0/1).
8. Arteriovenous invasion: absent.
9. Lymphovascular invasion: present, intratumoral.
10. Tumor border: infiltrative.
11. Microcalcification: present, non-tumoral.
12. Pathological TN category (AJCC 2017): ypT2N0(sn).

	Result	Intensity	Positive %
Estrogen receptor	Negative (0/8)	0	0
Progesterone receptor	Negative (0/8)	0	0
C-erbB2	Negative (0)		
Ki-67	Positive in 57% of tumor cells		

Lung metastasis.
Palliative chemotherapy (abraxane and atezolizumab → gemcitabine and cisplatin).

8 Case 8

8.1 Patient History and Progress

Female/56 years old, peri-menopause.

Screen detected a mass lesion on right breast 7 o'clock direction and left breast 4 o'clock direction.

No family history.

No comorbidities.

BRCA 1 and 2 mutation: Not detected.

8.2 Important Radiologic Findings

See Figs. 52, 53 and 54.

8.2.1 After Neoadjuvant Chemotherapy

See Figs. 55, 56 and 57.

8.3 Courses of Treatment

Neoadjuvant chemotherapy (#4 cycles of doxorubicin and cyclophosphamide + #4 cycles of paclitaxel) + Operation + Post-operative radiation therapy.

8.3.1 Operation

Bilateral breast conserving surgery, right sentinel lymph node biopsy (Figs. 58 and 59).

8.3.2 Pathology Report

<Right>

Microinvasive Ductal Carcinoma

1. Post-chemotherapy status.
2. Size of invasive component: <0.1 cm (ypT1mi).
3. Size of in situ component: 1.0 cm.
4. Histologic grade: not applicable.
5. Intraductal component: present, extratumoral (99%) (nuclear grade: high, necrosis: present, architectural pattern: cribriform/solid/comedo, extensive intraductal component: present).
6. Skin: no involvement of tumor.
7. Surgical margins:
   (a) Superior margin: 5 mm.
   (b) Inferior margin: 5 mm.
   (c) Medial margin: 20 mm.
   (d) Lateral margin: (see note 1).
   (e) Deep margin: 5 mm.
   (f) Superficial margin: 5 mm.
8. Lymph nodes: no metastasis in one axillary lymph node (ypN0(sn)) (sentinel LN: 0/1).
9. Arteriovenous invasion: absent.
10. Lymphovascular invasion: absent.

Fig. 52 Mammography (Feb. 2021): mediolateral oblique view shows an irregular isodense mass in the lower portion of the right breast. The mass is not identified on the craniocaudal view

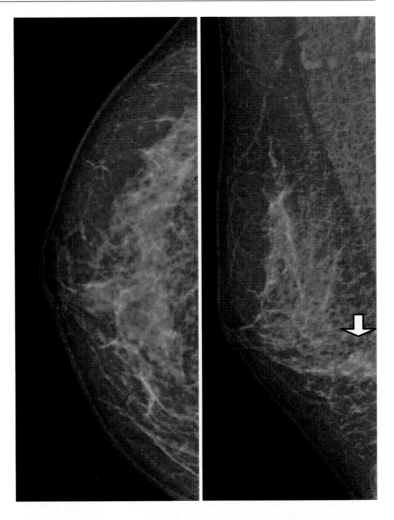

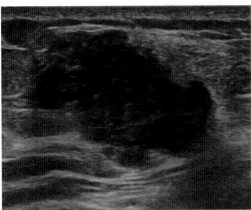

Fig. 53 Breast US (Feb. 2021): An irregular hypoechoic mass at the 7 o'clock direction of the right breast

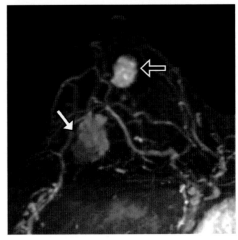

Fig. 54 Breast MRI (Feb. 2021): An irregular enhancing mass (white arrow) at the 7 o'clock direction of right breast. The other oval enhancing mass (black arrow) at the center was later confirmed as a benign fibroadenoma on excisional biopsy

Fig. 55 Mammography (Aug. 2021): mammography after treatment demonstrates no residual mass

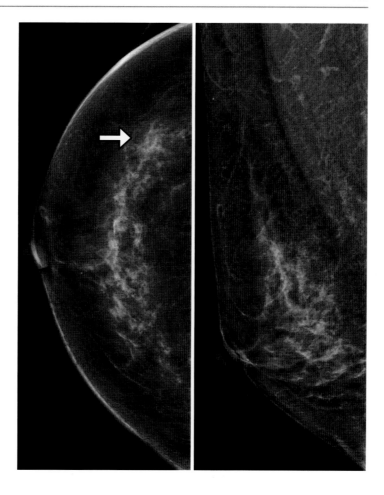

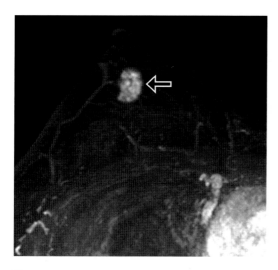

Fig. 56 Breast MRI (Aug. 2021): MRI after treatment demonstrates complete resolution of the malignant mass. There was no change in the oval benign mass (black arrow)

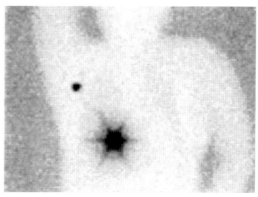

Fig. 57 Lymphoscintigraphy shows visualized sentinel lymph nodes in the right axilla

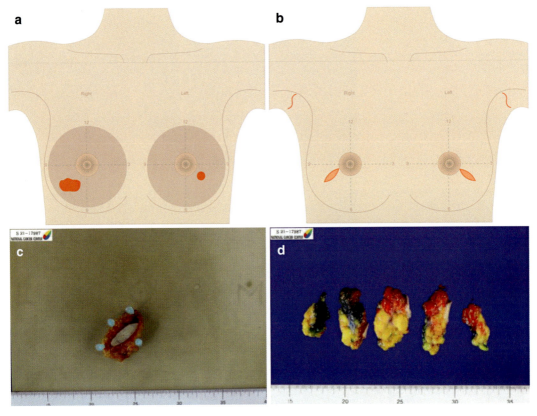

Fig. 58 (a) A schematic illustration of bilateral tumor location and (b) breast and axillary incision lines on both breast. (c) Gross pathology of lumpectomy (right) specimen. (d) The margins get marked and sliced with different colors on each direction

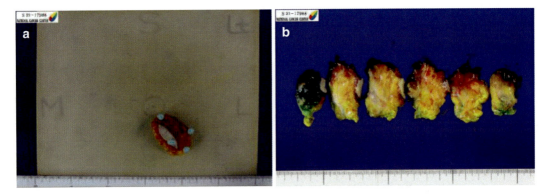

Fig. 59 (a) Gross pathology of lumpectomy (left) specimen. (b) The margins get marked and sliced with different colors on each direction

11. Tumor border: infiltrative.
12. Microcalcification: present, non-tumoral.
13. Pathological TN category (AJCC 2017): ypT1miN0(sn).

Note: 1. The lateral margin of the lumpectomy specimen (slide 7) is close to ductal carcinoma in situ (2 mm), but this margin submitted for frozen diagnosis (Fro 4) is free of tumor.
<Left>

Ductal Carcinoma In Situ
1. Post-chemotherapy status.
2. Size of tumor: 0.2 cm (ypTis).
3. Nuclear grade: high.
4. Necrosis: absent.
5. Architectural pattern: solid.
6. Skin: no involvement of tumor.
7. Surgical margins:
    (a) Superior margin: 20 mm.
    (b) Inferior margin: 10 mm.
    (c) Medial margin: 10 mm.
    (d) Lateral margin: 10 mm.
    (e) Deep margin: 2 mm.
    (f) Superficial margin: 2 mm.
8. Microcalcification: present, tumoral/non-tumoral.
9. Pathological TN category (AJCC 2017): ypTis.

	Result	Intensity	Positive %
Estrogen receptor	Negative (0/8)	0	0
Progesterone receptor	Negative (0/8)	0	0
C-erbB2	Negative (1+)		
Ki-67	Positive in 10% of tumor cells		

9 Case 9

9.1 Patient History and Progress

Female/65 years old, post-menopause.
Screen detected mass lesion on right breast 10 o'clock direction.
No family history.

S/P right salpingectomy (due to ectopic pregnancy).

9.2 Important Radiologic Findings

See Figs. 60, 61, 62, 63 and 64.

9.3 Courses of Treatment

Operation + adjuvant chemotherapy (#4 cycles of docetaxel and cyclophosphamide) + Operation + Post-operative radiation therapy.

9.3.1 Operation
Right breast conserving surgery, sentinel lymph node biopsy, VATS RML lobectomy (Fig. 65).

9.3.2 Pathology Report
Invasive Ductal Carcinoma
1. Size of tumor: 2.3 cm (pT2).
2. Histologic grade: 3/3 (tubule formation: 3/3, nuclear pleomorphism: 3/3, mitotic count: 3/3, 8/HPF).
3. Intraductal component: present, intratumoral/extratumoral (10%) (nuclear grade: high, necrosis: absent, architectural pattern: solid, extensive intraductal component: absent).
4. Skin: no involvement of tumor.
5. Surgical margins:
    (a) Superior margin: 10 mm.
    (b) Inferior margin: 10 mm.
    (c) Medial margin: 5 mm.
    (d) Lateral margin: 10 mm.
    (e) Deep margin: <1 mm from invasive ductal carcinoma (slide 7).
    (f) Superficial margin: 2 mm.
6. Lymph nodes: no metastasis in four axillary lymph nodes (pN0(sn)) (sentinel LN: 0/1, non-sentinel LN: 0/2, intramammary LN: 0/1).
7. Arteriovenous invasion: absent.
8. Lymphovascular invasion: present, intratumoral.
9. Tumor border: infiltrative.

Fig. 60 Mammography (Jan. 2021): An irregular hyperdense mass in the upper outer quadrant of the right breast

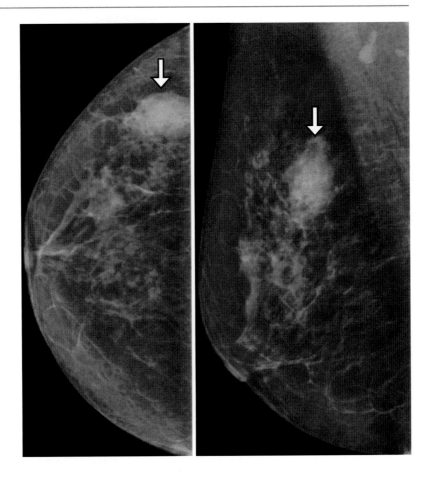

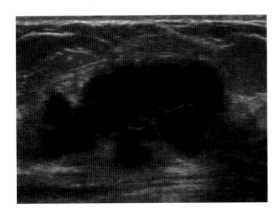

Fig. 61 Breast US (Jan. 2021): An irregular hypoechoic mass at the 10 o'clock direction of the right breast

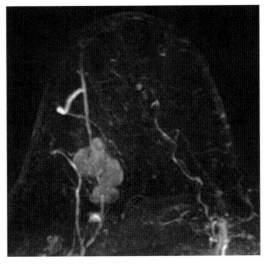

Fig. 62 Breast MRI (Jan. 2021): An irregular enhancing mass at the 10 o'clock direction of the right breast

Fig. 63 PET-CT shows (**a**) hypermetabolic mass in the right upper outer breast (mSUV = 15.1) and (**b**) irregular-shaped nodule with hypermetabolism in RML (mSUV = 4.3)

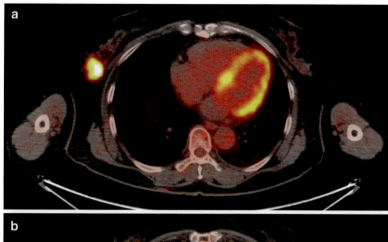

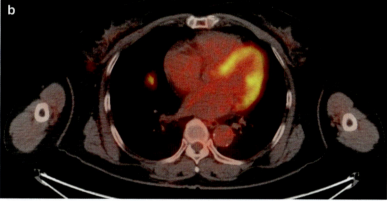

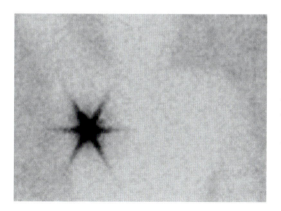

Fig. 64 Lymphoscintigraphy shows faintly visualized sentinel lymph node in Rt. axilla

	Result	Intensity	Positive %
Estrogen receptor	Negative (0/8)	0	0
Progesterone receptor	Negative (0/8)	0	0
C-erbB2	Negative (1+)		
Ki-67	Positive in 87% of tumor cells		

<Lung>

1. Localized chronic granulomatous inflammation with necrosis, suggestive of mycobacterial infection (see note).
2. Reactive hyperplasia in 5 regional lymph nodes (LN #10: 0/2, LN #11: 0/3).

10. Microcalcification: present, tumoral/non-tumoral.
11. Pathological TN category (AJCC 2017): pT2N0(sn).

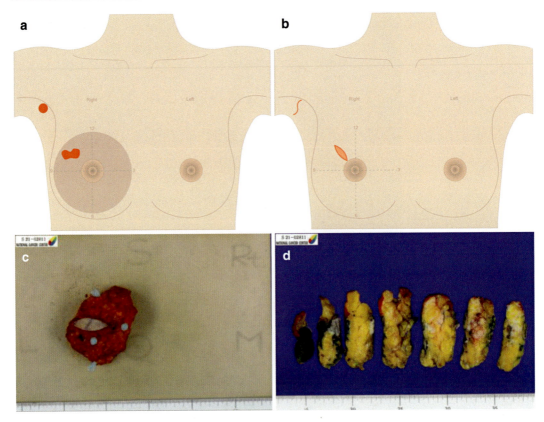

Fig. 65 (a) A schematic illustration of tumor location and lymph node metastasis. (b) breast and axillary incision lines. (c) Gross pathology of lumpectomy specimen. (d) The margins get marked and sliced with different colors on each direction

10 Case 10

10.1 Patient History and Progress

Female/56 years old, post-menopause.
Self-detected palpable mass lesion on right breast.
No family history.
Asthma.

10.2 Important Radiologic Findings

See Figs. 66, 67 and 68.

10.2.1 After Neoadjuvant Chemotherapy
See Figs. 69, 70, 71 and 72.

10.3 Courses of Treatment

Neoadjuvant chemotherapy (#4 cycles of doxorubicin and cyclophosphamide + #4 cycles of paclitaxel and cisplatin) + Operation + Post-operative radiation therapy + adagloxad simolenin plus capecitabine.

10.3.1 Operation
Right breast conserving surgery, sentinel lymph node biopsy (Fig. 73).

Fig. 66 Mammography (Feb. 2021): A round hyperdense mass at the 12 o'clock direction of the right breast. Enlarged lymph node in the right axilla

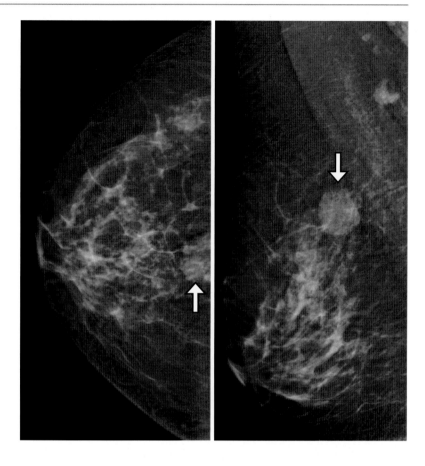

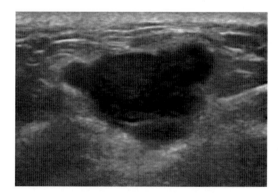

Fig. 67 Breast US (Feb. 2021): An irregular hypoechoic mass at the 12 o'clock direction of the right breast

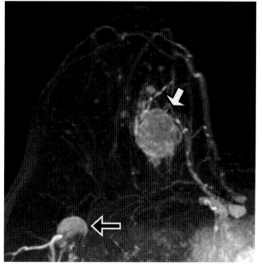

Fig. 68 Breast MRI (Feb. 2021): An irregular enhancing mass (white arrow) and associated enhancing foci at the 12 o'clock direction of the right breast. Enlarged lymph node (black arrow) in the right axilla

Fig. 69 Mammography (Aug. 2021): mammography after treatment demonstrates residual mass that is decreased in the longest diameter

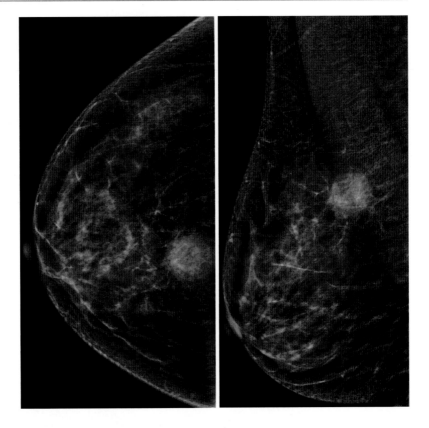

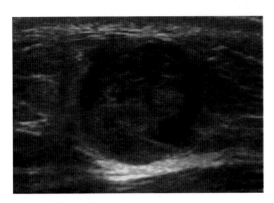

Fig. 70 Breast US (Aug. 2021): US after treatment demonstrates residual hypoechoic mass that is decreased in the longest diameter

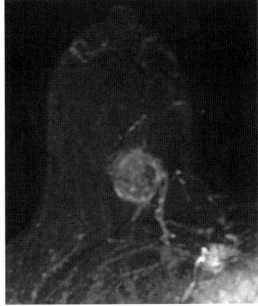

Fig. 71 Breast MRI (Aug. 2021): MRI after treatment demonstrates residual enhancing mass that is decreased in the longest diameter

HR(−) HER2(−) Breast Cancer

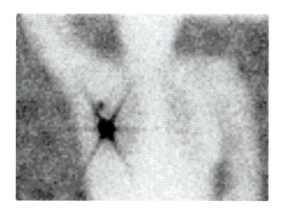

Fig. 72 Lymphoscintigraphy shows visualized sentinel lymph nodes in the right axilla

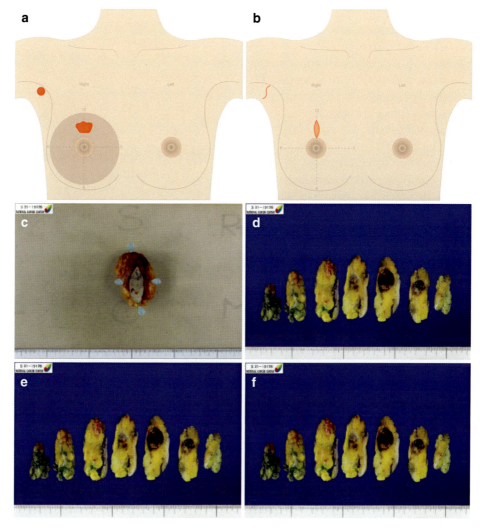

Fig. 73 (**a**) A schematic illustration of tumor location and lymph node metastasis and (**b**) breast and axillary incision lines. (**c**) Gross pathology of lumpectomy specimen. (**d**, **e**, **f**) The margins get marked and sliced with different colors on each direction

10.3.2 Pathology Report

Invasive Ductal Carcinoma

1. Post-chemotherapy status.
2. Size of tumor: 1.9 cm (ypT1c).
3. Histologic grade: 3/3 (tubule formation: 3/3, nuclear pleomorphism: 3/3, mitotic count: 3/3, 21/10HPF).
4. Intraductal component: absent.
5. Skin: no involvement of tumor.
6. Surgical margins:
   (a) Superior margin: 8 mm.
   (b) Inferior margin: 25 mm.
   (c) Medial margin: 10 mm.
   (d) Lateral margin: 20 mm.
   (e) Deep margin: <1 mm from invasive ductal carcinoma (slide 2).
   (f) Superficial margin: 3 mm.
7. Lymph nodes: no metastasis in three axillary lymph nodes (ypN0(sn)) (sentinel LN: 0/1, axillary LN: 0/2).
8. Arteriovenous invasion: absent.
9. Lymphovascular invasion: present, intratumoral.
10. Tumor border: infiltrative.
11. Microcalcification: present, non-tumoral.
12. Pathological TN category (AJCC 2017): ypT1cN0(sn).

	Result	Intensity	Positive %
Estrogen receptor	Negative (0/8)	0	0
Progesterone receptor	Negative (0/8)	0	0
C-erbB2	Negative (1+)		
Ki-67	Positive in 86% of tumor cells		

11 Case 11

11.1 Patient History and Progress

Female/50 years old, pre-menopause.

Screen detected mass lesion on upper outer portion of right breast.

Family history of breast cancer, mother and aunt (paternal).

No comorbidities.

BRCA 1 and 2 mutation: Not detected.

11.2 Important Radiologic Findings

See Figs. 74, 75, 76 and 77.

HR(−) HER2(−) Breast Cancer 613

Fig. 74 Mammography (Feb. 2021): An irregular hyperdense mass in the upper outer quadrant of right breast. Enlarged lymph nodes in the right axilla

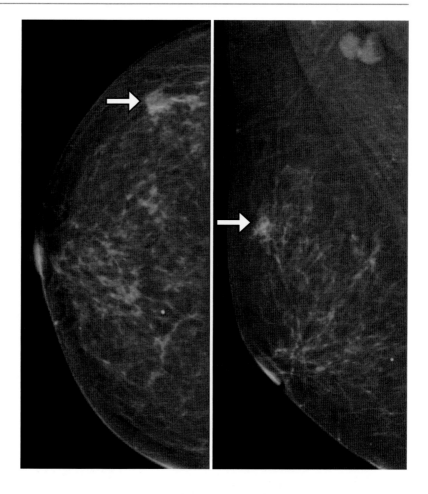

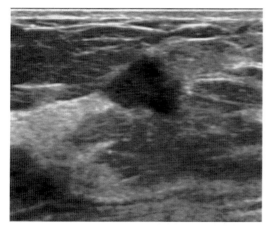

Fig. 75 Breast US (Feb. 2021): An irregular hypoechoic mass at the 10 o'clock direction of the right breast

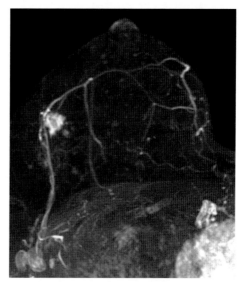

Fig. 76 Breast MRI (Feb. 2021): An irregular enhancing mass in the upper outer quadrant of the right breast. Enlarged lymph nodes in the right axilla

Fig. 77 PET-CT shows (**a**) a hypermetabolic nodule in right outer breast (mSUV = 3.3) and (**b**) hypermetabolic LNs in the right axilla, level I–II (mSUV = 3.7)

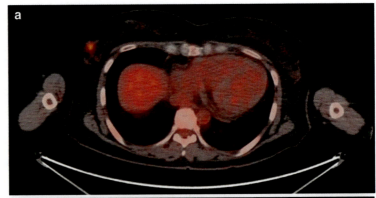

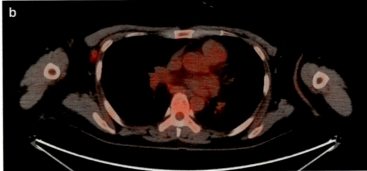

11.2.1 After Neoadjuvant Chemotherapy

See Figs. 78, 79, 80 and 81.

11.3 Courses of Treatment

Neoadjuvant chemotherapy (#4 cycles of doxorubicin and cyclophosphamide + #4 cycles of docetaxel) + Operation + Post-operative radiation therapy + Adjuvant capecitabine.

11.3.1 Operation

Right breast conserving surgery, sentinel lymph node biopsy (Fig. 82).

11.3.2 Pathology Report

Invasive Ductal Carcinoma

1. Post-chemotherapy status.
2. Size of tumor: 0.2 cm (ypT1a).
3. Histologic grade: 2/3 (tubule formation: 3/3, nuclear pleomorphism: 2/3, mitotic count: 1/3, 6/10HPF).
4. Intraductal component: absent.
5. Skin: no involvement of tumor.
6. Surgical margins:
   (a) Superior margin: 20 mm.
   (b) Inferior margin: 5 mm.
   (c) Medial margin: 10 mm.
   (d) Lateral margin: 20 mm.
   (e) Deep margin: 2 mm.
   (f) Superficial margin: 2 mm.
7. Lymph nodes: no metastasis in three axillary lymph nodes (ypN0(sn)) (sentinel LN: 0/3).
8. Arteriovenous invasion: absent.
9. Lymphovascular invasion: absent.
10. Tumor border: infiltrative.
11. Microcalcification: present, tumoral/non-tumoral.
12. Pathological TN category (AJCC 2017): ypT1aN0(sn).

	Result	Intensity	Positive %
Estrogen receptor	Negative (0/8)	0	0
Progesterone receptor	Negative (2/8)	1	<1%
C-erbB2	Negative (0)		
Ki-67	Positive in 2% of tumor cells		

Fig. 78 Mammography (Aug. 2021): Mammography after treatment demonstrates residual mass that is decreased in the longest diameter. A clip marker (arrow) was seen within the residual mass

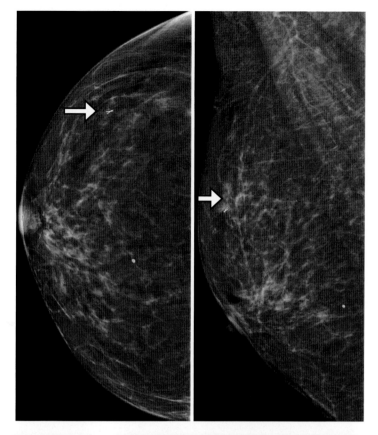

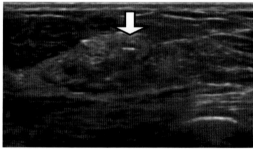

Fig. 79 Breast US (Aug. 2021): US after treatment demonstrates no residual mass. A clip marker (arrow) was seen at the tumor bed

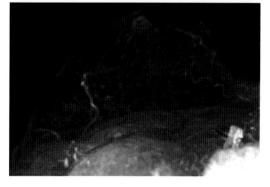

Fig. 80 Breast MRI (Aug. 2021): MRI after treatment shows complete resolution of enhancement in the right breast

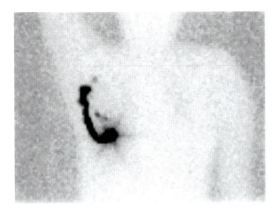

Fig. 81 Lymphoscintigraphy shows visualized sentinel lymph nodes in the right axilla

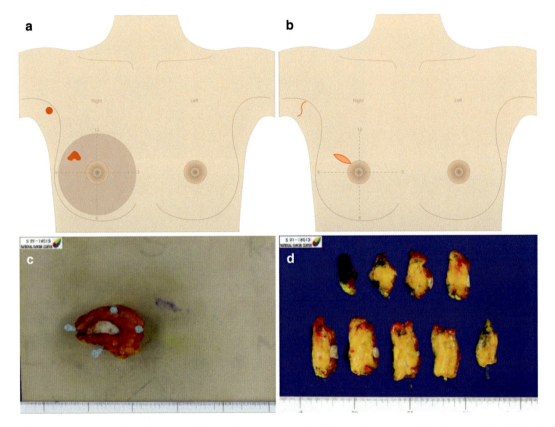

Fig. 82 (**a**) A schematic illustration of tumor location and lymph node metastasis and (**b**) breast and axillary incision lines. (**c**) Gross pathology of lumpectomy specimen. (**d**) The margins get marked and sliced with different colors on each direction

12 Case 12

12.1 Patient History and Progress

Female/47 years old, post-menopause.

Screen detected a mass lesion on right breast 10 o'clock direction.

Family history of breast cancer, aunt (maternal) and cousin.

Family history of ovarian cancer, aunt.

Lupus (follow-up), s/p bilateral salpingo-oophorectomy, s/p unilateral thyroidectomy.

BRCA 1 mutation carrier.

12.2 Important Radiologic Findings

See Figs. 83, 84 and 85.

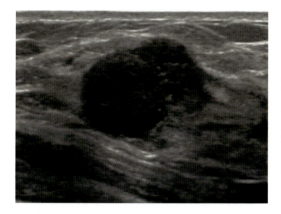

Fig. 83 Breast US (Mar. 2021): US shows an irregular hypoechoic mass at the 10 o'clock direction of the right breast

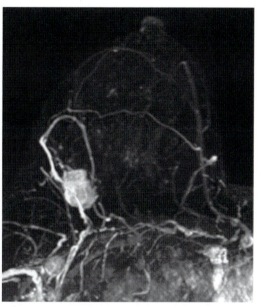

Fig. 84 Breast MRI (Mar. 2021): MRI shows an irregular enhancing mass at the 10 o'clock direction of the right breast

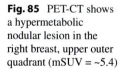

Fig. 85 PET-CT shows a hypermetabolic nodular lesion in the right breast, upper outer quadrant (mSUV = ~5.4)

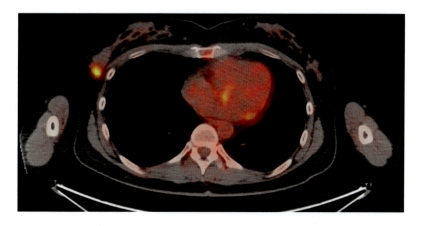

12.2.1 After Neoadjuvant Chemotherapy

See Figs. 86, 87 and 88.

12.3 Courses of Treatment

Neoadjuvant chemotherapy (#4 cycles of doxorubicin and cyclophosphamide + #4 cycles of docetaxel) + Operation + Adjuvant capecitabine.

12.3.1 Operation

Right nipple-areolar complex sparing mastectomy, sentinel lymph node biopsy, left prophylactic nipple-areolar complex sparing mastectomy, laparoscopic bilateral salpingo-oophorectomy (Figs. 89 and 90).

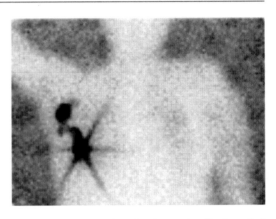

Fig. 88 Lymphoscintigraphy shows visualized sentinel lymph nodes in the right axilla

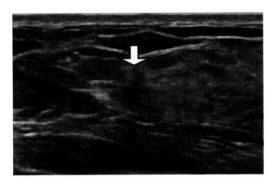

Fig. 86 Breast US (Aug. 2021): US after treatment demonstrates residual hypoechoic mass that is decreased in the longest diameter

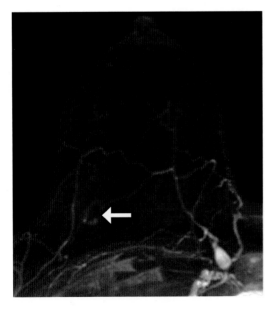

Fig. 87 Breast MRI (Aug. 2021): MRI after treatment demonstrates residual enhancing foci (white arrow)

12.3.2 Pathology Report

Invasive Ductal Carcinoma
1. Post-chemotherapy status.
2. Size of tumor: 0.5 cm (ypT1a).
3. Histologic grade: 2/3 (tubule formation: 3/3, nuclear pleomorphism: 3/3, mitotic count: 1/3, 1/10HPF).
4. Intraductal component: absent.
5. Surgical margins:
   (a) Deep margin: 2 mm.
   (b) Superficial margin: 8 mm.
6. Lymph nodes: no metastasis in three axillary lymph nodes (ypN0(sn)) (sentinel LN: 0/3).
7. Arteriovenous invasion: absent.
8. Lymphovascular invasion: present, intratumoral.
9. Tumor border: infiltrative.
10. Microcalcification: present, non-tumoral.
11. Pathological TN category (AJCC 2017): ypT1aN0(sn).

	Result	Intensity	Positive %
Estrogen receptor	Negative (0/8)	0	0
Progesterone receptor	Negative (0/8)	0	0
C-erbB2	Negative (0)		
Ki-67	Positive in 6% of tumor cells		

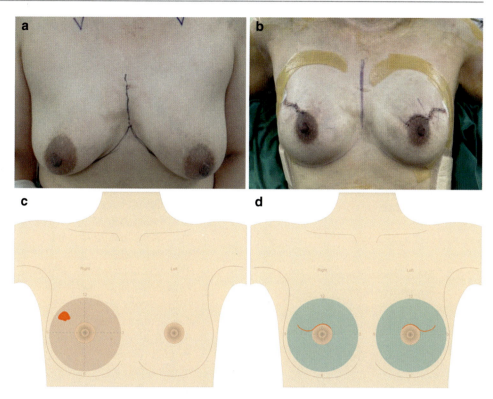

Fig. 89 (**a**) Preoperative and (**b**) immediate postoperative appearance. (**c**) A schematic illustration of tumor location and (**d**) incision lines on both breasts

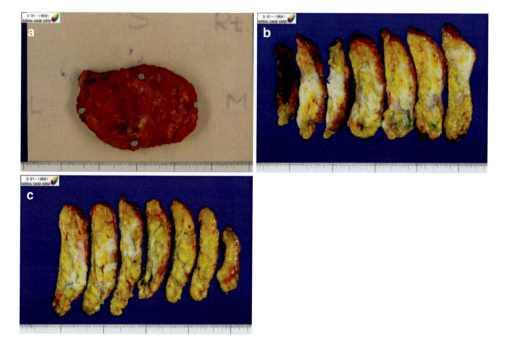

Fig. 90 (**a**) Gross pathology of mastectomy specimen. (**b**, **c**) The margins get marked and sliced with different colors on each direction

13 Case 13

13.1 Patient History and Progress

Female/67 years old, post-menopause.
Self-detected mass lesion on left breast.
No family history.
Hepatitis C virus carrier, arrhythmia.

13.2 Important Radiologic Findings

See Figs. 91, 92 and 93.

13.2.1 After Neoadjuvant Chemotherapy

See Figs. 94, 95, 96 and 97.

13.3 Courses of Treatment

Neoadjuvant chemotherapy (#4 cycles of doxorubicin and cyclophosphamide + #4 cycles of docetaxel) + Operation + Postoperative radiation therapy + Adjuvant capecitabine.

13.3.1 Operation

Left breast conserving surgery, sentinel lymph node biopsy (Fig. 98).

13.3.2 Pathology Report

Invasive Ductal Carcinoma

1. Post-chemotherapy status.
2. Size of tumor: 1.5 cm (ypT1c).
3. Histologic grade: 3/3 (tubule formation: 3/3, nuclear pleomorphism: 3/3, mitotic count: 2/3, 12/10HPF).
4. Intraductal component: present, intratumoral/extratumoral (5%) (nuclear grade: high, necrosis: absent, architectural pattern: solid, extensive intraductal component: absent).
5. Surgical margins:
   (a) Superior margin: 15 mm.
   (b) Inferior margin: 20 mm.
   (c) Medial margin: 5 mm (see note 1).
   (d) Lateral margin: 15 mm.
   (e) Deep margin: 3 mm.
   (f) Superficial margin: 10 mm.
6. Lymph nodes: no metastasis in two axillary lymph nodes (ypN0(sn)) (sentinel LN: 0/1, non-sentinel LN: 0/1).
7. Arteriovenous invasion: absent.
8. Lymphovascular invasion: present, intratumoral.
9. Tumor border: infiltrative.
10. Microcalcification: present, non-tumoral.
11. Pathological TN category (AJCC 2017): ypT1cN0 (sn).

	Result	Intensity	Positive %
Estrogen receptor	Negative (0/8)	0	0
Progesterone receptor	Negative (0/8)	0	0
C-erbB2	Negative (0)		
Ki-67	Positive in 16% of tumor cells		

HR(−) HER2(−) Breast Cancer 621

Fig. 91 Mammography (Feb. 2021): An irregular hyperdense mass at the upper outer quadrant of the left breast

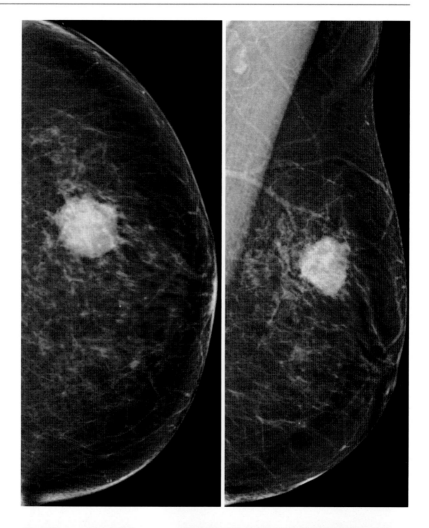

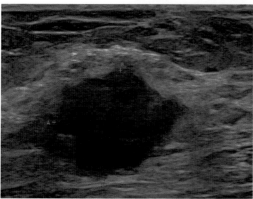

Fig. 92 Breast US (Feb. 2021): An irregular hypoechoic mass at the 1 o'clock direction of the left breast

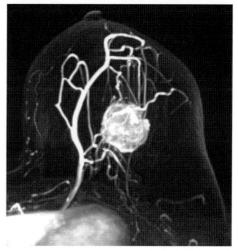

Fig. 93 Breast MRI (Feb. 2021): A round enhancing mass with irregular margins at the 1 o'clock direction of the left breast

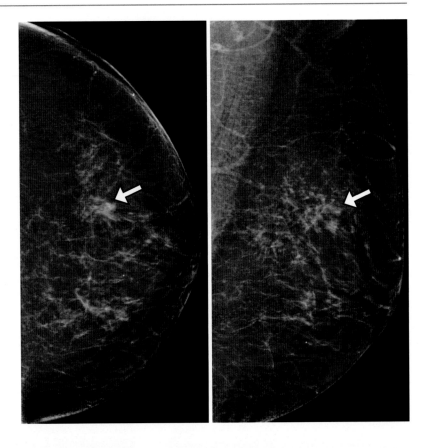

Fig. 94 Mammography (Aug. 2021): mammography after treatment demonstrates residual mass that is decreased in the longest diameter

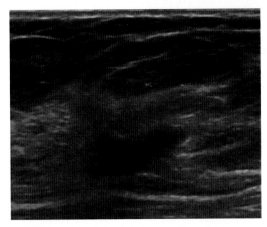

Fig. 95 Breast US (Aug. 2021): US after treatment demonstrates residual hypoechoic mass that is decreased in the longest diameter

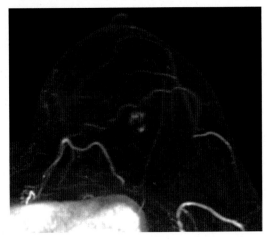

Fig. 96 Breast MRI (Aug. 2021): MRI after treatment demonstrates residual enhancing mass that is decreased in the longest diameter

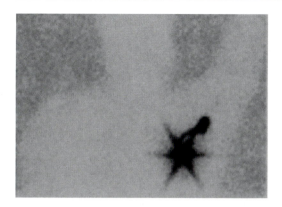

Fig. 97 Lymphoscintigraphy shows visualized sentinel lymph nodes in the left axilla

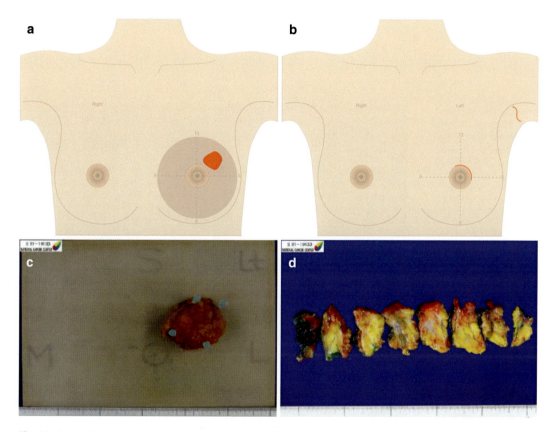

Fig. 98 (**a**) A schematic illustration of tumor location and (**b**) breast and axillary incision lines. (**c**) Gross pathology of lumpectomy specimen. (**d**) The margins get marked and sliced with different colors on each direction

14 Case 14

14.1 Patient History and Progress

Female/43 years old, pre-menopause.

Self-detected palpable mass lesion on right breast.

Family history of breast cancer, grandmother.

s/p Right breast, mammotome excision, s/p right ear, benign excision.

BRCA 1 and 2 mutation: Not detected.

14.2 Important Radiologic Findings

See Figs. 99, 100, 101 and 102.

14.3 Courses of Treatment

Operation + Adjuvant chemotherapy (#4 cycles of doxorubicin and cyclophosphamide + #12 cycles of paclitaxel) + Post-operative radiation therapy.

14.3.1 Operation

Right breast conserving surgery, sentinel lymph node biopsy (Fig. 103).

14.3.2 Pathology Report

Invasive Ductal Carcinoma

1. Size of tumor: 3.0 cm (pT2).
2. Histologic grade: 3/3 (tubule formation: 3/3, nuclear pleomorphism: 3/3, mitotic count: 3/3, 3/HPF).

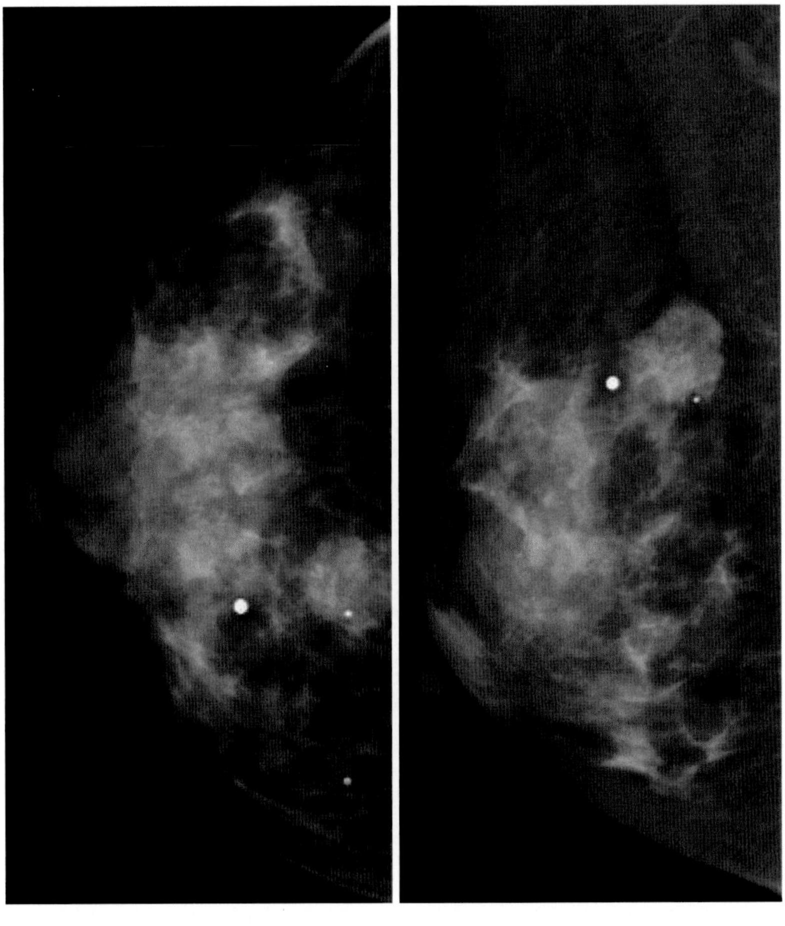

Fig. 99 Mammography (Feb. 2021): An irregular hyperdense mass in the upper outer quadrant of the right breast (marked by BB marker)

HR(−) HER2(−) Breast Cancer

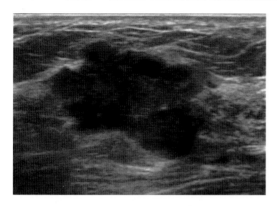

Fig. 100 Breast US (Feb. 2021): An irregular hypoechoic mass at the 12 o'clock direction of the right breast

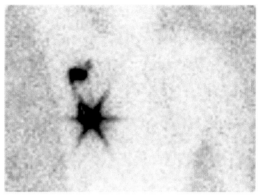

Fig. 102 Lymphoscintigraphy shows visualized sentinel lymph nodes in the right axilla

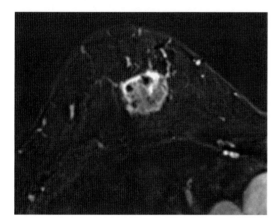

Fig. 101 Breast MRI (Fed. 2021): An irregular heterogeneous enhancing mass at the 12 o'clock direction of the right breast

3. Intraductal component: present, intratumoral/extratumoral (5%) (nuclear grade: high, necrosis: present, architectural pattern: solid/comedo, extensive intraductal component: absent).
4. Skin: no involvement of tumor.
5. Surgical margins:
   (a) Superior margin: 10 mm.
   (b) Inferior margin: 10 mm.
   (c) Medial margin: 10 mm.
   (d) Lateral margin: 10 mm.
   (e) Deep margin: 1 mm from invasive ductal carcinoma (slide 2).
   (f) Superficial margin: 2 mm.
6. Lymph nodes: no metastasis in two axillary lymph nodes (pN0(sn)) (sentinel LN: 0/2).
7. Arteriovenous invasion: absent.
8. Lymphovascular invasion: present, intratumoral.
9. Tumor border: infiltrative.
10. Microcalcification: present, tumoral/non-tumoral.
11. Pathological TN category (AJCC 2017): pT2N0(sn).

	Result	Intensity	Positive %
Estrogen receptor	Negative (0/8)	0	0
Progesterone receptor	Negative (0/8)	0	0
C-erbB2	Negative (1+)		
Ki-67	Positive in 56% of tumor cells		

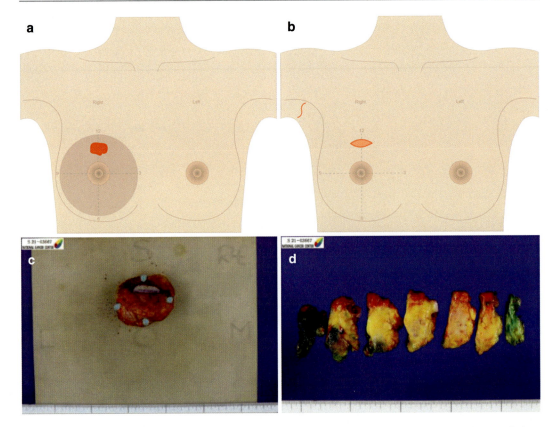

Fig. 103 (**a**) A schematic illustration of tumor location and (**b**) breast and axillary incision lines. (**c**) Gross pathology of lumpectomy specimen. (**d**) The margins get marked and sliced with different colors on each direction

15 Case 15

15.1 Patient History and Progress

Female/74 years old, post-menopause.

Self-detected bloody discharge on the nipple of the left breast.

No family history.

S/P hysterectomy (due to myoma), hypertension, s/p shoulder calcific tendinitis operation.

15.2 Important Radiologic Findings

See Figs. 104, 105 and 106.

15.3 Courses of Treatment

Operation + operation.

15.3.1 Operation

First operation: Jan. 2021 Left partial mastectomy (Fig. 107).

15.3.2 Pathology Report

1. Invasive Ductal Carcinoma.
   (a) Size of invasive component: 0.4 cm (pT1a).
   (b) Size of intraductal component: 4.0 cm.
   (c) Histologic grade: 3/3 (tubule formation: 3/3, nuclear pleomorphism: 3/3, mitotic count: 3/3, 30/10HPF).

HR(−) HER2(−) Breast Cancer 627

Fig. 104 Mammography (Nov. 2020): An about 1 cm round isodense mass (black arrow) in the outer portion of the left breast. The mass is not identified on the mediolateral oblique view. Segmental fine linear microcalcifications (white arrow) in the left upper outer quadrant

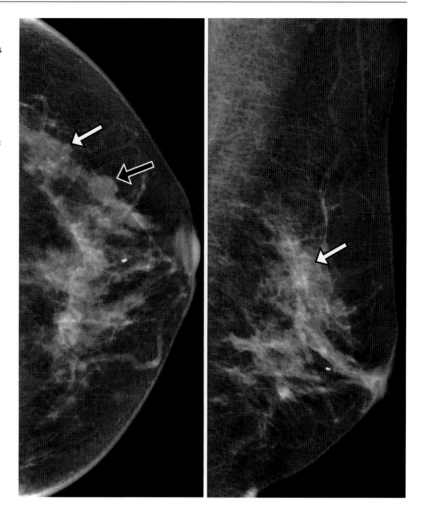

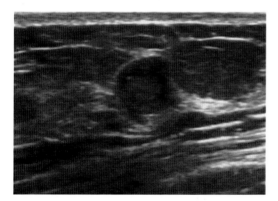

Fig. 105 Breast US (Nov. 2020): A round hypoechoic mass with angular margins at the 3 o'clock direction of the left breast

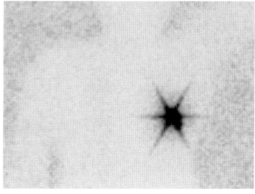

Fig. 106 Lymphoscintigraphy shows visualized sentinel lymph nodes in the left axilla

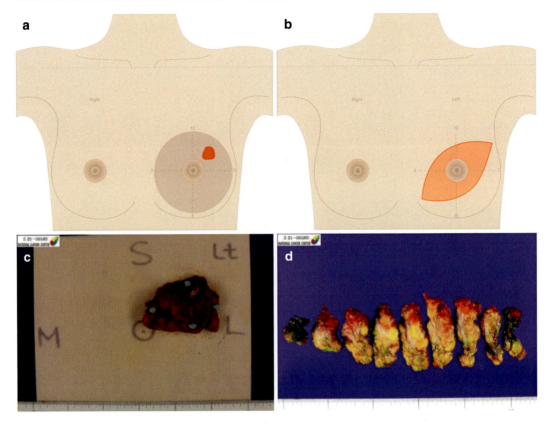

Fig. 107 (**a**) A schematic illustration of tumor location and (**b**) incision line on left breast. (**c**) Gross pathology of lumpectomy specimen. (**d**) The margins get marked and sliced with different colors on each direction

(d) Intraductal component: present, intratumoral/extratumoral (90%) (nuclear grade: high, necrosis: present, architectural pattern: solid/comedo, extensive intraductal component: present).
(e) Skin: no involvement of tumor.
(f) Surgical margins:
 - Superior margin: 30 mm.
 - Inferior margin: 5 mm.
 - Medial margin: 15 mm.
 - Lateral margin: <1 mm from ductal carcinoma in situ (slide 15).
 - Deep margin: positive for ductal carcinoma in situ (slides 4 and 14).
 - Superficial margin: <1 mm from ductal carcinoma in situ (slide 13).
(g) Arteriovenous invasion: absent.
(h) Lymphovascular invasion: absent.
(i) Tumor border: infiltrative.
(j) Microcalcification: present, tumoral.
(k) Pathological TN category (AJCC 2017): pT1aNx.

2. Intraductal papilloma with:
   (a) Usual ductal hyperplasia.
   (b) Apocrine metaplasia.
   (c) Epithelial displacement.

	Result	Intensity	Positive %
Estrogen receptor	Negative (2/8)	1	<1%
Progesterone receptor	Negative (2/8)	1	<1%
C-erbB2	Negative (1+)		
Ki-67	Positive in 23% of tumor cells		

15.3.3 Operation

Second operation: Feb. 2021 Left modified radical mastectomy, axillary lymph node sampling (Fig. 108).

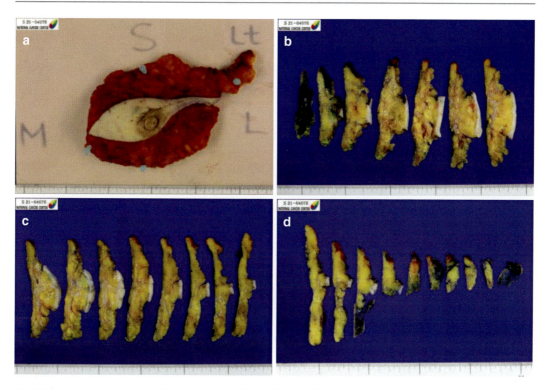

Fig. 108 (a) Gross pathology of lumpectomy specimen. (b, c, d) The margins get marked and sliced with different colors on each direction

15.3.4 Pathology Report
1. No residual carcinoma with foreign body reaction.
   (a) Post-excision status.
2. Intraductal papilloma with usual ductal hyperplasia.

16 Case 16

16.1 Patient History and Progress

Female/42 years old, pre-menopause.

Self-detected palpable mass lesion on left breast.
No family history.
s/p Cholecystectomy, s/p appendectomy, s/p vocal cord operation.

16.2 Important Radiologic Findings

See Figs. 109, 110, 111 and 112.

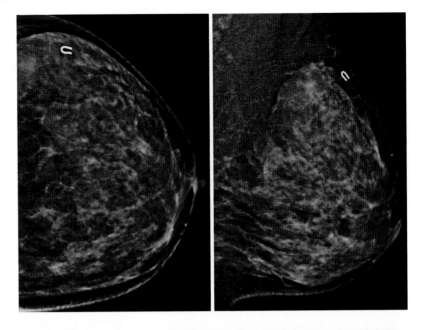

Fig. 109 Mammography (Aug. 2020): An irregular hyperdense mass with obscured margins in the upper outer quadrant of the left breast (marked by BB marker)

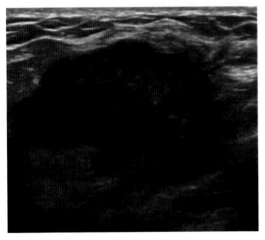

Fig. 110 Breast US (Aug. 2020): An irregular hypoechoic mass at the 1 o'clock direction of the left breast

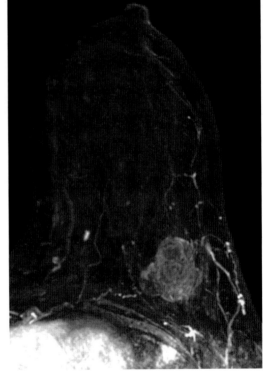

Fig. 111 Breast MRI (Aug. 2020): An irregular enhancing mass at the 1 o'clock direction of the left breast

Fig. 112 PET-CT shows (**a**) known left breast cancer with hypermetabolism (mSUV = 22.7) and (**b**) left axillary LN metastasis, level III

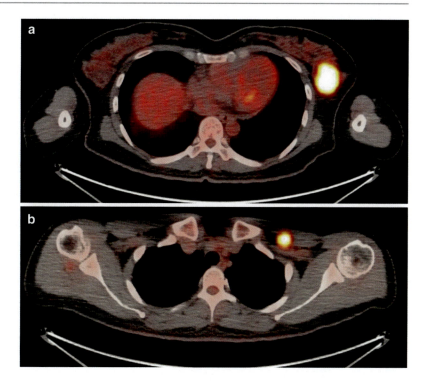

16.2.1 After Neoadjuvant Chemotherapy

See Figs. 113, 114, 115 and 116.

16.3 Courses of Treatment

Neoadjuvant chemotherapy (#4 cycles of doxorubicin and cyclophosphamide + #4 cycles of docetaxel) + Operation + Postoperative radiation therapy.

16.3.1 Operation

Left breast conserving surgery, axillary lymph node sampling (Fig. 117).

16.3.2 Pathology Report

No residual tumor with foamy histiocytic collection

1. Post-chemotherapy status.
2. Lymph nodes: no metastasis in six axillary lymph nodes (ypN0) (sentinel LN: 0/2, non-sentinel LN: 0/4).
3. Microcalcification: present, non-tumoral.

	Result	Intensity	Positive %
Estrogen receptor	Negative (0/8)	0	0
Progesterone receptor	Negative (0/8)	0	0
C-erbB2	Equivocal (2+)		
Ki-67	Positive in 88% of tumor cells		
SISH	Negative		

Fig. 113 Mammography DBT C-view (Feb. 2021): Mammography after treatment demonstrates no residual mass

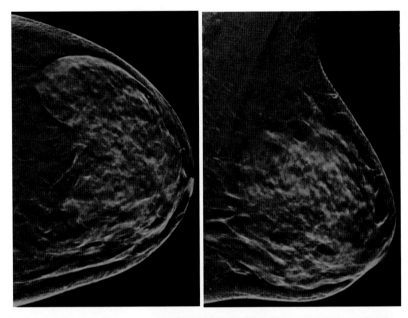

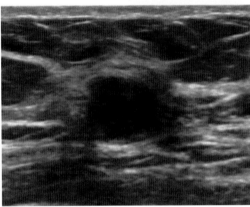

Fig. 114 Breast US (Feb. 2021): US after treatment demonstrates residual hypoechoic mass that is decreased in the longest diameter

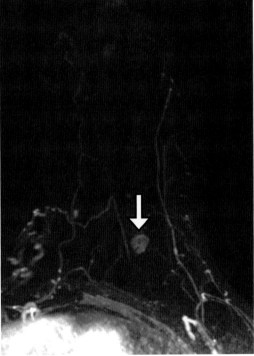

Fig. 115 Breast MRI (Feb. 2021): MRI after treatment demonstrates residual enhancing mass (white arrow) that is decreased in the longest diameter

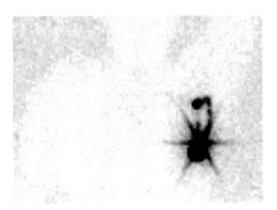

Fig. 116 Lymphoscintigraphy shows visualized sentinel lymph nodes in the left axilla

HR(−) HER2(−) Breast Cancer

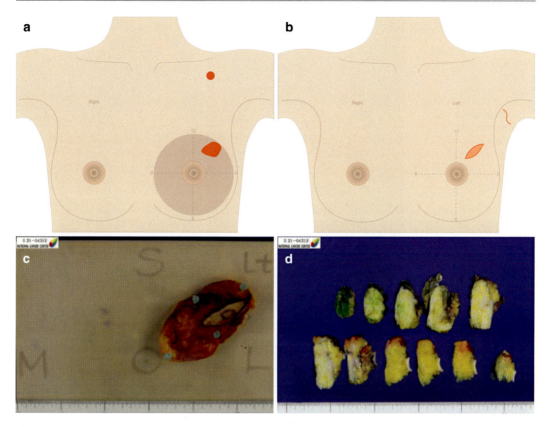

Fig. 117 (**a**) A schematic illustration of tumor location and (**b**) breast and axillary incision lines. (**c**) Gross pathology of lumpectomy specimen. (**d**) The margins get marked and sliced with different colors on each direction

17 Case 17

17.1 Patient History and Progress

Female/70 years old, post-menopause.

Screen detected mass at the upper outer quadrant of the left breast.

Family history of breast cancer, niece.

h/o Tuberculosis, s/p appendectomy, s/p myomectomy.

BRCA 1 and 2 mutation: Not tested.

17.2 Important Radiologic Findings

See Figs. 118, 119, 120 and 121.

17.3 Courses of Treatment

Operation + Adjuvant chemotherapy (#2 cycles of doxorubicin and cyclophosphamide, refuse) + Post-operative radiation therapy.

17.3.1 Operation
Left breast conserving surgery, sentinel lymph node biopsy (Fig. 122).

17.3.2 Pathology Report

Invasive Ductal Carcinoma
1. Size of tumor: 1.3 cm (pT1c).
2. Histologic grade: 3/3 (tubule formation: 3/3, nuclear pleomorphism: 3/3, mitotic count: 3/3, 5/HPF).

Fig. 118 Mammography: An irregular hyperdense mass at the upper outer quadrant of the left breast. The other circumscribed oval mass at the inner portion was identified as a cyst on ultrasound

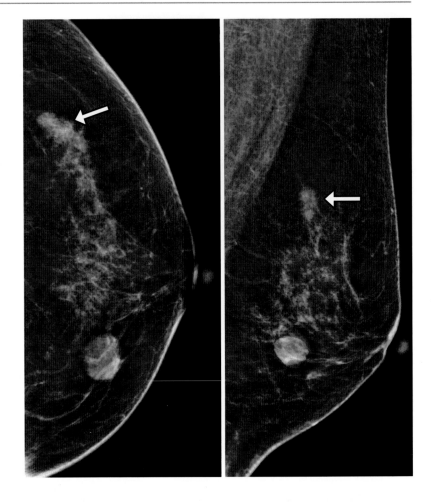

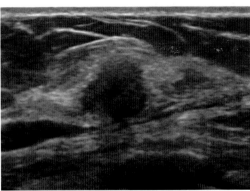

Fig. 119 Breast US: An irregular hypoechoic mass with microlobulated margins at the 2 o'clock direction of the left breast

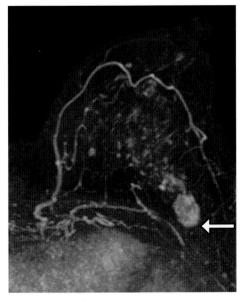

Fig. 120 Breast MRI: An oval enhancing mass in the upper outer quadrant of the left breast

HR(–) HER2(–) Breast Cancer

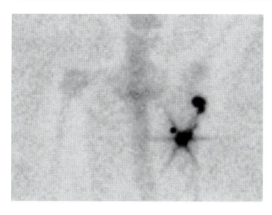

Fig. 121 Lymphoscintigraphy shows visualized sentinel lymph nodes in the left axilla

3. Intraductal component: present, intratumoral/extratumoral (10%) (nuclear grade: high, necrosis: present, architectural pattern: solid/comedo, extensive intraductal component: absent).
4. Skin: no involvement of tumor.
5. Surgical margins:
   (a) Superior margin: 10 mm.
   (b) Inferior margin: (see note).
   (c) Medial margin: 10 mm.
   (d) Lateral margin: 10 mm.
   (e) Deep margin: 2 mm.
   (f) Superficial margin: 2 mm.

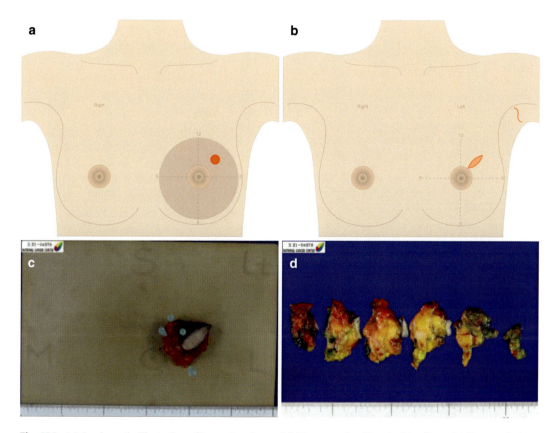

Fig. 122 (**a**) A schematic illustration of tumor location and (**b**) breast and axillary incision lines. (**c**) Gross pathology of lumpectomy specimen. (**d**) The margins get marked and sliced with different colors on each direction

6. Lymph nodes: no metastasis in one axillary lymph node (pN0(sn)) (sentinel LN: 0/1).
7. Arteriovenous invasion: absent.
8. Lymphovascular invasion: present, intratumoral.
9. Tumor border: infiltrative.
10. Microcalcification: present, tumoral/non-tumoral.
11. Pathological TN category (AJCC 2017): pT1cN0(sn).

Note: 1. The inferior margin of the lumpectomy specimen (slides 4 and 5) is close to invasive ductal carcinoma (3 mm) and ductal carcinoma in situ (<1 mm), but this margin submitted for frozen diagnosis (Fro 2) is free of tumor.

	Result	Intensity	Positive %
Estrogen receptor	Negative (0/8)	0	0
Progesterone receptor	Negative (0/8)	0	0
C-erbB2	Equivocal (2+)		
Ki-67	Positive in 12% of tumor cells		

18 Case 18

18.1 Patient History and Progress

Female/57 years old, post-menopause.

Self-detected palpable mass lesion and skin change on left breast.

Family history of breast cancer, aunt (paternal).

No comorbidities.

BRCA 1 and 2 mutation: Not detected.

18.2 Important Radiologic Findings

See Figs. 123, 124 and 125.

18.2.1 After Neoadjuvant Chemotherapy

See Figs. 126, 127, 128 and 129.

18.3 Courses of Treatment

Neoadjuvant chemotherapy (#4 cycles of doxorubicin and cyclophosphamide + #4 cycles of paclitaxel) + Operation + Post-operative radiation therapy + Adjuvant capecitabine.

18.3.1 Operation

Left breast conserving surgery, sentinel lymph node biopsy (Fig. 130).

18.3.2 Pathology Report

1. Invasive Ductal Carcinoma.
   (a) Post-chemotherapy status.
   (b) Size of tumor: 0.7 cm (ypT1b).
   (c) Histologic grade: 3/3 (tubule formation: 3/3, nuclear pleomorphism: 3/3, mitotic count: 3/3, 95/10HPF).
   (d) Intraductal component: absent.
   (e) Skin and nipple: no involvement of tumor.
   (f) Surgical margins:
     • Superior margin: 20 mm.
     • Inferior margin: 20 mm.
     • Medial margin: 10 mm.
     • Lateral margin: 10 mm.
     • Deep margin: 1.5 mm from invasive ductal carcinoma (slide 2).
     • Superficial margin: 15 mm.
   (g) Lymph nodes: no metastasis in three axillary lymph nodes (ypN0(sn)) (sentinel LN: 0/3).
   (h) Arteriovenous invasion: absent.
   (i) Lymphovascular invasion: absent.
   (j) Tumor border: infiltrative.
   (k) Microcalcification: present, non-tumoral.
   (l) Pathological TN category (AJCC 2017): ypT1bN0(sn).
2. Sclerosing adenosis with microcalcification.

Note: 1. A few isolated tumor cells are present only in the permanent section of Fro 7 for immunohistochemical staining.

	Result	Intensity	Positive %
Estrogen receptor	Negative (0/8)	0	0
Progesterone receptor	Negative (0/8)	0	0
C-erbB2	Negative (0)		
Ki-67	Positive in 63% of tumor cells		

Fig. 123 Mammography (Mar. 2021): An irregular hyperdense mass in the upper portion of the left breast

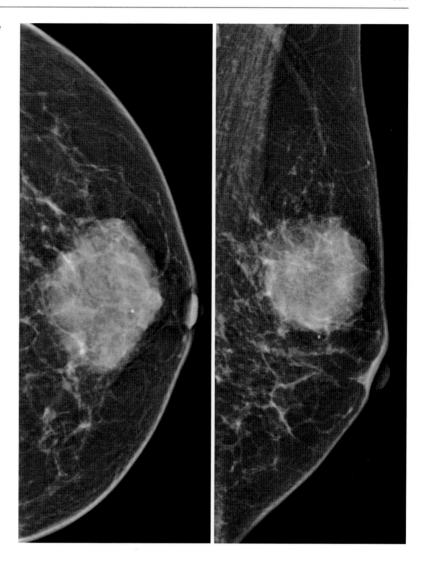

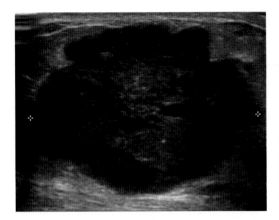

Fig. 124 Breast US (Mar. 2021): An irregular hypoechoic mass at the 12 o'clock direction of the left breast

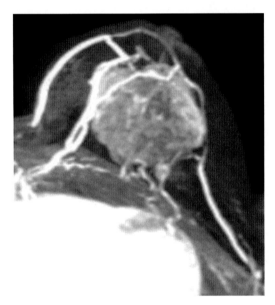

Fig. 125 Breast MRI (Mar. 2021): An irregular enhancing mass at the 12 o'clock direction of the left breast

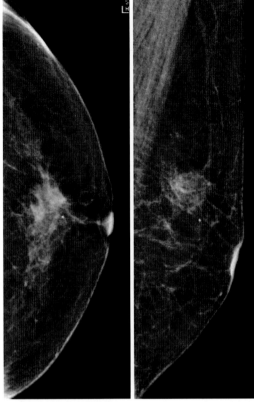

Fig. 126 Mammography (Sep. 2021): mammography after treatment demonstrates residual mass that is decreased in the longest diameter

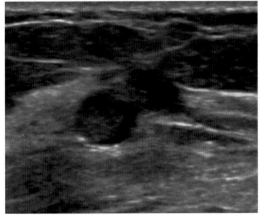

Fig. 127 Breast US (Sep. 2021): US after treatment demonstrates residual hypoechoic mass that is decreased in the longest diameter

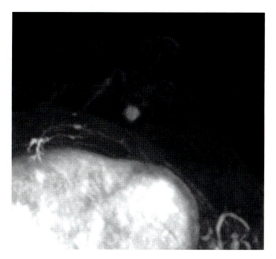

Fig. 128 Breast MRI (Sep. 2021): MRI after treatment demonstrates residual enhancing mass that is decreased in the longest diameter

Fig. 129 Lymphoscintigraphy shows visualized sentinel lymph nodes in the left axilla

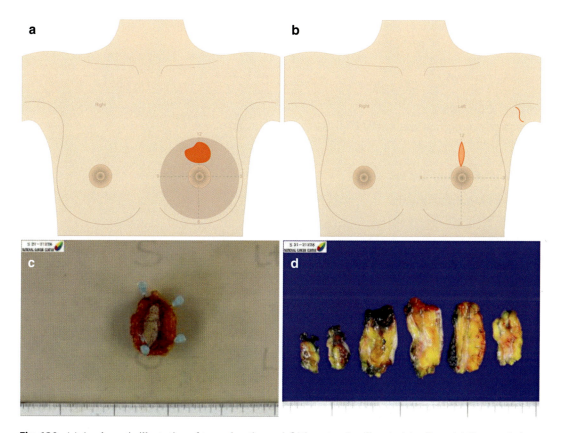

Fig. 130 (**a**) A schematic illustration of tumor location and (**b**) breast and axillary incision lines. (**c**) Gross pathology of lumpectomy specimen. (**d**) The margins get marked and sliced with different colors on each direction

19 Case 19

19.1 Patient History and Progress

Female/63 years old, post-menopause.

Screen detected mass lesion on right breast 10 o'clock direction.

No family history.

Hepatitis B virus carrier, h/o Tuberculosis.

19.2 Important Radiologic Findings

See Figs. 131, 132 and 133.

19.3 Courses of Treatment

Operation + adjuvant chemotherapy (#4 cycles of doxorubicin and cyclophosphamide + #3 cycles of paclitaxel-stop d/t drug-induced pneumonitis) + Post-operative radiation therapy.

19.3.1 Operation

Right breast conserving surgery (NAUTILUS trial: sentinel lymph node biopsy skip arm) (Fig. 134).

19.3.2 Pathology Report

Invasive Ductal Carcinoma

1. Size of tumor: 2.2 cm (pT2).
2. Histologic grade: 3/3 (tubule formation: 3/3, nuclear pleomorphism: 3/3, mitotic count: 3/3, 4/HPF).
3. Intraductal component: present, intratumoral/extratumoral (20%) (nuclear grade: high, necrosis: present, architectural pattern: solid/comedo, extensive intraductal component: absent).
4. Skin: no involvement of tumor.
5. Surgical margins:
   (a) Superior margin: 10 mm.
   (b) Inferior margin: 10 mm.
   (c) Medial margin: 10 mm.
   (d) Lateral margin: 10 mm.
   (e) Deep margin: 2 mm.
   (f) Superficial margin: 2 mm.
6. Arteriovenous invasion: absent.
7. Lymphovascular invasion: absent.
8. Tumor border: infiltrative.
9. Microcalcification: present, tumoral/nontumoral.
10. Pathological TN category (AJCC 2017): pT2Nx.

	Result	Intensity	Positive %
Estrogen receptor	Negative (0/8)	0	0
Progesterone receptor	Negative (0/8)	0	0
C-erbB2	Negative (1+)		
Ki-67	Positive in 91% of tumor cells		

HR(−) HER2(−) Breast Cancer

Fig. 131 Mammography (Mar. 2021): A round hyperdense mass with microlobulated margins in the upper outer quadrant of the right breast (marked by BB marker)

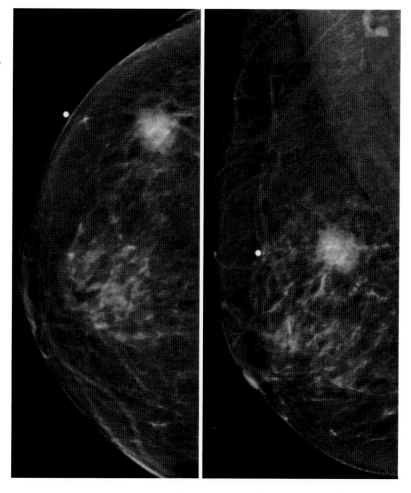

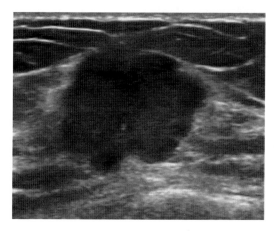

Fig. 132 Breast US (Mar. 2021): An irregular hypoechoic mass with echogenic halo at the 10 o'clock direction of the right breast

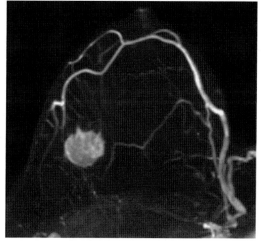

Fig. 133 Breast MRI (Mar. 2021): A round enhancing mass with irregular margins at the 10 o'clock direction of the right breast

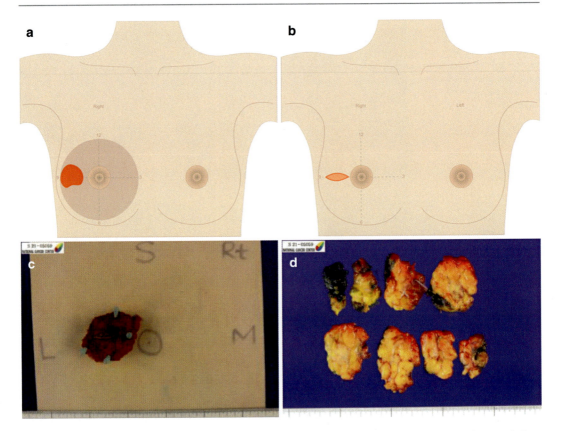

Fig. 134 (**a**) A schematic illustration of tumor location and (**b**) breast and axillary incision lines. (**c**) Gross pathology of lumpectomy specimen. (**d**) The margins get marked and sliced with different colors on each direction

20 Case 20

20.1 Patient History and Progress

Female/59 years old, post-menopause.

Screen detected mass lesion on left breast 9:30 o'clock direction.

Family history of breast cancer, aunt (maternal).

No comorbidities.
BRCA 1 and 2 mutation: Not detected.

20.2 Important Radiologic Findings

See Figs. 135, 136, 137 and 138.

HR(–) HER2(–) Breast Cancer   643

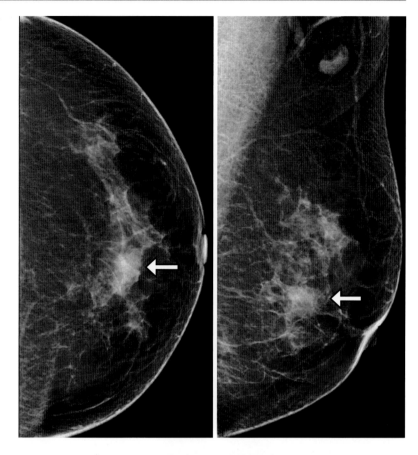

Fig. 135 Mammography (Aug. 2020): An irregular hyperdense mass in the center portion of the left breast

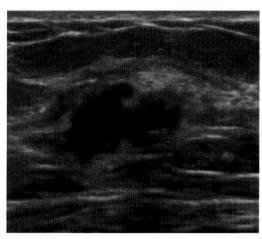

Fig. 136 Breast US (Aug. 2020): An irregular hypoechoic mass with microlobulated margins in the left subareolar area. Enlarged LN of left axilla level I and interpectoral space (level II)

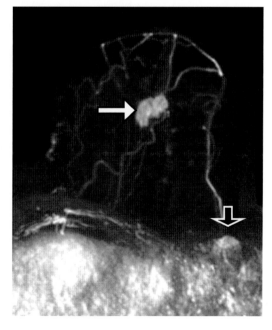

Fig. 137 Breast MRI (Aug. 2020): An irregular enhancing mass in the center portion of the left breast. Enlarged lymph node (black arrow) in the left axilla

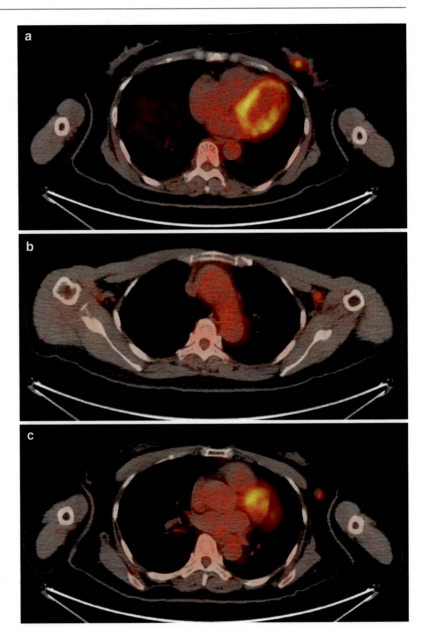

Fig. 138 PET-CT shows (**a**) a hypermetabolic lesion in the left upper inner breast (mSUV = 4.5), (**b**) hypermetabolic LNs in the left axilla level II, and (**c**) hypermetabolic LNs in the left axilla, level I

20.2.1 After Neoadjuvant Chemotherapy

See Figs. 139, 140, 141 and 142.

20.3 Courses of Treatment

Neoadjuvant chemotherapy (#4 cycles of doxorubicin and cyclophosphamide + #4 cycles of docetaxel) + Operation + Postoperative radiation therapy.

20.3.1 Operation

Left breast conserving surgery, axillary lymph node sampling (Fig. 143).

20.3.2 Pathology Report

No residual tumor with stromal fibrosis

Fig. 139 Mammography (Mar. 2021): mammography after treatment demonstrates residual mass that is decreased in the longest diameter

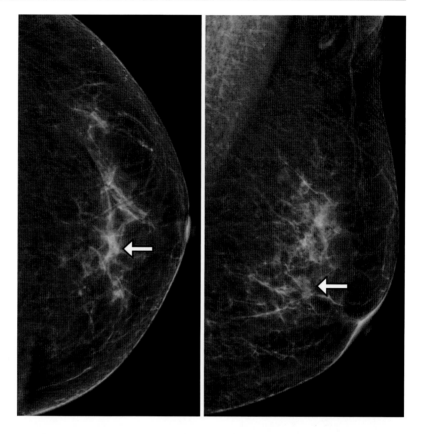

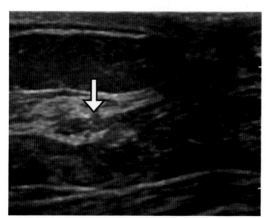

Fig. 140 Breast US (Mar. 2021): US after treatment demonstrates residual isoechoic mass that is decreased in the longest diameter

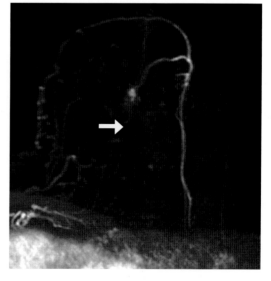

Fig. 141 Breast MRI (Mar. 2021): MRI after treatment demonstrates residual enhancing mass (white arrow) that is decreased in the longest diameter and decrease in size of the previously enlarged lymph node in the left axilla

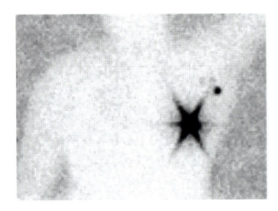

Fig. 142 Lymphoscintigraphy shows visualized sentinel lymph nodes in the left axilla

1. Post-chemotherapy status.
2. Lymph nodes: no metastasis in seven axillary lymph nodes (ypN0) (sentinel LN: 0/1, non-sentinel LN: 0/6).
3. Microcalcification: present, tumoral/non-tumoral.

	Result	Intensity	Positive %
Estrogen receptor	Negative (0/8)	0	0
Progesterone receptor	Negative (0/8)	0	0
C-erbB2	Negative (1+)		
Ki-67	Positive in 46% of tumor cells		

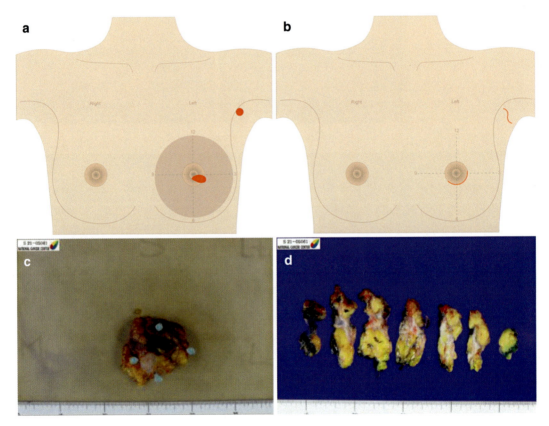

Fig. 143 (a) A schematic illustration of tumor location and axillary lymph node metastasis and (b) breast and axillary incision lines on left breast. (c) Gross pathology of lumpectomy specimen. (d) The margins get marked and sliced with different colors on each direction

21 Case 21

21.1 Patient History and Progress

Female/50 years old, pre-menopause.

Screen detected mass lesion on left breast 1 o'clock direction.

No family history.

No comorbidities.

BRCA 1 and 2 mutation: Not detected, STK11 VUS (variant of uncertain).

21.2 Important Radiologic Findings

See Figs. 144, 145, 146 and 147.

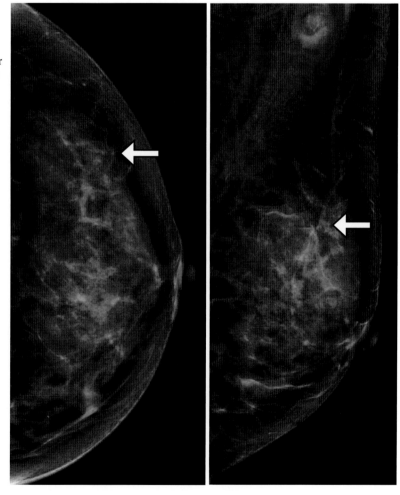

Fig. 144 Mammography (Mar. 2021): grouped microcalcifications with subtle architectural distortion in left upper outer quadrant. Enlarged LN, left axilla

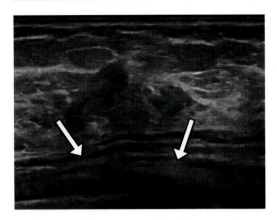

Fig. 145 Breast US (Mar. 2021): An irregular mass at the 2 o'clock direction of the left breast

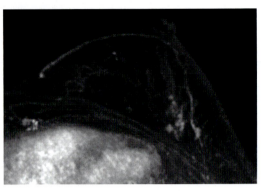

Fig. 146 Breast MRI (Mar. 2021): focal heterogeneous non-mass enhancement at the left upper outer quadrant

Fig. 147 PET-CT shows (**a**) hypermetabolic lesions in Lt. breast (mSUV = 2.9), (**b**) hypermetabolic lesions in Lt. axillary LNs level II, and (**c**) hypermetabolic lesions in Lt. axillary LNs level I

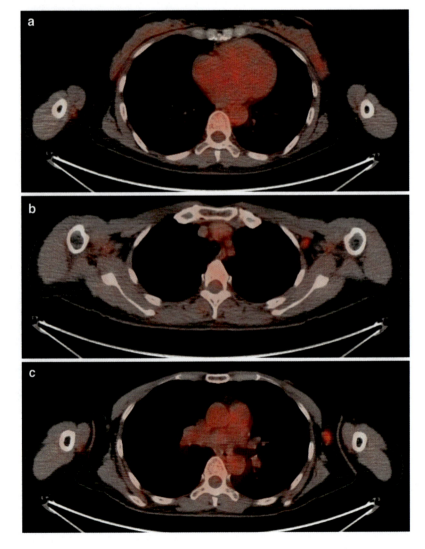

21.2.1 After Neoadjuvant Chemotherapy

See Figs. 148, 149, 150 and 151.

21.3 Courses of Treatment

Neoadjuvant chemotherapy (#4 cycles of doxorubicin and cyclophosphamide + #4 cycles of docetaxel) + Operation + Post-operative radiation therapy + Letrozole 2.5 mg + Adjuvant capecitabine.

21.3.1 Operation

Left breast conserving surgery, axillary lymph node dissection (Fig. 152).

21.3.2 Pathology Report

Microinvasive Ductal Carcinoma

1. Post-chemotherapy status.
2. Size of invasive component: <0.1 cm (ypT1mi).
3. Size of intraductal component: 2.0 cm.
4. Histologic grade: not applicable.
5. Intraductal component: present, intratumoral/extratumoral (>95%) (nuclear grade: high, necrosis: present, architectural pattern: cribriform/solid/comedo, extensive intraductal component: present).
6. Skin: no involvement of tumor.
7. Surgical margins:

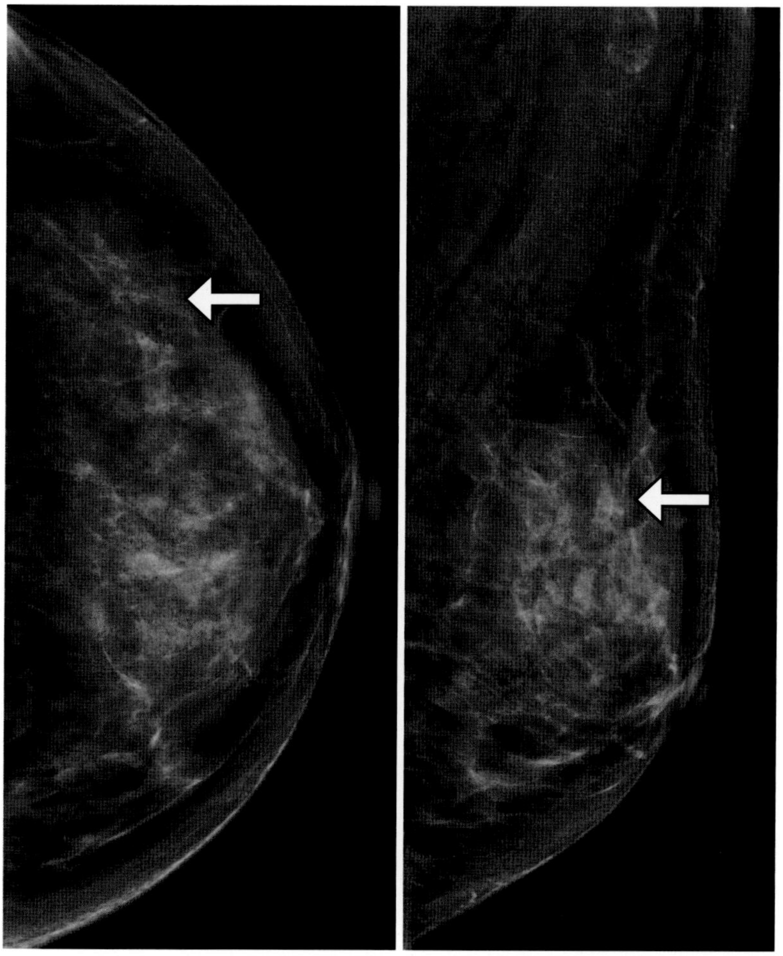

Fig. 148 Mammography (Oct. 2021): mammography after treatment demonstrates residual microcalcifications in the left upper outer quadrant

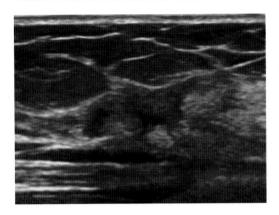

Fig. 149 Breast US (Oct. 2021): US after treatment demonstrates residual hypoechoic mass that is decreased in the longest diameter

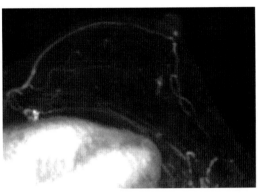

Fig. 150 Breast MRI (Oct. 2021): MRI after treatment demonstrates residual enhancing foci and non-mass enhancement that is decreased in the longest diameter

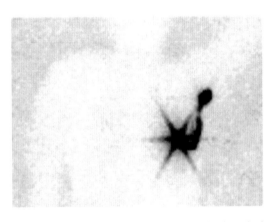

Fig. 151 Lymphoscintigraphy shows visualized sentinel lymph nodes in the left axilla

(a) Superior margin: positive for ductal carcinoma in situ (Fro 1) (see note).
(b) Inferior margin: 5 mm.
(c) Medial margin: 5 mm.
(d) Lateral margin: 5 mm.
(e) Deep margin: 2 mm.
(f) Superficial margin: <1 mm from invasive ductal carcinoma (slide 5).

8. Lymph nodes:
   (a) Metastasis in two out of six axillary lymph nodes (ypN1a(sn)) (sentinel LN: 2/2, axillary LN: 0/4).
   (b) Perinodal extension: absent.
   (c) Size of metastatic carcinoma: 3 mm.
9. Arteriovenous invasion: absent.
10. Lymphovascular invasion: present, peritumoral.
11. Tumor border: infiltrative.
12. Microcalcification: absent.
13. Pathological TN category (AJCC 2017): ypT1miN1a(sn).

Note: 1. Ductal carcinoma in situ is present only in the permanent section of Fro 1.

	Result	Intensity	Positive %
Estrogen receptor	Weak (3/8)	1	1–10%
Progesterone receptor	Negative (0/8)	0	0
C-erbB2	Negative (0)		
Ki-67	Positive in 52% of tumor cells		

HR(−) HER2(−) Breast Cancer

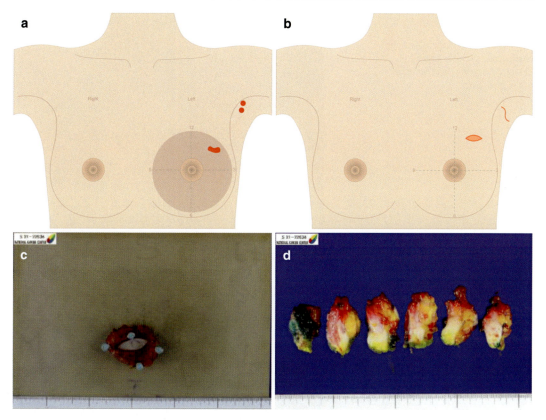

Fig. 152 (**a**) A schematic illustration of tumor location and axillary lymph node metastasis. (**b**) Breast and axillary incision lines on left breast. (**c**) Gross pathology of lumpectomy specimen. (**d**) The margins get marked and sliced with different colors on each direction

22　Case 22

22.1　Patient History and Progress

Female/57 years old, post-menopause.

Self-detected palpable mass lesion on right breast.

Family history of breast cancer, uncle (paternal).

s/p retinal detachments operation.

BRCA 1 and 2 mutation: Not detected, PALB2 PV, STK11 VUS (variant of uncertain).

22.2　Important Radiologic Findings

See Figs. 153, 154, 155 and 156.

Fig. 153 Mammography (Mar. 2021): An oval hyperdense mass in the upper outer quadrant of the right breast. Enlarged lymph nodes in the right axilla

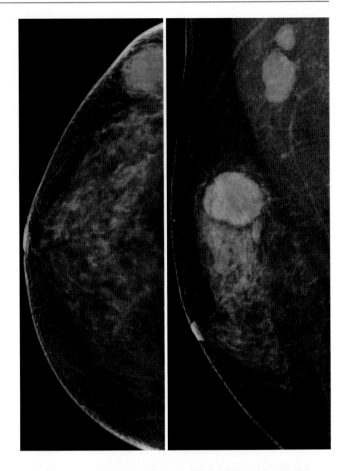

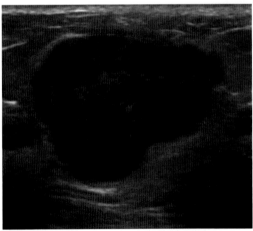

Fig. 154 Breast US (Mar. 2021): An irregular hypoechoic mass at the 10 o'clock direction of the right breast

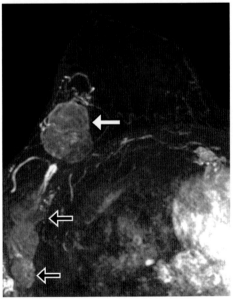

Fig. 155 Breast MRI (Mar. 2021): An irregular enhancing mass (white arrow) at the 10 o'clock direction of the right breast. Multiple enlarged lymph nodes (black arrow) in the right axilla

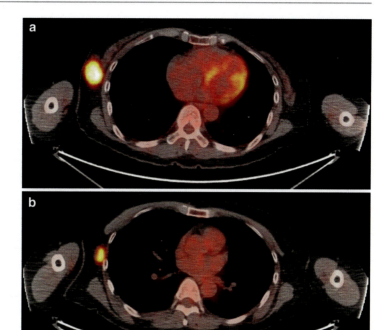

Fig. 156 PET-CT shows (**a**) hypermetabolic mass in right breast, upper outer quadrant (mSUV = ~10.8) and (**b**) hypermetabolic lymph nodes in right axilla level I area (mSUV = ~8.3)

22.2.1 After Neoadjuvant Chemotherapy

See Figs. 157, 158, 159 and 160.

22.3 Courses of Treatment

Neoadjuvant chemotherapy (#4 cycles of doxorubicin and cyclophosphamide + #4 cycles of docetaxel) + Operation + Postoperative radiation therapy + Adjuvant capecitabine.

22.3.1 Operation

Right breast conserving surgery, sentinel lymph node biopsy (Fig. 161).

22.3.2 Pathology Report

Invasive Ductal Carcinoma
1. Post-chemotherapy status.
2. Size of tumor: 0.9 cm (ypT1b).
3. Histologic grade: 3/3 (tubule formation: 3/3, nuclear pleomorphism: 3/3, mitotic count: 3/3, 11/10HPF).
4. Intraductal component: absent.
5. Skin: no involvement of tumor.
6. Surgical margins:
   - (a) Superior margin: 25 mm.
   - (b) Inferior margin: 20 mm.
   - (c) Medial margin: 5 mm.
   - (d) Lateral margin: 10 mm.
   - (e) Deep margin: 5 mm.
   - (f) Superficial margin: 10 mm.
7. Lymph nodes:
   - (a) Metastasis in two out of three axillary lymph nodes (ypN1a(sn)) (sentinel LN: 2/3).
   - (b) Perinodal extension: absent.
   - (c) Size of metastatic carcinoma: 5 mm.
8. Arteriovenous invasion: absent.
9. Lymphovascular invasion: absent.
10. Tumor border: infiltrative.
11. Microcalcification: absent.
12. Pathological TN category (AJCC 2017): ypT1bN1a(sn).

	Result	Intensity	Positive %
Estrogen receptor	Negative (2/8)	1	<1%
Progesterone receptor	Negative (0/8)	0	0
C-erbB2	Negative (1+)		
Ki-67	Positive in 12% of tumor cells		

Fig. 157 Mammography (Sep. 2021): mammography after treatment demonstrates residual mass that is decreased in the longest diameter. A clip marker (black arrow) was seen within the residual mass

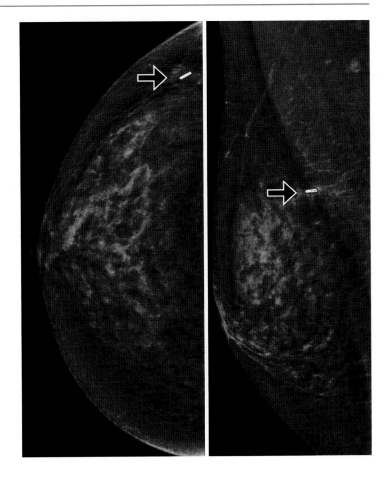

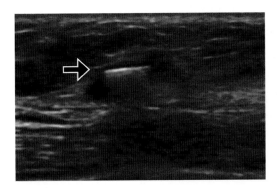

Fig. 158 Breast US (Sep. 2021): US after treatment demonstrates residual hypoechoic mass that is decreased in the longest diameter. A clip marker (arrow) was seen within the residual mass

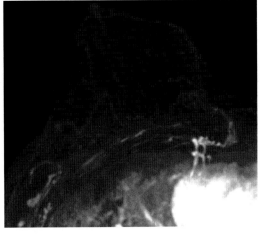

Fig. 159 Breast MRI (Sep. 2021): MRI after treatment shows complete resolution of enhancement in the right breast

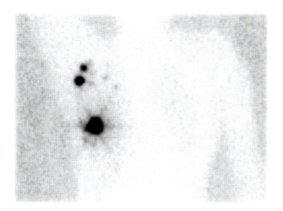

Fig. 160 Lymphoscintigraphy shows visualized sentinel lymph nodes in the right axilla

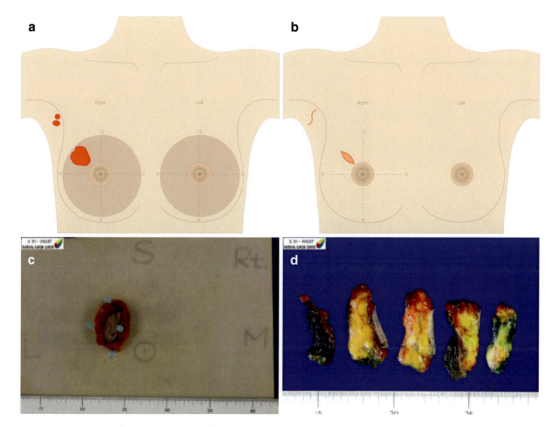

Fig. 161 (a) A schematic illustration of tumor location and axillary lymph node metastasis. (b) Breast and axillary incision lines on right breast. (c) Gross pathology of lumpectomy specimen. (d) The margins get marked and sliced with different colors on each direction

23 Case 23

23.1 Patient History and Progress

Female/56 years old, post-menopause.
Self-detected mass lesion on right breast.
Family history of breast cancer, aunt (maternal).
s/p Right knee fracture operation.
BRCA 1 and 2 mutation: Not detected, POLD1 VUS (variant of uncertain).

23.2 Important Radiologic Findings

See Figs. 162, 163 and 164.

23.2.1 After Neoadjuvant Chemotherapy

See Figs. 165, 166, 167 and 168.

23.3 Courses of Treatment

Neoadjuvant chemotherapy (#4 cycles of doxorubicin and cyclophosphamide + #4 cycles of docetaxel) + Operation + Postoperative radiation therapy.

23.3.1 Operation

Right breast conserving surgery, sentinel lymph node biopsy (Fig. 169).

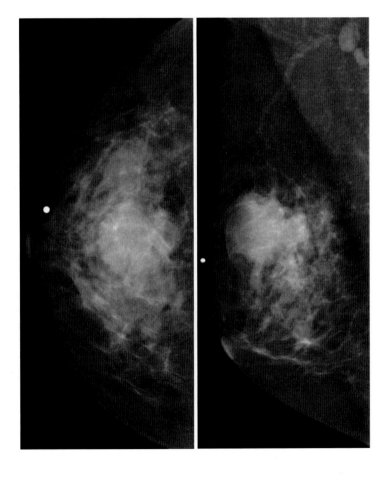

Fig. 162 Mammography (Aug. 2020): An irregular hyperdense mass in the upper portion of the right breast (marked by BB marker). Enlarged lymph nodes in the right axilla

HR(−) HER2(−) Breast Cancer

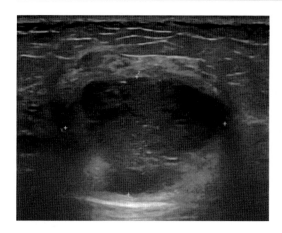

Fig. 163 Breast US (Aug. 2020): An irregular hypoechoic mass at the 12 o'clock direction of the right breast

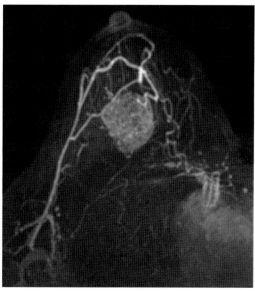

Fig. 164 Breast MRI (Aug. 2020): An irregular heterogeneous enhancing mass at the 12 o'clock direction of the right breast

Fig. 165 Mammography (Mar. 2021): mammography after treatment demonstrates no residual mass. A clip marker (white arrow) was seen at the tumor bed

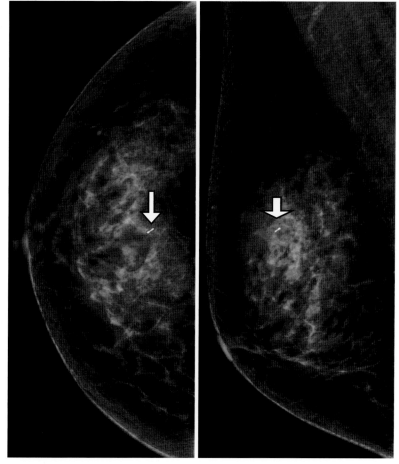

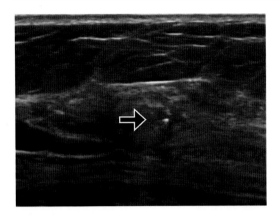

Fig. 166 Breast US (Mar. 2021): US after treatment demonstrates residual hypoechoic mass that is decreased in the longest diameter. A clip marker (arrow) was seen around the residual mass

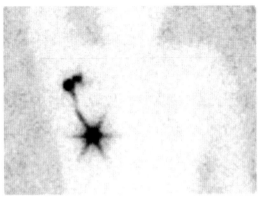

Fig. 168 Lymphoscintigraphy shows visualized sentinel lymph nodes in the right axilla

23.3.2 Pathology Report

No residual tumor with foamy histiocytic collection

1. Post-chemotherapy status.
2. Lymph nodes: no metastasis in one axillary lymph node (ypN0(sn)) (sentinel LN: 0/1).

Note: Histologic mapping has been done.

	Result	Intensity	Positive %
Estrogen receptor	Negative (0/8)	0	0
Progesterone receptor	Negative (0/8)	0	0
C-erbB2	Negative (1+)		
Ki-67	Positive in 74% of tumor cells		

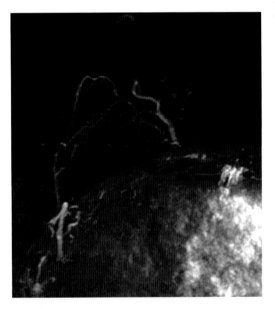

Fig. 167 Breast MRI (Mar. 2021): MRI after treatment shows complete resolution of enhancement in the right breast

HR(−) HER2(−) Breast Cancer

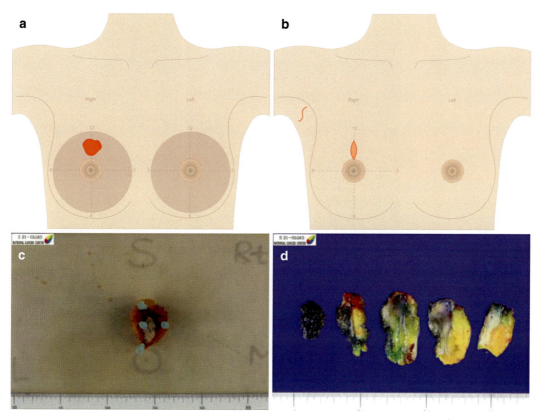

Fig. 169 (**a**) A schematic illustration of tumor location and (**b**) breast and axillary incision lines on right breast. (**c**) Gross pathology of lumpectomy specimen. (**d**) The margins get marked and sliced with different colors on each direction

24 Case 24

24.1 Patient History and Progress

Female/44 years old, pre-menopause.
  Self-detected mass lesion on right breast.
  Family history of breast cancer, aunt (paternal).
  Family history of ovarian cancer, sister.
  No comorbidities.
  BRCA 1 and 2 mutation: Not detected, EPCAM and MLH1 VUS (variant of uncertain).

24.2 Important Radiologic Findings

See Figs. 170, 171 and 172.

24.2.1 After Neoadjuvant Chemotherapy

See Figs. 173, 174, 175 and 176.

24.3 Courses of Treatment

Neoadjuvant chemotherapy (#4 cycles of doxorubicin and cyclophosphamide + #4 cycles of paclitaxel) + Operation + Postoperative radiation therapy + Adjuvant capecitabine.

24.3.1 Operation
Right breast conserving surgery, sentinel lymph node biopsy (Fig. 177).

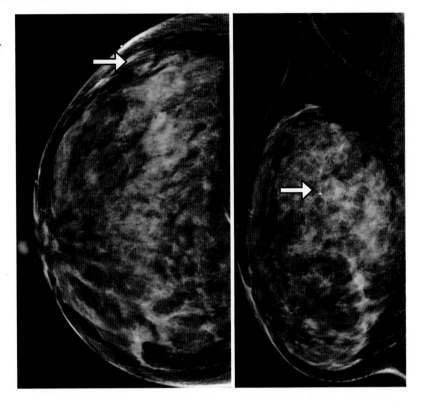

Fig. 170 Mammography (Apr. 2021): An oval isodense mass in the upper outer quadrant of right breast (marked by BB marker)

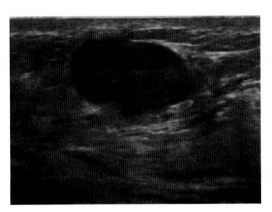

Fig. 171 Breast US (Apr. 2021): An oval hypoechoic mass at the 10 o'clock direction of the right breast

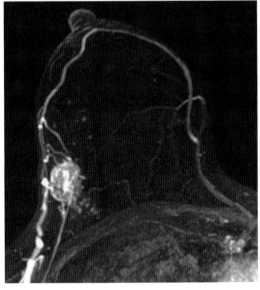

Fig. 172 Breast MRI (Apr. 2021): An irregular heterogeneous enhancing mass with associated non-mass enhancement in the upper outer quadrant of the right breast

HR(−) HER2(−) Breast Cancer   661

Fig. 173 Mammography (Sep. 2021): An irregular hyperdense mass in the upper outer quadrant of the right breast, showing interval increase in size

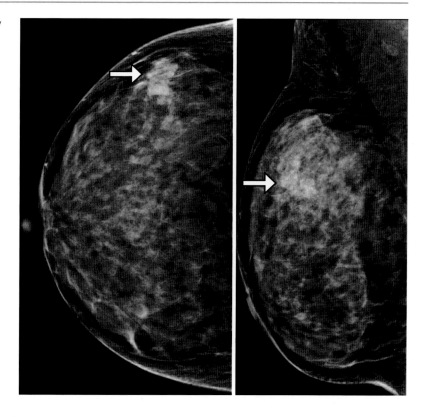

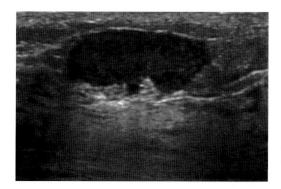

Fig. 174 Breast US (Sep. 2021): US after treatment demonstrates the irregular hypoechoic mass that is increased in the longest diameter

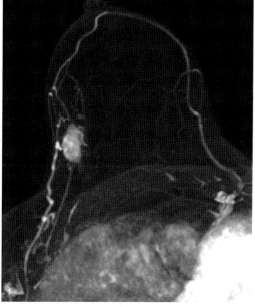

Fig. 175 Breast MRI (Sep. 2021): MRI after treatment demonstrates enhancing mass that is increased in the longest diameter

24.3.2 Pathology Report

Invasive Ductal Carcinoma
1. Post-chemotherapy status.
2. Size of tumor: 2.7 cm (ypT2).

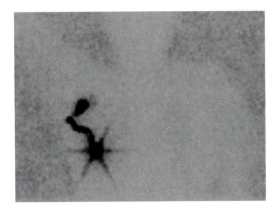

Fig. 176 Lymphoscintigraphy shows visualized sentinel lymph nodes in the right axilla

3. Histologic grade: 3/3 (tubule formation: 3/3, nuclear pleomorphism: 3/3, mitotic count: 3/3, 54/10HPF).
4. Intraductal component: present, intratumoral/extratumoral (5%) (nuclear grade: high, necrosis: absent, architectural pattern: micropapillary, extensive intraductal component: absent).
5. Skin: no involvement of tumor.
6. Surgical margins:
   (a) Superior margin: (see note).
   (b) Inferior margin: 15 mm.
   (c) Medial margin: 10 mm.
   (d) Lateral margin: 20 mm.
   (e) Deep margin: 10 mm.
   (f) Superficial margin: 2.5 mm.
7. Lymph nodes: no metastasis in three axillary lymph nodes (ypN0(sn)) (sentinel LN: 0/3).

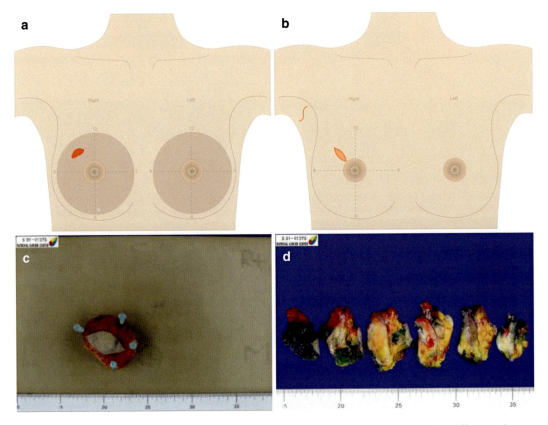

Fig. 177 (a) A schematic illustration of tumor location and (b) breast and axillary incision lines on right breast. (c) Gross pathology of lumpectomy specimen. (d) The margins get marked and sliced with different colors on each direction

HR(−) HER2(−) Breast Cancer 663

8. Arteriovenous invasion: absent.
9. Lymphovascular invasion: absent.
10. Tumor border: infiltrative.
11. Microcalcification: present, non-tumoral.
12. Pathological TN category (AJCC 2017): ypT2N0(sn).

Note: 1. The superior margin of the lumpectomy specimen (slide 3) is positive for invasive ductal carcinoma, but this margin submitted for frozen diagnosis (Fro 1) is free of tumor.

	Result	Intensity	Positive %
Estrogen receptor	Negative (0/8)	0	0
Progesterone receptor	Negative (0/8)	0	0
C-erbB2	Negative (0)		
Ki-67	Positive in 54% of tumor cells		

25 Case 25

25.1 Patient History and Progress

Female/70 years old, post-menopause.

Screen detected mass lesion on left breast 2 o'clock direction.

Family history of breast cancer, cousin (paternal).

Macular degeneration.

BRCA 1 and 2 mutation: Not tested.

25.2 Important Radiologic Findings

See Figs. 178, 179 and 180.

25.3 After Neoadjuvant Chemotherapy

See Figs. 181, 182, 183 and 184.

25.4 Courses of Treatment

Neoadjuvant chemotherapy (#4 cycles of doxorubicin and cyclophosphamide + #4 cycles of docetaxel) + Operation + Post-operative radiation therapy + Adjuvant capecitabine.

25.4.1 Operation

Left breast conserving surgery, sentinel lymph node biopsy (Fig. 185).

25.4.2 Pathology Report

Invasive Ductal Carcinoma with (a) focal squamous differentiation, (b) focal papillary pattern.

1. Post-chemotherapy status.
2. Size of tumor: 1.2 cm (ypT1c).
3. Histologic grade: 2/3 (tubule formation: 3/3, nuclear pleomorphism: 3/3, mitotic count: 1/3, <1/10HPF).
4. Intraductal component: present, intratumoral/extratumoral (15%) (nuclear grade: high, necrosis: absent, architectural pattern: papillary, extensive intraductal component: absent).
5. Skin: no involvement of tumor.
6. Surgical margins:
   (a) Superior margin: 10 mm.
   (b) Inferior margin: 15 mm.
   (c) Medial margin: 10 mm.
   (d) Lateral margin: 35 mm.
   (e) Deep margin: 6 mm.
   (f) Superficial margin: 15 mm.
7. Lymph nodes: no metastasis in two axillary lymph nodes (ypN0(sn)) (sentinel LN: 0/1, non-sentinel LN: 0/1).
8. Arteriovenous invasion: absent.
9. Lymphovascular invasion: absent.
10. Tumor border: infiltrative.
11. Microcalcification: absent.
12. Pathological TN category (AJCC 2017): ypT1cN0(SN).

	Result	Intensity	Positive %
Estrogen receptor	Negative (0/8)	0	0
Progesterone receptor	Negative (0/8)	0	0
C-erbB2	Negative (0)		
Ki-67	Positive in 28% of tumor cells		

Fig. 178 Mammography (Apr. 2021): An irregular isodense mass in the upper outer quadrant of the left breast

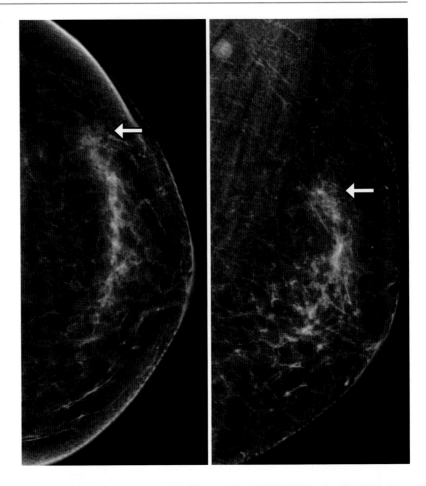

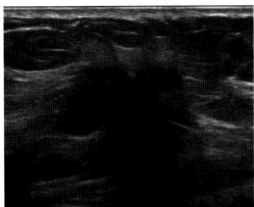

Fig. 179 Breast US (Apr. 2021): An irregular hypoechoic mass at the 2 o'clock direction of the left breast

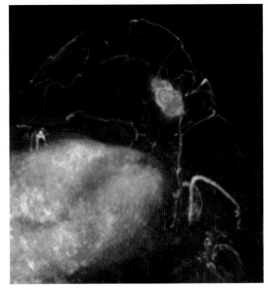

Fig. 180 Breast MRI (Apr. 2021): An irregular enhancing mass at the 2 o'clock direction of the left breast

Fig. 181 Mammography (Oct. 2021): mammography after treatment demonstrates the residual mass that is decreased in the longest diameter

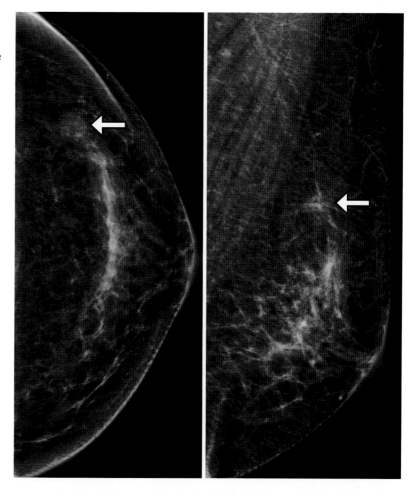

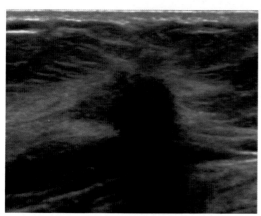

Fig. 182 Breast US (Oct. 2021): US after treatment demonstrates the residual hypoechoic mass that is decreased in the longest diameter

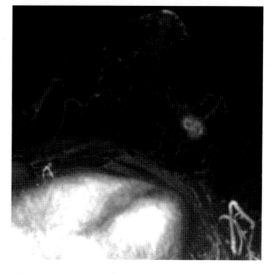

Fig. 183 Breast MRI (Oct. 2021): MRI after treatment demonstrates the residual enhancing mass that is decreased in the longest diameter

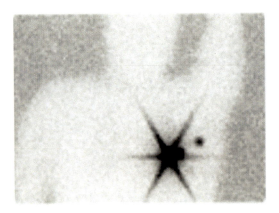

Fig. 184 Lymphoscintigraphy shows visualized sentinel lymph nodes in the left axilla

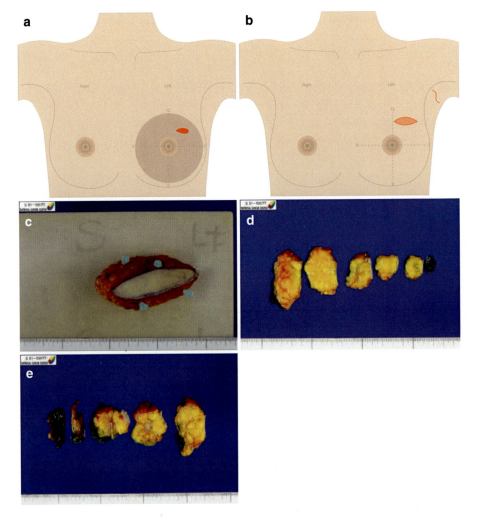

Fig. 185 (a) A schematic illustration of tumor location and (b) breast and axillary incision lines on left breast. (c) Gross pathology of lumpectomy specimen. (d, e) The margins get marked and sliced with different colors on each direction

26 Case 26

26.1 Patient History and Progress

Female/53 years old, post-menopause.

Self-detected mass lesion on right breast.
Family history of breast cancer, grandmother.
Family history of ovarian cancer, sister.
S/P appendectomy, s/p bilateral salpingo-oophorectomy, s/p left shoulder operation.
BRCA 1 mutation carrier.

26.2 Important Radiologic Findings

See Figs. 186, 187 and 188.

Breast, right, needle biopsy: Invasive ductal carcinoma, histologic grade 3 with medullary pattern.

	Result	Intensity	Positive %
Estrogen receptor	Negative (0/8)	0	0
Progesterone receptor	Negative (0/8)	0	0
C-erbB2	Negative (1+)		
Ki-67	Positive in 51% of tumor cells		

Breast, left, needle biopsy: Invasive ductal carcinoma, histologic grade 3.

	Result	Intensity	Positive %
Estrogen receptor	Negative (2/8)	1	<1%
Progesterone receptor	Negative (0/8)	0	0
C-erbB2	Equivocal (2+)		
Ki-67	Positive in 39% of tumor cells		
SISH	Tumor heterogeneity		

26.2.1 After Neoadjuvant Chemotherapy

See Figs. 189, 190, 191 and 192.

26.3 Courses of Treatment

Neoadjuvant chemotherapy (#4 cycles of doxorubicin and cyclophosphamide + #3 cycles of docetaxel + Trastuzumab) + Operation + Adjuvant capecitabine + Trastuzumab.

26.3.1 Operation

Robotic bilateral nipple-areolar complex sparing mastectomy, bilateral sentinel lymph node biopsy (Figs. 193, 194 and 195).

26.3.2 Pathology Report

<Right>

No residual tumor with stromal fibrosis
1. Post-chemotherapy status.
2. Lymph nodes: no metastasis in two axillary lymph nodes (ypN0(sn)) (sentinel LN: 0/2).

<Left>

Invasive Ductal Carcinoma
1. Post-chemotherapy status.
2. Size of tumor: 1.8 cm (ypT1c).
3. Histologic grade: 2/3 (tubule formation: 3/3, nuclear pleomorphism: 2/3, mitotic count: 1/3, <1/10HPF).
4. Intraductal component: present, intratumoral (60%) (nuclear grade: high, necrosis: absent, architectural pattern: solid, extensive intraductal component: present).
5. Surgical margins:
   (a) Deep margin: 1 mm from ductal carcinoma in situ (slide 3).
   (b) Superficial margin: 13 mm.
6. Lymph nodes:
   (a) Metastasis in one out of eight axillary lymph nodes (ypN1mi) (see note) (sentinel LN: 1/2, non-sentinel LN: 0/6).
   (b) Perinodal extension: absent.
   (c) Size of metastatic carcinoma: 0.5 mm.
7. Arteriovenous invasion: absent.
8. Lymphovascular invasion: present, intratumoral.
9. Tumor border: infiltrative.

Fig. 186 Mammography (Apr. 2021): An irregular hyperdense mass in the upper outer quadrant of the right breast

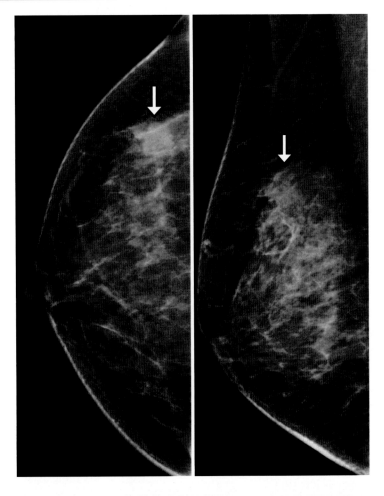

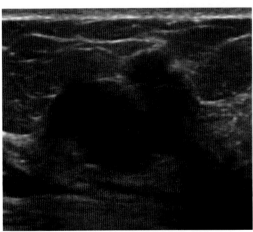

Fig. 187 Breast US (Apr. 2021): An irregular hypoechoic mass at the 10 o'clock direction of the right breast

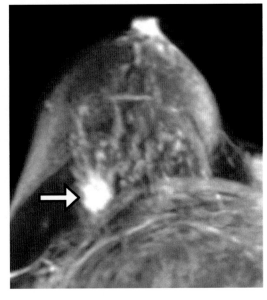

Fig. 188 Breast MRI (Apr. 2021): An irregular enhancing mass at the 10 o'clock direction of the right breast

HR(−) HER2(−) Breast Cancer 669

Fig. 189 Mammography (Oct. 2021): mammography after treatment demonstrates no residual mass

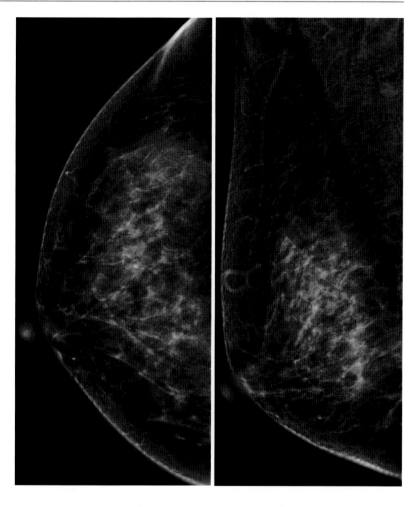

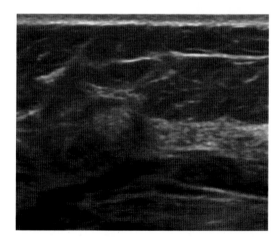

Fig. 190 Breast US (Oct. 2021): US after treatment demonstrates no residual mass

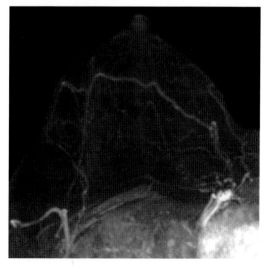

Fig. 191 Breast MRI (Jun. 2021): MRI after treatment shows complete resolution of enhancement in the right breast

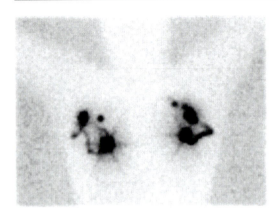

Fig. 192 Lymphoscintigraphy shows visualized sentinel lymph nodes in both axilla

10. Microcalcification: present, non-tumoral.
11. Pathological TN category (AJCC 2017): ypT1cN1mi.

Note: 1. Micrometastasis is present only in the permanent section of Fro 3.

	Result	Intensity	Positive %
Estrogen receptor	Negative (0/8)	0	0
Progesterone receptor	Negative (0/8)	0	0
C-erbB2	Negative (0)		
Ki-67	Positive in 1% of tumor cells		

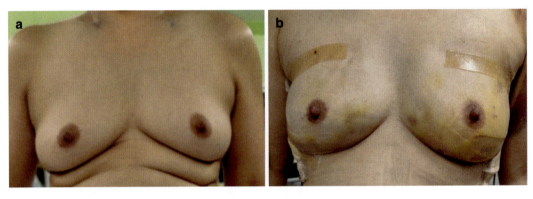

Fig. 193 (a) Preoperative and (b) postoperative appearance

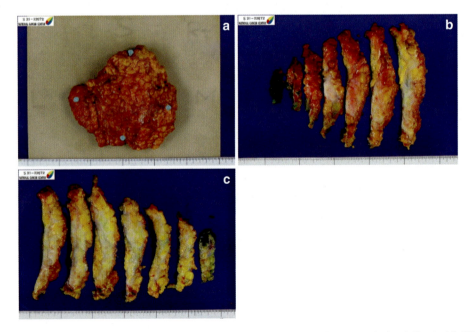

Fig. 194 (a) Gross pathology of mastectomy (right) specimen. (b, c) The margins get marked and sliced with different colors on each direction

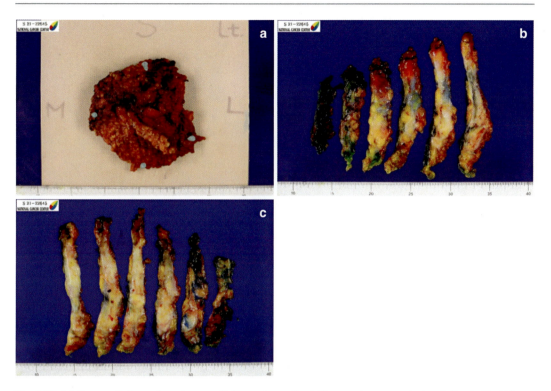

Fig. 195 (**a**) Gross pathology of mastectomy (left) specimen. (**b, c**) The margins get marked and sliced with different colors on each direction

27 Case 27

27.1 Patient History and Progress

Female/36 years old, pre-menopause.

Self-detected palpable mass lesion on left breast.

Family history of breast cancer, aunt (maternal).

No comorbidities.

BRCA 1 and 2 mutation: Not detected, RAD50 VUS (variant of uncertain).

27.2 Important Radiologic Findings

See Figs. 196, 197, 198 and 199.

Fig. 196 Mammography (May. 2021): An irregular hyperdense mass in the upper outer quadrant of left breast (marked by BB marker). Enlarged lymph nodes in the left axilla

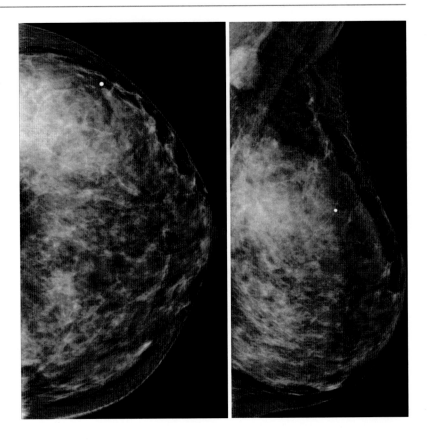

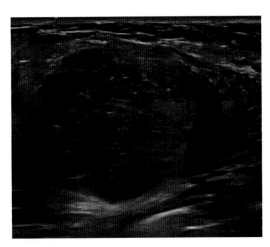

Fig. 197 Breast US (May. 2021): An irregular hypoechoic mass at the 2 o'clock direction of the left breast

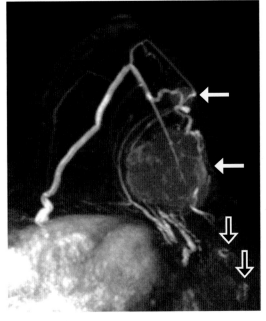

Fig. 198 Breast MRI (May. 2021): Two irregular enhancing masses at the 2 o'clock direction of left breast. Multiple enlarged lymph nodes in the left axilla

HR(−) HER2(−) Breast Cancer

Fig. 199 PET-CT shows (**a**) a hypermetabolic mass in the left breast parenchyma, upper outer quadrant (mSUV = ~12.4) and (**b**) hypermetabolic lymph nodes in the left axilla level I area (mSUV = ~6.7)

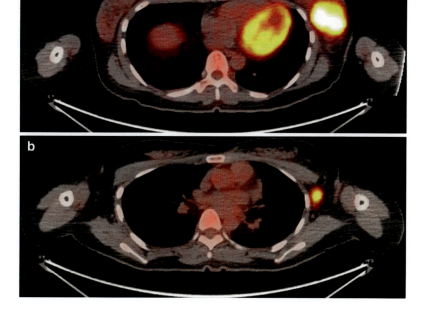

27.2.1 After Neoadjuvant Chemotherapy

See Figs. 200, 201 and 202.

27.3 Courses of Treatment

Neoadjuvant chemotherapy (#4 cycles of doxorubicin and cyclophosphamide + #4 cycles of docetaxel) + Operation + Postoperative radiation therapy + Adjuvant capecitabine.

27.3.1 Operation

Left breast conserving surgery, axillary lymph node sampling (Fig. 203).

27.3.2 Pathology Report

Invasive Ductal Carcinoma
1. Post-chemotherapy status.
2. Size of tumor: 2.8 cm (ypT2).
3. Histologic grade: 3/3 (tubule formation: 3/3, nuclear pleomorphism: 3/3, mitotic count: 3/3, 14/10HPF).
4. Intraductal component: absent.
5. Skin: no involvement of tumor.
6. Surgical margins:
   (a) Superior margin: 5 mm.
   (b) Inferior margin: 5 mm.
   (c) Medial margin: 5 mm.
   (d) Lateral margin: 5 mm.
   (e) Deep margin: 2 mm.
   (f) Superficial margin: 2 mm.
7. Lymph nodes: no metastasis in three axillary lymph nodes (ypN0(i+)(sn)) (sentinel LN: 0/2, axillary LN: 0/1).
8. Arteriovenous invasion: absent.
9. Lymphovascular invasion: present, intratumoral.
10. Tumor border: infiltrative.
11. Microcalcification: present, tumoral/non-tumoral.
12. Pathological TN category (AJCC 2017): ypT2N0(i+)(sn).

Note: 1. A few isolated tumor cells are present only in the permanent section of Fro 6 for immunohistochemical staining.

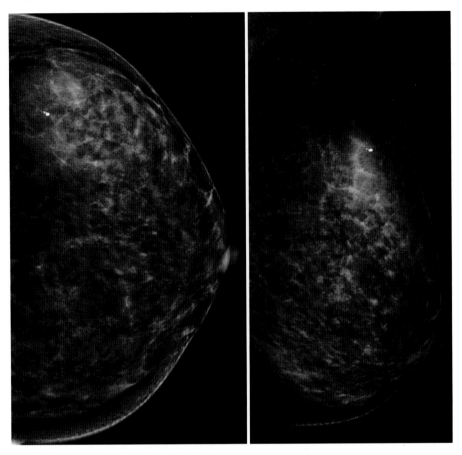

Fig. 200 Mammography (Nov. 2021): mammography after treatment demonstrates residual mass that is decreased in the longest diameter. A clip marker (black arrow) was seen within the residual mass

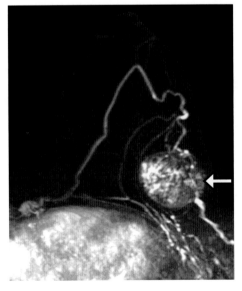

Fig. 201 Breast MRI (Nov . 2021): MRI after treatment demonstrates residual enhancing mass (white arrow) that is decreased in the longest diameter

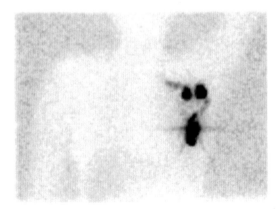

Fig. 202 Lymphoscintigraphy shows visualized sentinel lymph nodes in the left axilla

HR(−) HER2(−) Breast Cancer

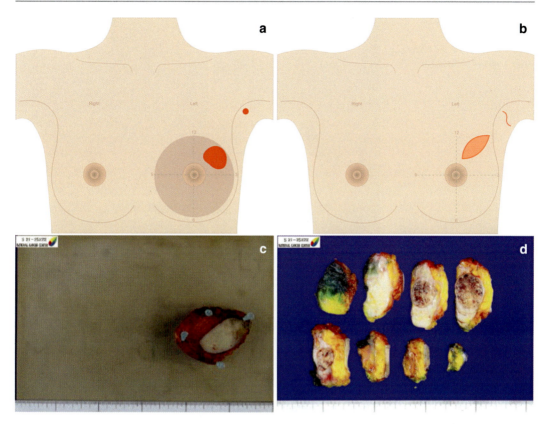

Fig. 203 (**a**) A schematic illustration of tumor location and lymph node metastasis. (**b**) Breast and axillary incision lines on left breast. (**c**) Gross pathology of lumpectomy specimen. (**d**) The margins get marked and sliced with different colors on each direction

	Result	Intensity	Positive %
Estrogen receptor	Negative (0/8)	0	0
Progesterone receptor	Negative (0/8)	0	0
C-erbB2	Negative (1+)		
Ki-67	Positive in 89% of tumor cells		

28 Case 28

28.1 Patient History and Progress

Female/57 years old, post-menopause.
 Self-detected palpable mass lesion on right.
 No family history.
 S/P right neck excision (due to lymphadenitis).

28.2 Important Radiologic Findings

See Figs. 204, 205 and 206.

28.3 Courses of Treatment

Operation + Post-operative radiation therapy (Adjuvant chemotherapy refuse).

28.3.1 Operation

Right breast conserving surgery (Fig. 207).

28.3.2 Pathology Report

Malignant Adenomyoepithelioma (Epithelial-Myoepithelial Carcinoma)
 1. Size of tumor: 2.0 cm (pT1c).

Fig. 204 Mammography (Sep. 2020): An irregular hyperdense mass in the upper outer quadrant of the right breast

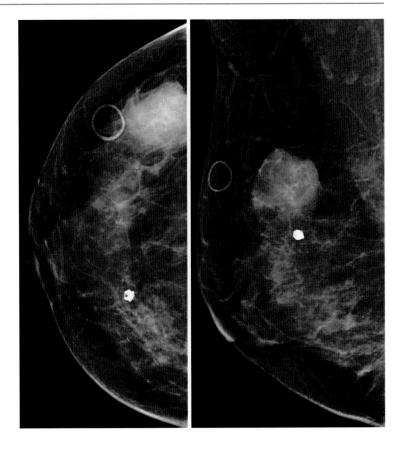

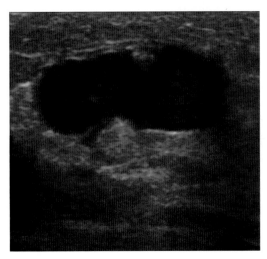

Fig. 205 Breast US (Sep. 2020): An irregular hypoechoic mass in the upper outer quadrant of the right breast

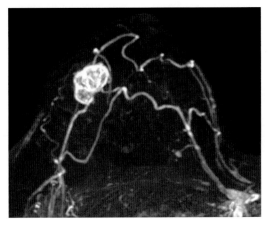

Fig. 206 Breast MRI (Apr. 2021): An irregular enhancing mass in the upper outer quadrant of the right breast

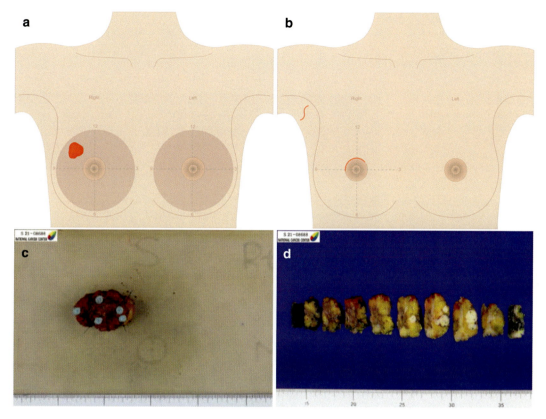

Fig. 207 (**a**) A schematic illustration of tumor location. (**b**) Breast and axillary incision lines on right breast. (**c**) Gross pathology of lumpectomy specimen. (**d**) The margins get marked and sliced with different colors on each direction

2. Histologic grade: 3/3 (tubule formation: 3/3, nuclear pleomorphism: 2/3, mitotic count: 3/3, 23/10HPF).
3. Intraductal component: absent.
4. Skin: no involvement of tumor.
5. Surgical margins:
   (a) Superior margin: 10 mm.
   (b) Inferior margin: 10 mm.
   (c) Medial margin: 15 mm.
   (d) Lateral margin: 25 mm.
   (e) Deep margin: 9 mm.
   (f) Superficial margin: <1 mm from epithelial-myoepithelial carcinoma (slides 2 and 7).
6. Arteriovenous invasion: absent.
7. Lymphovascular invasion: absent.
8. Tumor border: pushing.
9. Microcalcification: present, non-tumoral.
10. Pathological TN category (AJCC 2017): pT1c.

	Result	Intensity	Positive %
Estrogen receptor	Negative (0/8)	0	0
Progesterone receptor	Negative (0/8)	0	0
C-erbB2	Negative (0)		
Ki-67	Positive in 18% of tumor cells		

29 Case 29

29.1 Patient History and Progress

Female/27 years old, pre-menopause.
    Self-detected mass lesion on left breast.
    No family history.
    No comorbidities.
    BRCA 1 and 2 mutation: Not detected.

29.2 Important Radiologic Findings

See Figs. 208, 209, 210 and 211.

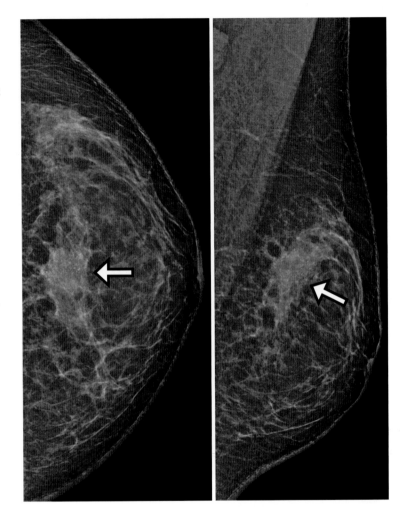

Fig. 208 Mammography (May. 2021): An irregular hyperdense mass with fine pleomorphic microcalcifications in the upper center portion of the left breast

HR(−) HER2(−) Breast Cancer

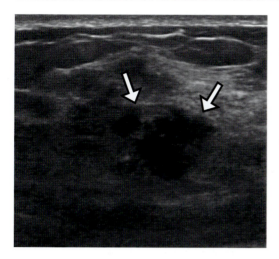

Fig. 209 Breast US (May. 2021): An irregular hypoechoic mass with microcalcifications at the 11 o'clock direction of the left breast

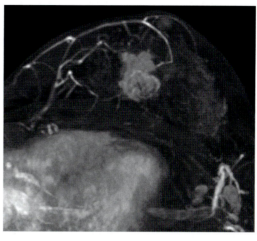

Fig. 210 Breast MRI (May. 2021): An irregular enhancing mass at the 11 o'clock direction of the left breast. Multiple enlarged lymph nodes in the left axilla

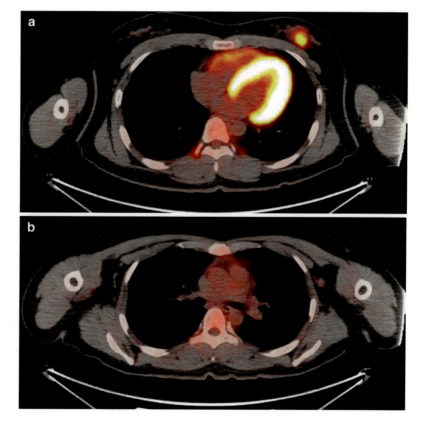

Fig. 211 PET-CT shows (**a**) a hypermetabolic mass in left breast (mSUV = 7.3) and (**b**) a few prominent LNs on the left axilla level I (mSUV = 1.3)

29.2.1 After Neoadjuvant Chemotherapy

See Figs. 212, 213 and 214.

29.3 Courses of Treatment

Neoadjuvant chemotherapy (#4 cycles of doxorubicin and cyclophosphamide + #4 cycles of docetaxel) + Operation + Post-operative radiation therapy + Adjuvant capecitabine.

29.3.1 Operation

Left breast conserving surgery, axillary lymph node dissection (Fig. 215).

29.3.2 Pathology Report

Microinvasive Ductal Carcinoma

1. Post-chemotherapy status.
2. Size of tumor: <0.1 cm (ypT1mi).
3. Histologic grade: not applicable.
4. Intraductal component: absent.
5. Skin: no involvement of tumor.
6. Surgical margins:
    (a) Superior margin: 10 mm.
    (b) Inferior margin: 10 mm.
    (c) Medial margin: 10 mm.
    (d) Lateral margin: 10 mm.
    (e) Deep margin: 2 mm.
    (f) Superficial margin: 2 mm.
7. Lymph nodes: no metastasis in six axillary lymph nodes (ypN0) (sentinel LN: 0/3, non-sentinel LN: 0/3).
8. Arteriovenous invasion: absent.
9. Lymphovascular invasion: absent.
10. Tumor border: infiltrative.
11. Microcalcification: present, tumoral/non-tumoral.
12. Pathological TN category (AJCC 2017): ypT1miN0.

	Result	Intensity	Positive %
Estrogen receptor	Negative (0/8)	0	0
Progesterone receptor	Negative (0/8)	0	0
C-erbB2	Negative (1+)		
Ki-67	Positive in 43% of tumor cells		

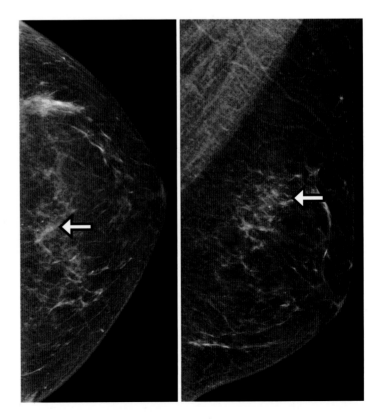

Fig. 212 Mammography (Nov. 2021): mammography after treatment demonstrates residual microcalcifications

HR(−) HER2(−) Breast Cancer

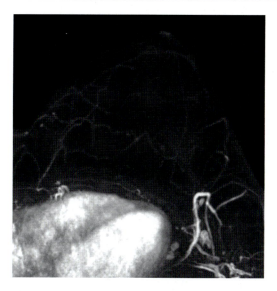

Fig. 213 Breast MRI (Nov. 2021): MRI after treatment shows complete resolution of enhancement in the left breast

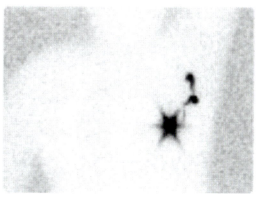

Fig. 214 Lymphoscintigraphy shows visualized sentinel lymph nodes in the left axilla

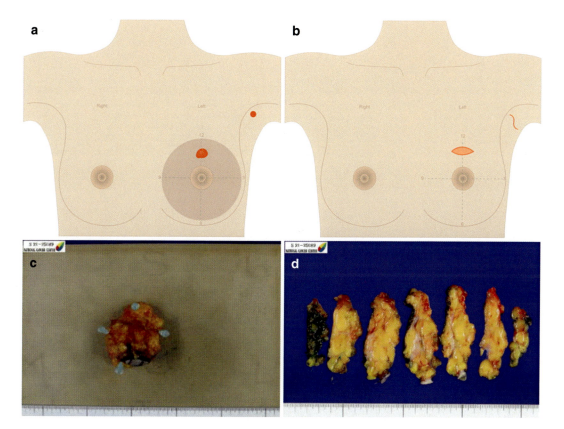

Fig. 215 (**a**) A schematic illustration of tumor location and lymph node metastasis. (**b**) Breast and axillary incision lines on left breast. (**c**) Gross pathology of lumpectomy specimen. (**d**) The margins get marked and sliced with different colors on each direction

30 Case 30

30.1 Patient History and Progress

Female/69 years old, post-menopause.

Self-detected palpable mass lesion on left breast.

No family history.

h/o Tuberculosis, s/p thoracic vertebra compression fracture.

30.2 Important Radiologic Findings

See Figs. 216, 217 and 218.

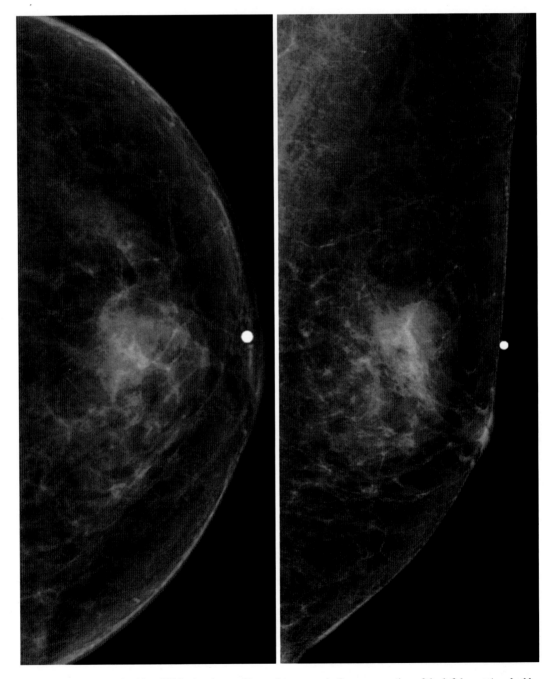

Fig. 216 Mammography (Apr. 2021): An obscured hyperdense mass in the upper portion of the left breast (marked by BB marker)

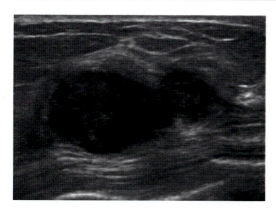

Fig. 217 Breast US (Apr. 2021): An irregular hypoechoic mass at the 12 o'clock direction of the left breast

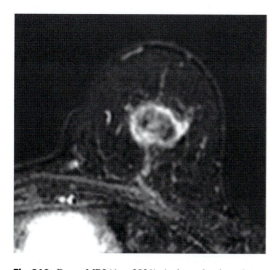

Fig. 218 Breast MRI (Apr. 2021): An irregular rim enhancing mass at the 12 o'clock direction of the left breast

30.2.1 After Neoadjuvant Chemotherapy

See Figs. 219, 220, 221, 222 and 223.

30.3 Courses of Treatment

Neoadjuvant chemotherapy (#2 cycles of doxorubicin and cyclophosphamide + #3 cycles of paclitaxel) + Operation + Adjuvant capecitabine.

30.3.1 Operation

Left modified radical mastectomy, sentinel lymph node biopsy (Fig. 224).

30.3.2 Pathology Report

Invasive Ductal Carcinoma
1. Post-chemotherapy status.
2. Size of tumor: 3.5 cm (ypT2).
3. Histologic grade: 3/3 (tubule formation: 3/3, nuclear pleomorphism: 3/3, mitotic count: 3/3, 4/1HPF).
4. Intraductal component: present, extratumoral (5%) (nuclear grade: high, necrosis: absent, architectural pattern: solid, extensive intraductal component: absent).
5. Skin and nipple: no involvement of tumor.
6. Surgical margins:
   (a) Deep margin: 1 mm from invasive ductal carcinoma (slide 6).
   (b) Superficial margin: 2 mm.

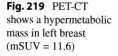
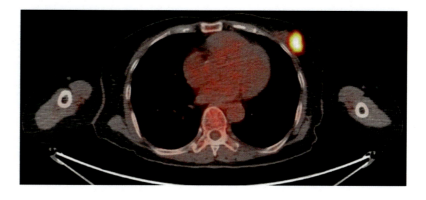

Fig. 219 PET-CT shows a hypermetabolic mass in left breast (mSUV = 11.6)

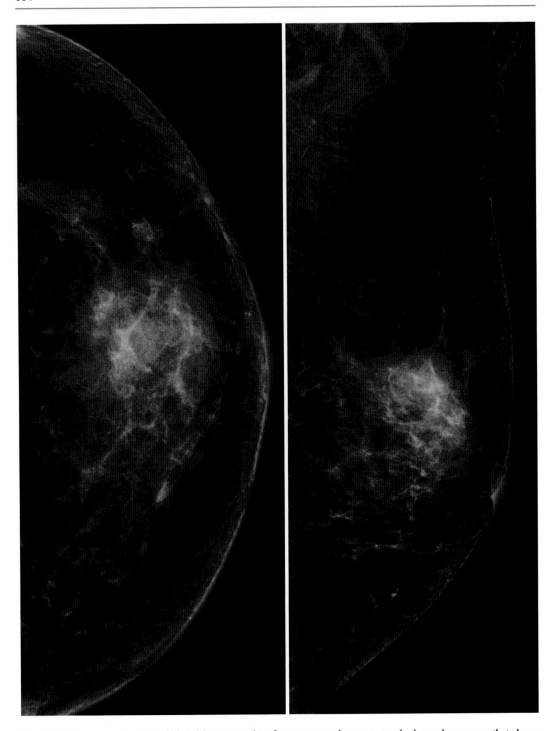

Fig. 220 Mammography (Aug. 2021): Mammography after treatment demonstrates the hyperdense mass that shows interval increase in size

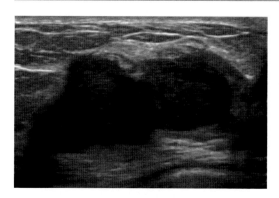

Fig. 221 Breast US (Aug. 2021): US after treatment demonstrates the irregular hypoechoic mass that is increased in the longest diameter

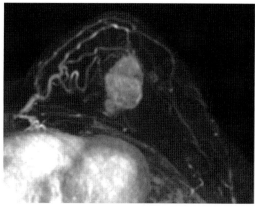

Fig. 222 Breast MRI (Aug. 2021): MRI after treatment demonstrates the irregular enhancing mass that is increased in the longest diameter

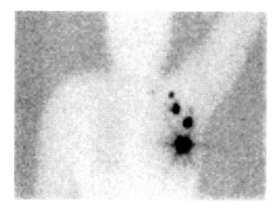

Fig. 223 Lymphoscintigraphy shows visualized sentinel lymph nodes in the left axilla

7. Lymph nodes: no metastasis in two axillary lymph nodes (ypN0(sn)) (sentinel LN: 0/2).
8. Arteriovenous invasion: absent.
9. Lymphovascular invasion: present, intratumoral.
10. Tumor border: infiltrative.
11. Microcalcification: present, tumoral/non-tumoral.
12. Pathological TN category (AJCC 2017): ypT2N0(sn).

	Result	Intensity	Positive %
Estrogen receptor	Negative (0/8)	0	0
Progesterone receptor	Negative (0/8)	0	0
C-erbB2	Equivocal (2+), SISH (−)		
Ki-67	Positive in 86% of tumor cells		

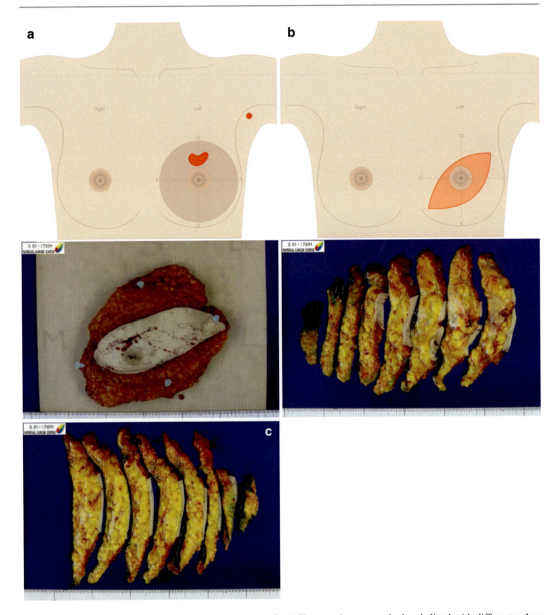

Fig. 224 (**a**) Gross pathology of mastectomy specimen. (**b, c**) The margins get marked and sliced with different colors on each direction

31 Case 31

31.1 Patient History and Progress

Female/41 years old, pre-menopause.
  Self-detected mass lesion on right breast.
  No family history.
  No comorbidities.

BRCA 1 and 2 mutation: Not detected, STK11 VUS (variant of uncertain).

31.2 Important Radiologic Findings

See Figs. 225, 226, 227 and 228.

Fig. 225 Mammography (Oct. 2020): An obscured mass in the upper outer quadrant of the right breast

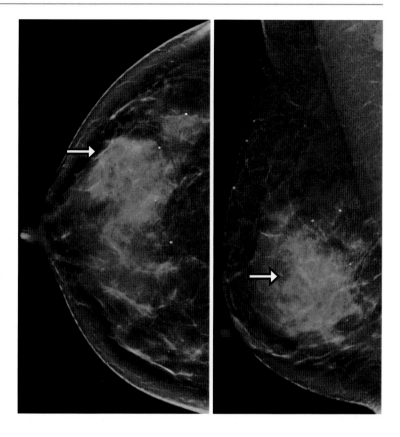

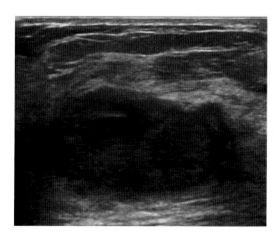

Fig. 226 Breast US (Oct. 2020): An irregular heterogeneous echoic mass with posterior acoustic enhancement at the 9 o'clock direction of the right breast

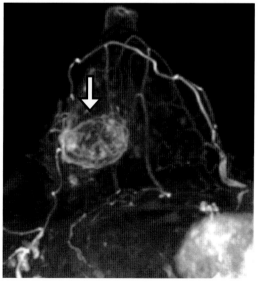

Fig. 227 Breast MRI (Oct. 2020): An irregular rim enhancing mass at the 9 o'clock direction of the right breast

Fig. 228 PET-CT shows (**a**) hypermetabolic necrotic mass in the right upper outer breast (mSUV = 6.1) and (**b**) small LN with subtle uptake in the right axilla level I (mSUV = 0.9)

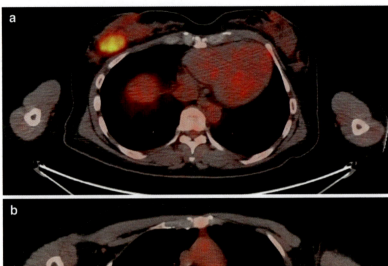
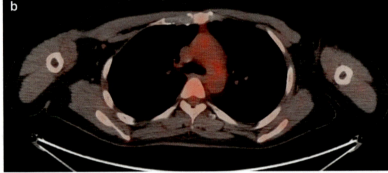

31.2.1 After Neoadjuvant Chemotherapy

See Figs. 229, 230, 231 and 232.

31.3 Courses of Treatment

Neoadjuvant chemotherapy (#4 cycles of doxorubicin and cyclophosphamide + #4 cycles of docetaxel) + Operation + Postoperative radiation therapy + Adjuvant capecitabine.

31.3.1 Operation

Right breast conserving surgery, axillary lymph node sampling (Fig. 233).

31.3.2 Pathology Report

Invasive Ductal Carcinoma
1. Post-chemotherapy status.
2. Size of tumor: 0.9 cm (ypT1b).
3. Histologic grade: 3/3 (tubule formation: 3/3, nuclear pleomorphism: 3/3, mitotic count: 3/3, 18/10HPF).
4. Intraductal component: absent.
5. Skin: no involvement of tumor.
6. Surgical margins:
    (a) Superior margin: 38 mm.
    (b) Inferior margin: 21 mm.
    (c) Medial margin: 20 mm.
    (d) Lateral margin: 15 mm.
    (e) Deep margin: 6 mm.
    (f) Superficial margin: 22 mm.
7. Lymph nodes: no metastasis in five axillary lymph nodes (ypN0(sn)) (sentinel LN: 0/3, non-sentinel LN: 0/2).

HR(−) HER2(−) Breast Cancer

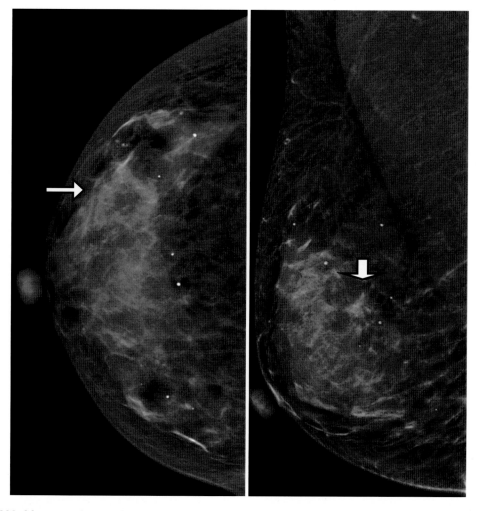

Fig. 229 Mammography (Apr. 2021): mammography after treatment demonstrates residual mass that is decreased in the longest diameter

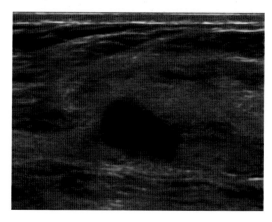

Fig. 230 Breast US (Apr. 2021): US after treatment demonstrates residual hypoechoic mass that is decreased in the longest diameter

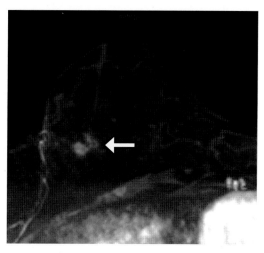

Fig. 231 Breast MRI (Apr. 2021): MRI after treatment demonstrates residual enhancing mass (white arrow) that is decreased in the longest diameter

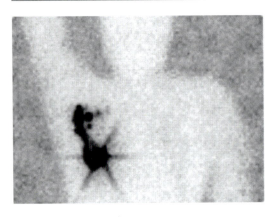

8. Arteriovenous invasion: absent.
9. Lymphovascular invasion: absent.
10. Tumor border: infiltrative.
11. Microcalcification: absent.
12. Pathological TN category (AJCC 2017): ypT1bN0(sn).

	Result	Intensity	Positive %
Estrogen receptor	Negative (0/8)	0	0
Progesterone receptor	Negative (0/8)	0	0
C-erbB2	Negative (0)		
Ki-67	Positive in 75% of tumor cells		

Fig. 232 Lymphoscintigraphy shows visualized sentinel lymph nodes in the right axilla

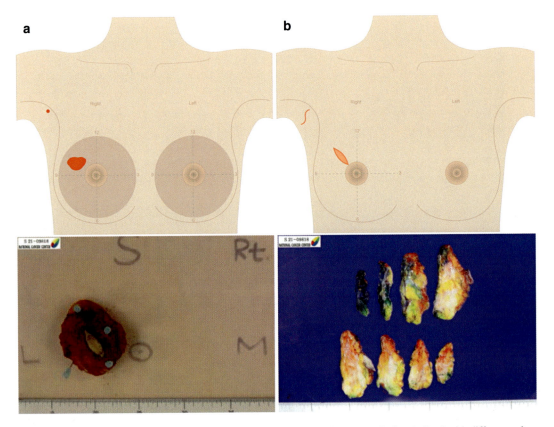

Fig. 233 (a) Gross pathology of lumpectomy specimen. (b) The margins get marked and sliced with different colors on each direction

32 Case 32

32.1 Patient History and Progress

Female/49 years old, pre-menopause.
  Self-detected mass lesion on left breast.
  Family history of breast cancer, aunt and cousin (paternal).
  Family history of prostate cancer, father.
  Hyperthyroidism.
  BRCA 1 and 2 mutation: Not detected.

32.2 Important Radiologic Findings

See Figs. 234, 235, 236 and 237.

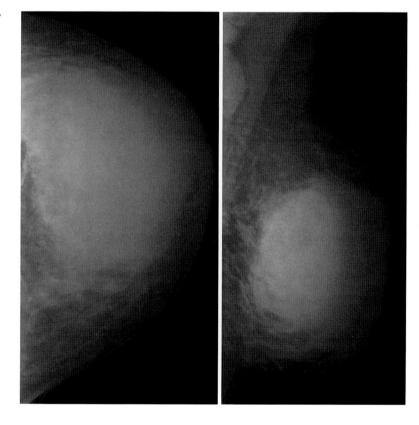

Fig. 234 Mammography (Nov. 2020): A huge hyperdense mass in left breast. Enlarged lymph node in the left axilla

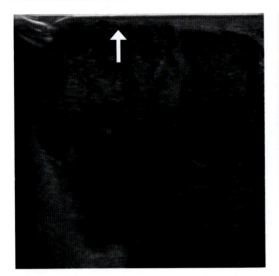

Fig. 235 Breast US (Nov. 2020): A huge irregular heterogeneous echoic mass with direct skin invasion (white arrow) in the left breast

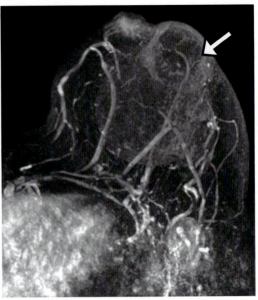

Fig. 236 Breast MRI (Nov. 2020): A huge irregular heterogeneous enhancing mass in the left breast

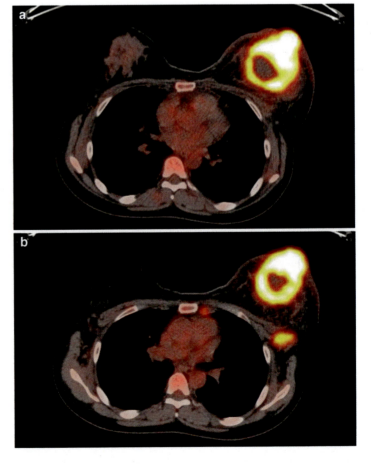

Fig. 237 PET-CT shows (**a**) large hypermetabolic necrotic mass in the left whole breast with skin invasion (mSUV = 23.6) and (**b**) multiple metastatic lymph nodes in the left axilla level I–III and the left internal mammary area

32.2.1 After Neoadjuvant Chemotherapy

See Figs. 238, 239, 240 and 241.

32.3 Courses of Treatment

Neoadjuvant chemotherapy (#4 cycles of doxorubicin and cyclophosphamide + #4 cycles of docetaxel) + Operation + Post-operative radiation therapy + Adjuvant capecitabine.

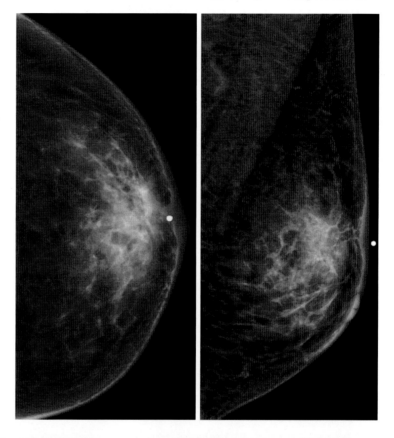

Fig. 238 Mammography (Apr. 2021): mammography after treatment demonstrates the residual mass that is decreased in the longest diameter (marked by BB marker)

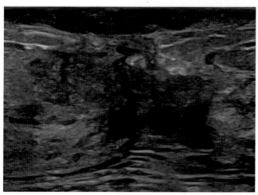

Fig. 239 Breast US (Apr. 2021): US after treatment demonstrates the residual mass that is decreased in the longest diameter

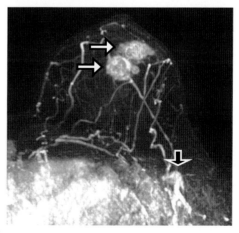

Fig. 240 Breast MRI (Apr. 2021): MRI after treatment demonstrates the residual enhancing masses (white arrow) that is decreased in the longest diameter

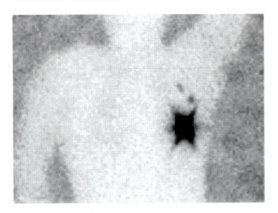

Fig. 241 Lymphoscintigraphy shows visualized sentinel lymph nodes in the left axilla

32.3.1 Operation

Left modified radical mastectomy, axillary lymph node dissection (Fig. 242).

32.3.2 Pathology Report

Invasive Ductal Carcinoma

1. Post-chemotherapy status.
2. Size of tumor: 2.7 cm (ypT2).
3. Histologic grade: 3/3 (tubule formation: 3/3, nuclear pleomorphism: 3/3, mitotic count: 3/3, 20/10HPF).
4. Intraductal component: absent.
5. Skin: dermal involvement of tumor.

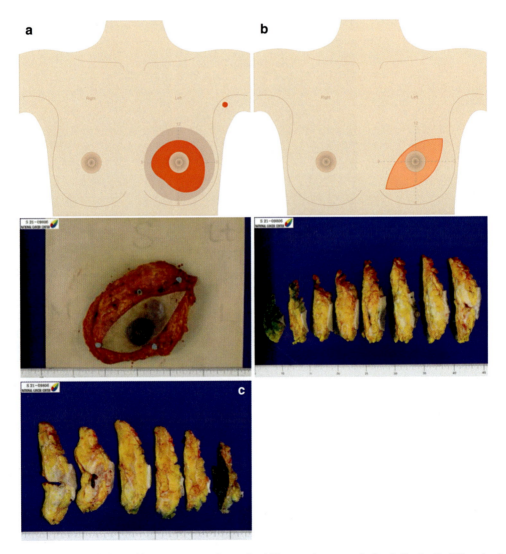

Fig. 242 (**a**) Gross pathology of lumpectomy specimen. (**b**, **c**) The margins get marked and sliced with different colors on each direction

6. Nipple: no involvement of tumor.
7. Surgical margins:
   (a) Deep margin: 22 mm.
   (b) Superficial margin: 7 mm.
8. Lymph nodes: no metastasis in 14 axillary lymph nodes (ypN0) (sentinel LN: 0/1, non-sentinel LN: 0/13).
9. Arteriovenous invasion: absent.
10. Lymphovascular invasion: absent.
11. Tumor border: infiltrative.
12. Microcalcification: absent.
13. Pathological TN category (AJCC 2017): ypT2N0.

	Result	Intensity	Positive %
Estrogen receptor	Negative (0/8)	0	0
Progesterone receptor	Negative (0/8)	0	0
C-erbB2	Negative (0)		
Ki-67	Positive in 75% of tumor cells		

33　Case 33

33.1　Patient History and Progress

Female/52 years old, post-menopause.
Screen detected mass lesion on left breast 11 o'clock direction.
No family history.
s/p cervical cancer (stage 0).
BRCA 1 and 2 mutation: Not detected.

33.2　Important Radiologic Findings

See Figs. 243, 244, 245 and 246.

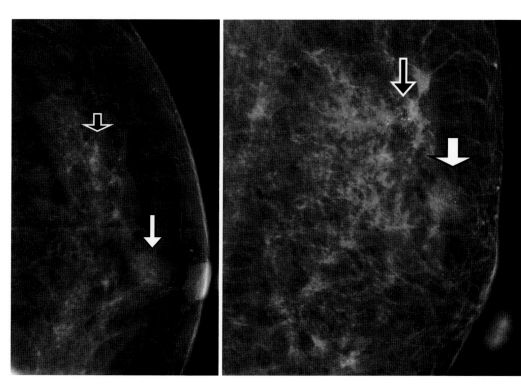

Fig. 243 Mammography (May. 2021): An irregular isodense mass (white arrow) with microcalcifications at 12 o'clock direction of left breast. Associated fine pleomorphic microcalcifications with focal asymmetries (black arrow) in the upper outer quadrant of the left breast

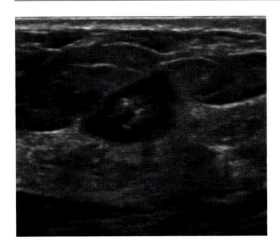

Fig. 244 Breast US (May. 2021): An irregular hypoechoic mass with microcalcifications at 12 o'clock direction of left breast

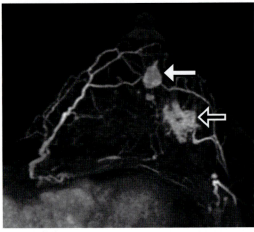

Fig. 245 Breast MRI (May. 2021): An irregular enhancing mass (white arrow) at the 12 o'clock direction of the left breast. Associated non-mass enhancement (black arrow) in the upper outer quadrant of the left breast

Fig. 246 PET-CT shows a hypermetabolic lesion in the left breast (mSUV = 3.8)

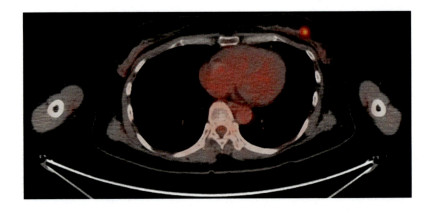

33.2.1 After Neoadjuvant Chemotherapy

See Figs. 247, 248, 249 and 250.

33.3 Courses of Treatment

Neoadjuvant chemotherapy (#4 cycles of doxorubicin and cyclophosphamide + #4 cycles of docetaxel) + Operation + Post-operative radiation therapy.

33.3.1 Operation

Left breast conserving surgery, sentinel lymph node biopsy (Fig. 251).

33.3.2 Pathology Report

Atypical ductal hyperplasia, focal

1. Post-chemotherapy status.
2. Lymph nodes: no metastasis in one axillary lymph node (ypN0(sn)) (sentinel LN: 0/1).

	Result	Intensity	Positive %
Estrogen receptor	Negative (0/8)	0	0
Progesterone receptor	Negative (0/8)	0	0
C-erbB2	Negative (1+)		
Ki-67	Positive in 61% of tumor cells		

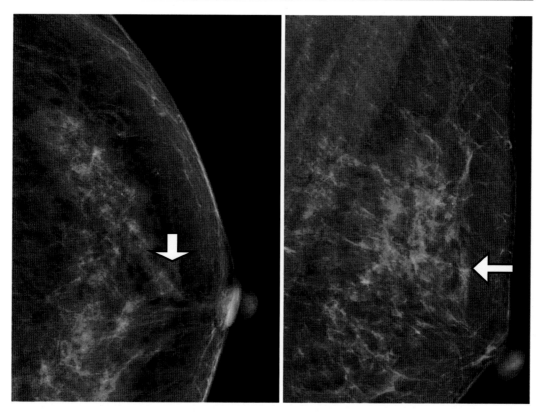

Fig. 247 Mammography (Nov. 2021): mammography after treatment demonstrates residual mass that is decreased in size

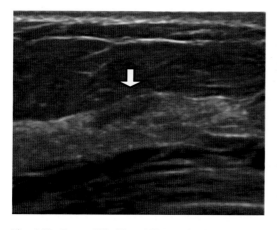

Fig. 248 Breast US (Nov. 2021): US after treatment demonstrates residual isoechoic mass that is decreased in the longest diameter

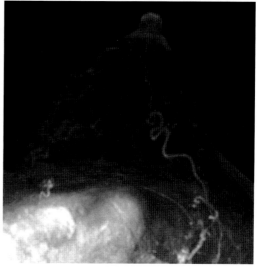

Fig. 249 Breast MRI (Nov. 2021): MRI after treatment shows complete resolution of enhancement in the left breast

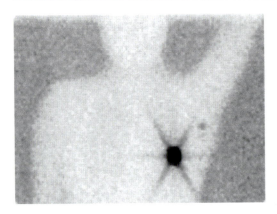

Fig. 250 Lymphoscintigraphy shows visualized sentinel lymph nodes in the left axilla

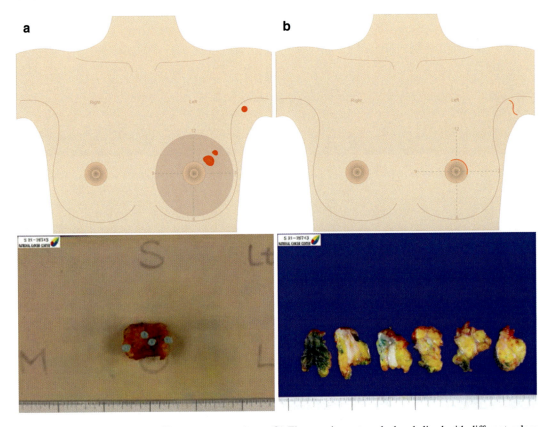

Fig. 251 (a) Gross pathology of lumpectomy specimen. (b) The margins get marked and sliced with different colors on each direction

34 Case 34

34.1 Patient History and Progress

Female/79 years old, post-menopause.

Screen detected mass lesion on left breast 12 o'clock direction.

No family history.

S/P paraffin injection, s/p appendectomy, s/p hysterectomy, s/p hemicolectomy (colon cancer).

S/P radical total gastrostomy (advanced gastric cancer).

BRCA 1 and 2 mutation: Not detected, BARD1 VUS (variant of uncertain).

34.2 Important Radiologic Findings

See Figs. 252, 253, and 254.

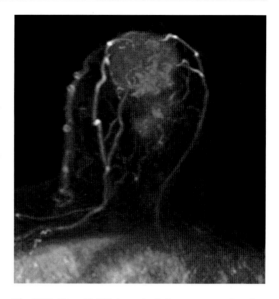

Fig. 253 Breast MRI: irregular heterogeneous enhancing masses in the upper portion of the left breast

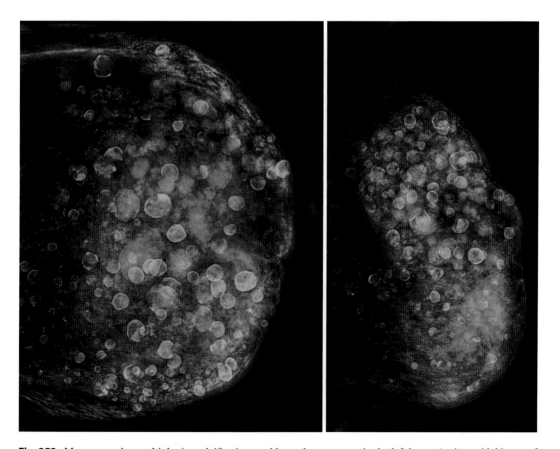

Fig. 252 Mammography: multiple rim calcifications and hyperdense masses in the left breast (patient with history of foreign body injection for cosmetic augmentation

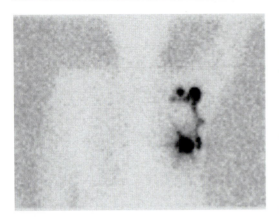

Fig. 254 Lymphoscintigraphy shows visualized sentinel lymph nodes in the left axilla

34.3 Courses of Treatment

Operation + Adjuvant chemotherapy (#1 cycles of docetaxel and cyclophosphamide, stop d/t mucositis).

34.3.1 Operation

Left modified radical mastectomy, sentinel lymph node biopsy (Fig. 255).

34.3.2 Pathology Report

Invasive Ductal Carcinoma associated with paraffinoma

1. Size of tumor: 3.0 cm (pT2).

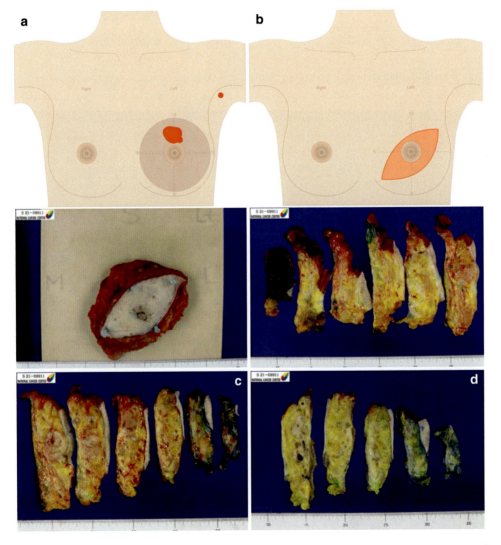

Fig. 255 (a) Gross pathology of lumpectomy specimen. (b, c, d) The margins get marked and sliced with different colors on each direction

HR(−) HER2(−) Breast Cancer

2. Histologic grade: 3/3 (tubule formation: 3/3, nuclear pleomorphism: 3/3, mitotic count: 2/3, 8/10HPF).
3. Intraductal component: absent.
4. Skin and nipple: no involvement of tumor.
5. Surgical margins:
   (a) Deep margin: 10 mm.
   (b) Superficial margin: 21 mm.
6. Lymph nodes: no metastasis in five axillary lymph nodes (pN0(sn)) (sentinel LN: 0/5).
7. Arteriovenous invasion: absent.
8. Lymphovascular invasion: absent.
9. Tumor border: infiltrative.
10. Microcalcification: absent.
11. Pathological TN category (AJCC 2017): pT2N0(sn).

	Result	Intensity	Positive %
Estrogen receptor	Negative (0/8)	0	0
Progesterone receptor	Negative (0/8)	0	0
C-erbB2	Negative (0)		
Ki-67	Positive in 23% of tumor cells		

35 Case 35

35.1 Patient History and Progress

Female/75 years old, post-menopause.

Screen detected mass lesion on left breast 2 o'clock direction.

No family history.

Hypertension, Hyperlipidemia, s/p hysterectomy, arrhythmia (s/p operation).

35.2 Important Radiologic Findings

See Figs. 256, 257 and 258.

35.3 Courses of Treatment

Operation + Adjuvant chemotherapy (#4 cycles of doxorubicin and cyclophosphamide) + Post-operative radiation therapy.

35.3.1 Operation

Left breast conserving surgery (nautilus trial: sentinel lymph node biopsy skip arm) (Fig. 259).

35.3.2 Pathology Report

Invasive Ductal Carcinoma with apocrine differentiation

1. Size of tumor: 1.1 cm (pT1c).
2. Histologic grade: 3/3 (tubule formation: 3/3, nuclear pleomorphism: 3/3, mitotic count: 2/3, 6/10HPF).
3. Intraductal component: present, extratumoral (10%) (nuclear grade: high, necrosis: present, architectural pattern: cribriform/solid/comedo, extensive intraductal component: absent).
4. Skin: no involvement of tumor.
5. Surgical margins:
   (a) Superior margin: 8 mm.
   (b) Inferior margin: 13 mm.
   (c) Medial margin: (see note).
   (d) Lateral margin: 15 mm.
   (e) Deep margin: 2 mm.
   (f) Superficial margin: 15 mm.
6. Arteriovenous invasion: absent.
7. Lymphovascular invasion: absent.
8. Tumor border: infiltrative.
9. Microcalcification: present, tumoral/non-tumoral.
10. Pathological TN category (AJCC 2017): pT1cNx.

Note: 1. The medial margin of the lumpectomy specimen (slide 5) is close to ductal carcinoma in situ (2 mm), but this margin submitted for frozen diagnosis (Fro 3) is free of tumor.

	Result	Intensity	Positive %
Estrogen receptor	Negative (0/8)	0	0
Progesterone receptor	Negative (0/8)	0	0
C-erbB2	Equivocal (2+)		
Ki-67	Positive in 7% of tumor cells		

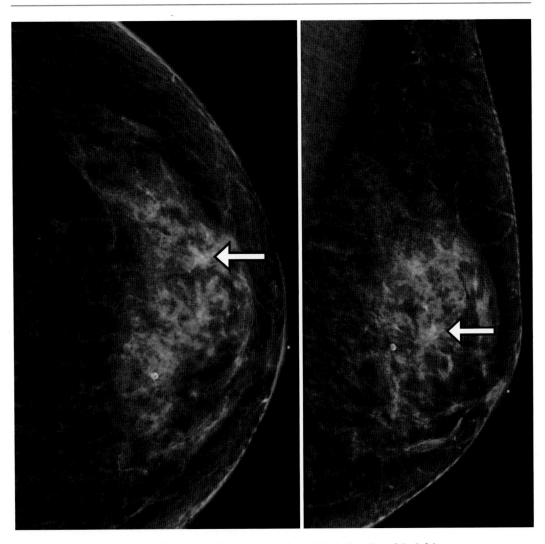

Fig. 256 Mammography (May 2021): A focal asymmetry at the 3 o'clock direction of the left breast

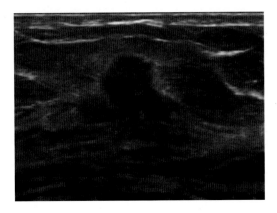

Fig. 257 Breast US (May. 2021): An irregular hypoechoic mass with echogenic halo at the 3 o'clock direction of the left breast

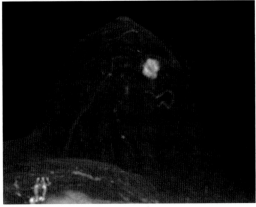

Fig. 258 Breast MRI (May. 2021): An irregular enhancing mass at the 3 o'clock direction of the left breast

HR(−) HER2(−) Breast Cancer

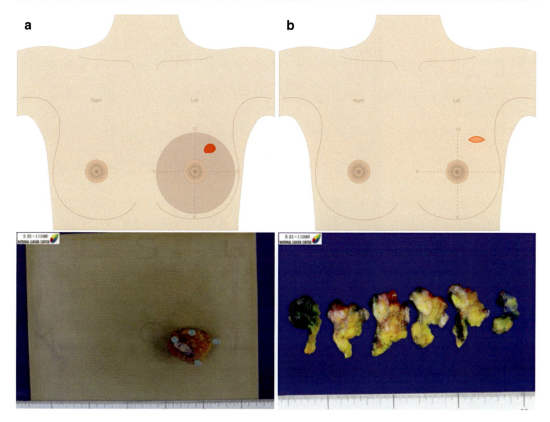

Fig. 259 (**a**) Gross pathology of lumpectomy specimen. (**b**) The margins get marked and sliced with different colors on each direction

36 Case 36

36.1 Patient History and Progress

Female/46 years old, pre-menopause.

Self-detected palpable mass lesion on left axillary.

Family history of breast cancer, aunt (maternal).

Hepatitis B virus carrier.

BRCA 1 and 2 mutation: Not detected, RET VUS (variant of uncertain).

36.2 Important Radiologic Findings

See Figs. 260, 261, 262 and 263.

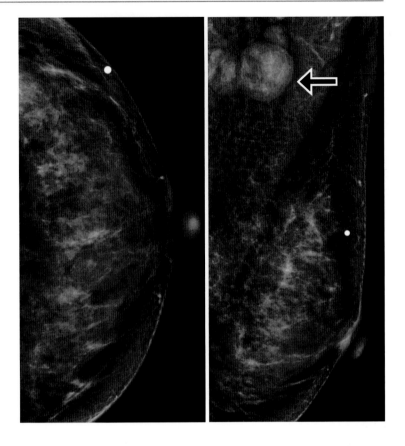

Fig. 260 Mammography (Jun. 2021): A focal asymmetry with microcalcifications in the upper outer quadrant of left breast (marked by BB marker). Multiple lymph nodes (black arrow) in left axilla

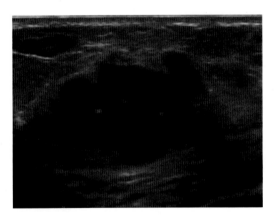

Fig. 261 Breast US (Jun. 2021): An irregular hypoechoic mass with microcalcifications at the 2 o'clock direction of the left breast

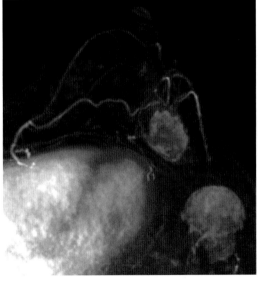

Fig. 262 Breast MRI (Jun. 2021): An irregular enhancing mass at the 2 o'clock direction of the left breast. Enlarged lymph nodes in the left axilla

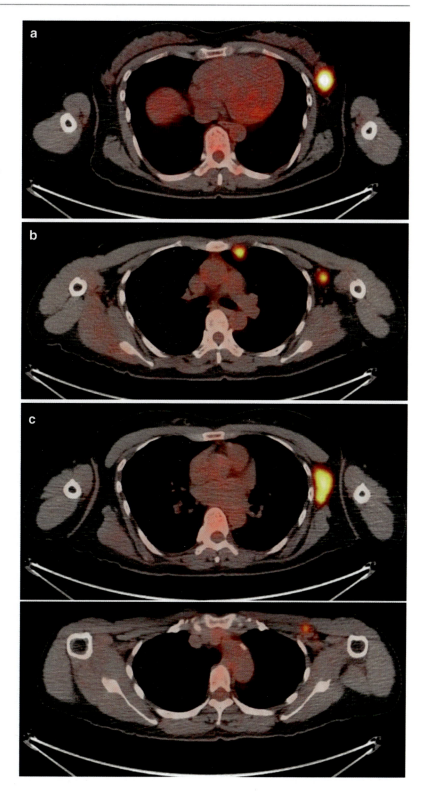

Fig. 263 PET-CT shows (**a**) hypermetabolic mass in the left breast (mSUV = 13.4), (**b**) an enlarged hypermetabolic lymph node in left internal mammary area (mSUV = 6.7), and (**c**) hypermetabolic lymph node in the left axilla level I–III (mSUV = 8.7)

36.2.1 After Neoadjuvant Chemotherapy

See Figs. 264, 265 and 266.

36.3 Courses of Treatment

Neoadjuvant chemotherapy (#4 cycles of doxorubicin and cyclophosphamide + #4 cycles of docetaxel) + Operation + Post-operative radiation therapy.

36.3.1 Operation

Left breast conserving surgery, sentinel lymph node biopsy (Fig. 267).

36.3.2 Pathology Report

1. No residual tumor with foamy histiocytic collection.
    (a) Post-chemotherapy status.
    (b) Lymph nodes: no metastasis in two axillary lymph nodes (ypN0(sn)) (sentinel LN: 0/2).
    (c) Related slides: S21–10541, S21–10544.
2. Adenomyoepithelial hyperplasia with microcalcification.

	Result	Intensity	Positive %
Estrogen receptor	Negative (0/8)	0	0
Progesterone receptor	Negative (0/8)	0	0
C-erbB2	Negative (0)		
Ki-67	Positive in 66% of tumor cells		

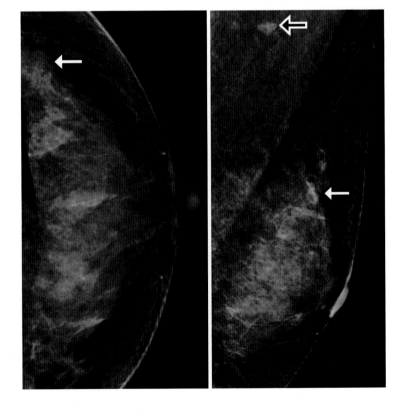

Fig. 264 Mammography (Nov. 2021): mammography after treatment demonstrates residual mass that is decreased in size. Decrease in size of previously enlarged lymph nodes in the left axilla (black arrow)

HR(−) HER2(−) Breast Cancer

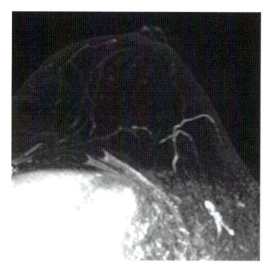

Fig. 265 Breast MRI (Nov. 2021): MRI after treatment shows complete resolution of enhancement in the left breast

Fig. 266 Lymphoscintigraphy shows visualized sentinel lymph nodes in the left axilla

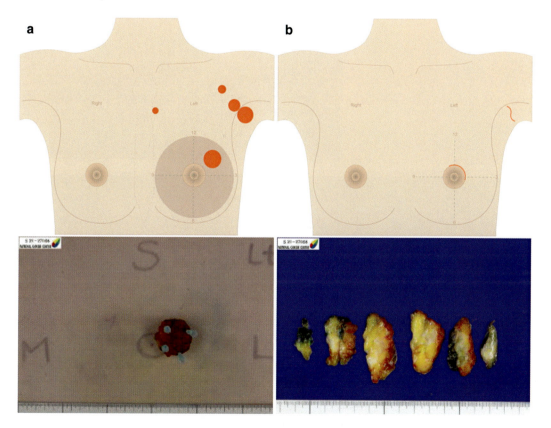

Fig. 267 (**a**) Gross pathology of lumpectomy specimen. (**b**) The margins get marked and sliced with different colors on each direction

37 Case 37

37.1 Patient History and Progress

Female/46 years old, pre-menopause.
Self-detected palpable mass lesion on right breast.
Family history of breast cancer, aunt (maternal).
s/p myomectomy.
BRCA 1 and 2 mutation: Not detected.

37.2 Important Radiologic Findings

See Figs. 268, 269, 270 and 271.

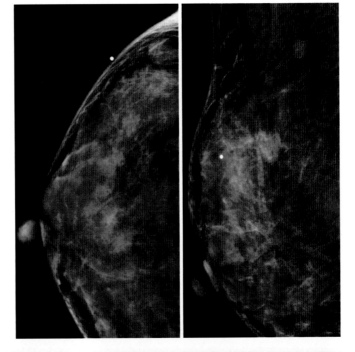

Fig. 268 Mammography (Jun. 2021): An irregular hyperdense mass with microcalcifications in the upper outer quadrant of the right breast (marked by BB marker)

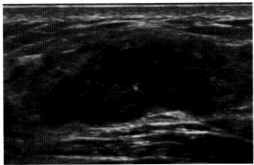

Fig. 269 Breast US (Jun. 2021): An irregular hypoechoic mass with microcalcification at the 10 o'clock direction of the right breast

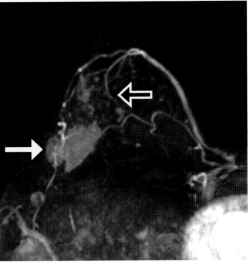

Fig. 270 Breast MRI (Jun. 2021): An irregular enhancing masses (white arrow) with associated heterogeneous non-mass enhancement (black arrow) in the upper outer quadrant of the right breast

Fig. 271 PET-CT shows (**a**) hypermetabolic lesions in the right breast (mSUV = 8.0) and (**b**) hypermetabolic LNs in the right axilla, level I (mSUV = 9.4)

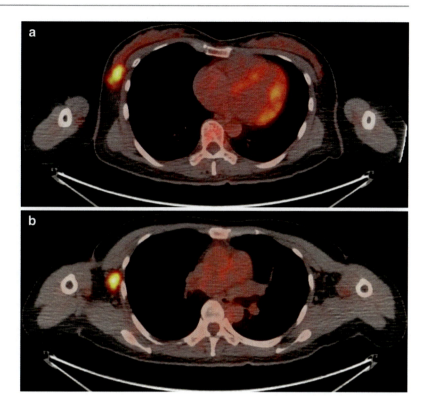

37.2.1 After Neoadjuvant Chemotherapy

See Figs. 272, 273, 274 and 275.

37.3 Courses of Treatment

Neoadjuvant chemotherapy (#4 cycles of doxorubicin and cyclophosphamide + #4 cycles of docetaxel) + Operation + Postoperative radiation therapy + Adjuvant capecitabine.

37.3.1 Operation

Right breast conserving surgery, sentinel lymph node biopsy (Fig. 276).

37.3.2 Pathology Report

Invasive Ductal Carcinoma
1. Post-chemotherapy status.
2. Size of invasive component: up to 0.3 cm, multifocal (ypT1a).
3. Size of intraductal component: 2.0 cm.
4. Histologic grade: 3/3 (tubule formation: 3/3, nuclear pleomorphism: 3/3, mitotic count: 2/3, 3/HPF).
5. Intraductal component: present, intratumoral/extratumoral (80%) (nuclear grade: high, necrosis: present, architectural pattern: papillary/micropapillary/cribriform/solid/comedo, extensive intraductal component: absent/present).
6. Skin: no involvement of tumor.
7. Surgical margins:
    (a) Superior margin: 20 mm.
    (b) Inferior margin: 5 mm.
    (c) Medial margin: (see note).
    (d) Lateral margin: 5 mm.
    (e) Deep margin: 2 mm.
    (f) Superficial margin: 2 mm.
8. Lymph nodes:
    (a) metastasis in two out of six axillary lymph nodes (ypN1a) (sentinel LN: 1/1, axillary LN: 0/4, intramammary LN: 1/1),
    (b) perinodal extension: present,
    (c) size of metastatic carcinoma: 4 mm.
9. Arteriovenous invasion: absent.

Fig. 272 Mammography (Dec. 2021): Mammography after treatment demonstrates residual mass that is decreased in the longest diameter

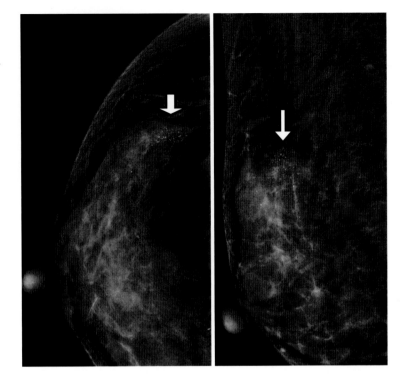

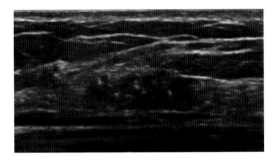

Fig. 273 Breast US (Dec. 2021): US after treatment demonstrates residual hypoechoic mass with microcalcifications that is decreased in the longest diameter

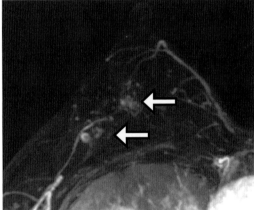

Fig. 274 Breast MRI (Dec. 2021): MRI after treatment demonstrates residual non-mass enhancement (white arrows)

HR(−) HER2(−) Breast Cancer

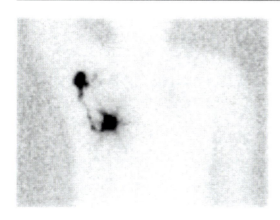

Fig. 275 Lymphoscintigraphy shows visualized sentinel lymph nodes in the right axilla

10. Lymphovascular invasion: present, intratumoral/peritumoral.
11. Tumor border: infiltrative.
12. Microcalcification: present, tumoral/non-tumoral.
13. Pathological TN category (AJCC 2017): ypT1aN1a.

	Result	Intensity	Positive %
Estrogen receptor	Weak (3/8)	1	1%–10%
Progesterone receptor	Negative (0/8)	0	0
C-erbB2	Negative (1+)		
Ki-67	Positive in 29% of tumor cells		

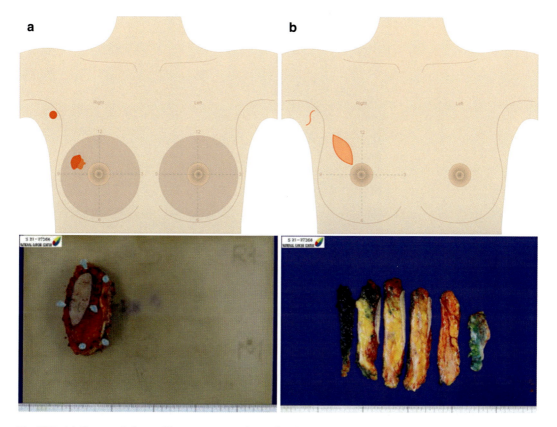

Fig. 276 (a) Gross pathology of lumpectomy specimen. (b) The margins get marked and sliced with different colors on each direction

38 Case 38

38.1 Patient History and Progress

Female/52 years old, post-menopause.

Self-detected palpable mass lesion on right breast.

No family history.

s/p bilateral salpingo-oophorectomy.
BRCA 1 mutation carrier.

38.2 Important Radiologic Findings

See Figs. 277, 278, 279 and 280.

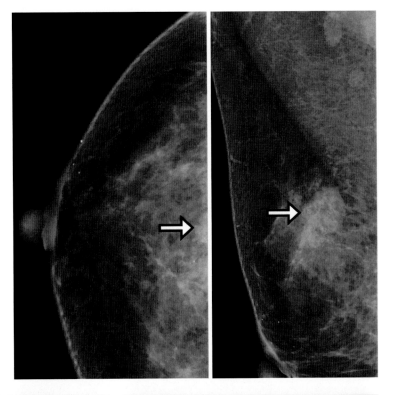

Fig. 277 Mammography (Jun. 2021): An irregular hyperdense mass with fine pleomorphic in the upper portion of the right breast

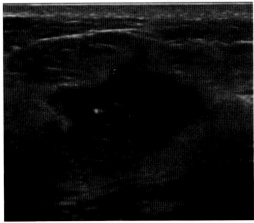

Fig. 278 Breast US (Jun. 2021): An irregular hypoechoic mass with microcalcification at the 12 o'clock direction of the right breast

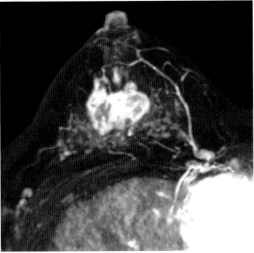

Fig. 279 Breast MRI (Jun. 2021): An irregular enhancing mass at the 12 o'clock direction of the right breast

Fig. 280 PET-CT shows hypermetabolic mass in the right upper breast (mSUV = 11.1)

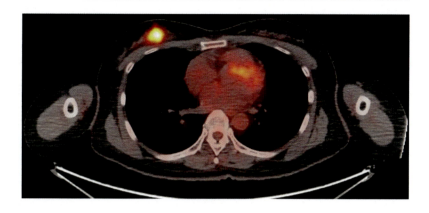

38.2.1 After Neoadjuvant Chemotherapy

See Figs. 281, 282, 283 and 284.

38.3 Courses of Treatment

Neoadjuvant chemotherapy (#4 cycles of doxorubicin and cyclophosphamide + #4 cycles of docetaxel) + Operation + Post-operative radiation therapy.

38.3.1 Operation

Bilateral nipple-areolar complex sparing mastectomy + implant reconstruction, sentinel lymph node biopsy (right) (Figs. 285 and 286).

38.3.2 Pathology Report

No residual tumor with stromal degeneration

1. Post-chemotherapy status.
2. Lymph nodes: no metastasis in one axillary lymph node (ypN0(sn)) (sentinel LN: 0/1).
3. Microcalcification: present.

	Result	Intensity	Positive %
Estrogen receptor	Negative (0/8)	0	0
Progesterone receptor	Negative (0/8)	0	0
C-erbB2	Negative (1+)		
Ki-67	Positive in 62% of tumor cells		

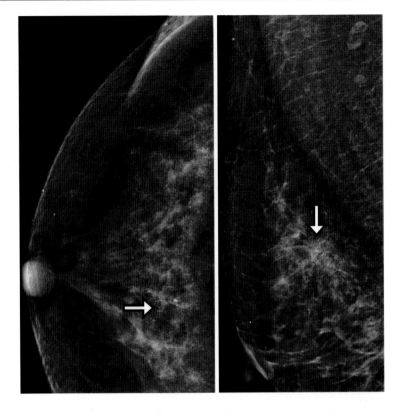

Fig. 281 Mammography (Dec. 2021): mammography after treatment demonstrates residual mass that is decreased in the longest diameter

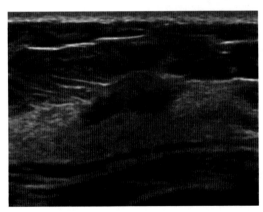

Fig. 282 Breast US (Dec. 2021): US after treatment demonstrates residual hypoechoic mass that is decreased in the longest diameter

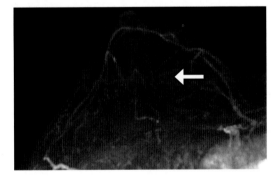

Fig. 283 Breast MRI (Dec. 2021): MRI after treatment demonstrates the residual non-mass enhancement (white arrow)

HR(−) HER2(−) Breast Cancer

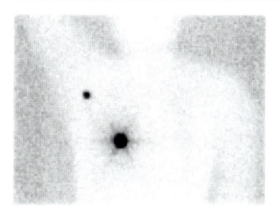

Fig. 284 Lymphoscintigraphy shows visualized sentinel lymph nodes in the right axilla

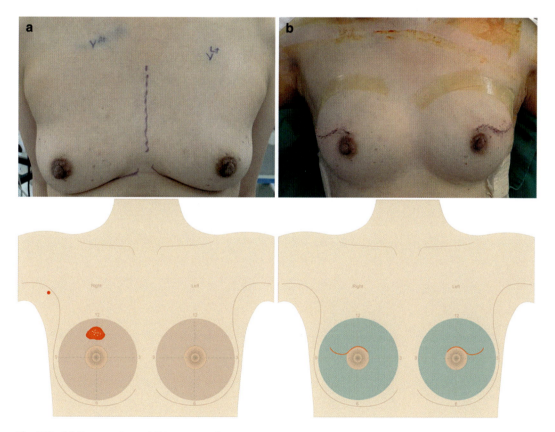

Fig. 285 (**a**) Preoperative and (**b**) postoperative appearance

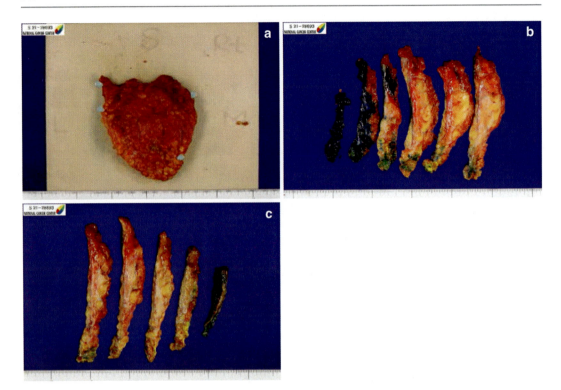

Fig. 286 (**a**) Gross pathology of mastectomy (right) specimen. (**b, c**) The margins get marked and sliced with different colors on each direction

Local Recurrence

Yunju Kim, Eun-Gyeong Lee, Ran Song, and Eun Sook Lee

1 Case 1

1.1 Patient History and Progress

Female/41 years old, pre-menopause.

Screen detected mass lesion on lower medial and lower outer portion of right breast.

Family history of breast cancer, maternal aunt. No comorbidities.

BRCA 1 and 2 mutation: Not detected.

1.2 Courses of Treatment

Right breast IDC → Neoadjuvant chemotherapy → Operation → Adjuvant therapy → **Right breast recurrence (IDC)**.

1.2.1 Primary Treatment

See Figs. 1, 2, 3 and 4.

Neoadjuvant Chemotherapy

Neoadjuvant chemotherapy #4 cycles of doxorubicin and cyclophosphamide followed by #4 cycles of docetaxel and trastuzumab.

Operation

Sep. 2012 Right breast conserving surgery, sentinel lymph node biopsy (Fig. 5).

Pathology Report

Invasive Ductal Carcinoma
1. Post-chemotherapy status.
2. Size of tumor: 0.4 cm (ypT1a).

Y. Kim
Department of Pathology, National Cancer Center, Goyang, Gyeonggi, Republic of Korea
e-mail: radkyj@ncc.re.kr

E.-G. Lee · R. Song
Division of Surgery, Center for Breast Cancer, National Cancer Center, Goyang, Republic of Korea
e-mail: bnf333@ncc.re.kr; thdfks37@ncc.re.kr

E. S. Lee (✉)
Center for Breast Cancer, National Cancer Center, Goyang, Kyonggi-do, Republic of Korea
e-mail: eslee@ncc.re.kr

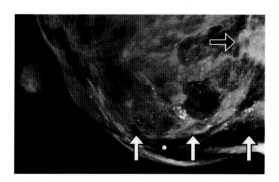

Fig. 1 Right mammography (Mar. 2012): Segmental fine pleomorphic microcalcifications (white arrows) with an irregular mass (black arrow) at lower breast. US-CNB = IDC

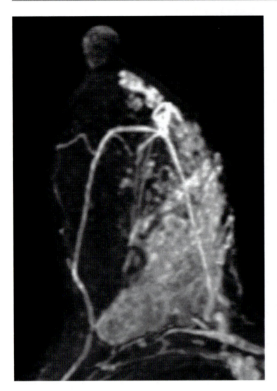

Fig. 2 Right MRI (Mar. 2012): Segmental clustered ring non-mass enhancement at lower breast

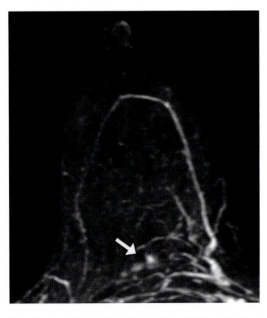

Fig. 3 Post-NAC right MRI (Sep. 2012): Residual enhancing foci at lower central breast

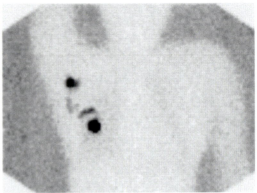

Fig. 4 Lymphoscintigraphy shows visualized sentinel lymph nodes in the right axilla

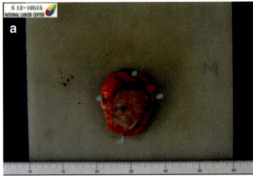

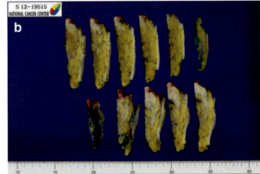

Fig. 5 (**a**) Gross pathology of lumpectomy specimen. (**b**) The margins get marked and sliced with different colors on each direction

3. Histologic grade: 2/3 (tubule formation: 3/3, nuclear pleomorphism: 3/3, mitotic count: 1/3, 1/10HPF).
4. Intraductal component: present, intratumoral/extratumoral (10%) (nuclear grade: high,

necrosis: absent, architectural pattern: cribriform, extensive intraductal component: absent).
5. Skin: no involvement of tumor.
6. Surgical margins:
   (a) Superior margin: 40 mm.
   (b) Inferior margin: 30 mm.
   (c) Medial margin: 5 mm.
   (d) Lateral margin: 15 mm.
   (e) Deep margin: 1 mm from invasive ductal carcinoma.
7. Lymph nodes: no metastasis in two axillary lymph nodes (ypN0(sn)) (sentinel LN: 0/2).
8. Vascular invasion: absent.
9. Lymphatic invasion: present, intratumoral.
10. Tumor border: infiltrative.
11. Microcalcification: present, tumoral/non-tumoral.
12. Pathologic stage (AJCC 2010): ypT1aN0(sn).

	Result	Intensity	Positive %
Estrogen receptor	Weak (2/7)	1	<10%
Progesterone receptor	Negative (0/7)	0	0
C-erbB2	Positive (3+)		
Ki-67	Positive in 7% of tumor cells		

Adjuvant Therapy

Postoperative radiation therapy.

Trastuzumab for 1 year + Tamoxifen 20 mg/day for 8.9 years.

1.2.2 Treatments After Recurrence

See Figs. 6, 7 and 8.

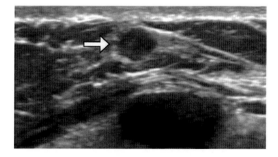

Fig. 6 Right US for routine surveillance (Jun. 2021): A new oval hypoechoic mass at lower inner breast. US-CNB = IDC

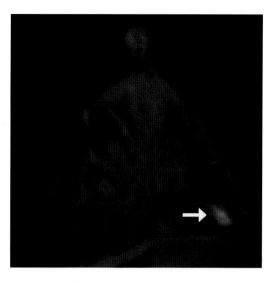

Fig. 7 Right MRI (Jul. 2021): A small enhancing mass (white arrow = proven IDC) at lower inner breast

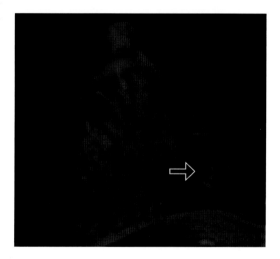

Fig. 8 Post-NAC right MRI (Dec. 2021): Nearly disappeared index tumor at lower inner breast. An artifact related to the inserted clip (black arrow)

Neoadjuvant Therapy

Neoadjuvant chemotherapy #6 cycles of docetaxel and trastuzumab and pertuzumab.

Operation

Dec. 2021 Right breast conserving surgery (Fig. 9).

Pathology Report

No residual tumor with stromal degeneration.

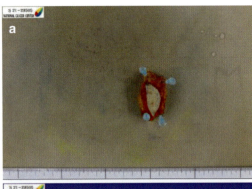

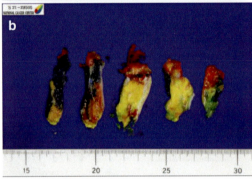

Fig. 9 (a) Gross pathology of lumpectomy specimen. (b) The margins get marked and sliced with different colors on each direction

1. Post-chemotherapy status.
2. Post-lumpectomy status.

	Result	Intensity	Positive %
Estrogen receptor	Negative (2/8)	1	<1%
Progesterone receptor	Negative (0/8)	0	0
C-erbB2	Positive (3+)		
Ki-67	Positive in 18% of tumor cells		

Adjuvant Therapy
Postoperative radiation therapy.
  Trastuzumab and pertuzumab.

2 Case 2

2.1 Patient History and Progress

Female/54 years old, peri-menopause.

Screen detected mass lesion on left breast 2 o'clock direction.
  No family history.
  No comorbidities.

2.2 Courses of Treatment

Left breast IDC → Operation → Adjuvant therapy → **Left breast recurrence (IDC).**

2.2.1 Primary Treatment
See Fig. 10.

Operation
Nov. 2008 Left breast conserving surgery, sentinel lymph node biopsy (outside).

Pathology Report

Invasive Ductal Carcinoma
1. Size of tumor: 0.4 cm (pT1a).
2. Lymph nodes: no metastasis in three axillary lymph nodes (pN0(sn)) (sentinel LN: 0/3).
3. Pathologic stage (AJCC 2010): pT1aN0(sn).

	Result	Intensity	Positive %
Estrogen receptor	Negative		
Progesterone receptor	Negative		
C-erbB2	Positive		

Adjuvant Therapy
Postoperative radiation therapy.

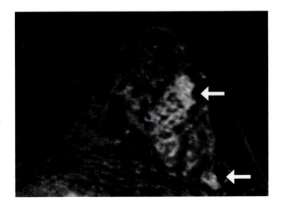

Fig. 10 Left MRI (2008): Irregular enhancing masses with non-mass enhancement at upper outer breast

Local Recurrence

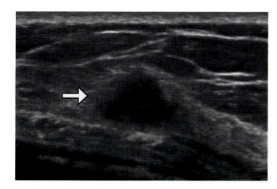

Fig. 11 Left US for evaluation of a palpable lump (2018): An irregular hypoechoic mass at the symptomatic area of upper inner breast. US-CNB = IDC

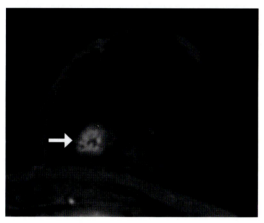

Fig. 12 Left MRI (2018): An irregular enhancing mass at upper inner breast

2.2.2 Treatments After Recurrence
See Figs. 11 and 12.

Operation

Feb. 2018 Left nipple-areolar complex sparing mastectomy with immediate implant reconstruction, sentinel lymph node biopsy (Fig. 13).

Pathology Report

Invasive Ductal Carcinoma, clinically recurrent
1. Post-lumpectomy status.
2. Size of tumor: 0.8 cm (rpT1b).
3. Histologic grade: 3/3 (tubule formation: 3/3, nuclear pleomorphism: 3/3, mitotic count: 3/3, 27/10HPF).
4. Intraductal component: absent, extratumoral (20%) (nuclear grade: high, necrosis: absent, architectural pattern: micropapillary/cribriform, extensive intraductal component: absent).
5. Surgical margins:
   (a) Deep margin: 1.5 mm.
   (b) Superficial margin: 7 mm.
6. Lymph nodes: no metastasis in one axillary lymph node (rpN0(sn)) (sentinel LN: 0/1).
7. Arteriovenous invasion: absent.
8. Lymphovascular invasion: absent.
9. Tumor border: infiltrative.
10. Microcalcification: present, tumoral.
11. Pathologic stage (AJCC 2017): rpT1bN0(sn).

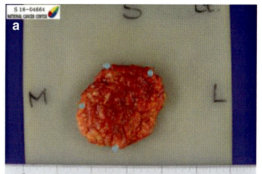
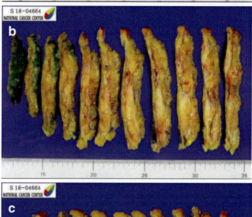
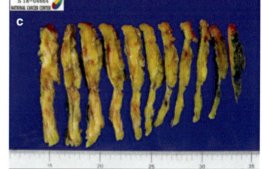

Fig. 13 (**a**) Gross pathology of mastectomy specimen. (**b, c**) The margins get marked and sliced with different colors on each direction

	Result	Intensity	Positive %
Estrogen receptor	Negative (0/8)	0	0
Progesterone receptor	Negative (0/8)	0	0
C-erbB2	Positive (3+)		
Ki-67	Positive in 50% of tumor cells		

Adjuvant Therapy

Adjuvant chemotherapy #4 cycles of docetaxel with concurrent trastuzumab for 2 years.

3 Case 3

3.1 Patient History and Progress

Female/47 years old, pre-menopause.
Screen detected microcalcification on upper portion of left breast.
Family history of colon cancer, father.
No comorbidities.

3.2 Courses of Treatment

Left breast IDC + DCIS → Operation → Left breast recurrence (DCIS).

See Figs. 14 and 15.

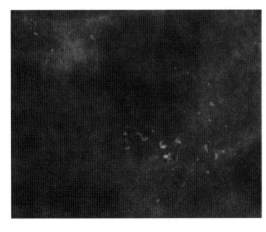

Fig. 14 Left magnification view (2018): Multifocal fine pleomorphic microcalcifications at upper central breast. Excisional biopsy = DCIS, high grade

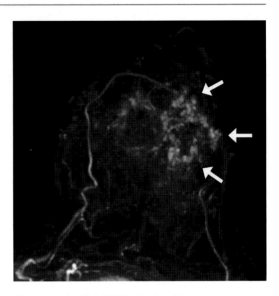

Fig. 15 Left MRI (2018): Regional heterogeneous non-mass enhancement at upper breast

3.2.1 Operation

First Operation (Aug. 2018) Left breast mass excision (Fig. 16).

3.2.2 Pathology Report

Ductal Carcinoma In Situ

1. Size of tumor: 1.5 cm.
2. Nuclear grade: high.
3. Necrosis: present.
4. Architectural pattern: solid/comedo.
5. Surgical margins:
    (a) Superior margin: 2 mm (slide 6).
    (b) Inferior margin: 1.5 mm (slide 6).
    (c) Medial margin: 10 mm.
    (d) Lateral margin: <1 mm (slide 7).
    (e) Deep margin: 2 mm.
6. Microcalcification: present, tumoral/non-tumoral.

	Result	Intensity	Positive %
Estrogen receptor	Negative (0/8)	0	0
Progesterone receptor	Negative (2/8)	1	<1%
C-erbB2	Positive (3+)		
Ki-67	Positive in 35% of tumor cells		

Local Recurrence

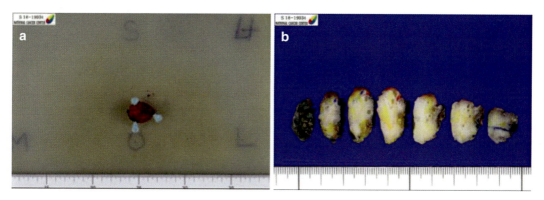

Fig. 16 (**a**) Gross pathology of breast mass excision specimen. (**b**) The margins get marked and sliced with different colors on each direction

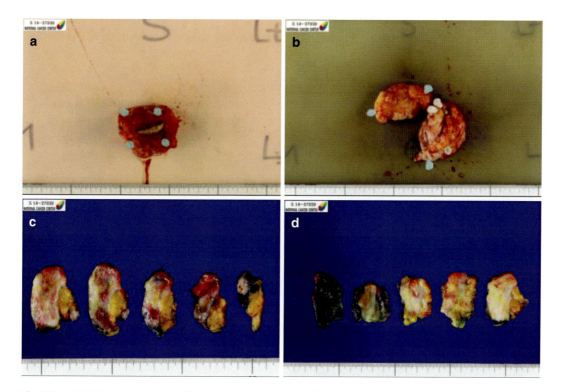

Fig. 17 (**a**, **b**) Gross pathology of wide excision specimen. (**c**, **d**) The margins get marked and sliced with different colors on each direction

3.2.3 Operation

Second Operation (Dec. 2018) Left breast wide excision (Fig. 17).

3.2.4 Pathology Report

Invasive Ductal Carcinoma
1. Post-excision status.
2. Size of invasive component: 0.2 cm (pT1a).
3. Size of intraductal component: 3.5 cm.
4. Histologic grade: 2/3 (tubule formation: 3/3, nuclear pleomorphism: 3/3, mitotic count: 1/3, <1/10HPF).
5. Intraductal component: present, extratumoral (99%) (nuclear grade: high, necrosis: present, architectural pattern: micropapillary/cribriform/solid/comedo, extensive intraductal component: present).

6. Skin: no involvement of tumor.
7. Surgical margins:
   (a) Superior margin: (see note 1).
   (b) Inferior margin: (see note 2).
   (c) Medial margin: 15 mm.
   (d) Lateral margin: (see note 3).
   (e) Deep margin: <1 mm from ductal carcinoma in situ (slide 14).
   (f) Superficial margin: 2 mm.
8. Arteriovenous invasion: absent.
9. Lymphovascular invasion: absent.
10. Tumor border: infiltrative.
11. Microcalcification: present, tumoral.
12. Pathological TN category (AJCC 2017): pT1a.

	Result	Intensity	Positive %
Estrogen receptor	Negative (0/8)	0	0
Progesterone receptor	Negative (0/8)	0	0
C-erbB2	Positive (3+)		
Ki-67	Positive in 65% of tumor cells		

3.3 Treatments After Recurrence

See Figs. 18, 19 and 20.

3.3.1 Operation

Dec. 2021 Left nipple-areolar complex sparing mastectomy with immediate implant reconstruction, sentinel lymph node biopsy (Fig. 21).

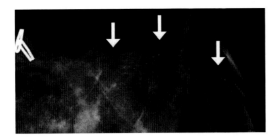

Fig. 18 Left mammography for routine surveillance (2021): Newly developed linear microcalcifications at the op bed

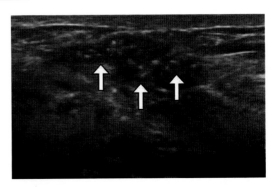

Fig. 19 Left US (2021): A focal hypoechoic lesion with echogenic microcalcifications at the op bed. US-CNB = DCIS, high grade

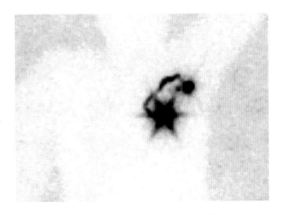

Fig. 20 Lymphoscintigraphy shows visualized sentinel lymph nodes in the left axilla

3.3.2 Pathology Report

Ductal Carcinoma In Situ
1. Post-excision status.
2. Size of tumor: 1.5 cm (rpTis).
3. Nuclear grade: high.
4. Necrosis: present.
5. Architectural pattern: micropapillary.
6. Skin: no involvement of tumor.
7. Surgical margins:
   (a) Deep margin: 2 mm.
   (b) Superficial margin: 2 mm.
8. Lymph nodes: no metastasis in one axillary lymph node (pN0(sn)) (sentinel LN:0/1).

Local Recurrence

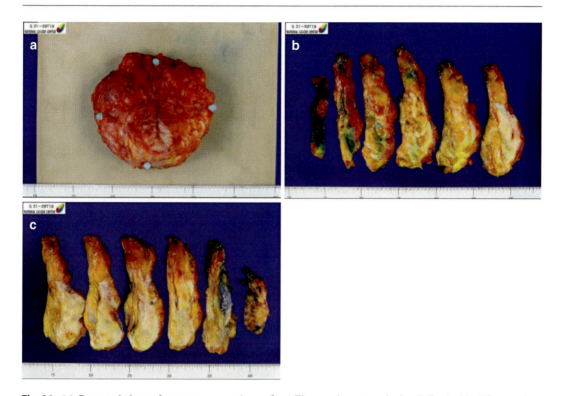

Fig. 21 (**a**) Gross pathology of mastectomy specimen. (**b**, **c**) The margins get marked and sliced with different colors on each direction

9. Microcalcification: present, tumoral/non-tumoral.
10. Pathological TN category (AJCC 2017): rpTisN0(sn).

	Result	Intensity	Positive %
Estrogen receptor	Negative (0/8)	0	0
Progesterone receptor	Negative (0/8)	0	0
C-erbB2	Positive (3+)		
Ki-67	Positive in 19% of tumor cells		

4 Case 4

4.1 Patient History and Progress

Female/41 years old, pre-menopause.

Screen detected mass lesion on left breast 1 and 2 o'clock direction.

Outside result of biopsy: Ductal carcinoma in situ.

No family history.

No comorbidities.
BRCA 1 and 2 mutation: Not detected.

4.2 Courses of Treatment

Left breast Invasive cribriform carcinoma → Operation → Adjuvant therapy → Left chest wall recurrence (IDC).

4.2.1 Primary Treatment
See Figs. 22, 23 and 24.

Operation

Jul. 2017 Left nipple-areolar complex sparing mastectomy with immediate implant reconstruction, sentinel lymph node biopsy (Figs. 25 and 26).

Pathology Report

Invasive Cribriform Carcinoma

1. Size of invasive component: 1.5 cm and 0.5 cm (pT1c).
2. Size of intraductal component: 7.0 cm.

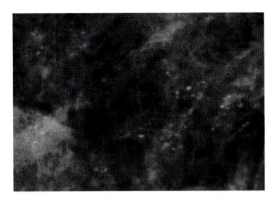

Fig. 22 Left mammography (May 2017): Amorphous and fine pleomorphic microcalcifications at upper breast. US-CNB = DCIS

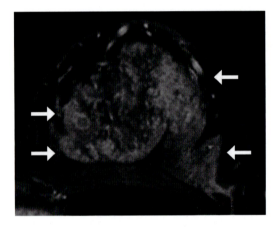

Fig. 23 Left MRI (Jun. 2017): Clumped non-mass enhancement at upper breast

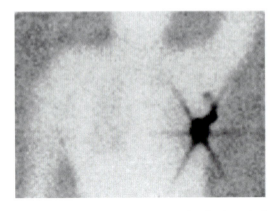

Fig. 24 Lymphoscintigraphy shows visualized sentinel lymph nodes in the left axilla

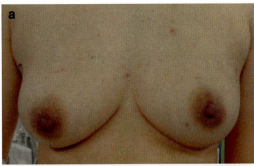

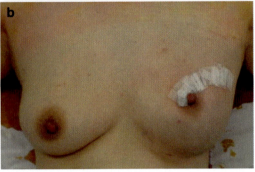

Fig. 25 (**a**) Preoperative and (**b**) immediate postoperative appearance

3. Histologic grade: 2/3 (tubule formation: 3/3, nuclear pleomorphism: 2/3, mitotic count: 1/3, 6/10HPF).
4. Intraductal component: present, intratumoral/extratumoral (90%) (nuclear grade: low, necrosis: present, architectural pattern: papillary/cribriform/solid/comedo, extensive intraductal component: present).
5. Skin: no involvement of tumor.
6. Surgical margins:
    (a) Deep margin: <1 mm from ductal carcinoma in situ (slides 4 and 15).
    (b) Superficial margin: positive for ductal carcinoma in situ (slides 5 and 10).
7. Lymph nodes: no metastasis in two axillary lymph nodes (pN0(sn)) (sentinel LN: 0/2)
8. Arteriovenous invasion: absent.
9. Lymphovascular invasion: absent.
10. Tumor border: infiltrative.
11. Microcalcification: present, tumoral.
12. Pathologic stage (AJCC 2010): pT1c(m) N0(sn).

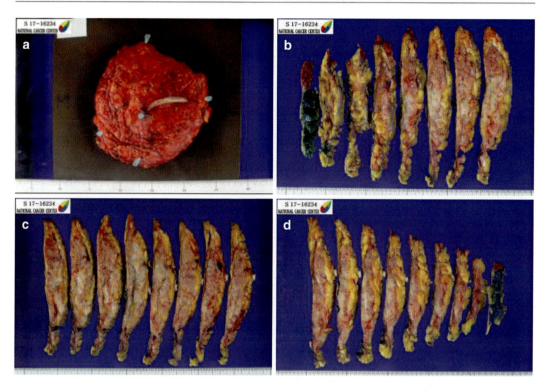

Fig. 26 (**a**) Gross pathology of mastectomy specimen. (**b, c, d**) The margins get marked and sliced with different colors on each direction

Invasive Lobular Carcinoma

1. Size of tumor: 0.4 cm.
2. Histologic grade: 2/3 (tubule formation: 3/3, nuclear pleomorphism: 2/3, mitotic count: 1/3, 2/10HPF).
3. In situ component: present, extratumoral (30%).
4. Arteriovenous invasion: absent.
5. Lymphovascular invasion: absent.
6. Tumor border: infiltrative.

	Result	Intensity	Positive %
Estrogen receptor	Strong (7/8)	2	>2/3
Progesterone receptor	Strong (7/8)	2	>2/3
C-erbB2	Negative (0)		
Ki-67	Positive in 18% of tumor cells		

Adjuvant Therapy
Tamoxifen 20 mg/day for 1.2 years.

4.2.2 Treatments After Recurrence
See Figs. 27 and 28.

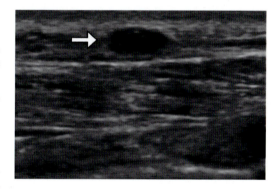

Fig. 27 US for evaluation of a palpable lump at anterior chest wall (Oct. 2018): An oval hypoechoic mass at the symptomatic area of upper inner left chest. US-CNB = IDC

Operation
Nov. 2018 Left simple mastectomy, implant removal (Fig. 29).

Pathology Report

Invasive Ductal Carcinoma
1. Post-nipple-sparing mastectomy status.
2. Size of tumor: 0.7 cm (rpT1b).

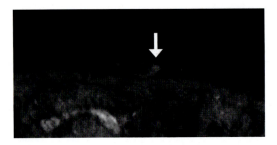

Fig. 28 MRI (Oct. 2018): An enhancing mass (white arrow = proven IDC) at subcutaneous layer of anterior chest wall

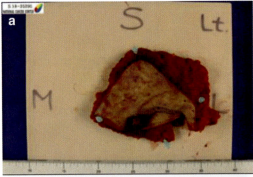

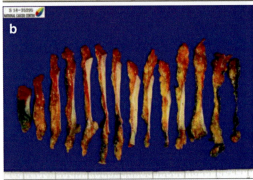

Fig. 29 (a) Gross pathology of mastectomy specimen. (b) The margins get marked and sliced with different colors on each direction

3. Histologic grade: 2/3 (tubule formation: 3/3, nuclear pleomorphism: 2/3, mitotic count: 1/3, 2/10HPF).
4. Intraductal component: present, intratumoral (10%) (nuclear grade: low, necrosis: present, architectural pattern: cribriform/comedo, extensive intraductal component: absent).
5. Skin and nipple: no involvement of tumor.
6. Surgical margins: deep margin: 3 mm.
7. Arteriovenous invasion: absent.
8. Lymphovascular invasion: absent.
9. Tumor border: infiltrative.
10. Microcalcification: present, tumoral.
11. Pathological TN category (AJCC 2017): rpT1b.

	Result	Intensity	Positive %
Estrogen receptor	Strong (8/8)	3	>2/3
Progesterone receptor	Strong (8/8)	3	>2/3
C-erbB2	Equivocal (2+) (SISH negative)		
Ki-67	Positive in 15% of tumor cells		

Adjuvant Therapy

Plan for tamoxifen with goserelin.

5 Case 5

5.1 Patient History and Progress

Female/69 years old, post-menopause.

Screen detected mass lesion on left breast 2 o'clock direction.

No family history.

No other history of disease, operation, or medication.

BRCA 1 VUS (variant of uncertain).

5.2 Courses of Treatment

Left breast IDC → Operation → Adjuvant therapy → Right breast recurrence (IDC).

5.2.1 Primary Treatment

See Figs. 30, 31 and 32.

Operation

Jan. 2006 Left breast conserving surgery, sentinel lymph node biopsy (Fig. 33).

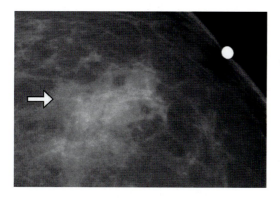

Fig. 30 Left mammography (2006): An irregular palpable mass at outer breast. US-CNB = IDC

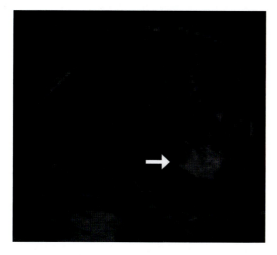

Fig. 31 Left MRI (2006): An irregular enhancing mass at outer breast

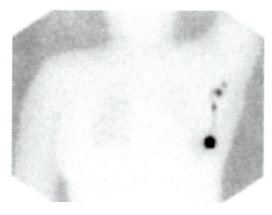

Fig. 32 Lymphoscintigraphy shows visualized sentinel lymph nodes in the left axilla

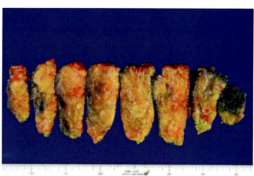

Fig. 33 Gross pathology of lumpectomy specimen. The margins get marked and sliced with different colors on each direction

Pathology Report

Invasive Ductal Carcinoma

1. Size of tumor: 2.0 cm (pT1c).
2. Histologic grade: 3/3 (tubule formation: 3/3, nuclear pleomorphism: 3/3, mitotic count: 2/3)
3. Ductal carcinoma in situ: present, intratumoral/extratumoral (30%) (nuclear grade: high, necrosis: present, architectural pattern: comedo, extensive intraductal component: present).
4. Skin: no involvement of tumor.
5. Surgical margins:
   (a) Superior margin: 10 mm.
   (b) Inferior margin: 30 mm.
   (c) Medial margin: 30 mm.
   (d) Lateral margin: 40 mm.
   (e) Deep margin: 2 mm.
6. Lymph nodes: no metastasis in 4 axillary lymph nodes (pN0(sn)) (sentinel LN: 0/4).
7. Vascular invasion: absent.
8. Lymphatic invasion: present, intratumoral.
9. Tumor border: infiltrative.
10. Microcalcification: present, tumoral/non-tumoral.
11. Pathologic staging: pT1cN0(sn).

	Result	Intensity	Positive %
Estrogen receptor	Negative (0/7)	0	0
Progesterone receptor	Negative (0/7)	0	0
C-erbB2	Negative (1+)		
Ki-67	Positive in 20% of tumor cells		

Adjuvant Therapy

Adjuvant chemotherapy #6 cycles of fluorouracil and doxorubicin and cyclophosphamide.

Postoperative radiation therapy.

5.2.2 Treatments After Recurrence

See Figs. 34, 35 and 36.

Operation

Aug. 2017 Right breast conserving surgery, sentinel lymph node biopsy (Fig. 37).

Pathology Report

Invasive Ductal Carcinoma

1. Size of tumor: 0.8 cm (pT1b).
2. Histologic grade: 2 (tubule formation: 3/3, nuclear pleomorphism: 2/3, mitotic count: 1/3, <1/10HPF).
3. Intraductal component: absent.
4. Skin: no involvement of tumor.
5. Surgical margins:
   (a) Superior margin: 30 mm.
   (b) Inferior margin: 40 mm.
   (c) Medial margin: 35 mm.
   (d) Lateral margin: 35 mm.

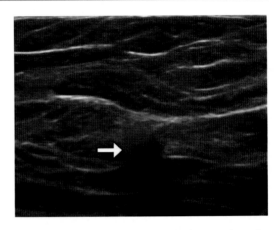

Fig. 35 Targeted right US (2016): An irregular hypoechoic mass at the corresponding area of the asymmetry. US-CNB = IDC

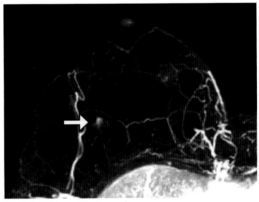

Fig. 36 Right MRI (2017): An irregular enhancing mass (white arrow = proven IDC)

   (e) Deep margin: 16 mm.
   (f) Superficial margin: 20 mm.
6. Lymph nodes: no metastasis in two axillary lymph nodes (pN0(sn)) (sentinel LN: 0/2).
7. Arteriovenous invasion: absent.
8. Lymphovascular invasion: absent.
9. Tumor border: infiltrative.
10. Microcalcification: present, non-tumoral.
11. Pathologic stage (AJCC 2010): pT1bN0(sn).

	Result	Intensity	Positive %
Estrogen receptor	Negative (8/8)	3	>2/3
Progesterone receptor	Negative (7/8)	2	>2/3
C-erbB2	Negative (0)		
Ki-67	Positive in 15% of tumor cells		

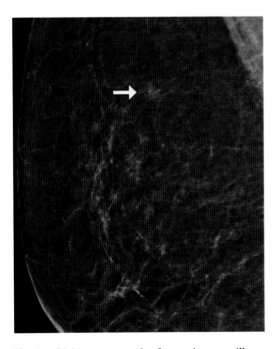

Fig. 34 Right mammography for routine surveillance (2016): A new developing asymmetry at upper breast

Local Recurrence

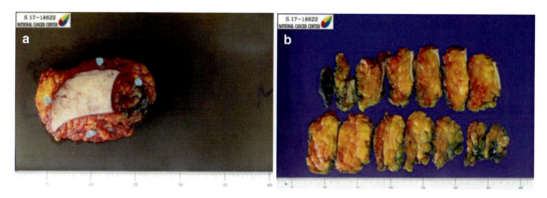

Fig. 37 (**a**) Gross pathology of lumpectomy specimen. (**b**) The margins get marked and sliced with different colors on each direction

Adjuvant Therapy
Postoperative radiation therapy.
    Tamoxifen 20 mg/day for 5 years.

6 Case 6

6.1 Patient History and Progress

Female/60 years old, post-menopause.
    Bloody nipple discharge on left breast.
    Screen detected mass lesion on right breast 6 o'clock direction and left breast 12 o'clock direction.
    No family history.
    Hypertension.

6.2 Courses of Treatment

Both breasts IDC→ Operation → Adjuvant therapy → **Left breast recurrence (IDC).**

6.2.1 Primary Treatment
See Figs. 38, 39, 40, 41, 42 and 43.

Operation
First Operation (Jul. 2010) Right breast conserving surgery, sentinel lymph node biopsy, left breast conserving surgery (Figs. 44 and 45).

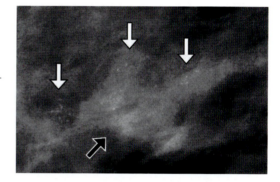

Fig. 38 Right mammography (2010): Regional amorphous microcalcifications (white arrows) with asymmetry (black arrow)

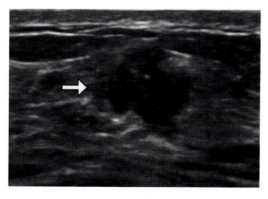

Fig. 39 Right US (2010): Irregular hypoechoic mass with echogenic microcalcifications. CNB = IDC

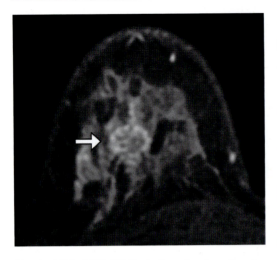

Fig. 40 Right MRI (2010): An irregular rim enhancing mass

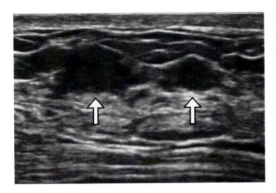

Fig. 41 Left US for evaluation of bloody nipple discharge (2010): Irregular hypoechoic masses at upper inner breast. Negative left mammography (not shown). US-CNB = Intraductal papillary carcinoma

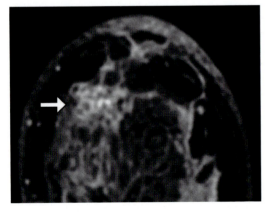

Fig. 42 Left MRI (2010): An irregular heterogeneously enhancing mass at upper breast

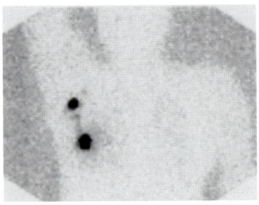

Fig. 43 Lymphoscintigraphy shows visualized sentinel lymph nodes in the right axilla

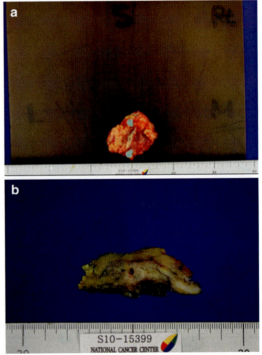

Fig. 44 (**a**) Gross pathology of right lumpectomy specimen. (**b**) The margins get marked and sliced with different colors on each direction

Pathology Report
<Right>

Invasive Ductal Carcinoma
1. Size of tumor: 1.2 cm (pT1c).
2. Histologic grade: 1/3 (tubule formation: 2/3, nuclear pleomorphism: 2/3, mitotic count: 1/3, 6/10HPF).

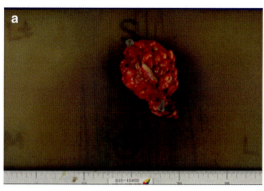 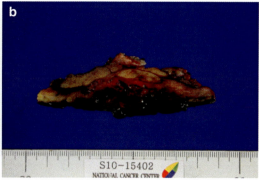

Fig. 45 (**a**) Gross pathology of left lumpectomy specimen. (**b**) The margins get marked and sliced with different colors on each direction

3. Intraductal component: present, intratumoral/extratumoral (40%) (nuclear grade: low, necrosis: present, architectural pattern: micropapillary, cribriform, and comedo, extensive intraductal component: present).
4. Skin: no involvement of tumor.
5. Surgical margins:
   (a) Superior margin: 5 mm.
   (b) Inferior margin: 4 mm from ductal carcinoma in situ (slide 2).
   (c) Medial margin: 10 mm.
   (d) Lateral margin: 10 mm.
   (e) Deep margin: 2 mm.
6. Lymph nodes: no metastasis in 2 axillary lymph nodes (pN0) (sentinel LN: 0/2).
7. Vascular invasion: absent.
8. Lymphatic invasion: present, intratumoral.
9. Tumor border: infiltrative.
10. Microcalcification: present, tumoral/non-tumoral.
11. Pathologic stage (AJCC 2010): pT1cN0(sn).

	Result	Intensity	Positive %
Estrogen receptor	Strong (7/7)	3	>2/3
Progesterone receptor	Strong (7/7)	3	>2/3
C-erbB2	Negative (1+)		
Ki-67	Positive in 20% of tumor cells		

<Left>

Invasive Ductal Carcinoma
1. Size of invasive carcinoma: 0.3 cm (pT1a).
2. Size of intraductal carcinoma: 3.0 cm.

3. Histologic grade: 1/3 (tubule formation: 2/3, nuclear pleomorphism: 1/3, mitotic count: 1/3, 5/10HPF).
4. Intraductal component: present, intratumoral/extratumoral (90%) (nuclear grade: low, necrosis: absent, architectural pattern: papillary and cribriform, extensive intraductal component: present).
5. Skin: no involvement of tumor.
6. Surgical margins:
   (a) Superior margin: 20 mm.
   (b) Inferior margin: 15 mm.
   (c) Medial margin: Positive for ductal carcinoma in situ (Fro 3).
   (d) Lateral margin: 10 mm.
   (e) Deep margin: 2 mm.
7. Vascular invasion: absent.
8. Lymphatic invasion: present, intratumoral.
9. Tumor border: infiltrative.
10. Microcalcification: present, tumoral/non-tumoral.
11. Pathologic stage (AJCC 2010): pT1a.

	Result	Intensity	Positive %
Estrogen receptor	Strong (7/7)	3	>2/3
Progesterone receptor	Strong (7/7)	3	>2/3
C-erbB2	Negative (1+)		
Ki-67	Positive in 5% of tumor cells		

Operation
Second Operation (Aug. 2010) Left breast wide excision, sentinel lymph node biopsy (Fig. 46).

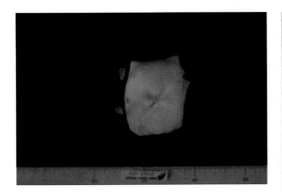

Fig. 46 Gross pathology of left breast wide excision specimen

Pathology Report
No residual tumor with foreign body reaction.
1. Post-lumpectomy status.
2. No metastasis in 1 lymph node (pN0(sn)) (left sentinel LN: 0/1).

Adjuvant Therapy
Postoperative radiation therapy.
  Tamoxifen 20 mg/day for 5 years.

6.2.2 Treatments After Recurrence
See Figs. 47, 48 and 49.

Operation
First Operation (Mar. 2022) Left breast conserving surgery (Fig. 50).

Pathology Report

Invasive Ductal Carcinoma associated with papillary carcinoma in situ
1. Post-lumpectomy status.
2. Size of tumor: 0.6 cm (rpT1b).
3. Histologic grade: 2/3 (tubule formation: 3/3, nuclear pleomorphism: 2/3, mitotic count: 1/3, 6/10HPF).
4. Intraductal component: present, intratumoral/extratumoral (30%) (nuclear grade: low, necrosis: absent, architectural pattern: papillary/cribriform, extensive intraductal component: absent).
5. Skin: no involvement of tumor.

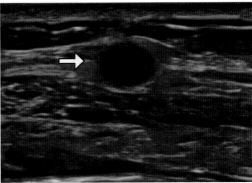

Fig. 47 Left US for routine surveillance (2022): A new hypoechoic mass at inner central breast. US-CNB = Papillary carcinoma in situ, low grade

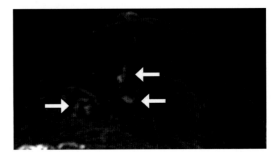

Fig. 48 Left MRI (2022): Multiple enhancing foci at the OP bed of upper inner breast

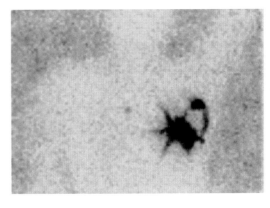

Fig. 49 Lymphoscintigraphy shows visualized sentinel lymph nodes in the left axilla

6. Surgical margins:
   (a) Superior margin: 5 mm.
   (b) Inferior margin: 10 mm.

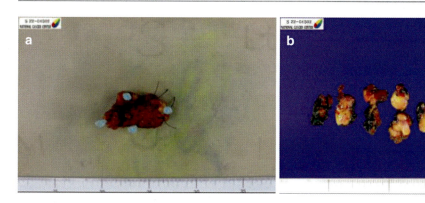

Fig. 50 (**a**) Gross pathology of mastectomy specimen. (**b**) The margins get marked and sliced with different colors on each direction

    (c) Medial margin: (see note 2).
    (d) Lateral margin: 10 mm.
    (e) Deep margin: 2 mm.
    (f) Superficial margin: 2 mm.
7. Arteriovenous invasion: absent.
8. Lymphovascular invasion: absent.
9. Tumor border: infiltrative.
10. Microcalcification: present, tumoral/non-tumoral.
11. Pathological TN category (AJCC 2017): rpT1b.

Note: 1. Invasive ductal carcinoma is present only in the permanent section of Fro 4.

2. The medial margin of the lumpectomy specimen (slide 9) is close to invasive ductal carcinoma (1 mm), but this margin submitted for frozen diagnosis (Fro 3) is free of tumor.

	Result	Intensity	Positive %
Estrogen receptor	Strong (8/8)	3	>2/3
Progesterone receptor	Strong (8/8)	3	1/3–2/3
C-erbB2	Negative (1+) (IDC) Equivocal (2+) (DCIS)		
Ki-67	Positive in 1% of tumor cells		

Operation
Second Operation (Apr. 2022) Left sentinel lymph node biopsy.

Pathology Report
No metastasis in two axillary lymph nodes (sentinel LN: 0/1, non-sentinel LN: 0/1).
1. Post-lumpectomy status.

Adjuvant Therapy
Letrozole 2.5 mg/day for 5 years.

7 Case 7

7.1 Patient History and Progress

Female/42 years old, pre-menopause.
    Screen detected mass lesion on left breast 4 o'clock direction.
    Family history of breast cancer, mother.
    No comorbidities.
    BRCA 1 and 2 mutation: Not detected.

7.2 Courses of Treatment

Left breast microinvasive ductal carcinoma + DCIS → Operation → Adjuvant therapy → Right breast recurrence (DCIS).

7.2.1 Primary Treatment
See Figs. 51, 52 and 53.

Operation
First Operation (Jan. 2019) Left breast conserving surgery, sentinel lymph node biopsy (Fig. 54).

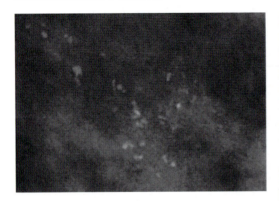

Fig. 51 Left magnification view (2018): Fine pleomorphic microcalcifications at outer breast. US-CNB = DCIS, high grade

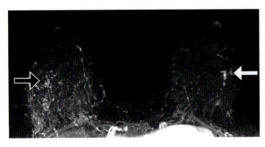

Fig. 52 MRI (2019): Linear non-mass enhancement at outer left breast (white arrow = proven DCIS). Benign appearing enhancing foci at outer right breast (black arrow)

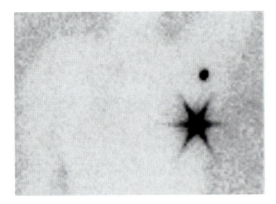

Fig. 53 Lymphoscintigraphy shows visualized sentinel lymph nodes in the left axilla

Pathology Report

Microinvasive Ductal Carcinoma

1. Size of invasive component: <0.1 cm (pT1mi).

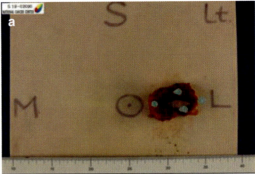

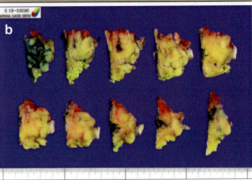

Fig. 54 (**a**) Gross pathology of lumpectomy specimen. (**b**) The margins get marked and sliced with different colors on each direction

2. Size of intraductal component: 4.0 cm.
3. Histologic grade: 3/3 (tubule formation: 3/3, nuclear pleomorphism: 3/3, mitotic count: 3/3, 3/HPF).
4. Intraductal component: present, intratumoral/extratumoral (99%) (nuclear grade: high, necrosis: present, architectural pattern: micropapillary/cribriform, extensive intraductal component: present).
5. Skin: no involvement of tumor.
6. Surgical margins:
   (a) Superior margin: 5 mm.
   (b) Inferior margin: 15 mm.
   (c) Medial margin: 10 mm.
   (d) Lateral margin: positive for ductal carcinoma in situ (Fro 6) (see note).
   (e) Deep margin: 2 mm.
   (f) Superficial margin: 2 mm.
7. Lymph nodes: no metastasis in one axillary lymph node (pN0(sn)) (sentinel LN: 0/1).
8. Arteriovenous invasion: absent.
9. Lymphovascular invasion: absent.

10. Tumor border: infiltrative.
11. Microcalcification: present, tumoral/non-tumoral.
12. Pathological TN category (AJCC 2017): pT1miN0(sn).

Note: 1. Ductal carcinoma in situ is present only in the permanent section of Fro 6.

	Result	Intensity	Positive %
Estrogen receptor	Strong (7/8)	3	1/3–2/3
Progesterone receptor	Negative (0/8)	0	0
C-erbB2	Positive (3+)		
Ki-67	Positive in 41% of tumor cells		

Operation
Second Operation (Feb. 2019) Left breast wide excision (Fig. 55).

Pathology Report
1. Ductal carcinoma in situ, residual.
   (a) Status post-lumpectomy status for microinvasive ductal carcinoma (S19–2090).
   (b) Nuclear grade: high.
   (c) Necrosis: absent.
   (d) Architectural pattern: cribriform.
   (e) Microcalcification: absent.
   (f) Resection margin:
      • Lateral: (see note).
2. Foreign body reaction with fat necrosis.

Note: The lateral margin of the wide excision specimen (slide 1) is close to ductal carcinoma in situ (<1 mm), but this margin submitted for frozen diagnosis (Fro 1) is free of tumor.

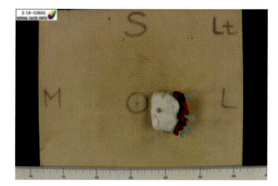

Fig. 55 Gross pathology of breast wide excision specimen

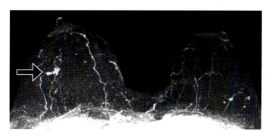

Fig. 56 MRI for routine FU (2022): Linear non-mass enhancement at the same site of previous enhancing foci of outer right breast (black arrow)

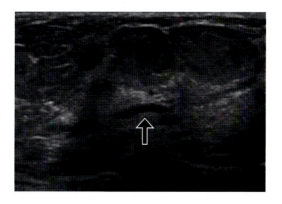

Fig. 57 MRI-directed right US (2022): Focal ductal dilatation at the corresponding area of the MRI abnormality. US-CNB = PCIS, low grade

Adjuvant Therapy
Postoperative radiation therapy.
Tamoxifen 20 mg/day for 3 years.

7.2.2 Treatments After Recurrence
See Figs. 56 and 57.

Operation
Mar. 2022 Right breast conserving surgery (Fig. 58).

Pathology Report

Papillary Carcinoma In Situ
1. Size of tumor: 0.8 cm (pTis).
2. Nuclear grade: low.
3. Necrosis: absent.
4. Architectural pattern: papillary/solid.

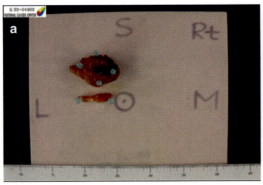
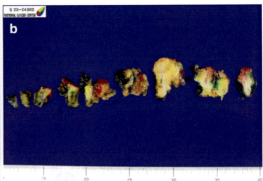

Fig. 58 (**a**) Gross pathology of lumpectomy specimen. (**b**) The margins get marked and sliced with different colors on each direction

5. Skin: no involvement of tumor.
6. Surgical margins:
   (a) Superior margin: (see note 1).
   (b) Inferior margin: 10 mm.
   (c) Medial margin: 5 mm.
   (d) Lateral margin: 20 mm.
   (e) Deep margin: 2 mm.
   (f) Superficial margin: <1 mm from ductal carcinoma in situ (slide 2).
7. Microcalcification: present, tumoral/non-tumoral.
8. Pathological TN category (AJCC 2017): pTis.

Note: 1. The superior margin of the lumpectomy specimen (slide 3) is close to ductal carcinoma in situ (3 mm), but this margin submitted for frozen diagnosis (Fro 1) is free of tumor.

	Result	Intensity	Positive %
Estrogen receptor	Strong (8/8)	3	>2/3
Progesterone receptor	Negative (2/8)	1	<1%
C-erbB2	Equivocal (2+)		
Ki-67	Positive in 2% of tumor cells		

Adjuvant Therapy
Plan for tamoxifen for 5 years.

8 Case 8

8.1 Patient History and Progress

Female/48 years old, pre-menopause.
Screen detected mass lesion on right breast 12 o'clock direction and left 6 o'clock direction.
Family history of breast cancer, maternal aunt.
No comorbidities.
BRCA 1 and 2 mutation: Not detected.

8.2 Courses of Treatment

Right breast IDC/Left breast intraductal papilloma, sclerosing → Operation → Adjuvant therapy → **Left breast recurrence (DCIS).**

8.2.1 Primary Treatment
See Figs. 59 and 60.

Operation
First Operation (Feb. 2021) Both breast mass excision (Figs. 61 and 62).

Pathology Report
<Right>

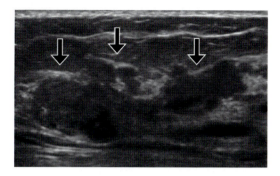

Fig. 59 Right US for evaluation of bloody nipple discharge (Jan. 2021): Multiple irregular hypoechoic masses at upper breast. US-CNB = ADH involving sclerosing adenosis

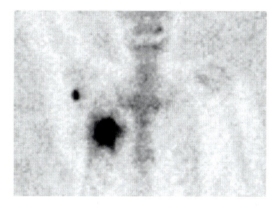

Fig. 60 Lymphoscintigraphy shows visualized sentinel lymph nodes in the right axilla

1. Invasive Ductal Carcinoma involving sclerosing adenosis.
   (a) Size of tumor: 1.5 cm (pT1c).
   (b) Histologic grade: 2/3 (tubule formation: 3/3, nuclear pleomorphism: 2/3, mitotic count: 1/3, 8/10HPF).
   (c) Intraductal component: present, intratumoral/extratumoral (70%) (nuclear grade: low, necrosis: present, architectural pattern: cribriform/solid, extensive intraductal component: present).
   (d) Skin: no involvement of tumor.
   (e) Surgical margins:
   - Superior margin: 2 mm from ductal carcinoma in situ (slide 7).
   - Inferior margin: 2 mm from ductal carcinoma in situ (slide MG4).
   - Medial margin: 2 mm from invasive ductal carcinoma (slide 6).
   - Lateral margin: 2 mm from ductal carcinoma in situ (slide 9).
   - Deep margin: 2 mm.
   - Superficial margin: 2 mm.
   (f) Arteriovenous invasion: absent.
   (g) Lymphovascular invasion: present, intratumoral.
   (h) Tumor border: infiltrative.

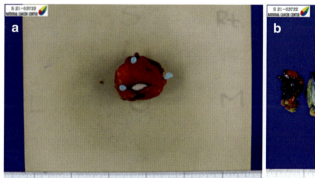
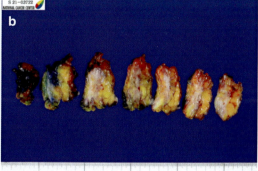

Fig. 61 (**a**) Gross pathology of right breast mass excision specimen. (**b**) The margins get marked and sliced with different colors on each direction

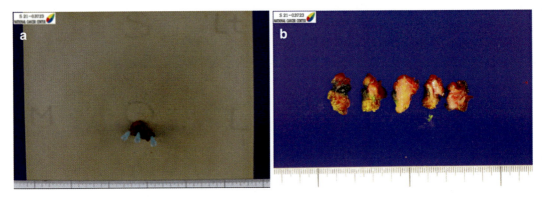

Fig. 62 (**a**) Gross pathology of left breast mass excision specimen. (**b**) The margins get marked and sliced with different colors on each direction

    (i) Microcalcification: present, tumoral/non-tumoral.
    (j) Pathological TN category (AJCC 2017): pT1c.
2. Intraductal papilloma.
3. Sclerosing adenosis with microcalcification.

	Result	Intensity	Positive %
Estrogen receptor	Strong (8/8)	3	>2/3
Progesterone receptor	Strong (8/8)	3	>2/3
C-erbB2	Negative (1+) (IDC) Equivocal (2+) (DCIS)		
Ki-67	Positive in 24% of tumor cells		

<Left>

1. Intraductal papilloma with usual ductal hyperplasia
2. Sclerosing adenosis with microcalcification.

Operation
Second Operation (Mar. 2021) Right axillary lymph node sampling.

Pathology Report
No metastasis in eight axillary lymph nodes (right sentinel LN: 0/2, right axillary LN: 0/6).
1. Post-excision status.

Adjuvant Therapy
Postoperative radiation therapy.
    Tamoxifen 20 mg/day for 0.8 year.

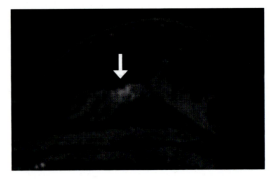

Fig. 63 Left MRI for routine surveillance (Jan. 2022): Focal non-mass enhancement at upper inner breast

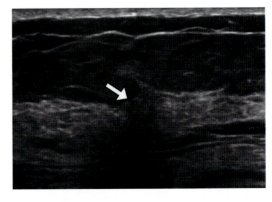

Fig. 64 MRI-directed left US (Jan. 2022): An isoechoic lesion with indistinct margins at the corresponding area of the MRI abnormality. US-CNB = ADH involving sclerosing papilloma

8.2.2 Treatments After Recurrence
See Figs. 63 and 64.

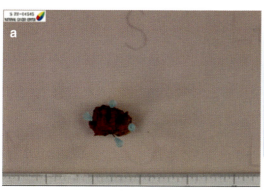 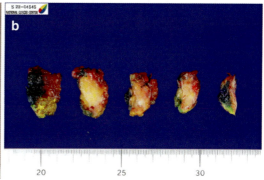

Fig. 65 (**a**) Gross pathology of lumpectomy specimen. (**b**) The margins get marked and sliced with different colors on each direction

Operation

Mar. 2022 Left breast conserving surgery (Fig. 65).

Pathology Report

1. Ductal Carcinoma In Situ involving sclerosing adenosis.
   (a) Size of tumor: 0.8 cm (pTis).
   (b) Nuclear grade: low.
   (c) Necrosis: absent.
   (d) Architectural pattern: micropapillary/cribriform.
   (e) Surgical margins:
      - Superior margin: <1 mm from ductal carcinoma in situ (slide 2).
      - Inferior margin: 10 mm.
      - Medial margin: 5 mm.
      - Lateral margin: 10 mm.
      - Deep margin: 2 mm.
      - Superficial margin: 2 mm.
   (f) Microcalcification: present, tumoral/non-tumoral.
2. Intraductal papilloma with usual ductal hyperplasia.

	Result	Intensity	Positive %
Estrogen receptor	Strong (8/8)	3	>2/3
Progesterone receptor	Negative (2/8)	1	<1%
C-erbB2	Equivocal (2+)		
Ki-67	Positive in 1% of tumor cells		

Adjuvant Therapy

Plan for tamoxifen for 5 years.

9 Case 9

9.1 Patient History and Progress

Female/51 years old, pre-menopause.
　Screen detected mass lesion on right breast 12 o'clock direction.
　Outside result of biopsy: Mucinous carcinoma.
　Family history of colon cancer, father.
　No comorbidities.
　BRCA 1 and 2 mutation: Not detected.

9.2 Courses of Treatment

Right breast mucinous carcinoma → Operation → Adjuvant therapy → **Left breast recurrence (IDC + DCIS)**/Right breast ADH.

9.2.1 Primary Treatment

See Figs. 66, 67 and 68.

Operation

May 2013 Right breast conserving surgery, sentinel lymph node biopsy (Fig. 69).

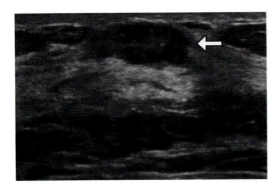

Fig. 66 Right US for evaluation of a palpable lump (2013): An isoechoic mass with microlobulated margins at subareolar area. US-CNB = Mucinous carcinoma

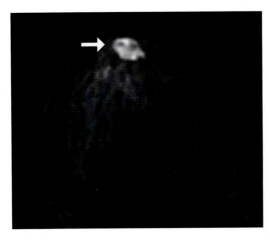

Fig. 67 T2-weighed right MRI (2013): An oval mass with high T2 signal intensity at subareolar area

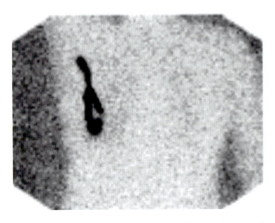

Fig. 68 Lymphoscintigraphy shows visualized sentinel lymph nodes in the right axilla

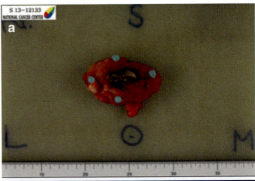

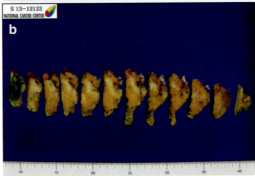

Fig. 69 (**a**) Gross pathology of lumpectomy specimen. (**b**) The margins get marked and sliced with different colors on each direction

Pathology Report

Mucinous Carcinoma

1. Size of tumor: 1.5 cm (pT1c).
2. Histologic grade: 1/3 (tubule formation: 2/3, nuclear pleomorphism: 2/3, mitotic count: 1/3, 7/10HPF).
3. Intraductal component: absent.
4. Skin: no involvement of tumor.
5. Surgical margins:
    (a) Superior margin: 10 mm.
    (b) Inferior margin: 15 mm.
    (c) Medial margin: 15 mm.
    (d) Lateral margin: 20 mm.
    (e) Deep margin: 12 mm.
    (f) Superficial margin: 3 mm.
6. Lymph nodes: no metastasis in one axillary lymph node (pN0(sn)) (sentinel LN: 0/1).
7. Vascular invasion: absent.
8. Lymphatic invasion: absent.
9. Tumor border: infiltrative.

Local Recurrence

10. Microcalcification: absent.
11. Pathologic stage (AJCC 2010): pT1cN0(sn).

	Result	Intensity	Positive %
Estrogen receptor	Strong (8/8)	3	>2/3
Progesterone receptor	Strong (8/8)	3	>2/3
C-erbB2	Negative (0)		
Ki-67	Positive in 13% of tumor cells		

Adjuvant Therapy
Postoperative radiation therapy.
Tamoxifen 20 mg/day for 5 years.

9.2.2 Treatments After Recurrence
See Figs. 70, 71, 72 and 73.

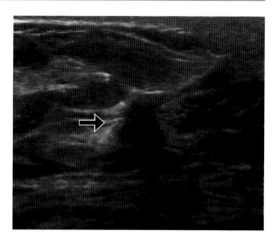

Fig. 72 MRI-directed right US (2021): A hypoechoic mass with non-parallel orientation at the corresponding area of the MRI abnormality

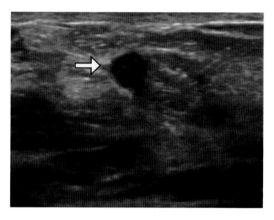

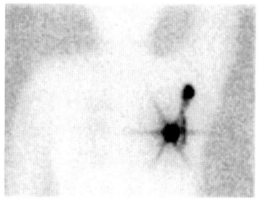

Fig. 73 Lymphoscintigraphy shows visualized sentinel lymph nodes in the left axilla

Fig. 70 Left US for routine surveillance (2021): A new hypoechoic mass with angular margins at lower outer breast. US-CNB = IDC

Fig. 71 MRI (2021): An enhancing mass in the left breast (white arrow = proven IDC). Another enhancing mass in the right breast (black arrow)

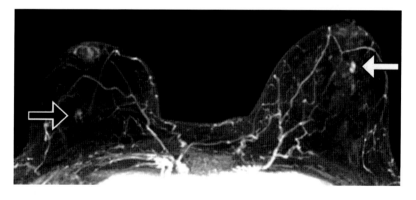

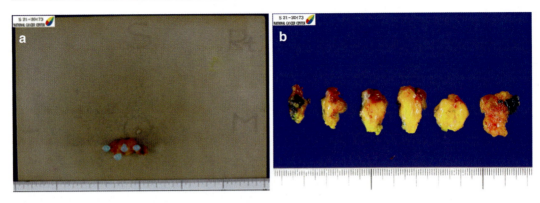

Fig. 74 (**a**) Gross pathology of right lumpectomy specimen. (**b**) The margins get marked and sliced with different colors on each direction

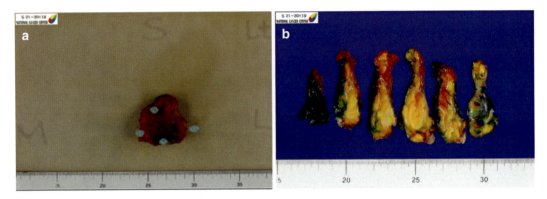

Fig. 75 (**a**) Gross pathology of left lumpectomy specimen. (**b**) The margins get marked and sliced with different colors on each direction

Operation

Sep. 2021 Left breast conserving surgery, sentinel lymph node biopsy, right breast conserving surgery (Figs. 74 and 75).

Pathology Report

<Right>

Atypical ductal hyperplasia involving intraductal papilloma with marked cautery artifact.

<Left>

Ductal Carcinoma In Situ, residual

1. Size of tumor: up to 0.2 cm.
2. Nuclear grade: low.
3. Necrosis: absent.
4. Architectural pattern: micropapillary.
5. Skin: no involvement of tumor.
6. Surgical margins:
    (a) Superior margin: 15 mm.
    (b) Inferior margin: 5 mm.
    (c) Medial margin: 10 mm.
    (d) Lateral margin: 10 mm.
    (e) Deep margin: 5 mm.
    (f) Superficial margin: 1 mm from ductal carcinoma in situ (slide 5).
7. Lymph nodes: no metastasis in one axillary lymph node (pN0(sn)) (sentinel LN: 0/1)
8. Microcalcification: present, tumoral.

Note: 1. In the previous biopsy specimen (S21–18409), invasive ductal carcinoma measures at least 0.5 cm in greatest dimension.

	Result	Intensity	Positive %
Estrogen receptor	Strong (8/8)	3	>2/3
Progesterone receptor	Strong (8/8)	3	>2/3
C-erbB2	Negative (1+)		
Ki-67	Positive in 8% of tumor cells		

Adjuvant Therapy

Postoperative radiation therapy.

Letrozole 2.5 mg/day for 5 years with goserelin.

10 Case 10

10.1 Patient History and Progress

Female/42 years old, pre-menopause.

Screen detected mass lesion on right breast 5 o'clock direction.

Outside result of biopsy: Invasive ductal carcinoma.

No family history.

s/p myomectomy.

10.2 Courses of Treatment

Right breast IDC→ Operation → Adjuvant therapy → **Right breast recurrence (IDC).**

10.2.1 Primary Treatment
See Figs. 76, 77 and 78.

Operation
Jul. 2018 Right nipple-areolar complex sparing mastectomy with immediate implant reconstruction, sentinel lymph node biopsy, left breast augmentation (Figs. 79 and 80).

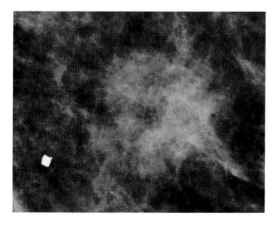

Fig. 76 Right mammography (2018): An irregular palpable mass at lower inner breast. US-CNB = IDC

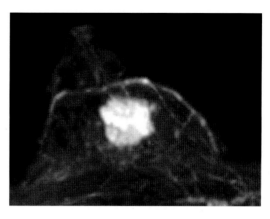

Fig. 77 Right MRI (2018): An irregular enhancing mass

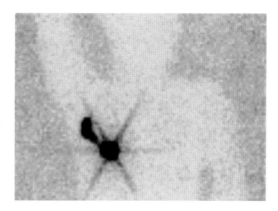

Fig. 78 Lymphoscintigraphy shows visualized sentinel lymph nodes in the right axilla

Pathology Report
1. Invasive ductal carcinoma.
    (a) Size of tumor: 1.8 cm (pT1c).
    (b) Histologic grade: 2/3 (tubule formation: 3/3, nuclear pleomorphism: 2/3, mitotic count: 1/3, 5/10HPF).
    (c) Intraductal component: present, intratumoral/extratumoral (10%) (nuclear grade: low, necrosis: present, architectural pattern: cribriform/solid, extensive intraductal component: absent).
    (d) Skin: no involvement of tumor.
    (e) Surgical margins:

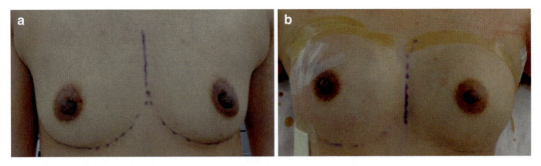

Fig. 79 (**a**) Preoperative and (**b**) immediate postoperative appearance

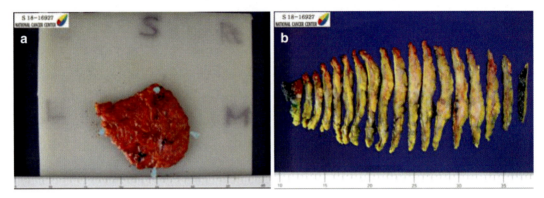

Fig. 80 (**a**) Gross pathology of mastectomy specimen. (**b**) The margins get marked and sliced with different colors on each direction

- Deep margin: <1 mm from invasive ductal carcinoma (slide 3).
- Superficial margin: (see note 1).
  (f) Lymph nodes:
  - Metastasis in one out of five axillary lymph nodes (pN1mi(sn)) (see note 2) (sentinel LN: 1/4, non-sentinel LN: 0/1).
  - Perinodal extension: absent.
  - Size of metastatic carcinoma: 1.2 mm.
  (g) Arteriovenous invasion: absent.
  (h) Lymphovascular invasion: present, intratumoral/peritumoral.
  (i) Tumor border: infiltrative.
  (j) Microcalcification: present, non-tumoral.
  (k) Pathological TN category (AJCC 2017): pT1cN1mi(sn).
2. Intraductal papilloma.

Note: 1. The superficial margin of the lumpectomy specimen (slide 3) is close to ductal carcinoma in situ (<1 mm), but this margin submitted for frozen diagnosis (Fro 2) is free of tumor.

2. Micrometastasis is present only in the permanent section of Fro 3.

	Result	Intensity	Positive %
Estrogen receptor	Strong (7/8)	2	>2/3
Progesterone receptor	Strong (7/8)	2	>2/3
C-erbB2	Negative (1+)		
Ki-67	Positive in 5% of tumor cells		

Adjuvant Therapy

Tamoxifen 20 mg/day for 3.5 years.

10.2.2 Treatments After Recurrence

See Figs. 81 and 82.

Operation

Mar. 2022 Right breast wide excision, excisional biopsy of right second intercostal space mass, implant change (Figs. 83 and 84).

Local Recurrence

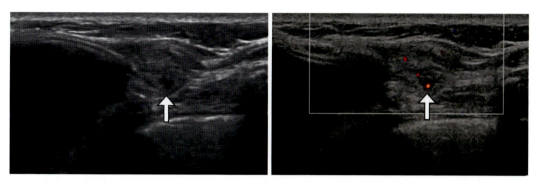

Fig. 81 Right US for routine surveillance (2022): Heterogeneous non-mass lesion with mild vascularity at lower periphery of the implant-reconstructed breast. US-CNB = IDC

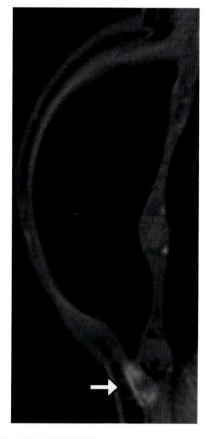

Fig. 82 Right MRI (2022): An enhancing mass at lower periphery of the implant-reconstructed breast

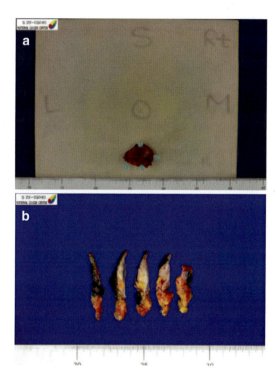

Fig. 83 (**a**) Gross pathology of wide excision specimen. (**b**) The margins get marked and sliced with different colors on each direction

Plan for postoperative radiation therapy.
Plan for letrozole with goserelin.

Adjuvant Therapy

Adjuvant chemotherapy #4 cycles of doxorubicin and cyclophosphamide followed by #4 cycles of docetaxel.

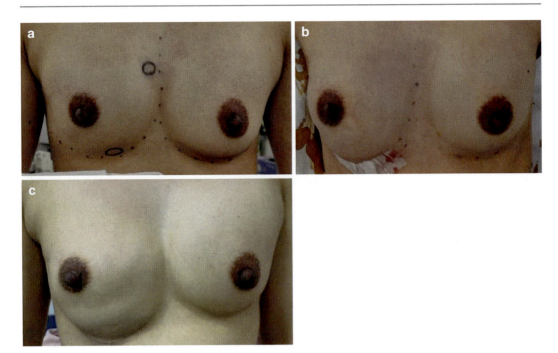

Fig. 84 (**a**) Preoperative, (**b**) immediate postoperative, and (**c**) late follow-up appearance

11　Case 11

11.1　Patient History and Progress

Female/45 years old, post-menopause.

Screen detected mass lesion on right breast 10 o'clock direction.

No family history.

S/P bilateral salpingo-oophorectomy (right ovary borderline tumor).

BRCA 1 and 2 mutation: Not detected.

11.2　Courses of Treatment

Right breast IDC → Operation → Adjuvant therapy → **Right breast recurrence (IDC).**

11.2.1　Primary Treatment

Operation
Nov. 2008 Right breast conserving surgery, sentinel lymph node biopsy (outside).

Pathology Report

Invasive Ductal Carcinoma
1. Size of tumor: 1.3 cm (pT1c).
2. Lymph nodes: no metastasis in four axillary lymph nodes (pN0(sn)) (sentinel LN: 0/4).
3. Pathologic stage (AJCC 2010): pT1cN0(sn).

	Result	Intensity	Positive %
Estrogen receptor	Positive		
Progesterone receptor	Positive		
C-erbB2	Negative		
Ki-67	Positive in 5–10% of tumor cells		

Adjuvant Therapy
Adjuvant chemotherapy #4 cycles of doxorubicin and cyclophosphamide.

Postoperative radiation therapy.

Tamoxifen 20 mg/day for 1.8 years.

11.2.2　Treatments After Recurrence
See Figs. 85, 86 and 87.

Local Recurrence

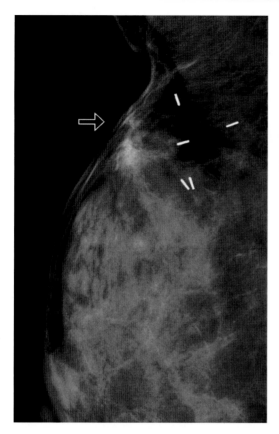

Fig. 85 Right mammography for routine surveillance (2013): Benign postoperative changes at upper periphery

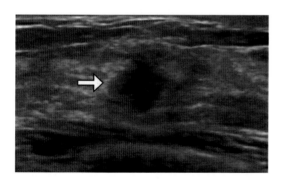

Fig. 86 Right US for routine surveillance (2013): A new irregular hypoechoic mass at subareolar area. US-CNB = IDC

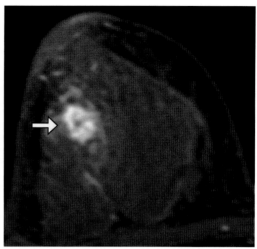

Fig. 87 Right MRI (2013): An irregular enhancing mass at subareolar area

Operation
Sep. 2013 Right nipple-areolar complex sparing mastectomy with immediate implant reconstruction, sentinel lymph node biopsy (Fig. 88).

Pathology Report

Invasive Ductal Carcinomas (×2)
1. Post-chemotherapy status.
2. Post-lumpectomy status.
3. Size of tumor: 0.8 cm and 0.3 cm (ypT1b).
4. Histologic grade: 2/3 (tubule formation: 2/3, nuclear pleomorphism: 2/3, mitotic count: 2/3, 12/10HPF).
5. Intraductal component: present, intratumoral/intratumoral (10%) (nuclear grade: low, necrosis: absent, architectural pattern: cribriform, extensive intraductal component: absent).
6. Skin: no involvement of tumor.
7. Surgical margins:
   (a) Deep margin: 6 mm.
   (b) Superficial margin: 10 mm.

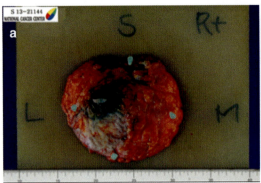 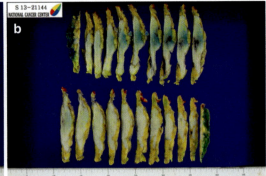

Fig. 88 (**a**) Gross pathology of mastectomy specimen. (**b**) The margins get marked and sliced with different colors on each direction

8. Lymph nodes: no metastasis in one axillary lymph node (ypN0)(sn) (sentinel LN: 0/1).
9. Vascular invasion: absent.
10. Lymphatic invasion: absent.
11. Tumor border: infiltrative.
12. Microcalcification: absent.
13. Pathologic stage (AJCC 2010): ypT1bN0(sn).

	Result	Intensity	Positive %
Estrogen receptor	Strong (7/8)	2	>2/3
Progesterone receptor	Strong (8/8)	3	>2/3
C-erbB2	Equivocal (2+) (SISH negative)		
Ki-67	Positive in 21% of tumor cells		

Adjuvant Therapy

Tamoxifen 20 mg/day for 5 years with goserelin.

12 Case 12

12.1 Patient History and Progress

Female/55 years old, peri-menopause.
  Screen detected mass lesion on right breast 9 o'clock direction.
  Family history of prostate cancer, father.
  s/p hysterectomy, HPV infection.

12.2 Courses of Treatment

Right breast DCIS → Operation → **Right breast recurrence (microinvasive ductal carcinoma).**

12.2.1 Primary Treatment

See Figs. 89, 90 and 91.

Operation

Aug. 2007 Right breast conserving surgery, sentinel lymph node biopsy (Fig. 92).

Pathology Report

Ductal carcinoma in situ

1. Size of tumor: 2.3 cm (pTis).
2. Nuclear grade: low.
3. Necrosis: absent.
4. Architectural pattern: cribriform, solid and papillary.
5. Skin: no involvement of tumor.
6. Surgical margins:
    (a) Superior margin: 20 mm.
    (b) Inferior margin: 20 mm.
    (c) Medial margin: 30 mm.
    (d) Lateral margin: 50 mm.
    (e) Deep margin: 2 mm.
7. Lymph nodes: no metastasis in 5 axillary lymph nodes (pN0(sn)) (sentinel LN: 0/4, right intramammary LN (Fro 6): 0/1).

Local Recurrence 751

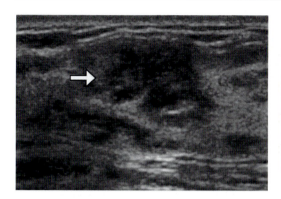

Fig. 89 Right US for evaluation of a palpable lump (2007): An irregular hypoechoic mass at outer central breast. US-CNB = DCIS, high grade

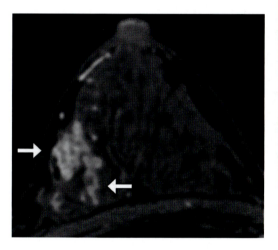

Fig. 90 Right MRI (2007): Clumped non-mass enhancement at outer central breast

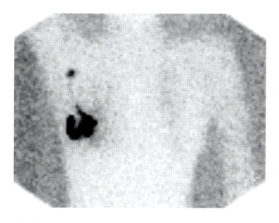

Fig. 91 Lymphoscintigraphy shows visualized sentinel lymph nodes in the right axilla

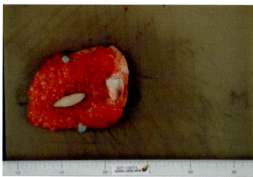

Fig. 92 Gross pathology of lumpectomy specimen

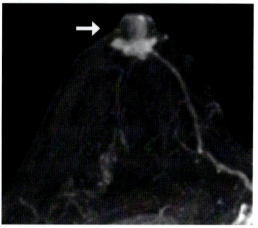

Fig. 93 Right MRI (2017): Strongly enhanced nipple-areolar complex. Biopsy = DCIS, low grade

8. Microcalcification: present, tumoral/non-tumoral.
9. Pathologic staging: pTisN0(sn).

	Result	Intensity	Positive %
Estrogen receptor	Strong (7/7)	3	>2/3
Progesterone receptor	Strong (6/7)	3	1/3–2/3
C-erbB2	Equivocal (2+)		
Ki-67	Positive in 10% of tumor cells		

12.2.2 Treatments After Recurrence
See Fig. 93.

Operation
Sep. 2017 Right total mastectomy with tissue expander insertion (Figs. 94 and 95).

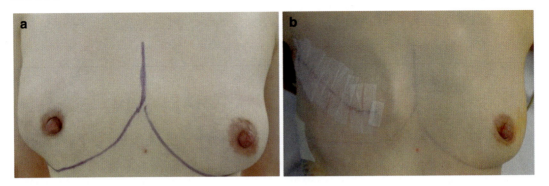

Fig. 94 (**a**) Preoperative and (**b**) immediate postoperative appearance

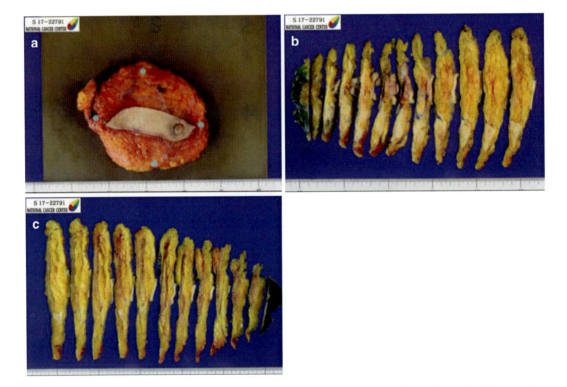

Fig. 95 (**a**) Gross pathology of mastectomy specimen. (**b**, **c**) The margins get marked and sliced with different colors on each direction

Pathology Report
1. Microinvasive Ductal Carcinoma involving lactiferous duct.
    (a) Post-lumpectomy status.
    (b) Size of invasive component: <0.1 cm (pT1mi(Paget)).
    (c) Size of intraductal component: 1.3 cm.
    (d) Histologic grade: 2/3 (tubule formation: 3/3, nuclear pleomorphism: 2/3, mitotic count: 1/3, 6/10HPF).
    (e) Intraductal component: present, intratumoral/extratumoral (99%) (nuclear grade: low, necrosis: present, architectural pattern: micropapillary/cribriform, extensive intraductal component: present).
    (f) Nipple: involvement of lactiferous duct (slide 10).
    (g) Skin: no involvement of tumor.
    (h) Surgical margins:

- Deep margin: 3 mm.
- Superficial margin: 4 mm.
  (i) Arteriovenous invasion: absent.
  (j) Lymphovascular invasion: absent.
  (k) Tumor border: infiltrative.
  (l) Microcalcification: present, tumoral.
  (m) Pathologic stage (AJCC 2010): pT1mi(Paget).
2. Lobular carcinoma in situ, 0.3 cm.

	Result	Intensity	Positive %
Estrogen receptor	Strong (8/8)	3	>2/3
Progesterone receptor	Intermediate (6/8)	2	1/3–2/3
C-erbB2	Equivocal (2+)		
Ki-67	Positive in 13% of tumor cells		

Adjuvant Therapy
Tamoxifen 20 mg/day for 5 years.

13 Case 13

13.1 Patient History and Progress

Female/42 years old, pre-menopause.

Screen detected mass lesion on right breast 3 o'clock direction and bloody discharge from right nipple.

Outside result of biopsy: Ductal carcinoma in situ.

No family history.
No comorbidities.
BRCA 1 and 2 mutation: not detected.

13.2 Courses of Treatment

Right breast microinvasive ductal carcinoma → Operation → **Right breast recurrence (DCIS).**

13.2.1 Primary Treatment
See Figs. 96, 97 and 98.

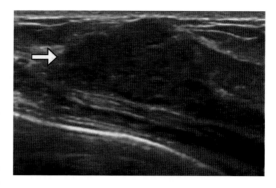

Fig. 96 Right US (2016): Multiple hypoechoic lesions with indistinct margins (partly shown). US-CNB = DCIS, high grade

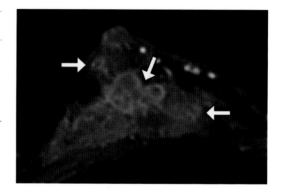

Fig. 97 Right MRI (2016): Multifocal clustered ring non-mass enhancement

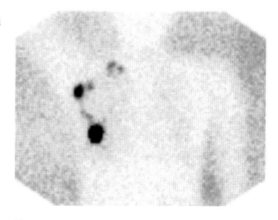

Fig. 98 Lymphoscintigraphy shows visualized sentinel lymph nodes in the right axilla

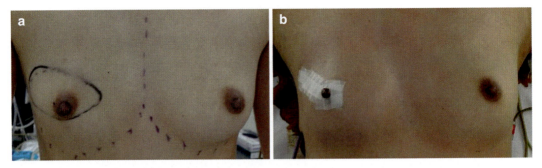

Fig. 99 (**a**) Preoperative and (**b**) immediate postoperative appearance

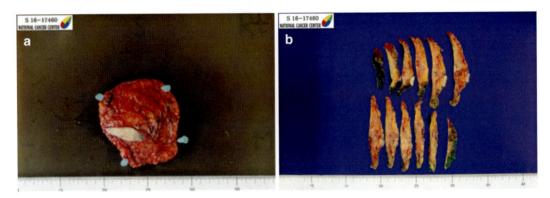

Fig. 100 (**a**) Gross pathology of mastectomy specimen. (**b**) The margins get marked and sliced with different colors on each direction

Operation

Jul. 2016 Right nipple-areolar complex sparing mastectomy with immediate implant reconstruction, sentinel lymph node biopsy (Figs. 99 and 100).

Pathology Report

Microinvasive Ductal Carcinoma

1. Size of invasive component: <0.1 cm (pT1mi).
2. Size of intraductal component: 4.5 cm.
3. Histologic grade: 3/3 (tubule formation: 3/3, nuclear pleomorphism: 3/3, mitotic count: 2/3, 11/HPF).
4. Intraductal component: present, intratumoral/extratumoral (98%) (nuclear grade: high, necrosis: present, architectural pattern: micropapillary/cribriform, extensive intraductal component: present).
5. Skin: no involvement of tumor.
6. Surgical margins:
   (a) Deep margin: <1 mm from ductal carcinoma in situ (slide 3).
   (b) Superficial margin: <1 mm from ductal carcinoma in situ (slide 10).
7. Lymph nodes: no metastasis in three axillary lymph nodes (pN0(sn)) (sentinel LN: 0/3)
8. Arteriovenous invasion: absent.
9. Lymphovascular invasion: absent.
10. Tumor border: infiltrative.
11. Microcalcification: present, tumoral/non-tumoral.
12. Pathologic stage (AJCC 2010): pT1miN0(sn).

	Result	Intensity	Positive %
Estrogen receptor	Negative (0/8)	0	0
Progesterone receptor	Negative (0/8)	0	0
C-erbB2	Positive (3+)		
Ki-67	Positive in 35% of tumor cells		

13.2.2 Treatments After Recurrence
See Fig. 101.

Operation
Aug. 2019 Right nipple excision, implant removal (Fig. 102).

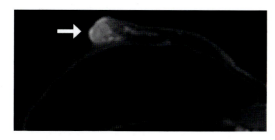

Fig. 101 Right MRI for evaluation of bloody discharge and eczema of the nipple (2019): Strongly enhanced nipple of the implant-reconstructed breast. Punch biopsy = Paget's disease

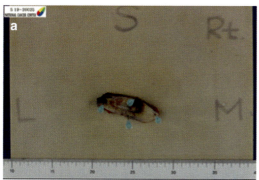

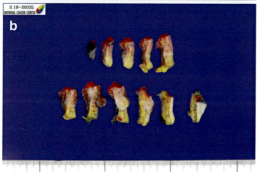

Fig. 102 (**a**) Gross pathology of nipple excision specimen. (**b**) The margins get marked and sliced with different colors on each direction

Pathology Report
Ductal Carcinoma In Situ
1. Post-nipple-sparing mastectomy status.
2. Size of tumor: 1.0 cm (rpTis(Paget)).
3. Nuclear grade: high.
4. Necrosis: present.
5. Architectural pattern: micropapillary/cribriform/comedo.
6. Nipple: involvement of lactiferous duct with Paget's disease.
7. Surgical margins:
    (a) Superior margin: 5 mm.
    (b) Inferior margin: 5 mm.
    (c) Medial margin: 5 mm.
    (d) Lateral margin: 5 mm.
    (e) Deep margin: 2 mm.
    (f) Superficial margin: 2 mm.
8. Microcalcification: present, tumoral.
9. Pathological TN category (AJCC 2017): rpTis.

	Result	Intensity	Positive %
Estrogen receptor	Negative (0/8)	0	0
Progesterone receptor	Negative (2/8)	1	<1%
C-erbB2	Positive (3+)		
Ki-67	Positive in 19% of tumor cells		

14 Case 14

14.1 Patient History and Progress

Female/72 years old, post-menopause.

Screen detected mass lesion on right breast 1 o'clock direction and left 9 o'clock direction.

No family history.

Diabetes mellitus.

BRCA 1 and 2 mutation: Not detected, ATM and POLE VUS (variant of uncertain).

14.2 Courses of Treatment

Right breast infiltrating ductal carcinoma → Operation → Left breast recurrence (IDC).

14.2.1 Primary Treatment
See Figs. 103 and 104.

Operation
Aug. 2003 Right breast conserving surgery, axillary lymph node dissection, left breast mass excision.

Pathology Report
<Right>

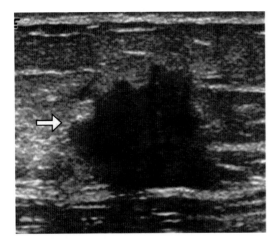

Fig. 103 Right US (2003): An irregular hypoechoic mass. US-CNB = IDC

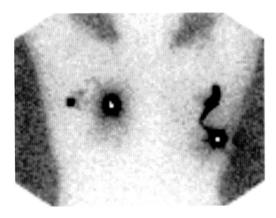

Fig. 104 Lymphoscintigraphy shows visualized sentinel lymph nodes in both axilla

Infiltrating Ductal Carcinoma
1. Size of tumor: 2 cm (pT1c).
2. Histologic grade: 2/3 (tubule formation: 2/3, nuclear pleomorphism: 2/3, mitotic count: 2/3).
3. Ductal carcinoma in situ: present, intratumoral (5%) (nuclear grade: low, necrosis: absent, architectural pattern: solid, extensive intraductal component: absent).
4. Skin: no involvement of tumor.
5. Surgical margins: clear
   (a) Superior margin: 30 mm.
   (b) Inferior margin: 35 mm.
   (c) Medial margin: 35 mm.
   (d) Lateral margin: 25 mm.
   (e) Deep margin: 10 mm.
6. Lymph nodes:
   (a) Metastasis in 2 out of 22 axillary lymph nodes (pN1a) (sentinel LN: 1/2, axillary LN: 1/20).
   (b) Perinodal extension: absent.
   (c) Size of metastatic carcinoma: 6 mm.
7. Vascular invasion: absent.
8. Lymphatic invasion: absent.
9. Tumor border: infiltrative.
10. Microcalcification: absent.
11. Pathologic staging: pT1cN1a.

	Result	Intensity	Positive %
Estrogen receptor	Intermediate (5/7)	2	1/3–2/3
Progesterone receptor	Weak (2/7)	1	<10%
C-erbB2	Equivocal (2+)		
Ki-67	Positive in 2% of tumor cells		

<Left>
Ductal hyperplasia with organizing hematoma.

Adjuvant Therapy
Adjuvant chemotherapy #6 cycles of fluorouracil and doxorubicin and cyclophosphamide.
Postoperative radiation therapy.
Tamoxifen 20 mg/day for 1.7 years followed by anastrozole 1 mg/day for 1 year followed by tamoxifen 20 mg/day for 2.3 years.

14.2.2 Treatments After Recurrence
See Figs. 105, 106 and 107.

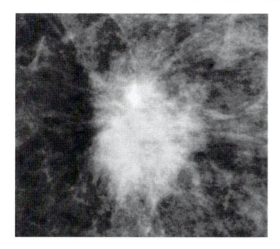

Fig. 105 Left mammography (2021): An irregular hyperdense mass

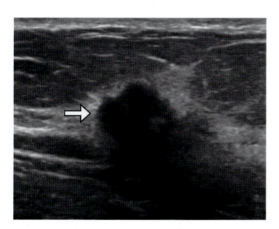

Fig. 106 Left US (2021): A hypoechoic mass with microlobulated margins. US-CNB = IDC

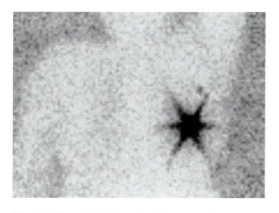

Fig. 107 Lymphoscintigraphy shows visualized sentinel lymph nodes in the left axilla

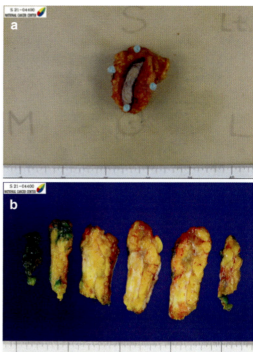

Fig. 108 (**a**) Gross pathology of lumpectomy specimen. (**b**) The margins get marked and sliced with different colors on each direction

Operation
Mar. 2021 Left breast conserving surgery, sentinel lymph node biopsy (Fig. 108).

Pathology Report
Invasive Ductal Carcinoma
1. Size of tumor: 1.1 cm (pT1c).
2. Histologic grade: 2/3 (tubule formation: 2/3, nuclear pleomorphism: 2/3, mitotic count: 2/3, 11/10HPF).
3. Intraductal component: present, intratumoral/extratumoral (20%) (nuclear grade: low, necrosis: absent, architectural pattern: cribriform, extensive intraductal component: absent).
4. Skin: no involvement of tumor.
5. Surgical margins:
   (a) Superior margin: 10 mm.
   (b) Inferior margin: 10 mm.
   (c) Medial margin: 10 mm.
   (d) Lateral margin: 10 mm.

(e) Deep margin: 2 mm.
(f) Superficial margin: 2 mm.
6. Lymph nodes: no metastasis in one axillary lymph node (pN0(sn)) (sentinel LN: 0/1).
7. Arteriovenous invasion: absent.
8. Lymphovascular invasion: absent.
9. Tumor border: infiltrative.
10. Microcalcification: present, tumoral/non-tumoral.
11. Pathological TN category (AJCC 2017): pT1cN0(sn).

	Result	Intensity	Positive %
Estrogen receptor	Weak (4/8)	2	1–10%
Progesterone receptor	Weak (4/8)	2	1–10%
C-erbB2	Negative (0)		
Ki-67	Not informative		

Adjuvant Therapy
Postoperative radiation therapy.
Anastrozole 1 mg/day for 5 years.

15 Case 15

15.1 Patient History and Progress

Female/63 years old, post-menopause.
Self-detected mass lesion on right breast 9 o'clock direction.
Family history of breast cancer, mother.
Hypertension, s/p Left leg fracture operation.
BRCA 1 and 2 mutation: Not detected.

15.2 Courses of Treatment

Right breast IDC → Operation → Adjuvant therapy →**Left breast and axillary lymph node recurrence (IDC)** → **Left axillary lymph node recurrence.**

15.2.1 Primary Treatment
See Figs. 109 and 110.

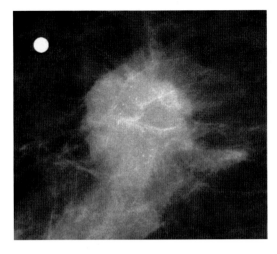

Fig. 109 Right mammography (Apr. 2012): An irregular palpable mass with microcalcifications. US-CNB = IDC

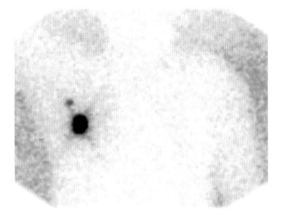

Fig. 110 Lymphoscintigraphy shows visualized sentinel lymph nodes in the left axilla

Operation
May 2012 Right totQAal mastectomy, axillary lymph node dissection (Fig. 111).

Pathology Report
Invasive Ductal Carcinomas (×2).
1. Size of tumor: 2.1 cm, 0.7 cm (pT2(m)).
2. Histologic grade: 2 (tubule formation: 2/3, nuclear pleomorphism: 3/3, mitotic count: 1/3, 8/10HPF).

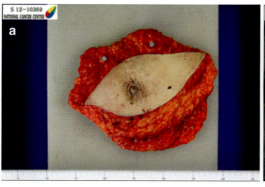 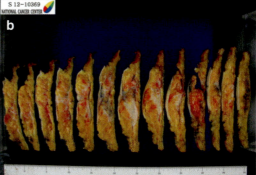

Fig. 111 (**a**) Gross pathology of mastectomy specimen. (**b**) The margins get marked and sliced with different colors on each direction

3. Intraductal component: present, intratumoral/extratumoral (3%) (nuclear grade: high, necrosis: present, architectural pattern: comedo and cribriform, extensive intraductal component: absent).
4. Skin and nipple: no involvement of tumor.
5. Surgical margins: free from tumor.
   (a) Deep margin: 5 mm.
   (b) Superficial margin: 15 mm.
6. Lymph nodes:
   (a) Metastasis in one out of nine axillary lymph nodes (pN1a) (sentinel LN: 1/1, axillary LN: 0/8).
   (b) Perinodal extension: absent.
   (c) Size of metastatic carcinoma: 5 mm.
7. Vascular invasion: absent.
8. Lymphatic invasion: absent.
9. Neural invasion: present.
10. Tumor border: infiltrative.
11. Microcalcification: present, tumoral.
12. Pathologic stage (AJCC 2010): pT2(m)N1a.

	Result	Intensity	Positive %
Estrogen receptor	Strong (7/7)	3	>2/3
Progesterone receptor	Weak (3/7)	2	<10%
C-erbB2	Positive (3+)		
Ki-67	Positive in 29% of tumor cells		

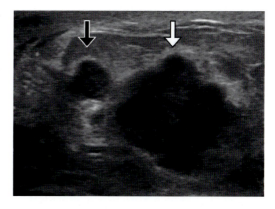

Fig. 112 Left US for evaluation of a palpable lump (Apr. 2021): An irregular palpable mass (white arrow) with an adjacent satellite mass (black arrow). US-CNB = IDC

Adjuvant Therapy
Adjuvant chemotherapy #4 cycles of doxorubicin and cyclophosphamide followed by #4 cycles of docetaxel and trastuzumab for 1 year.
Anastrozole 1 mg/day for 1.3 years.

15.2.2 Treatments After Recurrence
See Figs. 112, 113 and 114.

Neoadjuvant Chemotherapy
Neoadjuvant chemotherapy #2 cycles of cyclophosphamide and methotrexate and fluorouracil (stop d/t no response).

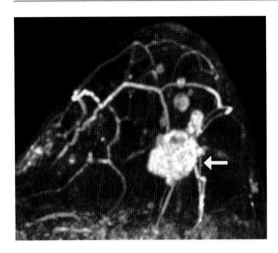

Fig. 113 Left MRI (Apr. 2021): An irregular index tumor (white arrow) with multiple satellite masses

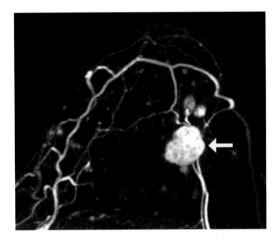

Fig. 114 Post-NAC left MRI (Jun. 2021): Minimally decreased size of the index tumor (white arrow) with multiple satellite masses

Operation (First Recurrence)

Jul. 2021 Left total mastectomy, axillary lymph node dissection (level I) (Fig. 115).

Pathology Report

Invasive Ductal Carcinoma

1. Post-chemotherapy status.
2. Size of tumor: 2.3 cm (ypT2).
3. Histologic grade: 2/3 (tubule formation: 3/3, nuclear pleomorphism: 2/3, mitotic count: 1/3, 6/10HPF).
4. Intraductal component: present, intratumoral/extratumoral (30%) (nuclear grade: low, necrosis: present, architectural pattern: solid/comedo, extensive intraductal component: present).
5. Skin: no involvement of tumor.
6. Surgical margins:
   (a) Deep margin: <1 mm from invasive ductal carcinoma (slide 7).
   (b) Superficial margin: 2 mm.
7. Lymph nodes:
   (a) Metastasis in one out of one axillary lymph node (ypN1a(sn)) (axillary LN (#A): 1/1, axillary LN (Fro 1): 0/0, axillary LN #2: 0/0).
   (b) Perinodal extension: present.
   (c) Size of metastatic carcinoma: 20 mm.
8. Arteriovenous invasion: absent.
9. Lymphovascular invasion: present, intratumoral.
10. Tumor border: infiltrative.
11. Microcalcification: present, tumoral/non-tumoral.
12. Pathological TN category (AJCC 2017): ypT2N1a(sn).

	Result	Intensity	Positive %
Estrogen receptor	Strong (8/8)	3	>2/3
Progesterone receptor	Strong (8/8)	3	>2/3
C-erbB2	Negative (1+)		
Ki-67	Positive in 41% of tumor cells		

Adjuvant Therapy

Adjuvant chemotherapy #4 cycles of cyclophosphamide and docetaxel.

Operation (Second Recurrence)

Oct. 2021 Left axillary lymph node dissection.

Pathology Report

1. Post-lumpectomy status.
2. Lymph nodes:
   (a) Metastasis in three out of five axillary lymph nodes (left axillary LN (Fro 1): 0/1, "left axillary LN": 3/4).

Local Recurrence

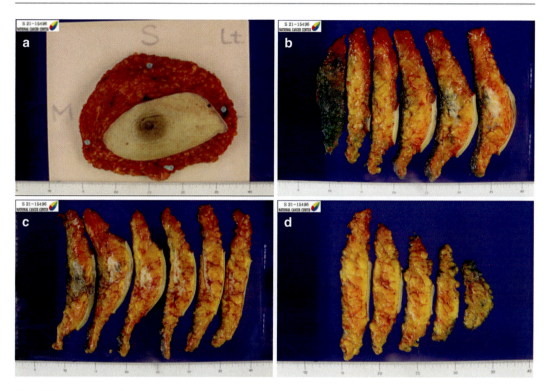

Fig. 115 (**a**) Gross pathology of mastectomy specimen. (**b, c, d**) The margins get marked and sliced with different colors on each direction

(b) Perinodal extension: present.
(c) Size of metastatic carcinoma: 5 mm.

	Result	Intensity	Positive %
Estrogen receptor	Strong (8/8)	3	>2/3
Progesterone receptor	Strong (8/8)	3	>2/3
C-erbB2	Negative (1+)		
Ki-67	Positive in 6% of tumor cells		

Adjuvant Therapy

Postoperative radiation therapy.
Letrozole 2.5 mg/day for 5 years.

16 Case 16

16.1 Patient History and Progress

Female/43 years old, pre-menopause.
 Screen detected mass lesion on left breast 7 o'clock direction.
 Outside result of biopsy: Ductal carcinoma in situ.
 No family history.
 No comorbidities.

16.2 Courses of Treatment

Left breast DCIS → Operation → Adjuvant therapy → **Left breast recurrence (DCIS).**

16.2.1 Primary Treatment

See Figs. 116 and 117.

Operation

Feb. 2014 Left breast conserving surgery (Fig. 118).

Pathology Report

Ductal Carcinoma In Situ
1. Size of tumor: 3.0 cm (pTis).
2. Nuclear grade: low.
3. Necrosis: present.
4. Architectural pattern: micropapillary/cribriform/comedo.

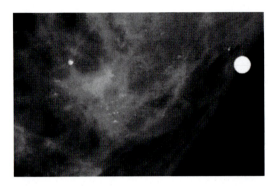

Fig. 116 Left mammography (2014): An irregular palpable mass with microcalcifications at lower central breast. US-CNB = DCIS, low grade

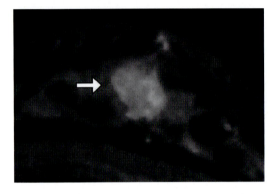

Fig. 117 Left MRI (2014): An irregular enhancing mass at lower central breast

5. Skin: no involvement of tumor.
6. Surgical margins:
   (a) Nipple margin: positive for atypical ductal hyperplasia (Fro 1) (see note 1).
   (b) Superior margin: (see note 2).
   (c) Inferior margin: 20 mm.
   (d) Medial margin: 5 mm.
   (e) Lateral margin: 15 mm.
   (f) Deep margin: 2 mm.
   (g) Superficial margin: 2 mm.
7. Microcalcification: present, tumoral/non-tumoral.
8. Pathologic stage (AJCC 2010): pTis.

Note: 1. Atypical ductal hyperplasia is present only in the permanent section of Fro 1.

2. The superior margin of the lumpectomy specimen (slide 1) is positive for ductal carcinoma in situ, but this margin submitted for frozen diagnosis (Fro 2) is free of tumor.

	Result	Intensity	Positive %
Estrogen receptor	Intermediate (6/8)	2	1/3–2/3
Progesterone receptor	Negative (0/8)	0	0
C-erbB2	Positive (3+)		
Ki-67	Positive in 36% of tumor cells		

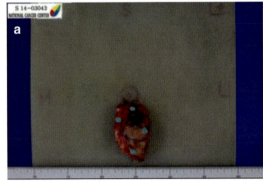 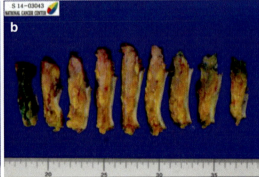

Fig. 118 (**a**) Gross pathology of lumpectomy specimen. (**b**) The margins get marked and sliced with different colors on each direction

Adjuvant Therapy
Postoperative radiation therapy.
   Tamoxifen 20 mg/day for 5 years.

16.2.2 Treatments After Recurrence
See Figs. 119 and 120.

Operation
Jan. 2019 Left nipple wide excision (Fig. 121).

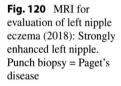

Fig. 119 Left US for evaluation of nipple eczema (2018): Increased vascularity in the nipple

Pathology Report
Ductal Carcinoma In Situ.
1. Post-lumpectomy status.
2. Size of tumor: 0.5 cm (rpTis).
3. Nuclear grade: high.
4. Necrosis: absent.
5. Architectural pattern: micropapillary/cribriform.
6. Skin and nipple: Paget's disease.
7. Surgical margins:
    (a) Superior margin: 5 mm.
    (b) Inferior margin: 5 mm.
    (c) Medial margin: 5 mm.
    (d) Lateral margin: 5 mm.
    (e) Deep margin: 2 mm.
    (f) Superficial margin: 2 mm.
8. Microcalcification: present, tumoral/non-tumoral.
9. Pathological TN category (AJCC 2017): rpTis(Paget).

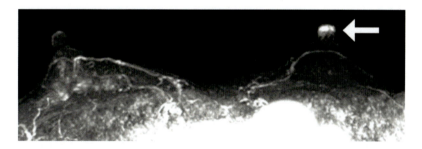

Fig. 120 MRI for evaluation of left nipple eczema (2018): Strongly enhanced left nipple. Punch biopsy = Paget's disease

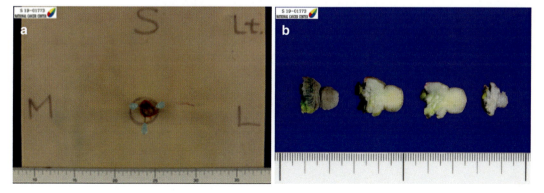

Fig. 121 (a) Gross pathology of nipple wide excision specimen. (b) The margins get marked and sliced with different colors on each direction

	Result	Intensity	Positive %
Estrogen receptor	Negative (2/8)	1	<1%
Progesterone receptor	Negative (0/8)	0	0
C-erbB2	Positive (3+)		
Ki-67	Positive in 58% of tumor cells		

17 Case 17

17.1 Patient History and Progress

Female/43 years old, pre-menopause.
Screen detected mass lesion on right breast 7 o'clock direction.
Outside result of mammotome biopsy: ductal carcinoma in situ.
No family history.
s/p Total thyroidectomy (thyroid cancer).
BRCA 2 VUS (variant of uncertain).

17.2 Courses of Treatment

Right breast DCIS → Operation → Adjuvant therapy → **Right breast recurrence (mucinous carcinoma).**

17.2.1 Primary Treatment
See Fig. 122.

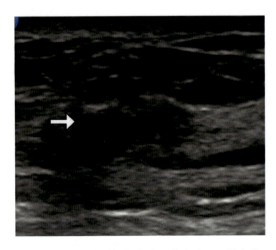

Fig. 122 Right US (2015): An isoechoic mass with indistinct margins at lower outer breast. US-VABE = DCIS, high grade

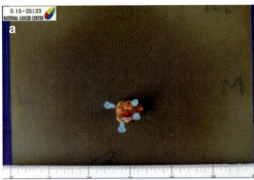

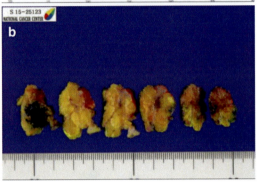

Fig. 123 (a) Gross pathology of lumpectomy specimen. (b) The margins get marked and sliced with different colors on each direction

Operation
Nov. 2015 Right breast conserving surgery (Fig. 123).

Pathology Report

Ductal Carcinoma In Situ
1. Post-excisional biopsy status.
2. Size of tumor: 1.5 cm, residual.
3. Nuclear grade: high.
4. Necrosis: present.
5. Architectural pattern: cribriform/solid/comedo.
6. Skin: no involvement of tumor.
7. Surgical margins:
    (a) Superior margin: 5 mm.
    (b) Inferior margin: 7 mm.
    (c) Medial margin: 15 mm.
    (d) Lateral margin: (see note).
    (e) Deep margin: 2 mm.
    (f) Superficial margin: 8 mm.
8. Microcalcification: present, tumoral/non-tumoral.

Note: 1. The lateral margin of the lumpectomy specimen (slide 7) is close to ductal carcinoma in situ (<1 mm), but this margin submitted for frozen diagnosis (Fro 5) is free of tumor.

	Result	Intensity	Positive %
Estrogen receptor	Negative (0/8)	0	0
Progesterone receptor	Negative (0/8)	0	0
C-erbB2	Positive (3+)		
Ki-67	Positive in 56% of tumor cells		

Adjuvant Therapy
Postoperative radiation therapy.

17.2.2 Treatments After Recurrence
See Figs. 124, 125 and 126.

Operation
Jan. 2020 Right total mastectomy, sentinel lymph node biopsy, Left total mastectomy (Figs. 127 and 128).

Pathology Report
<Right>

Mucinous Carcinoma
1. Post-lumpectomy status.
2. Size of tumor: 1.1 cm (rpT1c).
3. Histologic grade: 2/3 (tubule formation: 3/3, nuclear pleomorphism: 2/3, mitotic count: 1/3, <1/10HPF).

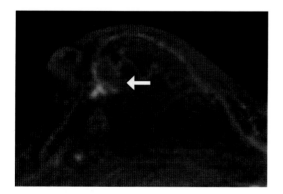

Fig. 124 Right MRI for routine surveillance (2019): A new focal non-mass enhancement at upper outer breast

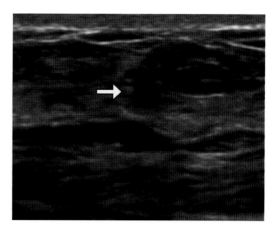

Fig. 125 MRI-directed right US (2019): An isoechoic mass with non-parallel orientation at the corresponding area of the MRI abnormality. US-CNB = Mucinous carcinoma

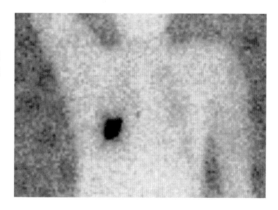

Fig. 126 Lymphoscintigraphy shows visualized sentinel lymph nodes in the right axilla

4. Intraductal component: present, extratumoral (5%) (nuclear grade: low, necrosis: present, architectural pattern: solid/comedo, extensive intraductal component: absent).
5. Skin and nipple: no involvement of tumor.
6. Surgical margins:
   (a) Deep margin: 10 mm.
   (b) Superficial margin: 4 mm.
7. Lymph nodes: no metastasis in five axillary lymph nodes (rpN0(sn)) (sentinel LN: 0/2, axillary LN: 0/2, intramammary LN: 0/1).
8. Arteriovenous invasion: absent.
9. Lymphovascular invasion: absent.
10. Tumor border: infiltrative.
11. Microcalcification: absent.

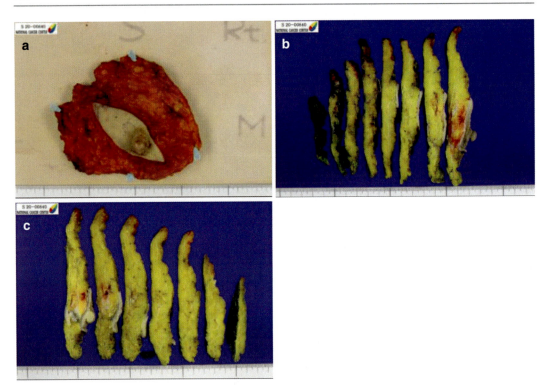

Fig. 127 (**a**) Gross pathology of right mastectomy specimen. (**b**, **c**) The margins get marked and sliced with different colors on each direction

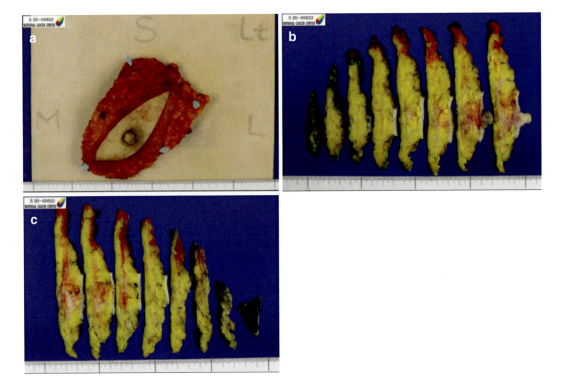

Fig. 128 (**a**) Gross pathology of left mastectomy specimen. (**b**, **c**) The margins get marked and sliced with different colors on each direction

12. Pathological TN category (AJCC 2017): rpT1cN0(sn).

	Result	Intensity	Positive %
Estrogen receptor	Intermediate (6/8)	2	1/3–2/3
Progesterone receptor	Weak (4/8)	2	1–10%
C-erbB2	Negative (0)		
Ki-67	Positive in 22% of tumor cells		

<Left>
1. Fibroadenoma.
2. Usual ductal hyperplasia with apocrine metaplasia.

Adjuvant Therapy
Tamoxifen 20 mg/day for 5 years.

18 Case 18

18.1 Patient History and Progress

Female/71 years old, post-menopause.
  Screen detected mass lesion on right breast.
  No family history.
  Diabetes mellitus, Grave's disease.
  BRCA 2 mutation carrier.

18.2 Courses of Treatment

Left breast IDC→ Operation → Adjuvant therapy → Right breast recurrence (IDC).

18.2.1 Primary Treatment

Operation
May 2001 Left modified radical mastectomy (outside).

Pathology Report
Invasive Ductal Carcinoma
1. Size of tumor: 3.0 cm (pT2).
2. Lymph nodes: two metastases in 24 axillary lymph nodes (pN1) (sentinel LN: 0/2, axillary LN: 0/2, intramammary LN: 0/1).
3. Pathological TN category: pT2N1.

	Result	Intensity	Positive %
Estrogen receptor	Negative	0	0
Progesterone receptor	Negative	0	0
C-erbB2	Negative (0)		
Ki-67	Positive in 70% of tumor cells		

Adjuvant Therapy
Adjuvant chemotherapy #4 cycles of doxorubicin and cyclophosphamide followed by #4 cycles of docetaxel.

18.2.2 Treatments After Recurrence
See Figs. 129, 130 and 131.

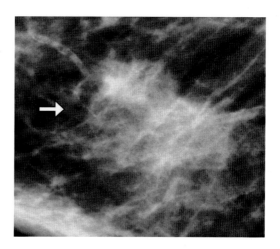

Fig. 129 Right mammography (2021): An irregular hyperdense mass at lower inner breast

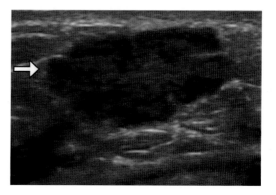

Fig. 130 Right US (2021): A hypoechoic mass with microlobulated margins at lower inner breast. US-CNB = IDC

Operation

Mar. 2021 Right total mastectomy, sentinel lymph node biopsy (Fig. 132).

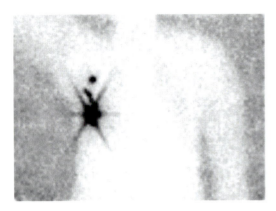

Fig. 131 Lymphoscintigraphy shows visualized sentinel lymph nodes in the right axilla

Pathology Report

Invasive Ductal Carcinoma

1. Post left mastectomy status.
2. Size of tumor: 1.6 cm (pT1c).
3. Histologic grade: 3/3 (tubule formation: 3/3, nuclear pleomorphism: 3/3, mitotic count: 3/3, 12/HPF).
4. Intraductal component: present, intratumoral/extratumoral (30%) (nuclear grade: high, necrosis: present, architectural pattern: micropapillary/comedo, extensive intraductal component: present).
5. Nipple: involvement of lactiferous duct.
6. Skin: no involvement of tumor.
7. Surgical margins:
   (a) Deep margin: 2 mm.
   (b) Superficial margin: 2 mm.
8. Lymph nodes:

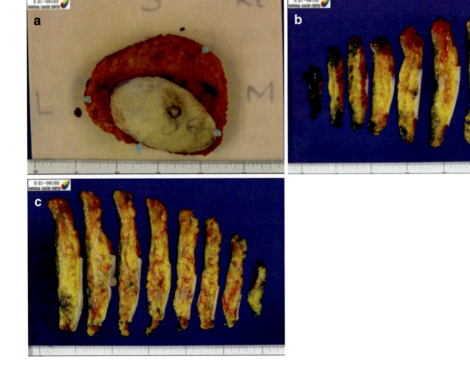

Fig. 132 (**a**) Gross pathology of mastectomy specimen. (**b, c**) The margins get marked and sliced with different colors on each direction

(a) Metastasis in one out of four axillary lymph nodes (pN1mi(sn)) (sentinel LN: 1/3, non-sentinel LN: 0/1).
(b) Perinodal extension: absent.
(c) Size of metastatic carcinoma: 0.8 mm.
9. Arteriovenous invasion: absent.
10. Lymphovascular invasion: present, intratumoral.
11. Tumor border: infiltrative.
12. Microcalcification: present, tumoral/non-tumoral.
13. Pathological TN category (AJCC 2017): pT1cN1mi(sn).

	Result	Intensity	Positive %
Estrogen receptor	Strong (8/8)	3	>2/3
Progesterone receptor	Strong (8/8)	3	>2/3
C-erbB2	Negative (1+)		
Ki-67	Positive in 80% of tumor cells		

Adjuvant Therapy

Anastrozole 1 mg/day (stop d/t low compliance).

19 Case 19

19.1 Patient History and Progress

Female/52 years old, pre-menopause.
Screen detected mass lesion on right breast subareolar area and left breast subareolar area.
No family history.
Hypertension.

19.2 Courses of Treatment

Left breast IDC → Adjuvant therapy.

19.2.1 Primary Treatment

See Figs. 133, 134, 135, 136 and 137.

Neoadjuvant Chemotherapy

Neoadjuvant chemotherapy #4 cycles of doxorubicin and cyclophosphamide followed by #4 cycles of docetaxel and trastuzumab.

Operation

May 2017 Left breast conserving surgery, axillary lymph node dissection, right breast conserving surgery (Figs. 138 and 139).

Pathology Report

<Right>
Complex sclerosing lesion with microcalcification.
<Left>

Invasive Ductal Carcinoma, associated with complex sclerosing lesion

1. Post-chemotherapy status.
2. Size of invasion component: 1.3 cm (ypT1c(m)).
3. Size of intraductal component: 1.6 cm.

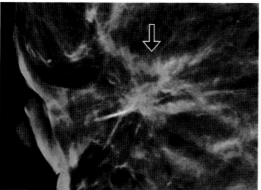 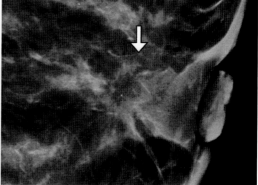

Fig. 133 Mammography (2016): Irregular masses with architectural distortion at both subareolar areas (white arrow = left, black arrow = right)

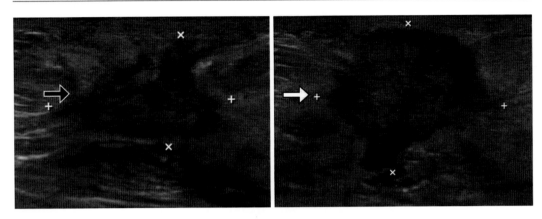

Fig. 134 US (2016): Irregular hypoechoic masses at both subareolar areas (white arrow = left, black arrow = right). US-CNB = Left IDC, Right ADH

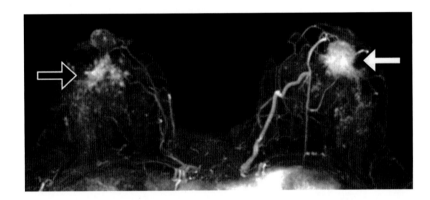

Fig. 135 MRI (2016): Irregular enhancing masses at both subareolar areas (white arrow = left, black arrow = right)

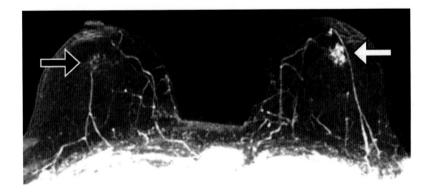

Fig. 136 Post-NAC MRI (2017): Decreased size of the masses at both subareolar areas (white arrow = left, black arrow = right)

4. Histologic grade: 2/3 (tubule formation: 3/3, nuclear pleomorphism: 2/3, mitotic count: 1/3, 4/10HPF).
5. Intraductal component: present, extratumoral (70%) (nuclear grade: low, necrosis: absent, architectural pattern: micropapillary/cribriform, extensive intraductal component: present).

6. Skin: no involvement of tumor.
7. Surgical margins:
   (a) Superior margin: 15 mm.
   (b) Inferior margin: 4 mm.
   (c) Medial margin: (see NOTE 1).
   (d) Lateral margin: 50 mm.
   (e) Deep margin: 7 mm.
   (f) Superficial margin: 14 mm.

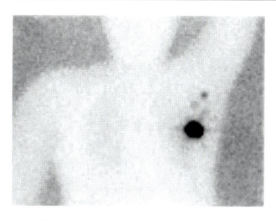

Fig. 137 Lymphoscintigraphy shows visualized sentinel lymph nodes in the left axilla

8. Lymph nodes:
   (a) Metastasis in two out of eight axillary lymph nodes (ypN1a(sn)) (sentinel LN: 2/2, axillary LN: 0/6).
   (b) Perinodal extension: present.
   (c) Size of metastatic carcinoma: 3 mm.
9. Arteriovenous invasion: absent.
10. Lymphovascular invasion: present, peritumoral.
11. Tumor border: infiltrative.
12. Microcalcification: present, tumoral/non-tumoral.
13. Pathologic stage (AJCC 2010): ypT1c(m) N1a(sn).

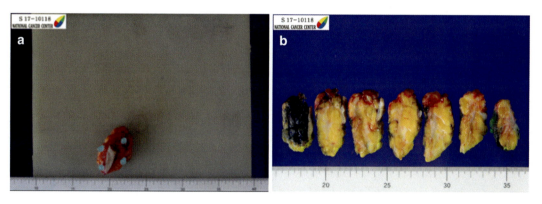

Fig. 138 (**a**) Gross pathology of right lumpectomy specimen. (**b**) The margins get marked and sliced with different colors on each direction

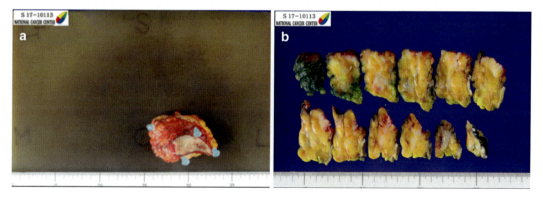

Fig. 139 (**a**) Gross pathology of left lumpectomy specimen. (**b**) The margins get marked and sliced with different colors on each direction

Note 1: The medial margin of the lumpectomy specimen (slide 4) is <1 mm from invasive ductal carcinoma, but this margin submitted for frozen diagnosis (Fro 6) is free of tumor.

	Result	Intensity	Positive %
Estrogen receptor	Weak (4/8)	2	1–10%
Progesterone receptor	Weak (4/8)	2	1–10%
C-erbB2	Positive (3+)		
Ki-67	Positive in 1% of tumor cells		

Adjuvant Therapy

Postoperative radiation therapy.
  Trastuzumab for 1 year.
  Tamoxifen 20 mg/day for 5 years.

20 Case 20

20.1 Patient History and Progress

Female/41 years old, pre-menopause.
  Screen detected mass lesion on right breast 12 o'clock direction.
  Outside result of biopsy: Ductal carcinoma in situ.
  No family history.
  s/p Right breast conserving surgery (Breast cancer), s/p parotidectomy, Panic disorder.
  BRCA 1 VUS (variant of uncertain), APC, and MSH2 VUS.

20.2 Courses of Treatment

Right breast DCIS → Operation → Adjuvant therapy → **Right breast recurrence (microinvasive ductal carcinoma).**

20.2.1 Primary Treatment
See Fig. 140.

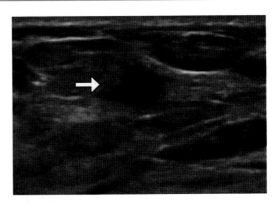

Fig. 140 Right US (2017): A hypoechoic mass with spiculated margins at inner central breast

Operation

Jul. 2017 Right breast conserving surgery, sentinel lymph node biopsy (outside).

Pathology Report

Ductal Carcinoma In Situ
1. Size of tumor: 1.2 cm.
2. Nuclear grade: high.
3. Necrosis: present, central.
4. Architectural pattern: comedo.
5. Skin: no involvement of tumor.
6. Surgical margins: uninvolved by DCIS distance from closest margin: 2 mm (specify margin: 9H).
7. Lymph nodes: no metastasis in five lymph nodes (pN0(sn)).
8. Lymphovascular invasion: not identified.
9. Perineural invasion: not identified.
10. Pathological TN category: pTisN0.

	Result	Intensity	Positive %
Estrogen receptor	Negative	0	0
Progesterone receptor	Negative	0	0
C-erbB2	Positive (3+)		
Ki-67	Positive in 35% of tumor cells		

Adjuvant Therapy
Postoperative radiation therapy.

20.2.2 Treatments After Recurrence
See Figs. 141, 142 and 143.

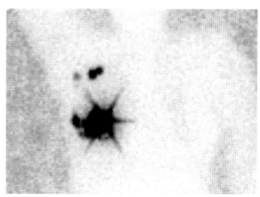

Fig. 143 Lymphoscintigraphy shows visualized sentinel lymph nodes in the right axilla

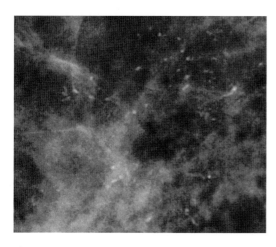

Fig. 141 Right mammography for routine surveillance (2021): Newly developed regional fine pleomorphic microcalcifications at upper central breast. Stereotactic VAB = DCIS, high grade

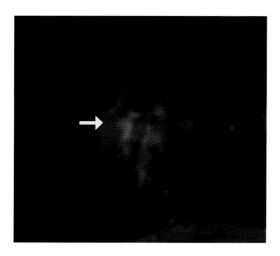

Fig. 142 Right MRI (2021): Regional heterogeneous non-mass enhancement at upper central breast

Operation
Jul. 2021 Right nipple-areolar complex sparing mastectomy with immediate implant reconstruction, sentinel lymph node biopsy (Figs. 144 and 145).

Pathology Report
1. Microinvasive Ductal Carcinoma
   (a) Size of invasive component: <0.1 cm (pT1mi).
   (b) Size of in situ component: 1.5 cm.
   (c) Histologic grade: not applicable.
   (d) Intraductal component: present, intratumoral/extratumoral (99%) (nuclear grade: high, necrosis: present, architectural pattern: micropapillary/cribriform/solid/comedo, extensive intraductal component: present).
   (e) Surgical margins:
      - Deep margin: 3 mm.
      - Superficial margin: 8 mm.
   (f) Lymph nodes: no metastasis in three axillary lymph nodes (pN0(sn)) (sentinel LN: 0/3).
   (g) Arteriovenous invasion: absent.

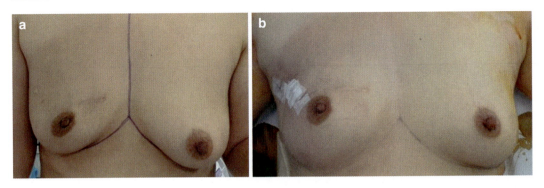

Fig. 144 (a) Preoperative and (b) immediate postoperative appearance

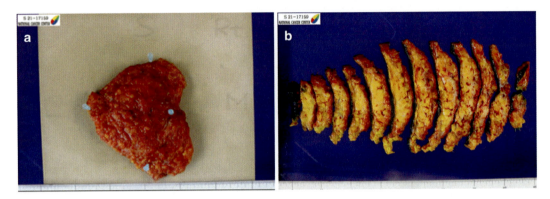

Fig. 145 (a) Gross pathology of mastectomy specimen. (b) The margins get marked and sliced with different colors on each direction

   (h) Lymphovascular invasion: absent.
   (i) Tumor border: infiltrative.
   (j) Microcalcification: present, tumoral/non-tumoral.
   (k) Pathological TN category (AJCC 2017): pT1miN0(sn).
   (l) Related slides: none.
2. Fibroadenoma.

	Result	Intensity	Positive %
Estrogen receptor	Negative (0/8)	0	0
Progesterone receptor	Weak (3/8)	2	<1%
C-erbB2	Positive (3+)		
Ki-67	Positive in 23% of tumor cells		

21 Case 21

21.1 Patient History and Progress

Female/55 years old, peri-menopause.
   Screen detected calcification on upper portion of right breast.
   Outside result of biopsy: suggestive ductal carcinoma in situ.
   No family history.
   S/p hysterectomy.

21.2 Courses of Treatment

Right breast DCIS→ → Operation → Right breast recurrence (DCIS).

21.2.1 Primary Treatment
See Fig. 146.

Operation
Jan. 2017 Right nipple-areolar complex sparing mastectomy with immediate implant reconstruction, sentinel lymph node biopsy (Figs. 147 and 148).

Pathology Report

Ductal Carcinoma In Situ
1. Size of tumor: 5.5 cm (pTis).
2. Nuclear grade: low.
3. Necrosis: present.

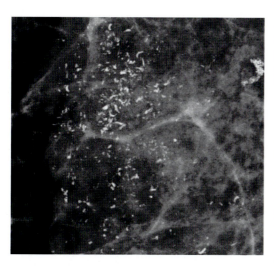

Fig. 146 Right magnification view (2017): Fine linear and pleomorphic microcalcifications at upper breast. US-CNB = DCIS, low grade

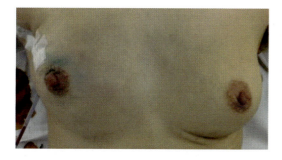

Fig. 147 Immediate postoperative appearance

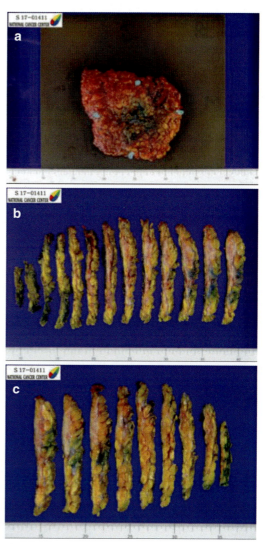

Fig. 148 (**a**) Gross pathology of mastectomy specimen. (**b**, **c**) The margins get marked and sliced with different colors on each direction

4. Architectural pattern: micropapillary/solid/comedo.
5. Skin: no involvement of tumor.
6. Surgical margins:
   (a) Deep margin: (see note).
   (b) Superficial margin: <1 mm from ductal carcinoma in situ (slide MG5).
7. Lymph nodes: no metastasis in two axillary lymph nodes (pN0(sn)) (sentinel LN: 0/2).

8. Microcalcification: present, tumoral/non-tumoral.
9. Pathologic stage (AJCC 2010): pTisN0(sn).

Note: 1. The deep margin of the mastectomy specimen (slide 7) is close to ductal carcinoma in situ (<1 mm), but this margin submitted for frozen diagnosis (Fro 4) is free of tumor.

	Result	Intensity	Positive %
Estrogen receptor	Intermediate (5/8)	2	10%-1/3
Progesterone receptor	Negative (0/8)	0	0
C-erbB2	Positive (3+)		
Ki-67	Positive in 22% of tumor cells		

21.2.2 Treatments After Recurrence
See Figs. 149 and 150.

Operation
Feb. 2020 Right nipple excision (Fig. 151).

Pathology Report

Ductal Carcinoma In Situ
1. Post-nipple-sparing mastectomy status.
2. Size of tumor: 1.1 cm (rpTis).
3. Nuclear grade: low.
4. Necrosis: absent.
5. Architectural pattern: solid.

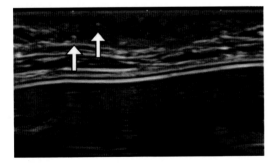

Fig. 149 Right US for routine surveillance (2020): Echogenic microcalcifications in the nipple-areolar complex of the implant-reconstructed breast

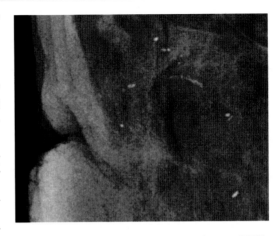

Fig. 150 Right magnification view (2020): Microcalcifications at subareolar area. US-CNB = DCIS, low grade

6. Skin and nipple: no involvement of tumor.
7. Surgical margins:
    (a) Superior margin: 5 mm.
    (b) Inferior margin: 11 mm.
    (c) Medial margin: 5 mm.
    (d) Lateral margin: 10 mm.
    (e) Deep margin: (see note).
    (f) Superficial margin: 2 mm.
8. Microcalcification: present, tumoral.
9. Pathological TN category (AJCC 2017): rpTis.

Note: 1. The deep margin of the lumpectomy specimen (slide 1) is close to ductal carcinoma in situ (<1 mm), but this margin submitted for frozen diagnosis (Fro 5) is free of tumor.

	Result	Intensity	Positive %
Estrogen receptor	Weak (4/8)	1	10%-1/3
Progesterone receptor	Negative (0/8)	0	0
C-erbB2	Positive (3+)		
Ki-67	Positive in 8% of tumor cells		

Adjuvant Therapy
Postoperative radiation therapy.

Local Recurrence

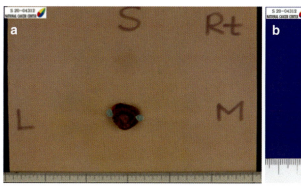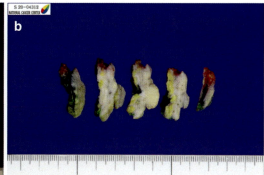

Fig. 151 (**a**) Gross pathology of nipple excision specimen. (**b**) The margins get marked and sliced with different colors on each direction

22 Case 22

22.1 Patient History and Progress

Female/80 years old, post-menopause.

Screen detected mass lesion on upper outer portion of Left breast.

Outside result of biopsy: Mucinous carcinoma.

No family history.

Dementia.

BRCA 1 and 2 mutation: No examination.

22.2 Courses of Treatment

Left breast mucinous carcinoma→ Adjuvant therapy → **Right breast recurrence (mucinous carcinoma).**

22.2.1 Primary Treatment
See Fig. 152.

Operation

Apr. 2007 Left breast mass excision (outside).

Pathology Report

Mucinous Carcinoma
1. Size of tumor: 2.0 cm.
2. Margin involved.

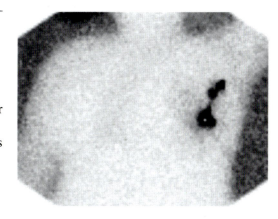

Fig. 152 Lymphoscintigraphy shows visualized sentinel lymph nodes in the left axilla

	Result	Intensity	Positive %
Estrogen receptor	Strong (7/8)	3	>2/3
Progesterone receptor	Weak (3/8)	1	10%-1/3
C-erbB2	Negative (0)		

Operation (2nd)

May 2007 Left breast conserving surgery, sentinel lymph node biopsy (Fig. 153).

Pathology Report

No residual carcinoma with foreign body reaction.
1. Post-excisional biopsy status.

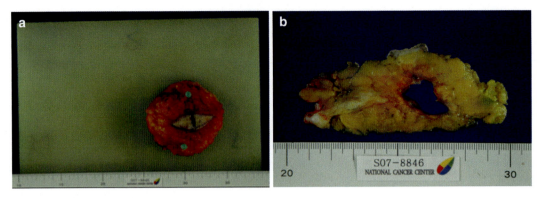

Fig. 153 (a) Gross pathology of lumpectomy specimen. (b) The margins get marked and sliced with different colors on each direction

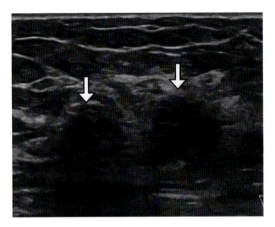

Fig. 154 Right US for evaluation of palpable lumps (2021): Hypoechoic masses with microlobulated margins. US-CNB = Mucinous carcinoma

Adjuvant Therapy
Adjuvant chemotherapy #4 cycles of doxorubicin and cyclophosphamide.
Postoperative radiation therapy.
Letrozole 2.5 mg/day 1.7 years, tamoxifen 20 mg/day for 2.2 years.

22.2.2 Treatments After Recurrence
See Fig. 154.
Letrozole 2.5 mg/day (rejection of surgical treatment).

23 Case 23

23.1 Patient History and Progress

Female/49 years old, pre-menopause.
Palpable mass lesion on left breast 2 o'clock direction.
Family history of breast cancer, maternal grandmother.
s/p Left breast conserving surgery (breast cancer), s/p Bilateral salpingo-oophorectomy.
BRCA 1 mutation carrier.

23.2 Courses of Treatment

Left breast medullary carcinoma → Operation → Adjuvant therapy → **Left breast recurrence (IDC)**/Right breast intraductal papilloma.

23.2.1 Primary Treatment

Operation
2003 Left breast conserving surgery, axillary lymph node dissection (outside).

Pathology Report
Medullary Carcinoma.

Adjuvant Therapy

Adjuvant chemotherapy #6 cycles of doxorubicin and cyclophosphamide.

Postoperative radiation therapy.

23.2.2 Treatments After Recurrence

See Figs. 155, 156 and 157.

Operation

Feb. 2019 Both nipple-areolar complex sparing mastectomy (Figs. 158 and 159).

Pathology Report

<Right>

1. Intraductal papilloma with:
   (a) sclerosing adenosis.
   (b) microcalcification.
2. Sclerosing adenosis.
3. Columnar cell hyperplasia.
4. Fibroadenomatous change.

<Left>

1. Invasive Ductal Carcinoma with focal papillary pattern.

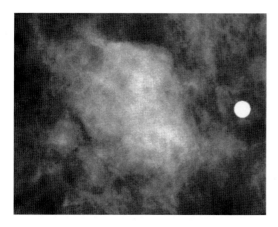

Fig. 155 Left mammography for evaluation of a palpable lump (2018): A hyperdense palpable mass at upper outer breast

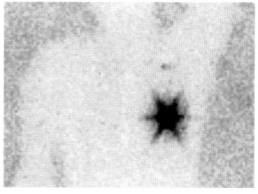

Fig. 157 Lymphoscintigraphy shows visualized sentinel lymph nodes in the left axilla

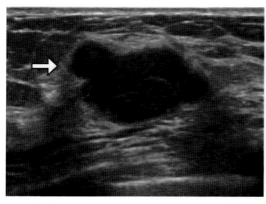

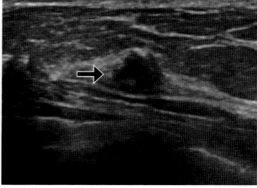

Fig. 156 Left US for evaluation of a palpable lump (2018): A hypoechoic palpable mass at upper outer breast (white arrow). US-CNB = IDC. Another hypoechoic mass at the op bed of lower inner breast (black arrow). US-CNB = IDC

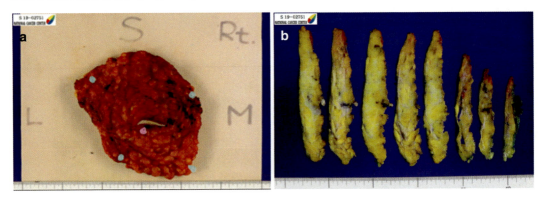

Fig. 158 (**a**) Gross pathology of right mastectomy specimen. (**b**) The margins get marked and sliced with different colors on each direction

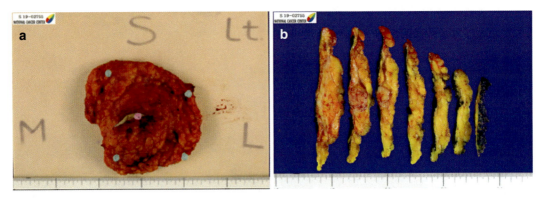

Fig. 159 (**a**) Gross pathology of left mastectomy specimen. (**b**) The margins get marked and sliced with different colors on each direction

- (a) Size of tumor: 1.9 cm (pT1c(2)).
- (b) Histologic grade: 3/3 (tubule formation: 3/3, nuclear pleomorphism: 3/3, mitotic count: 3/3, 11/HPF).
- (c) Intraductal component: present, extratumoral (5%) (nuclear grade: high, necrosis: absent, architectural pattern: papillary/solid, extensive intraductal component: absent).
- (d) Skin: no involvement of tumor.
- (e) Surgical margins:
  - Deep margin: (see note).
  - Superficial margin: 15 mm.
- (f) Lymph nodes: no lymph node identified.
- (g) Arteriovenous invasion: absent.
- (h) Lymphovascular invasion: absent.
- (i) Tumor border: infiltrative.
- (j) Microcalcification: absent.
- (k) Pathological TN category (AJCC 2017): pT1c.

2. Invasive Ductal Carcinoma.
- (a) Size of tumor: 0.6 cm.
- (b) Histologic grade: 2/3 (tubule formation: 3/3, nuclear pleomorphism: 2/3, mitotic count: 1/3, 1/10HPF).
- (c) Intraductal component: present, intratumoral/extratumoral (30%) (nuclear grade: low, necrosis: absent, architectural pattern: cribriform, extensive intraductal component: present).
- (d) Arteriovenous invasion: absent.
- (e) Lymphovascular invasion: absent.
- (f) Tumor border: infiltrative.

Note: 1. The deep margin of the lumpectomy specimen (slide 2) is close to invasive ductal carcinoma (<1 mm), but this margin separately submitted for permanent diagnosis (slide B) is free of tumor.

	Result	Intensity	Positive %
Estrogen receptor	Negative (2/8)	1	<1%
Progesterone receptor	Negative (0/8)	0	0
C-erbB2	Negative (1+)		
Ki-67	Positive in 48% of tumor cells		

Adjuvant Therapy

Adjuvant chemotherapy #4 cycles of cyclophosphamide and docetaxel.

24 Case 24

24.1 Patient History and Progress

Female/45 years old, pre-menopause.

Screen detected mass lesion on upper outer portion of left breast.

Outside result of biopsy: Invasive ductal carcinoma.

Family history of breast cancer, maternal aunt, another aunt.

No comorbidities.

BRCA 1 and 2 mutation: Not detected.

24.2 Courses of Treatment

Left breast IDC → Neoadjuvant chemotherapy → Operation → Adjuvant therapy → **Left chest wall recurrence (IDC).**

24.2.1 Primary Treatment
See Figs. 160, 161, 162 and 163.

Neoadjuvant Chemotherapy
#4 cycles of doxorubicin and cyclophosphamide followed by #4 cycles of docetaxel.

Operation
Aug. 2019 Left modified radical mastectomy (Fig. 164).

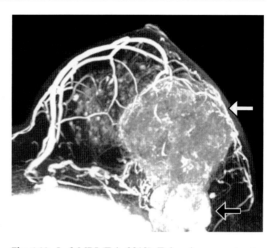

Fig. 160 Left MRI (Feb. 2019): Enhancing mass at outer breast (white arrow). Enlarged axillary LN (black arrow). US-CNB = IDC

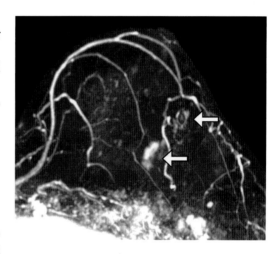

Fig. 161 Left MRI during NAC (May 2019): Decreased and fragmented malignant tumors

Pathology Report

Invasive Ductal Carcinoma
1. Post-chemotherapy status.
2. Size of tumor: 5.0 cm (ypT2).
3. Histologic grade: 3 (tubule formation: 3/3, nuclear pleomorphism: 3/3, mitotic count: 2/3, 16/10HPF).
4. Intraductal component: present, intratumoral/extratumoral (20%) (nuclear grade:

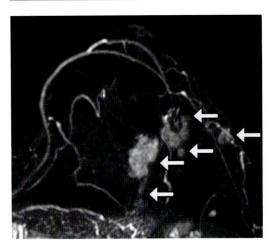

Fig. 162 Left MRI after completion of NAC (Aug. 2019): Increased number and size of malignant masses

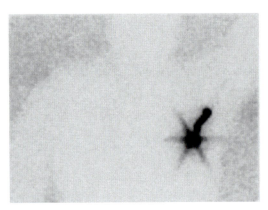

Fig. 163 Lymphoscintigraphy shows visualized sentinel lymph nodes in the left axilla

high, necrosis: present, architectural pattern: solid/comedo, extensive intraductal component: absent).
5. Skin and nipple: no involvement of tumor.
6. Surgical margins:
   (a) Deep margin: <1 mm from invasive ductal carcinoma (slides 2 and 8).
   (b) Superficial margin: 20 mm.
7. Lymph nodes: no metastasis in 17 axillary lymph nodes (ypN0) (sentinel LN: 0/6, non-sentinel LN: 0/11).
8. Arteriovenous invasion: present, intratumoral.

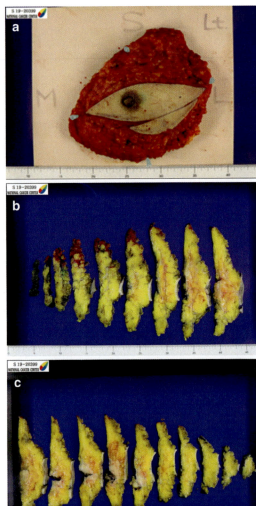

Fig. 164 (a) Gross pathology of mastectomy specimen. (b, c) The margins get marked and sliced with different colors on each direction

9. Lymphovascular invasion: present, intratumoral.
10. Tumor border: infiltrative.
11. Microcalcification: present, tumoral/non-tumoral.
12. Pathological TN category (AJCC 2017): ypT2N0.

	Result	Intensity	Positive %
Estrogen receptor	Negative (0/8)	0	0
Progesterone receptor	Negative (0/8)	0	0
C-erbB2	Equivocal (2+) (SISH negative)		
Ki-67	Positive in 46% of tumor cells		

Adjuvant Therapy

Postoperative radiation therapy.

Adjuvant chemotherapy #8 cycles of capecitabine.

24.2.2 Treatments After Recurrence

See Figs. 165 and 166.

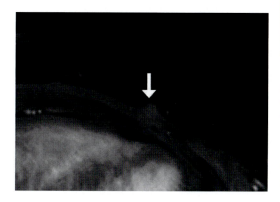

Fig. 165 MRI for routine surveillance (Aug. 2021): An enhancing mass at left anterior chest wall

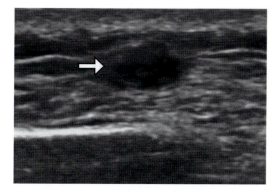

Fig. 166 MRI-directed left US (Aug. 2021): A hypoechoic mass at the corresponding area of the MRI abnormality. US-CNB = IDC

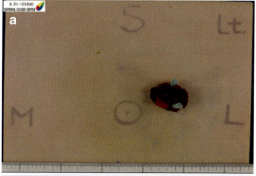

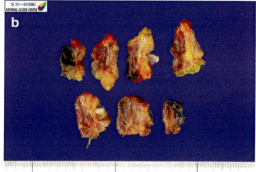

Fig. 167 (**a**) Gross pathology of chest wall excision specimen. (**b**) The margins get marked and sliced with different colors on each direction

Operation

Sep. 2021 Left chest wall wide excision (Fig. 167).

Pathology Report

Invasive Ductal Carcinoma

1. Post-modified radical mastectomy status.
2. Size of tumor: 1.0 cm (rpT1b).
3. Histologic grade: 3/3 (tubule formation: 3/3, nuclear pleomorphism: 3/3, mitotic count: 3/3, 10/HPF).
4. Intraductal component: absent.
5. Skin: no involvement of tumor.
6. Surgical margins:
    (a) Superior margin: 8 mm.
    (b) Inferior margin: 10 mm.
    (c) Medial margin: 20 mm.
    (d) Lateral margin: 5 mm.
    (e) Deep margin: 9 mm.
    (f) Superficial margin: 3 mm.

7. Arteriovenous invasion: absent.
8. Lymphovascular invasion: absent.
9. Tumor border: infiltrative.
10. Microcalcification: absent.
11. Pathological TN category (AJCC 2017): rpT1b.

	Result	Intensity	Positive %
Estrogen receptor	Negative (0/8)	0	0
Progesterone receptor	Negative (0/8)	0	0
C-erbB2	Negative (1+)		
Ki-67	Positive in 72% of tumor cells		

Adjuvant Therapy
Adjuvant chemotherapy #8 cycles of paclitaxel.

25 Case 25

25.1 Patient History and Progress

Female/69 years old, post-menopause.
For chemotherapy after left breast cancer surgery.
No family history.
s/p Left breast conserving surgery, s/p total Thyroidectomy (thyroid cancer).
s/p Hysterectomy and bilateral salpingo-oophorectomy.

25.2 Courses of Treatment

Left breast IDC → Operation → Adjuvant therapy → Left breast recurrence (DCIS).

25.2.1 Primary Treatment

Operation
Nov. 2007 Left breast conserving surgery, axillary lymph node dissection (outside).

Pathology Report

Invasive Ductal Carcinoma
1. Size of tumor: 1.1 cm (pT1c).
2. Histologic grade: 3/3.
3. Lymph nodes: three metastases in fourteen axillary lymph nodes (pN1).

	Result	Intensity	Positive %
Estrogen receptor	Negative (0/7)	0	0
Progesterone receptor	Strong (6/7)	3	1/3–2/3
C-erbB2	Equivocal (2+) (SISH negative)		

Adjuvant Therapy
Adjuvant chemotherapy #4 cycles of doxorubicin and cyclophosphamide followed by #4 cycles of docetaxel.
Postoperative radiation therapy.
Letrozole 2.5 mg/day for 5 years.

25.2.2 Treatments After Recurrence
See Fig. 168.

Operation
Apr. 2020 Left breast wide excision (Fig. 169).

Pathology Report

Ductal Carcinoma In Situ with apocrine differentiation involving fibroadenoma
1. Post-lumpectomy status.
2. Size of tumor: 0.6 cm (rpTis).
3. Nuclear grade: low.
4. Necrosis: present.
5. Architectural pattern: cribriform/solid/comedo.

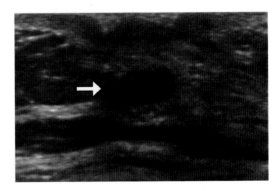

Fig. 168 Left US for routine surveillance (2020): A new oval hypoechoic mass. US-CNB = ADH involving FA

Local Recurrence

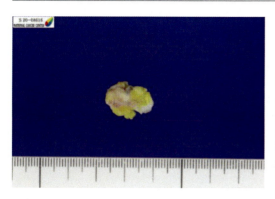

Fig. 169 Gross pathology of breast excision specimen

6. Surgical margins: <1 mm from the nearest margin (slide 1).
7. Microcalcification: present, non-tumoral.
8. Pathological TN category (AJCC 2017): rpTis.

	Result	Intensity	Positive %
Estrogen receptor	Negative (0/8)	0	0
Progesterone receptor	Negative (0/8)	0	0
C-erbB2	Equivocal (2+)		
Ki-67	Positive in 9% of tumor cells		

26 Case 26

26.1 Patient History and Progress

Female/40 years old, post-menopause.
Bloody nipple discharge from right breast.
Outside result of biopsy: Ductal carcinoma in situ.
No family history.
No comorbidities.
BRCA 1 and 2 mutation: Not detected.

26.2 Courses of Treatment

Right breast DCIS→ Operation → Adjuvant therapy → **Right breast recurrence (IDC).**

26.2.1 Primary Treatment

See Figs. 170 and 171.

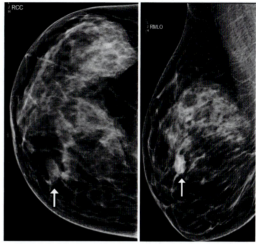

Fig. 170 Mammography: oval isodense mass in right breast

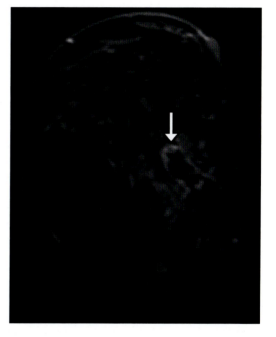

Fig. 171 MRI: vacuum-assisted breast excision status. Marginal enhancing lesion at the 3 o'clock location of right breast

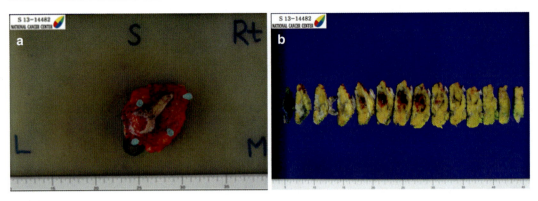

Fig. 172 (**a**) Gross pathology of lumpectomy specimen. (**b**) The margins get marked and sliced with different colors on each direction

Operation
Jun. 2013 Right breast conserving surgery (Fig. 172).

Pathology Report

Ductal Carcinoma In Situ
1. Post-excisional biopsy status.
2. Size of tumor: 2.0 cm, residual.
3. Nuclear grade: low.
4. Necrosis: absent.
5. Architectural pattern: cribriform and papillary.
6. Skin: no involvement of tumor.
7. Surgical margins:
   (a) Superior margin: 25 mm.
   (b) Inferior margin: 7 mm.
   (c) Medial margin: 30 mm.
   (d) Lateral margin: 20 mm.
   (e) Deep margin: 3 mm.
   (f) Superficial margin: 13 mm.
8. Microcalcification: absent.

	Result	Intensity	Positive %
Estrogen receptor	Strong (7/8)	2	>2/3
Progesterone receptor	Strong (8/8)	2	>2/3
C-erbB2	Negative (0)		
Ki-67	Positive in 5% of tumor cells		

Adjuvant Therapy
Postoperative radiation therapy.

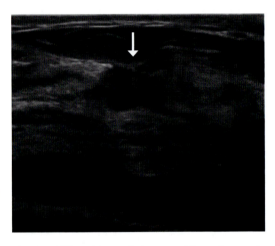

Fig. 173 US: oval hypoechoic mass with angular margin at the 10 o'clock location of right breast

26.2.2 Treatments After Recurrence
See Figs. 173 and 174.

Operation
Nov. 2021 Right nipple-areolar complex sparing mastectomy with immediate implant reconstruction (Fig. 175).

Pathology Report

Invasive Ductal Carcinoma
1. Post-lumpectomy status.
2. Size of tumor: 1.2 cm (rpT1c).
3. Histologic grade: 2/3 (tubule formation: 3/3, nuclear pleomorphism: 2/3, mitotic count: 2/3, 11/10HPF).

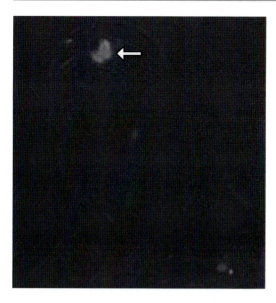

Fig. 174 MRI: irregular heterogeneous enhancing mass at the 10 o'clock location of right breast

4. Intraductal component: present, intratumoral/extratumoral (10%) (nuclear grade: low, necrosis: absent, architectural pattern: cribriform, extensive intraductal component: absent).
5. Skin: no involvement of tumor.
6. Surgical margins:
   (a) Deep margin: 2 mm.
   (b) Superficial margin: 2 mm.
7. Lymph nodes: not submitted.
8. Arteriovenous invasion: absent.
9. Lymphovascular invasion: present, intratumoral.
10. Tumor border: infiltrative.
11. Microcalcification: present, tumoral/non-tumoral.
12. Pathological TN category (AJCC 2017): rpT1c.

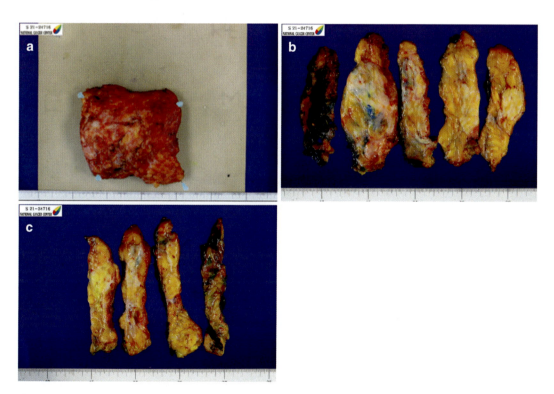

Fig. 175 (a) Gross pathology of mastectomy specimen. (b, c) The margins get marked and sliced with different colors on each direction

	Result	Intensity	Positive %
Estrogen receptor	Strong (8/8)	2	>2/3
Progesterone receptor	Strong (8/8)	2	>2/3
C-erbB2	Negative (1+)		
Ki-67	Positive in 11% of tumor cells		

Adjuvant Therapy
Anastrozole 1 mg/day.

27　Case 27

27.1　Patient History and Progress

Female/57 years old, post-menopause.
 Screen detected mass lesion on right breast 1 o'clock direction.
 Outside result of biopsy: Invasive ductal carcinoma.
 Family history of breast cancer, younger sister.
 No comorbidities.
 BRCA 1 and 2 mutation: Not detected.

27.2　Courses of Treatment

Right breast tubular carcinoma → Operation → Adjuvant therapy → **Left breast recurrence (IDC)**.

27.2.1　Primary Treatment
See Figs. 176, 177, 178 and 179.

Operation
Sep. 2013 Right breast conserving surgery, sentinel lymph node biopsy (Fig. 180).

Pathology Report
Tubular Carcinoma
1. Size of tumor: 1.5 cm (pT1c).
2. Histologic grade: 1/3 (tubule formation: 1/3, nuclear pleomorphism: 2/3, mitotic count: 1/3, 2/10HPF).

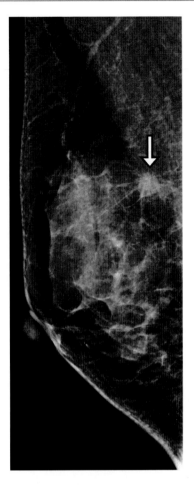

Fig. 176 Right MLO MG: spiculated hyperdense mass in right upper breast

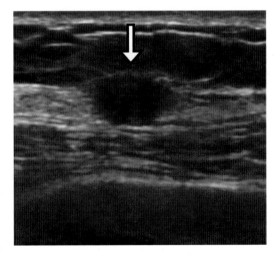

Fig. 177 US: spiculated oval hypoechoic mass at the 1 o'clock location of right breast

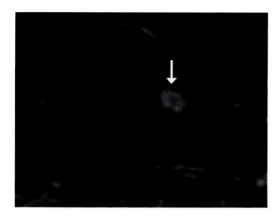

Fig. 178 MRI: irregular rim enhancing mass at the 1 o'clock location of right breast

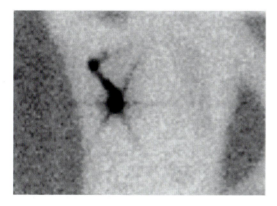

Fig. 179 Lymphoscintigraphy shows visualized sentinel lymph nodes in the right axilla

3. Intraductal component: present, intratumoral/extratumoral (5%) (nuclear grade: low, necrosis: absent, architectural pattern: cribriform, extensive intraductal component: absent).
4. Skin: no involvement of tumor.
5. Surgical margins:
   (a) Superior margin: 18 mm.
   (b) Inferior margin: 13 mm.
   (c) Medial margin: 10 mm.
   (d) Lateral margin: 10 mm.
   (e) Deep margin: 3 mm.
   (f) Superficial margin: 3 mm.
6. Lymph nodes: no metastasis in one axillary lymph nodes (pN0(sn)) (sentinel LN: 0/1).
7. Vascular invasion: absent.
8. Lymphatic invasion: absent.
9. Tumor border: infiltrative.
10. Microcalcification: present, tumoral.
11. Pathologic stage (AJCC 2010): pT1cN0(sn).

	Result	Intensity	Positive %
Estrogen receptor	Strong (8/8)	3	>2/3
Progesterone receptor	Strong (8/8)	3	>2/3
C-erbB2	Negative (1+)		
Ki-67	Positive in 11% of tumor cells		

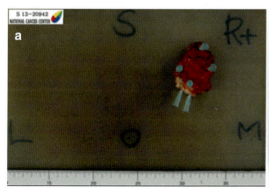
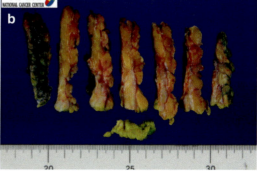

Fig. 180 (a) Gross pathology of lumpectomy specimen. (b) The margins get marked and sliced with different colors on each direction

Adjuvant Therapy

Postoperative radiation therapy.
  Tamoxifen 20 mg/day for 5 years.

27.2.2 Treatments After Recurrence

See Figs. 181, 182 and 183.

Operation

First Operation (Nov. 2021) Left breast conserving surgery, sentinel lymph node biopsy (Fig. 184).

Pathology Report

Invasive Ductal Carcinoma

1. Size of tumor: 0.3 cm (pT1a).
2. Histologic grade: 2/3 (tubule formation: 3/3, nuclear pleomorphism: 2/3, mitotic count: 1/3, 6/10HPF).
3. Intraductal component: present, intratumoral/extratumoral (50%) (nuclear grade: low, necrosis: absent, architectural pattern: micropapillary/cribriform, extensive intraductal component: present).
4. Skin: no involvement of tumor.
5. Surgical margins:
   (a) Superior margin: 10 mm.
   (b) Inferior margin: positive for invasive ductal carcinoma (Fro 7) (see note).
   (c) Medial margin: 10 mm.
   (d) Lateral margin: 10 mm.
   (e) Deep margin: <1 mm from ductal carcinoma in situ (slide 1).
   (f) Superficial margin: 2 mm.
6. Lymph nodes: no metastasis in two axillary lymph nodes (pN0(sn)) (sentinel LN: 0/2).
7. Arteriovenous invasion: absent.
8. Lymphovascular invasion: absent.
9. Tumor border: infiltrative.
10. Microcalcification: present, tumoral/non-tumoral.
11. Pathological TN category (AJCC 2017): pT1aN0(sn).

Note: 1. Invasive ductal carcinoma is focally present only in the permanent section of Fro 7.

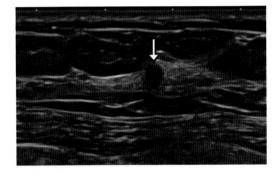

Fig. 181 US: Not parallel hypoechoic mass at the 1 o'clock location of left breast

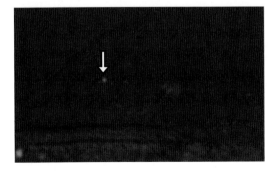

Fig. 182 MRI: An enhancing focus at the 1 o'clock location of left breast

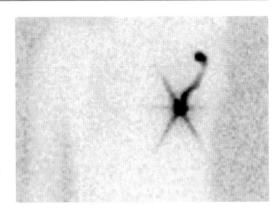

Fig. 183 Lymphoscintigraphy shows visualized sentinel lymph nodes in the left axilla

	Result	Intensity	Positive %
Estrogen receptor	Strong (8/8)	3	>2/3
Progesterone receptor	Intermediate (6/8)	3	10%-1/3
C-erbB2	Negative (1+)		
Ki-67	Positive in 2% of tumor cells		

Local Recurrence

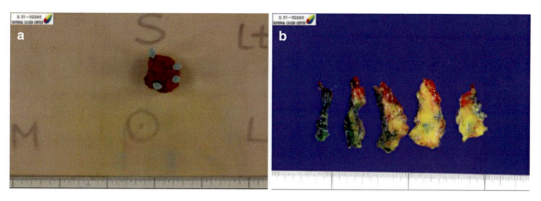

Fig. 184 (**a**) Gross pathology of lumpectomy specimen. (**b**) The margins get marked and sliced with different colors on each direction

Operation
Second Operation (Dec. 2021) Left breast wide excision.

Pathology Report
Atypical ductal hyperplasia

1. Post-lumpectomy status.

Adjuvant Therapy
Postoperative radiation therapy.

28 Case 28

28.1 Patient History and Progress

Female/50 years old, pre-menopause.
 Screen detected mass lesion on left breast 2 o'clock direction.
 Outside result of mammotome excision: Ductal carcinoma in situ.
 No family history.
 No comorbidities.

28.2 Courses of Treatment

Left breast DCIS → Operation → Adjuvant therapy → **Left breast recurrence (microinvasive ductal carcinoma).**

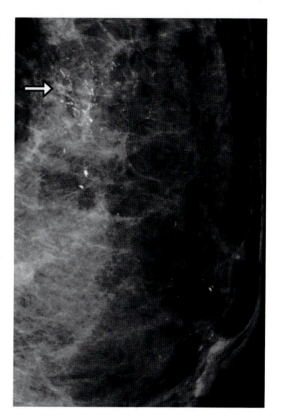

Fig. 185 MG: segmental fine linear or fine linear branching microcalcification with extension to left subareolar area

28.2.1 Primary Treatment
See Figs. 185, 186, 187 and 188.

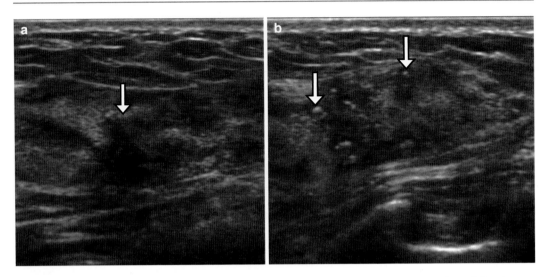

Fig. 186 (a) Irregular hypoechoic mass with indistinct margin. (b) Echogenic dots, suggesting microcalcifications

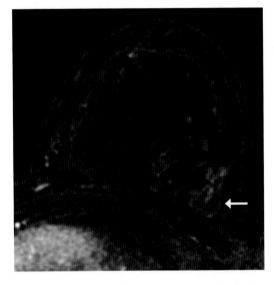

Fig. 187 MRI: regional heterogenous non-mass enhancement at the corresponding area of the microcalcifications on mammography

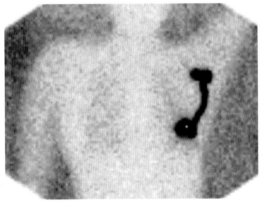

Fig. 188 Lymphoscintigraphy shows visualized sentinel lymph nodes in the left axilla

Operation

Aug. 2008 Left breast conserving surgery, axillary lymph node dissection (Fig. 189).

Pathology Report

Ductal carcinoma in situ

1. Post mammotome biopsy status.
2. Size of tumor: 2.0 cm, residual (pTis).
3. Nuclear grade: high.
4. Necrosis: present.
5. Architectural pattern: solid and comedo.
6. Skin: no involvement of tumor.
7. Surgical margins:
    (a) Superior margin: 10 mm.
    (b) Inferior margin: 10 mm.
    (c) Medial margin: 10 mm.
    (d) Lateral margin: 10 mm.
    (e) Deep margin: 2 mm.
8. Lymph nodes: no metastasis in 3 axillary lymph nodes (pN0(sn)) (sentinel LN: 0/3, axillary LN: 0/0).

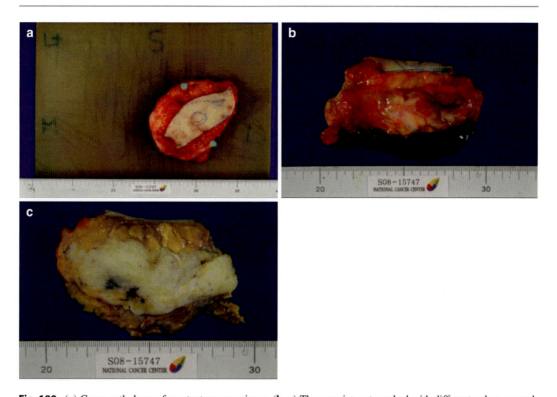

Fig. 189 (**a**) Gross pathology of mastectomy specimen. (**b, c**) The margins get marked with different colors on each direction

9. Microcalcification: present, tumoral/non-tumoral.
10. Pathologic staging: pTisN0(sn).

	Result	Intensity	Positive %
Estrogen receptor	Negative (0/7)	0	0
Progesterone receptor	Negative (0/7)	0	0
C-erbB2	Positive (3+)		
Ki-67	Positive in 10% of tumor cells		

Adjuvant Therapy
Postoperative radiation therapy.

28.2.2 Treatments After Recurrence
See Figs. 190, 191 and 192.

Operation
Apr. 2011 Left nipple-areolar complex sparing mastectomy with immediate implant reconstruction (Fig. 193).

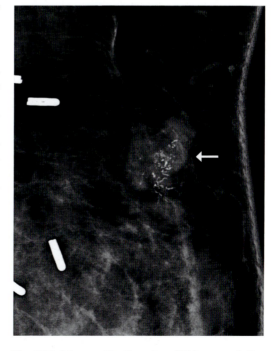

Fig. 190 Lt. magnification view (ML): grouped fine pleomorphic or fine linear microcalcifications

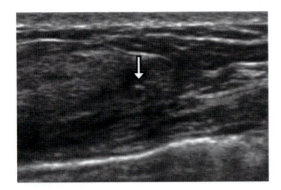

Fig. 191 US: echogenic dots, suggesting microcalcifications

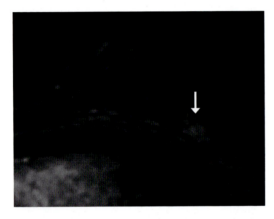

Fig. 192 MRI: Focal heterogeneous non-mass enhancement at the corresponding area of the microcalcifications on mammography

Pathology Report

Microinvasive Ductal Carcinoma

1. Size of tumor: 0.1 cm (pTis).
2. Histologic grade: 2/3 (tubule formation: 3/3, nuclear pleomorphism: 2/3, mitotic count: 1/3, not identified).
3. Intraductal component: present, intratumoral/extratumoral (90%) (nuclear grade: high, necrosis: present, architectural pattern: comedo, cribriform, and solid, extensive intraductal component: absent/present).
4. Skin: no involvement of tumor.
5. Surgical margins: (deep margin: 1 mm from ductal carcinoma in situ).
6. Vascular invasion: absent.
7. Lymphatic invasion: absent.
8. Tumor border: infiltrative.
9. Microcalcification: present, tumoral/non-tumoral.
10. Pathologic stage (AJCC 2010): pTisNx.

	Result	Intensity	Positive %
Estrogen receptor	Strong (7/7)	3	>2/3
Progesterone receptor	Strong (7/7)	3	>2/3
C-erbB2	Positive (2+)		
Ki-67	Positive in 25% of tumor cells		

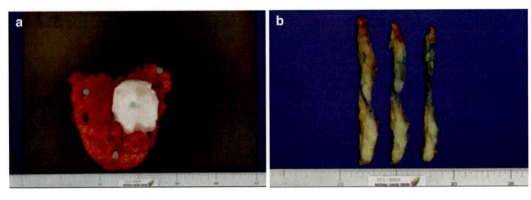

Fig. 193 (a) Gross pathology of mastectomy specimen. (b) The margins get marked and sliced with different colors on each direction

Adjuvant Therapy

Tamoxifen 20 mg/day for 6.5 years with goserelin.

29 Case 29

29.1 Patient History and Progress

Female/46 years old, pre-menopause.

Screen detected mass lesion on left breast 7:30 o'clock direction.

Outside result of biopsy: (1) Invasive ductal carcinoma, (2) Atypical ductal hyperplasia.

Family history of breast cancer, mother.

Asthma.

BRCA 1 VUS (variant of uncertain).

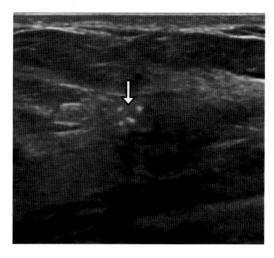

Fig. 195 US: echogenic dots, suggesting microcalcifications

29.2 Courses of Treatment

Left breast IDC→ Operation → Adjuvant therapy → **Left breast recurrence (IDC).**

29.2.1 Primary Treatment

See Figs. 194, 195, 196 and 197.

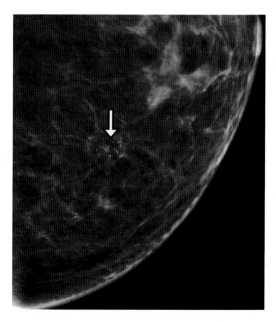

Fig. 194 Outside MG Lt. CC: Regional fine linear microcalcifications in left inner breast

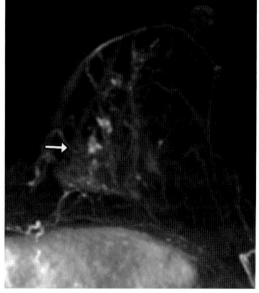

Fig. 196 MRI maximum intensity projection (MIP): segmental heterogeneous non-mass enhancement

Operation

Nov. 2017 Left nipple-areolar complex sparing mastectomy with immediate implant reconstruction, sentinel lymph node biopsy (Fig. 198).

Pathology Report

Invasive Ductal Carcinoma

1. Size of tumor: 3.0 cm (pT2).

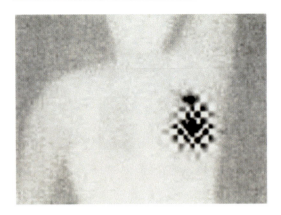

Fig. 197 Lymphoscintigraphy shows visualized sentinel lymph nodes in the left axilla

2. Histologic grade: 2/3 (tubule formation: 3/3, nuclear pleomorphism: 2/3, mitotic count: 2/3, 12/10HPF).
3. Intraductal component: present, intratumoral/extratumoral (20%) (nuclear grade: low, necrosis: present, architectural pattern: cribriform/solid/comedo, extensive intraductal component: present).
4. Skin: no involvement of tumor.
5. Surgical margins:
   (a) Deep margin: <1 mm from invasive ductal carcinoma (slide 2).
   (b) Superficial margin: <1 mm from ductal carcinoma in situ (slide 9).

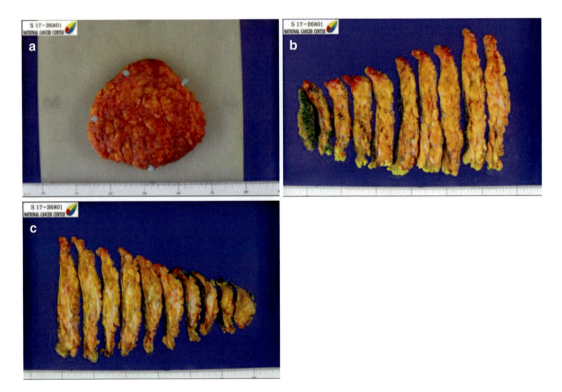

Fig. 198 (**a**) Gross pathology of mastectomy specimen. (**b**, **c**) The margins get marked and sliced with different colors on each direction

6. Lymph nodes: no metastasis in one axillary lymph node (pN0(sn)) (sentinel LN: 0/1).
7. Arteriovenous invasion: absent.
8. Extensive lymphovascular invasion: present, intratumoral/peritumoral.
9. Tumor border: infiltrative.
10. Microcalcification: present, tumoral/non-tumoral.
11. Pathologic stage (AJCC 2010): pT2N0(sn).

	Result	Intensity	Positive %
Estrogen receptor	Strong (8/8)	3	>2/3
Progesterone receptor	Negative (2/8)	1	<1%
C-erbB2	Equivocal (2+) (SISH negative)		
Ki-67	Positive in 11% of tumor cells		

Adjuvant Therapy

Adjuvant chemotherapy #4 cycles of cyclophosphamide and docetaxel.

Tamoxifen 20 mg/day for 3.6 years.

29.2.2 Treatments After Recurrence

See Figs. 199 and 200.

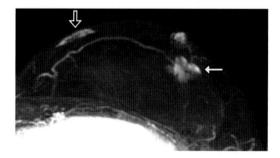

Fig. 199 MRI maximum intensity projection (MIP): 2.6 cm irregular heterogeneous enhancing mass (white arrow) in the subareolar area of left breast and enhancing lesion in the skin layer (black arrow)

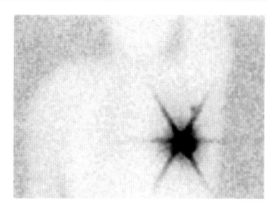

Fig. 200 Lymphoscintigraphy shows visualized sentinel lymph nodes in the left axilla

Operation

Nov. 2011 Left total mastectomy, sentinel lymph node biopsy, implant removal, right total mastectomy (Figs. 201 and 202).

Pathology Report

<Right>

Fibrocystic change.

<Left>

Invasive Ductal Carcinoma

1. Post-nipple-sparing mastectomy status.
2. Size of tumor: 2.0 cm and 1.8 cm (rpT1c(2)).
3. Histologic grade: 2/3 (tubule formation: 3/3, nuclear pleomorphism: 2/3, mitotic count: 2/3, 11/10HPF).
4. Intraductal component: absent.
5. Skin: dermal involvement of tumor.
6. Surgical margins:
   (a) Deep margin: positive for invasive ductal carcinoma (slide 1).
   (b) Superficial margin: 2 mm.
7. Lymph nodes: no metastasis in one axillary lymph node (rpN0(sn)) (sentinel LN: 0/1).

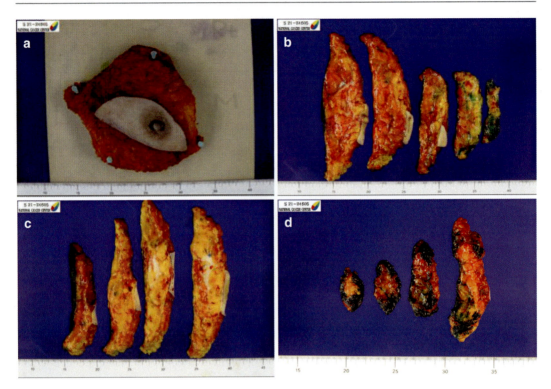

Fig. 201 (**a**) Gross pathology of right mastectomy specimen. (**b, c, d**) The margins get marked and sliced with different colors on each direction

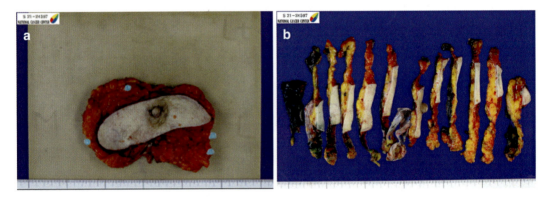

Fig. 202 (**a**) Gross pathology of left mastectomy specimen. (**b**) The margins get marked and sliced with different colors on each direction

8. Arteriovenous invasion: absent.
9. Lymphovascular invasion: present, intratumoral.
10. Tumor border: infiltrative.
11. Microcalcification: present, tumoral/non-tumoral.
12. Pathological TN category (AJCC 2017): rpT1cN0(sn).

	Result	Intensity	Positive %
Estrogen receptor	Strong (8/8)	3	>2/3
Progesterone receptor	Negative (2/8)	1	<1%
C-erbB2	Equivocal (2+) (SISH negative)		
Ki-67	Positive in 2% of tumor cells		

Adjuvant Therapy
Postoperative radiation therapy.
Letrozole 2.5 mg/day.

30   Case 30

30.1   Patient History and Progress

Female/89 years old, post-menopause.

Screen detected mass lesion on right breast 1 o'clock direction.

Outside result of biopsy: Invasive ductal carcinoma.

No family history.

Hypertension, Hypothyroidism, s/p Cardiac stent insertion (angina).

s/p Shoulder ligament rupture operation.

30.2   Courses of Treatment

Right breast IDC → Operation → Adjuvant therapy → **Left breast recurrence (IDC).**

30.2.1   Primary Treatment
See Figs. 203, 204, 205 and 206.

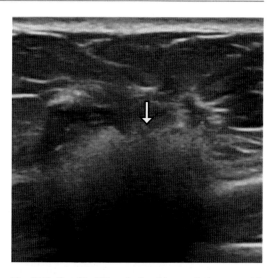

Fig. 204 Outside US: spiculated hypoechoic mass with indistinct margin

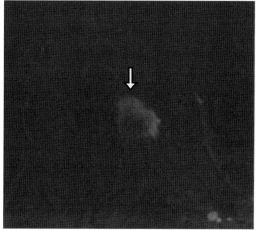

Fig. 205 MRI: spiculated heterogeneous enhancing mass at the 1 o'clock location of right breast

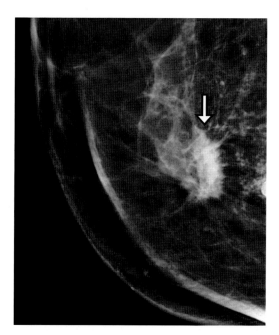

Fig. 203 Outside MG: spiculated hyperdense mass in the inner portion of right breast

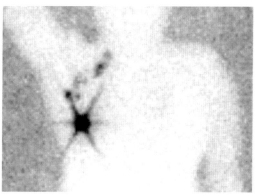

Fig. 206 Lymphoscintigraphy shows visualized sentinel lymph nodes in the right axilla

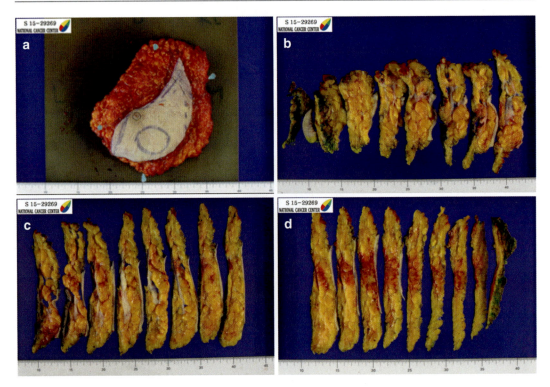

Fig. 207 (a) Gross pathology of mastectomy specimen. (b, c, d) The margins get marked and sliced with different colors on each direction

Operation
Dec. 2015 Right total mastectomy, axillary lymph node dissection (Fig. 207).

Pathology Report
Invasive Ductal Carcinoma
1. Size of tumor: 2.2 cm (pT2).
2. Histologic grade: 2/3 (tubule formation: 3/3, nuclear pleomorphism: 2/3, mitotic count: 1/3, 5/10HPF).
3. Intraductal component: present, intratumoral/extratumoral (5%) (nuclear grade: low, necrosis: present, architectural pattern: cribriform/solid, extensive intraductal component: absent).
4. Skin and nipple: no involvement of tumor.
5. No involvement of skeletal muscle.
6. Surgical margins:
    (a) Deep margin: 8 mm.
    (b) Superficial margin: 15 mm.
7. Lymph nodes:
    (a) metastasis in 1 out of 5 axillary lymph nodes (pN1a) (sentinel LN: 1/3, axillary LN: 0/2).
    (b) perinodal extension: present.
    (c) size of metastatic carcinoma: 11 mm.
8. Arteriovenous invasion: absent.
9. Lymphovascular invasion: present, peritumoral.
10. Tumor border: infiltrative.
11. Microcalcification: present, tumoral.
12. Pathologic stage (AJCC 2010): pT2N1a.

	Result	Intensity	Positive %
Estrogen receptor	Strong (8/8)	3	>2/3
Progesterone receptor	Weak (3/8)	1	1–10%
C-erbB2	Negative (1+)		
Ki-67	Positive in 11% of tumor cells		

Adjuvant Therapy
Anastrozole 1 mg/day for 4 years.

30.2.2 Treatments After Recurrence

See Figs. 208, 209 and 210.

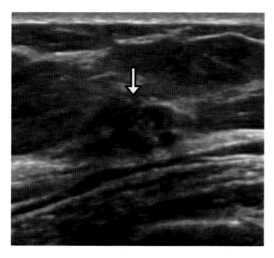

Fig. 208 US: irregular hypoechoic mass with indistinct margin at the 1 o'clock location of left breast

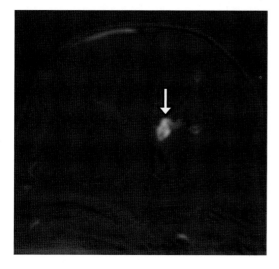

Fig. 209 MRI: irregular heterogeneous enhancing mass at the 1 o'clock location of left breast

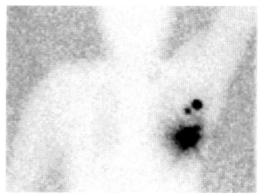

Fig. 210 Lymphoscintigraphy shows visualized sentinel lymph nodes in the left axilla

Operation

Feb. 2020 Left total mastectomy, sentinel lymph node biopsy (Fig. 211).

Pathology Report

Invasive Ductal Carcinoma

1. Size of tumor: 0.9 cm (pT1b).
2. Histologic grade: 2 (tubule formation: 3/3, nuclear pleomorphism: 3/3, mitotic count: 1/3, 3/10HPF).
3. Intraductal component: present, intratumoral/extratumoral (50%) (nuclear grade: high, necrosis: present, architectural pattern: comedo, extensive intraductal component: present).
4. Skin and nipple: no involvement of tumor.
5. Surgical margins:
   (a) Deep margin: 2 mm.
   (b) Superficial margin: 20 mm.
6. Lymph nodes: no metastasis in one axillary lymph nodes (pN0(sn)) (sentinel LN: 0/1).
7. Arteriovenous invasion: absent.
8. Lymphovascular invasion: absent.

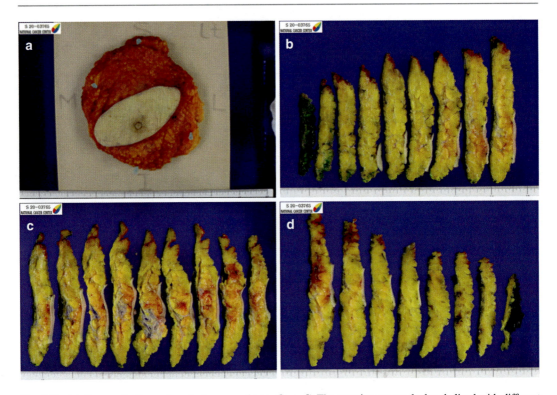

Fig. 211 (**a**) Gross pathology of mastectomy specimen. (**b, c, d**) The margins get marked and sliced with different colors on each direction

9. Tumor border: infiltrative.
10. Microcalcification: absent.
11. Pathological TN category (AJCC 2017): pT1bN0(sn).

	Result	Intensity	Positive %
Estrogen receptor	Negative (0/8)	0	0
Progesterone receptor	Negative (0/8)	0	0
C-erbB2	Equivocal (2+) (SISH negative)		
Ki-67	Positive in 6% of tumor cells		

31 Case 31

31.1 Patient History and Progress

Female/49 years old, pre-menopause.
Screen detected mass lesion on right breast 1 o'clock direction.
No family history.
No comorbidities.

31.2 Courses of Treatment

Right breast Papillary carcinoma in situ→ Operation → **Right breast recurrence (DCIS).**

31.2.1 Primary Treatment
See Figs. 212, 213, 214 and 215.

Operation
Jan. 2017 Right nipple-areolar complex sparing mastectomy with immediate implant reconstruction, sentinel lymph node biopsy, left nipple-areolar complex sparing mastectomy with immediate implant reconstruction (Figs. 216, 217 and 218).

Pathology Report
<Right>

Local Recurrence

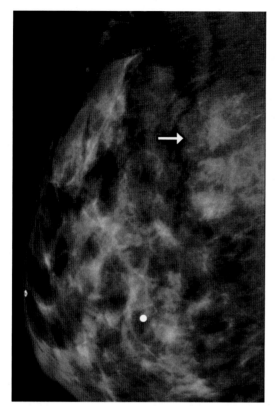

Fig. 212 Rt MLO MG: irregular hyperdense mass in right upper inner quadrant

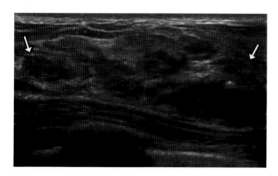

Fig. 213 US: irregular indistinct hypoechoic masses in right upper inner quadrant

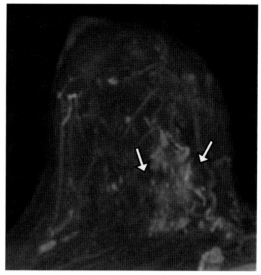

Fig. 214 MRI: regional heterogeneous non-mass enhancement in right upper inner quadrant (showing moderate background parenchymal enhancement)

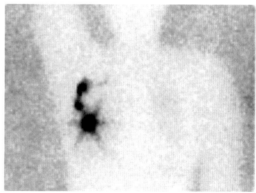

Fig. 215 Lymphoscintigraphy shows visualized sentinel lymph nodes in the right axilla

Papillary carcinoma in situ
1. Size of tumor: 5.0 cm (pTis).
2. Nuclear grade: low.
3. Necrosis: present.
4. Architectural pattern: papillary/cribriform.
5. Surgical margins:
   (a) Deep margin: <1 mm (slide 6).
   (b) Superficial margin: 0.08 mm (slide 2).
6. Lymph nodes: no metastasis in four axillary lymph nodes (pN0(sn)) (sentinel LN: 0/4).
7. Microcalcification: absent.
8. Pathologic stage (AJCC 2010): pTisN0(sn).

	Result	Intensity	Positive %
Estrogen receptor	Strong (7/8)	3	1/3–2/3
Progesterone receptor	Strong (8/8)	3	>2/3
C-erbB2	Equivocal (2+)		
Ki-67	Positive in 26% of tumor cells		

<Left>

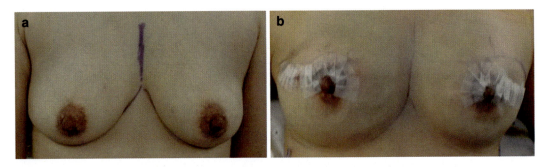

Fig. 216 (**a**) Preoperative and (**b**) immediate postoperative appearance

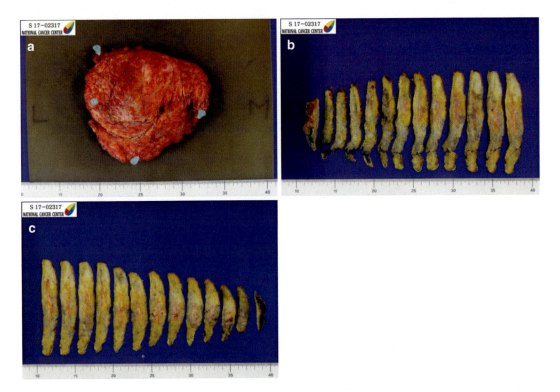

Fig. 217 (**a**) Gross pathology of right mastectomy specimen. (**b, c**) The margins get marked and sliced with different colors on each direction

Local Recurrence

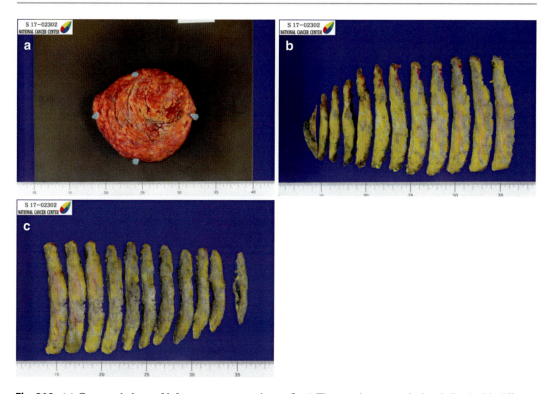

Fig. 218 (**a**) Gross pathology of left mastectomy specimen. (**b, c**) The margins get marked and sliced with different colors on each direction

1. Intraductal papillomas, multiple, up to 0.8 cm
2. Sclerosing adenosis with microcalcification.

31.2.2 Treatments After Recurrence
See Figs. 219 and 220.
Biopsy
Right 1 o'clock.
Ductal carcinoma in situ:

1. Nuclear grade: low.
2. Necrosis: absent.
3. Architectural pattern: papillary/cribriform.
4. Microcalcification: absent.

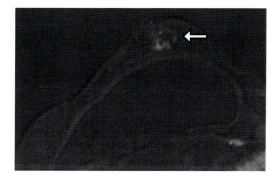

Fig. 219 Postop. MRI: Focal heterogeneous non-mass enhancement in right breast

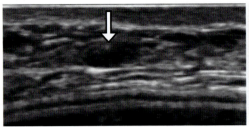 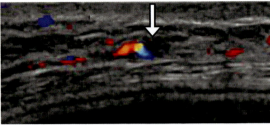

Fig. 220 US: microlobulated hypoechoic mass with increased vascularity

Closed follow-up due to rejection of surgical treatment.

32 Case 32

32.1 Patient History and Progress

Female/42 years old, pre-menopause.
Screen detected mass lesion on right breast 12 o'clock direction.
Outside result of lumpectomy: Ductal carcinoma in situ.
No family history.
No comorbidities.
BRCA 2 VUS (variant of uncertain).

32.2 Courses of Treatment

Right breast DCIS → Operation → Adjuvant therapy → **Right breast recurrence (tubular carcinoma + DCIS)**.

32.2.1 Primary Treatment

Operation
Aug. 2014 Right breast wide excision (outside).

Pathology Report
Ductal carcinoma in situ involving intraductal papilloma

1. Nuclear grade: low.
2. Necrosis: absent.
3. Architectural pattern: papillary/cribriform.

	Result	Intensity	Positive %
Estrogen receptor	Strong (8/8)	3	>2/3
Progesterone receptor	Strong (8/8)	3	>2/3
C-erbB2	Negative (1+)		
Ki-67	Positive in 10.8% of tumor cells		

Adjuvant Therapy
Postoperative radiation therapy.
Tamoxifen 20 mg/day for 2 years.

32.2.2 Treatments After Recurrence
See Figs. 221 and 222.

Operation
First Operation (Jul. 2019) Rt. breast excisional biopsy (Fig. 223).

Pathology Report
Tubular Carcinoma
1. Post-lumpectomy status.
2. Size of invasive component: 0.2 cm (rpT1a).
3. Size of intraductal component: 1.0 cm.
4. Histologic grade: 1/3 (tubule formation: 1/3, nuclear pleomorphism: 2/3, mitotic count: 1/3, 6/10HPF).
5. Intraductal component: present, intratumoral/extratumoral (90%) (nuclear grade: low, necrosis: present, architectural pattern: micropapillary/cribriform/comedo, extensive intraductal component: present).
6. Skin: no involvement of tumor.

Local Recurrence

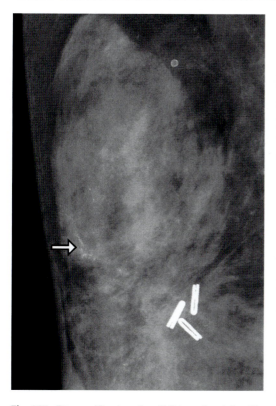

Fig. 221 Rt magnification view (ML): regional fine linear microcalcifications in right upper breast

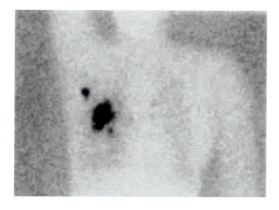

Fig. 222 Lymphoscintigraphy shows visualized sentinel lymph nodes in the left axilla

7. Surgical margins:
   (a) Superior margin: 10 mm.
   (b) Inferior margin: 10 mm.
   (c) Medial margin: <1 mm from tubular carcinoma (slide 5).
   (d) Lateral margin: 10 mm.

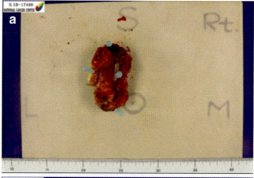

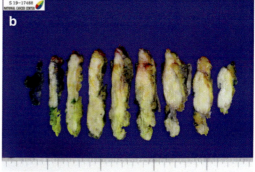

Fig. 223 (**a**) Gross pathology of breast excision specimen. (**b**) The margins get marked and sliced with different colors on each direction

   (e) Deep margin: 2 mm.
   (f) Superficial margin: 2 mm.
8. Arteriovenous invasion: absent.
9. Lymphovascular invasion: absent.
10. Tumor border: infiltrative.
11. Microcalcification: present, tumoral/non-tumoral.
12. Pathological TN category (AJCC 2017): rpT1a.

	Result	Intensity	Positive %
Estrogen receptor	Negative (2/8)	1	<1%
Progesterone receptor	Negative (2/8)	1	<1%
C-erbB2	Negative (1+)		
Ki-67	Positive in 7% of tumor cells		

Operation

Second Operation (Sep. 2019–09) Right nipple-areolar complex sparing mastectomy, sentinel lymph node biopsy (Fig. 224).

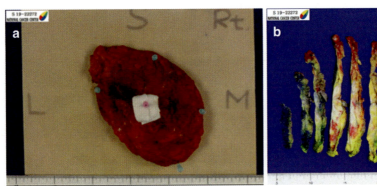
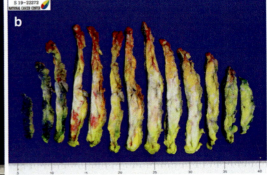

Fig. 224 (**a**) Gross pathology of mastectomy specimen. (**b**) The margins get marked and sliced with different colors on each direction

Pathology Report

Ductal Carcinoma In Situ, residual
1. Post-excision status.
2. Size of tumor: 0.2 cm.
3. Nuclear grade: low.
4. Necrosis: present.
5. Architectural pattern: cribriform/solid/comedo.
6. Surgical margins:
   (a) Nipple margin: (see note).
   (b) Deep margin: 3 mm.
   (c) Superficial margin: 2 mm.
7. Lymph nodes: no metastasis in one axillary lymph node (pN0(sn)) (sentinel LN: 0/1).
8. Microcalcification: absent.

Note: 1. Atypical ductal hyperplasia is present in the section of Fro 1.

33 Case 33

33.1 Patient History and Progress

Female/45 years old, pre-menopause.
Screen detected mass lesion on upper inner portion of left breast.
Outside result of biopsy: Invasive ductal carcinoma.
Family history of breast cancer, mother at her 50 years old.
S/P Hysterectomy, s/p bilateral breast augmentation.

33.2 Courses of Treatmaent

Left breast IDC → Neoadjuvant chemotherapy → Operation → Adjuvant therapy → **Left breast recurrence (IDC).**

33.2.1 Primary Treatment

See Figs. 225, 226, 227 and 228.

Neoadjuvant Chemotherapy

Neoadjuvant chemotherapy #6 cycles of trastuzumab and pertuzumab and docetaxel and carboplatin.

Operation

Oct. 2018 Left breast conserving surgery, sentinel lymph node biopsy (Fig. 229).

Pathology Report

Invasive Ductal Carcinoma
1. Post-chemotherapy status.
2. Size of tumor: 3.5 cm, 1.4 cm (ypT2(2)).
3. Histologic grade: 3/3 (tubule formation: 3/3, nuclear pleomorphism: 3/3, mitotic count: 3/3, 30/10HPF).
4. Intraductal component: present, extratumoral (10%) (nuclear grade: high, necrosis: present, architectural pattern: micropapillary/solid/comedo, extensive intraductal component: absent).
5. Skin: no involvement of tumor.

Local Recurrence 809

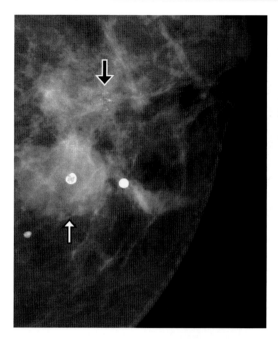

Fig. 225 Lt CC MG: Irregular hyperdense mass (white arrow) with associated fine pleomorphic microcalcifications (black arrow) in left upper inner quadrant

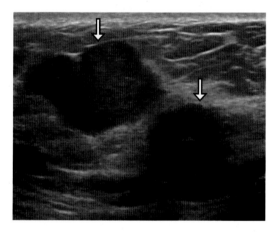

Fig. 226 US: irregular microlobulated hypoechoic masses at the 10 o'clock direction of left breast

6. Surgical margins:
   (a) Superior margin: 30 mm.
   (b) Inferior margin: 6 mm.

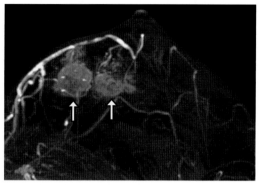

Fig. 227 MRI maximum intensity projection (MIP): irregular heterogeneous enhancing masses

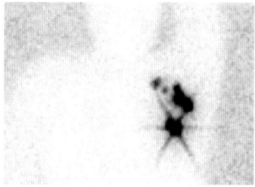

Fig. 228 Lymphoscintigraphy shows visualized sentinel lymph nodes in the left axilla

   (c) Medial margin: 15 mm.
   (d) Lateral margin: (see note 1).
   (e) Deep margin: 6 mm.
   (f) Superficial margin: <1 mm from invasive ductal carcinoma (slide 12).
7. Lymph nodes: no metastasis in 3 axillary lymph nodes (ypN0(sn)) (sentinel LN: 0/3).
8. Arteriovenous invasion: absent.
9. Lymphovascular invasion: present, intratumoral/peritumoral.
10. Tumor border: infiltrative.
11. Microcalcification: present, tumoral.
12. Pathological TN category (AJCC 2017): ypT2(2)N0(sn).

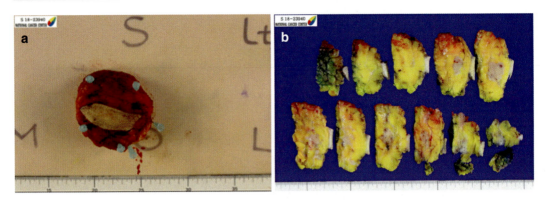

Fig. 229 (**a**) Gross pathology of lumpectomy specimen. (**b**) The margins get marked and sliced with different colors on each direction

Note: 1. The lateral margin of the lumpectomy specimen (slide 16) is close to ductal carcinoma in situ (1.5 mm), but this margin submitted for frozen diagnosis (Fro 7) is free of tumor.

	Result	Intensity	Positive %
Estrogen receptor	Negative (0/8)	0	0
Progesterone receptor	Negative (0/8)	0	0
C-erbB2	Positive (3+)		
Ki-67	Positive in 59% of tumor cells		

Adjuvant Therapy
Postoperative radiation therapy.
    Trastuzumab for 1 year.

33.2.2 Treatments After Recurrence
See Fig. 230.

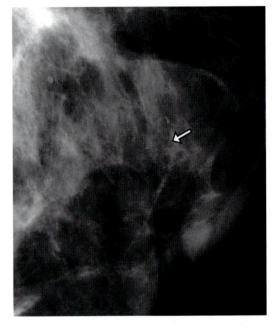

Fig. 230 Lt magnification view (ML): Regional amorphous microcalcifications in left subareolar area

Operation
First Operation (Nov. 2019) Left breast mass excision (Fig. 231).

Pathology Report
Invasive Ductal Carcinoma
1. Post-lumpectomy status.
2. Size of tumor: 1.8 cm (rpT1c).
3. Histologic grade: 3/3 (tubule formation: 3/3, nuclear pleomorphism: 3/3, mitotic count: 3/3, 22/10HPF).
4. Intraductal component: present, intratumoral (5%) (nuclear grade: high, necrosis: absent, architectural pattern: solid, extensive intraductal component: absent).
5. Surgical margins:
   (a) Superior margin: 15 mm.
   (b) Inferior margin: positive for invasive ductal carcinoma (slide 2).
   (c) Medial margin: 10 mm.
   (d) Lateral margin: positive for invasive ductal carcinoma (slide 4).
   (e) Deep margin: 1 mm from invasive ductal carcinoma (slide 3).
   (f) Superficial margin: 5 mm.

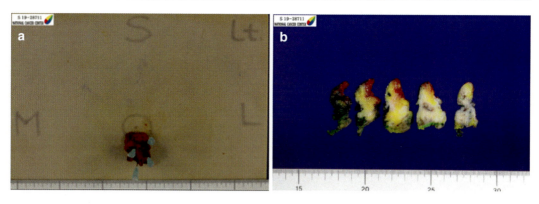

Fig. 231 (a) Gross pathology of breast mass excision specimen. (b) The margins get marked and sliced with different colors on each direction

6. Arteriovenous invasion: absent.
7. Lymphovascular invasion: absent.
8. Tumor border: infiltrative.
9. Microcalcification: present, tumoral.
10. Pathological TN category (AJCC 2017): rpT1cNx.

	Result	Intensity	Positive %
Estrogen receptor	Negative (0/8)	0	0
Progesterone receptor	Negative (0/8)	0	0
C-erbB2	Positive (3+)		
Ki-67	Positive in 27% of tumor cells		

Operation

Second Operation (Dec. 2019) Left breast wide excision (Fig. 232).

Pathology Report

Lateral Margin

Invasive Ductal Carcinoma, residual

1. Post-lumpectomy and excision status.
2. Size of tumor: 0.6 cm.
3. Histologic grade: 3/3 (tubule formation: 3/3, nuclear pleomorphism: 3/3, mitotic count: 3/3, 22/10HPF).
4. Intraductal component: present, intratumoral (20%) (nuclear grade: high, necrosis: absent, architectural pattern: solid, extensive intraductal component: absent).

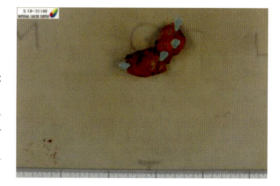

Fig. 232 Gross pathology of breast wide excision specimen

5. Surgical margins:
   (a) Lateral margin: (see note).
6. Vascular invasion: absent.
7. Lymphatic invasion: absent.
8. Tumor border: infiltrative.
9. Microcalcification: absent.

Inferior Margin

No residual tumor

1. Post-lumpectomy and excision status.

Note: The lateral margin of the lumpectomy specimen (slide 4) is close to ductal carcinoma in situ (4 mm), but this margin submitted for frozen diagnosis (Fro 2) is free of tumor.

Adjuvant Therapy

Chemotherapy #14 cycles of T-DM1 (trastuzumab emtansine).

34 Case 34

34.1 Patient History and Progress

Female/47 years old, pre-menopause.
　Screen detected microcalcification on upper outer portion of right breast.
　Family history of ovarian cancer mother.
　No comorbidities.
　BRCA 1 and 2 mutation: Not detected.

34.2 Courses of Treatment

Right breast IDC → Operation → Adjuvant therapy → **Right breast recurrence (IDC).**

34.2.1 Primary Treatment
See Figs. 233, 234 and 235.

Operation
Sep. 2019 Right breast conserving surgery (Fig. 236).

Pathology Report

Invasive Ductal Carcinoma
1. Size of invasive component: 0.7 cm (pT1b).

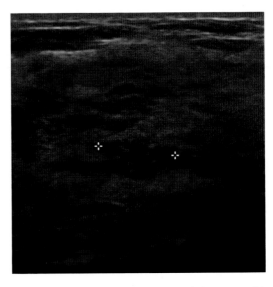

Fig. 234 US: microlobulated hypoechoic mass with echogenic dots (suggesting microcalcifications)

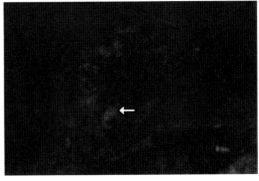

Fig. 235 MRI: oval homogeneous enhancing mass at the 11 o'clock direction of right breast

2. Size of intraductal component: 1.0 cm.
3. Histologic grade: 2/3 (tubule formation: 3/3, nuclear pleomorphism: 2/3, mitotic count: 1/3, 3/10HPF).
4. Intraductal component: present, extratumoral (60%) (nuclear grade: low, necrosis: present, architectural pattern: papillary/cribriform, extensive intraductal component: absent).
5. Skin: no involvement of tumor.
6. Surgical margins:
   (a) Superior margin: 28 mm.
   (b) Inferior margin: 12 mm.
   (c) Medial margin: 10 mm.
   (d) Lateral margin: 30 mm.

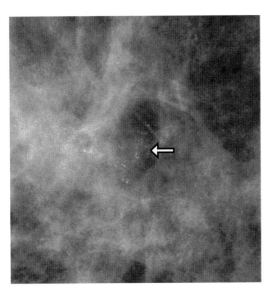

Fig. 233 Rt magnification view (ML): Grouped fine pleomorphic microcalcifications in right upper outer

Local Recurrence

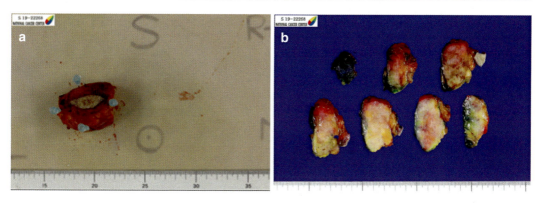

Fig. 236 (**a**) Gross pathology of lumpectomy specimen. (**b**) The margins get marked and sliced with different colors on each direction

   (e) Deep margin: <1 mm from ductal carcinoma in situ (slide 7).
   (f) Superficial margin: 13 mm.
7. Arteriovenous invasion: absent.
8. Lymphovascular invasion: absent.
9. Tumor border: infiltrative.
10. Microcalcification: present, non-tumoral.
11. Pathological TN category (AJCC 2017): pT1b.

	Result	Intensity	Positive %
Estrogen receptor	Intermediate (6/8)	2	1/3–2/3
Progesterone receptor	Strong (8/8)	3	>2/3
C-erbB2	Positive (3+)		
Ki-67	Positive in 53% of tumor cells		

Adjuvant Therapy
Postoperative radiation therapy.
   Tamoxifen 20 mg/day for 1.8 years.

34.2.2 Treatments After Recurrence
See Figs. 237 and 238.

Operation
Aug. 2021 Right nipple-areolar complex sparing mastectomy with immediate implant reconstruction (Fig. 239).

Pathology Report

Invasive Ductal Carcinoma
1. Post-lumpectomy status.

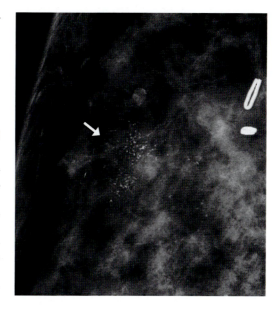

Fig. 237 Rt magnification view (ML): Regional fine pleomorphic microcalcifications in right upper outer quadrant

2. Size of tumor: 2.1 cm, multifocal (rpT2).
3. Histologic grade: 3/3 (tubule formation: 3/3, nuclear pleomorphism: 3/3, mitotic count: 3/3, 4/1HPF).
4. Intraductal component: present, intratumoral/extratumoral (50%) (nuclear grade: high, necrosis: present, architectural pattern: papillary/micropapillary/cribriform/solid/comedo, extensive intraductal component: present).
5. Skin: no involvement of tumor.
6. Surgical margins:

(a) Deep margin: <1 mm from ductal carcinoma in situ (slides 1 and 3).
(b) Superficial margin: positive for invasive ductal carcinoma (slide 5).
7. Arteriovenous invasion: absent.
8. Lymphovascular invasion: present, intratumoral.
9. Tumor border: infiltrative.
10. Microcalcification: present, tumoral/non-tumoral.
11. Pathological TN category (AJCC 2017): rpT2.

	Result	Intensity	Positive %
Estrogen receptor	Strong (7/8)	2	>2/3
Progesterone receptor	Strong (7/8)	3	1/3–2/3
C-erbB2	Positive (3+)		
Ki-67	Positive in 51% of tumor cells		

Adjuvant Therapy

Adjuvant chemotherapy #4 cycles of doxorubicin and cyclophosphamide.
Trastuzumab for 1 year.
Letrozole 2.5 mg/day.

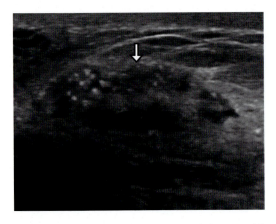

Fig. 238 US: indistinct heterogeneous echoic mass with microcalcifications at the 11 o'clock direction of right breast

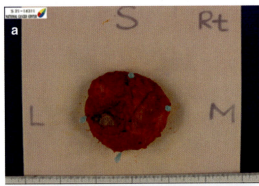
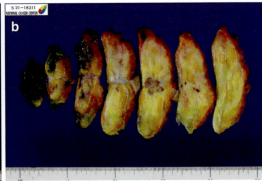
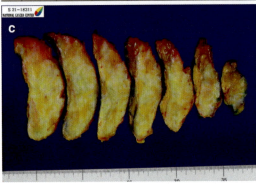

Fig. 239 (a) Gross pathology of mastectomy specimen. (b, c) The margins get marked and sliced with different colors on each direction

35 Case 35

35.1 Patient History and Progress

Female/53 years old, peri-menopause.

Screen detected mass lesion on left breast subareola.

No family history.

No comorbidities.

BRCA 1 and 2 mutation: Not detected.

35.2 Courses of Treatment

Right breast IDC → Neoadjuvant chemotherapy → Operation → Adjuvant therapy → **Right breast recurrence (DCIS).**

35.2.1 Primary Treatment

Operation

First Operation (Aug. 2004) Left breast conserving surgery, sentinel lymph node biopsy.

Pathology Report

Invasive Ductal Carcinoma

1. Size of invasive carcinoma: 0.4 cm (pT1a).
2. Size of intraductal carcinoma: 4 cm.
3. Histologic grade: 2/3 (tubule formation: 2/3, nuclear pleomorphism: 2/3, mitotic count: 2/3).
4. Ductal carcinoma in situ: present, intratumoral/extratumoral (95%) (nuclear grade: low, necrosis: present, architectural pattern: cribriform and comedo, extensive intraductal component: present).
5. Skin: no involvement of tumor.
6. Surgical margins:
   - (a) Superior margin: 20 mm.
   - (b) Inferior margin: (see note).
   - (c) Medial margin: 20 mm.
   - (d) Lateral margin: 10 mm.
   - (e) Deep margin: 10 mm.
7. Lymph nodes: no metastasis in 3 axillary lymph nodes (pN0(sn)) (sentinel LN: 0/3, axillary LN: 0/0).
8. Vascular invasion: absent.
9. Lymphatic invasion: absent.
10. Tumor border: infiltrative.
11. Microcalcification: present, tumoral.
12. Pathologic staging: pT1aN0(sn).

Note: Ductal carcinoma in situ is noted only in the permanent section of nipple margin (Fro 4) and inferior margin (Fro 5).

	Result	Intensity	Positive %
Estrogen receptor	Strong (6/7)	3	1/3–2/3
Progesterone receptor	Intermediate (5/7)	2	1/3–2/3
C-erbB2	Negative (1+)		
Ki-67	Positive in 5% of tumor cells		

Operation

Second Operation (Sep. 2004) Left breast wide excision.

Pathology Report

No residual carcinoma with foreign body reaction.

1. Post-lumpectomy status.

Adjuvant Therapy

Postoperative radiation therapy.

Tamoxifen 20 mg/day for 2 years.

35.2.2 Treatments After Recurrence

See Figs. 240 and 241.

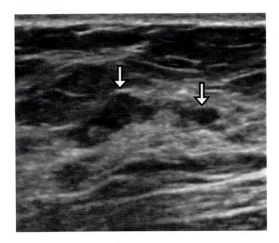

Fig. 240 OPD US: microlobulated hypoechoic masses

Fig. 241 MRI: focal heterogeneous non-mass enhancement

Operation

Mar. 2017 Right nipple-areolar complex sparing mastectomy with immediate implant reconstruction, Left breast augmentation with implant (Figs. 242 and 243).

Pathology Report

1. Ductal Carcinoma In Situ
   (a) Size of tumor: 2.0 cm (pTis).
   (b) Nuclear grade: low.
   (c) Necrosis: absent.
   (d) Architectural pattern: cribriform.
   (e) Surgical margins:
      - Deep margin: 7 mm.
      - Superficial margin: 6 mm.
   (f) Microcalcification: present, tumoral/non-tumoral.
   (g) Pathologic stage (AJCC 2010): pTisNx.
2. Sclerosing adenosis.

	Result	Intensity	Positive %
Estrogen receptor	Strong (8/8)	3	>2/3
Progesterone receptor	Strong (7/8)	3	1/3–2/3
C-erbB2	Equivocal (2+)		
Ki-67	Positive in 17% of tumor cells		

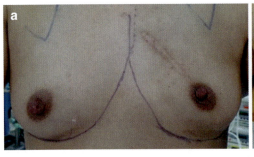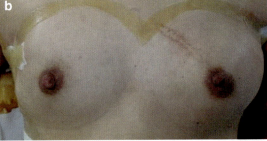

Fig. 242 (**a**) Preoperative and (**b**) immediate postoperative appearance

Local Recurrence

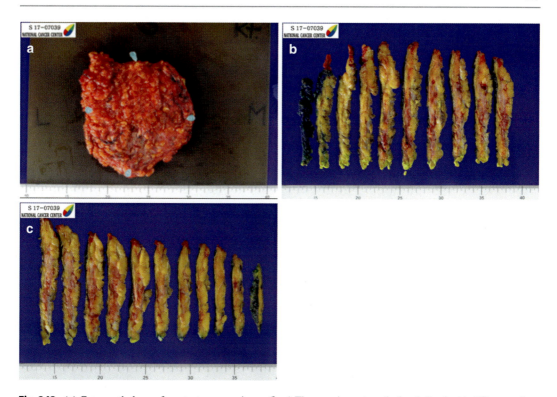

Fig. 243 (**a**) Gross pathology of mastectomy specimen. (**b, c**) The margins get marked and sliced with different colors on each direction

Adjuvant Therapy
Tamoxifen 20 mg/day for 0.3 year (self-cessation).

36 Case 36

36.1 Patient History and Progress

Female/48 years old, pre-menopause.
  Screen detected mass lesion on right breast 10 o'clock direction.
  Outside result of biopsy: Papillary carcinoma in situ.
  No family history.
  s/p bilateral breast augmentation.
  BRCA 1 and 2 mutation: Not detected.

36.2 Courses of Treatment

Right breast DCIS → Operation → **Left breast recurrence (DCIS).**

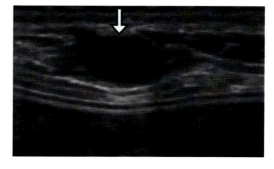

Fig. 244 O/S US: Oval hypoechoic mass with angular margin at the 9 o'clock direction of right breast

36.2.1 Primary Treatment
See Fig. 244.

Operation
Mar. 2016 Right breast conserving surgery (Fig. 245).

Pathology Report

Ductal Carcinoma In Situ
1. Post mammotome biopsy status.

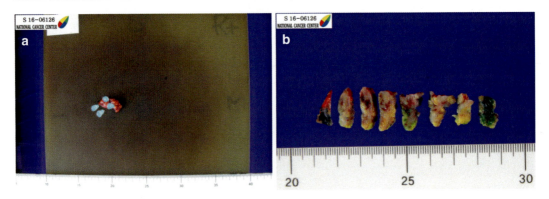

Fig. 245 (**a**) Gross pathology of lumpectomy specimen. (**b**) The margins get marked and sliced with different colors on each direction

2. Size of tumor: 0.2 cm, residual.
3. Nuclear grade: low.
4. Necrosis: absent/present.
5. Architectural pattern: cribriform.
6. Surgical margins:
   (a) Superior margin: (see note).
   (b) Inferior margin: 7 mm.
   (c) Medial margin: 4 mm from ductal carcinoma in situ.
   (d) Lateral margin: 8 mm.
   (e) Deep margin: 2 mm.
   (f) Superficial margin: 2 mm.
7. Microcalcification: absent.

Note: 1. The superior margin of the lumpectomy specimen (slide 4) is close to ductal carcinoma in situ (<1 mm), but this margin submitted for frozen diagnosis (Fro 1) is free of tumor.

	Result	Intensity	Positive %
Estrogen receptor	Strong (8/8)	3	>2/3
Progesterone receptor	Strong (8/8)	3	>2/3
C-erbB2	Negative (1+)		
Ki-67	Positive in 29% of tumor cells		

36.2.2 Treatments After Recurrence
See Fig. 246.

Operation
Jun. 2018 Left nipple-areolar complex sparing mastectomy (Figs. 247 and 248).

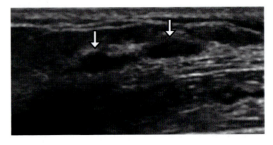

Fig. 246 US: microlobulated hypoechoic masses at the 1 o'clock direction of left breast

Pathology Report

Ductal Carcinoma In Situ
1. Size of tumor: 3.5 cm (pTis).
2. Nuclear grade: low.
3. Necrosis: absent.
4. Architectural pattern: papillary/cribriform/solid.
5. Skin: no involvement of tumor.
6. Surgical margins:
   (a) Deep margin: 2 mm.
   (b) Superficial margin: 2 mm.
7. Microcalcification: present, tumoral/non-tumoral.
8. Pathological TN category (AJCC 2017): pTis.

Axillary Tail: Ductal Carcinoma In Situ
1. Size of tumor: 0.3 cm.
2. Nuclear grade: low.
3. Necrosis: absent.
4. Architectural pattern: cribriform.
5. Surgical margin: involvement of superficial margin.

Local Recurrence

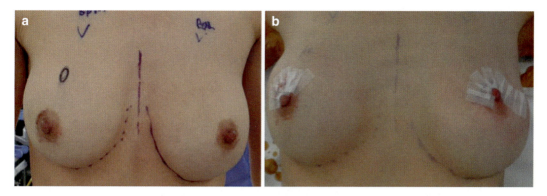

Fig. 247 (**a**) Preoperative and (**b**) immediate postoperative appearance

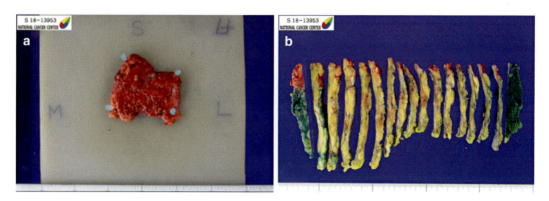

Fig. 248 (**a**) Gross pathology of mastectomy specimen. (**b**) The margins get marked and sliced with different colors on each direction

	Result	Intensity	Positive %
Estrogen receptor	Strong (8/8)	3	>2/3
Progesterone receptor	Strong (8/8)	3	>2/3
C-erbB2	Negative (0)		
Ki-67	Positive in 51% of tumor cells		

Adjuvant Therapy
Tamoxifen 20 mg/day for 5 years.

37 Case 37

37.1 Patient History and Progress

Female/43 years old, pre-menopause.
Screen detected mass lesion on left breast 7 o'clock direction.

Outside result of biopsy: ductal carcinoma in situ.
No family history.
No comorbidities.
BRCA 1 and 2 mutation: Not detected.

37.2 Courses of Treatment

Left breast DCIS→ Operation → Adjuvant therapy → **Left breast recurrence (DCIS).**

37.2.1 Primary Treatment
See Figs. 249, 250 and 251.

Operation
Feb. 2014 Left breast conserving surgery (Fig. 252).

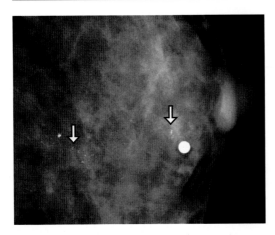

Fig. 249 Lt CC view: segmental fine pleomorphic or amorphous microcalcifications in left breast, palpable site

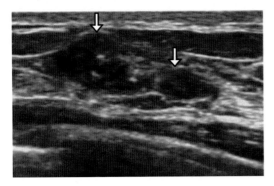

Fig. 250 US: microlobulated hypoechoic masses with microcalcifications

Fig. 251 MRI: irregular heterogeneous enhancing mass at the 6 o'clock direction of left breast

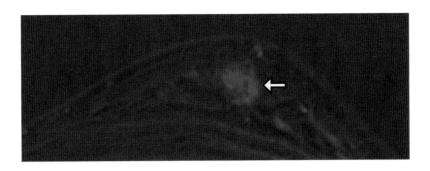

Pathology Report

Ductal Carcinoma In Situ

1. Size of tumor: 3.0 cm (pTis).
2. Nuclear grade: low.
3. Necrosis: present.
4. Architectural pattern: micropapillary/cribriform/comedo.
5. Skin: no involvement of tumor.
6. Surgical margins:
   (a) Nipple margin: positive for atypical ductal hyperplasia (Fro 1) (see note 1).
   (b) Superior margin: (see note 2).
   (c) Inferior margin: 20 mm.
   (d) Medial margin: 5 mm.
   (e) Lateral margin: 15 mm.
   (f) Deep margin: 2 mm.
   (g) Superficial margin: 2 mm.
7. Microcalcification: present, tumoral/non-tumoral.
8. Pathologic stage (AJCC 2010): pTis.

Note: 1. Atypical ductal hyperplasia is present only in the permanent section of Fro 1.

2. The superior margin of the lumpectomy specimen (slide 1) is positive for ductal carcinoma in situ, but this margin submitted for frozen diagnosis (Fro 2) is free of tumor.

Local Recurrence

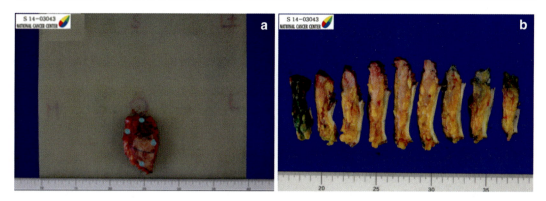

Fig. 252 (**a**) Gross pathology of lumpectomy specimen. (**b**) The margins get marked and sliced with different colors on each direction

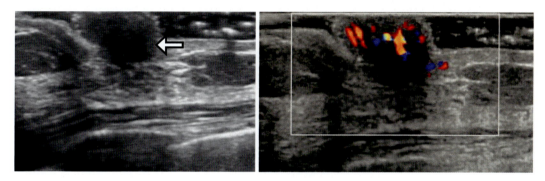

Fig. 253 US: indistinct hypoechoic mass with increased vascularity in left nipple

	Result	Intensity	Positive %
Estrogen receptor	Intermediate (6/8)	2	1/3–2/3
Progesterone receptor	Negative (0/8)	0	0
C-erbB2	Positive (3+)		
Ki-67	Positive in 36% of tumor cells		

Adjuvant Therapy
Postoperative radiation therapy.
  Tamoxifen 20 mg/day for 5 years.

37.2.2 Treatments After Recurrence
See Figs. 253 and 254.

Operation
Jan. 2019 Left nipple excision (Fig. 255).

Pathology Report

Ductal Carcinoma In Situ
1. Post-lumpectomy status.
2. Size of tumor: 0.5 cm (rpTis).
3. Nuclear grade: high.
4. Necrosis: absent.
5. Architectural pattern: micropapillary/cribriform.
6. Skin and nipple: Paget's disease.
7. Surgical margins:
    (a) Superior margin: 5 mm.
    (b) Inferior margin: 5 mm.
    (c) Medial margin: 5 mm.
    (d) Lateral margin: 5 mm.
    (e) Deep margin: 2 mm.
    (f) Superficial margin: 2 mm.

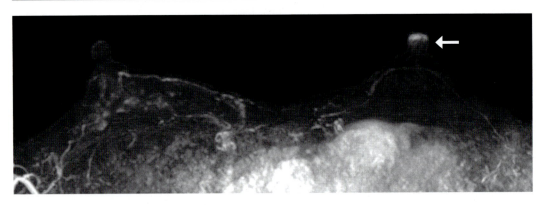

Fig. 254 MRI: asymmetric enhancement in the tip of left nipple

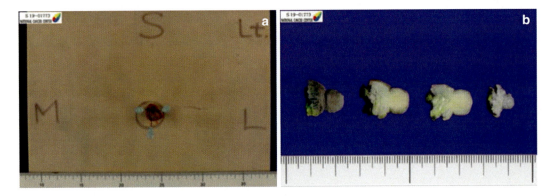

Fig. 255 (**a**) Gross pathology of nipple excision specimen. (**b**) The margins get marked and sliced with different colors on each direction

8. Microcalcification: present, tumoral/non-tumoral.
9. Pathological TN category (AJCC 2017): rpTis(Paget).

	Result	Intensity	Positive %
Estrogen receptor	Negative (2/8)	1	<1%
Progesterone receptor	Negative (0/8)	0	0
C-erbB2	Positive (3+)		
Ki-67	Positive in 58% of tumor cells		

38 Case 38

38.1 Patient History and Progress

Female/47 years old, pre-menopause.

Screen detected mass lesion on right breast 12 o'clock direction.

Outside result of Lumpectomy: Invasive ductal carcinoma.

No family history.

38.2 Courses of Treatment

Right breast IDC → Operation → Adjuvant therapy → **Right breast DCIS.**

38.2.1 Primary Treatment

Operation

Jun. 2012 Right breast conserving surgery, sentinel lymph node biopsy (outside).

Pathology Report

Invasive Ductal Carcinoma
1. Size of tumor: 0.9 cm (pT1b).
2. Lymph nodes: no metastasis in four axillary lymph nodes (pN0(sn)).
3. Pathological TN category: pT1bN0.

	Result	Intensity	Positive %
Estrogen receptor	Positive (6/8)		
Progesterone receptor	Positive (6/8)		
C-erbB2	Equivocal (2+)		

Adjuvant Therapy

Adjuvant chemotherapy #6 cycles of cyclophosphamide and methotrexate and fluorouracil.
Postoperative radiation therapy.
Tamoxifen 20 mg/day for 5 years.

38.2.2 Treatments After Recurrence

See Fig. 256.

Operation

Jul. 2021 Right breast conserving surgery (Fig. 257).

Pathology Report

Ductal Carcinoma In Situ
1. Size of tumor: 0.3 cm (pTis).
2. Nuclear grade: low.
3. Necrosis: absent.
4. Architectural pattern: cribriform/solid.
5. Skin: no involvement of tumor.
6. Surgical margins:
   (a) Superior margin: 5 mm.
   (b) Inferior margin: 2 mm (slides 3 and 4).

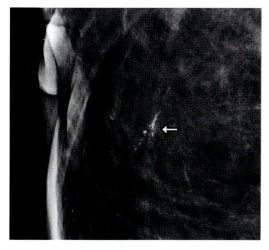

Fig. 256 Rt magnification view (ML): coarse heterogeneous microcalcifications with linear distribution in right lower inner quadrant

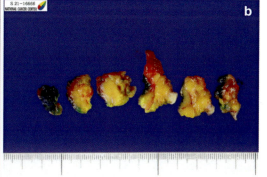

Fig. 257 (a) Gross pathology of lumpectomy specimen. (b) The margins get marked and sliced with different colors on each direction

(c) Medial margin: 10 mm.
(d) Lateral margin: 10 mm.
(e) Deep margin: 2 mm.
(f) Superficial margin: 2 mm.
7. Microcalcification: present, tumoral/non-tumoral.
8. Pathological TN category (AJCC 2017): pTis.

	Result	Intensity	Positive %
Estrogen receptor	Strong (8/8)	3	>2/3
Progesterone receptor	Strong (8/8)	3	>2/3
C-erbB2	Negative (1+)		
Ki-67	Positive in 8% of tumor cells		

Adjuvant Therapy
Postoperative radiation therapy.
 Tamoxifen 20 mg/day.

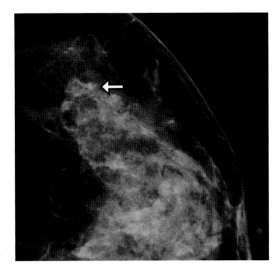

Fig. 258 Lt CC MG: subtle asymmetry in the outer portion of left breast

39 Case 39

39.1 Patient History and Progress

Female/42 years old, post-menopause.
 Bloody discharge from left nipple.
 No family history.

39.2 Courses of Treatment

Left breast IDC→ Operation → Adjuvant therapy → **Left breast recurrence (IDC).**

39.2.1 Primary Treatment
See Figs. 258, 259, 260 and 261.

Operation
Aug. 2013 Left skin sparing mastectomy with latissimus dorsi muscle flap reconstruction (Fig. 262).

Pathology Report
Invasive Ductal Carcinoma
1. Size of invasive tumor: 3 cm (pT2).
2. Size of intraductal component: 4.5 cm.

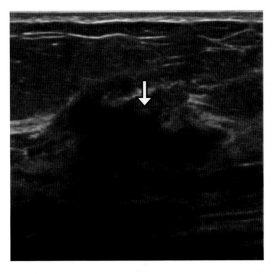

Fig. 259 US: irregular hypoechoic mass with angular margin at the 2 o'clock direction of left breast

3. Histologic grade: 1/3 (tubule formation: 3/3, nuclear pleomorphism: 1/3, mitotic count: 1/3, 7/10HPF).
4. Intraductal component: present, intratumoral/extratumoral (30%) (nuclear grade: low, necrosis: absent, architectural pattern: cribriform, extensive intraductal component: present).
5. Skin: no involvement of tumor.
6. Surgical margins:

Local Recurrence

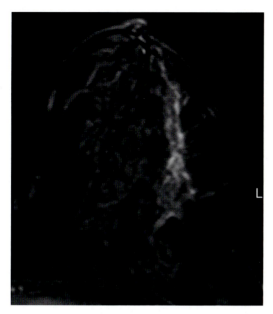

Fig. 260 MRI: segmental heterogeneous non-mass enhancement in the outer portion of left breast

Fig. 261 Lymphoscintigraphy shows visualized sentinel lymph nodes in the left axilla

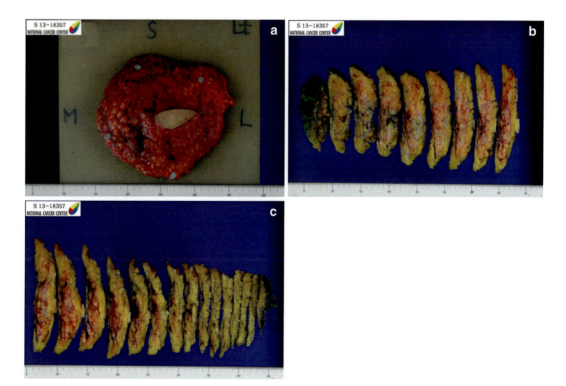

Fig. 262 (**a**) Gross pathology of mastectomy specimen. (**b, c**) The margins get marked and sliced with different colors on each direction

(a) Deep margin: 13 mm.
   (b) Superficial margin: 16 mm.
7. Lymph nodes:
   (a) Metastasis in 1 out of 10 axillary lymph nodes (pN1mi) (sentinel LN: 1/3, axillary LN: 0/7).
   (b) Perinodal extension: absent.
   (c) Size of metastatic carcinoma: 2 mm.
8. Vascular invasion: absent.
9. Lymphatic invasion: absent.
10. Tumor border: infiltrative.
11. Microcalcification: absent.
12. Pathologic stage (AJCC 2010): pT2N1mi.

	Result	Intensity	Positive %
Estrogen receptor	Strong (8/8)	3	>2/3
Progesterone receptor	Strong (8/8)	3	>2/3
C-erbB2	Negative (0)		
Ki-67	Positive in 26% of tumor cells		

Adjuvant Therapy

Tamoxifen 20 mg/day for 2.6 years with goserelin.

39.2.2 Treatments after Recurrence

See Figs. 263 and 264.

Operation

Jun. 2018 Left nipple wide excision (Fig. 265).

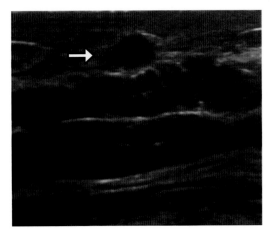

Fig. 263 US: microlobulated hypoechoic mass in left subareolar area

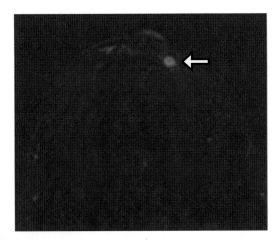

Fig. 264 MRI: round homogeneous enhancing mass in left subareolar area

Pathology Report

Invasive Ductal Carcinoma

1. Post-nipple-sparing mastectomy status.
2. Size of tumor: 0.3 cm, residual (see note).
3. Histologic grade: 2/3 (tubule formation: 3/3, nuclear pleomorphism: 2/3, mitotic count: 1/3, 7/10HPF).
4. Intraductal component: present, intratumoral/extratumoral (10%) (nuclear grade: low, necrosis: absent, architectural pattern: cribriform, extensive intraductal component: absent).
5. Skin and nipple: no involvement of tumor.
6. Surgical margins:
   (a) Superior margin: 10 mm.
   (b) Inferior margin: 5 mm.
   (c) Medial margin: 20 mm.
   (d) Lateral margin: 5 mm.
   (e) Deep margin: 2 mm.
   (f) Superficial margin: 2 mm.
7. Arteriovenous invasion: absent.
8. Lymphovascular invasion: present, intratumoral.
9. Tumor border: infiltrative.
10. Microcalcification: present, tumoral/non-tumoral.

Note: 1. In the previous biopsy specimen (S18–12629), invasive ductal carcinoma measures at least 0.4 cm in greatest dimension.

Local Recurrence

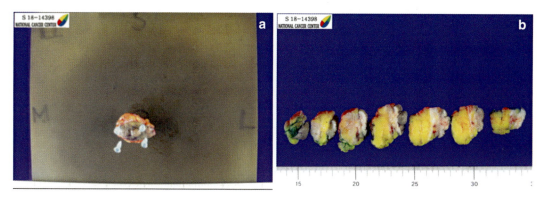

Fig. 265 (**a**) Gross pathology of nipple excision specimen. (**b**) The margins get marked and sliced with different colors on each direction

	Result	Intensity	Positive %
Estrogen receptor	Intermediate (5/8)	2	10%–1/3
Progesterone receptor	Strong (8/8)	3	>2/3
C-erbB2	Negative (1+)		
Ki-67	Positive in 14% of tumor cells		

Adjuvant Therapy

Postoperative radiation therapy.
Letrozole 2.5 mg/day for 5 years.

40 Case 40

40.1 Patient History and Progress

Female/60 years old, post-menopause.

Screen detected mass lesion on right breast 12 o'clock and 9 o'clock direction.

Outside result of biopsy: right breast 12 o'clock, Atypical ductal hyperplasia.

Right breast 9:30 o'clock, Fibrocystic change.

Family history of breast cancer, older sister and younger sister.

Hepatitis C virus carrier, Facet Joint Syndrome lumbosacral region, Dyspnea disorder.

BRCA 1 VUS (variant of uncertain).

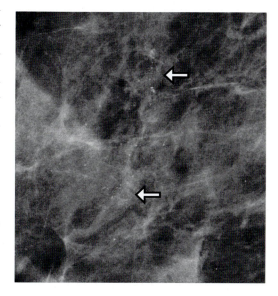

Fig. 266 Rt magnification view (ML): segmental fine pleomorphic microcalcifications in right upper outer quadrant

40.2 Courses of Treatment

Right breast DCIS→ Operation → Right breast recurrence (microinvasive ductal carcinoma).

40.2.1 Primary Treatment

See Fig. 266.

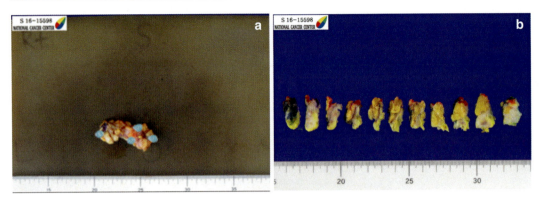

Fig. 267 (**a**) Gross pathology of breast excision specimen. (**b**) The margins get marked and sliced with different colors on each direction

Operation
Jul. 2016 Right breast mass excision (Fig. 267).

Pathology Report

Ductal Carcinoma In Situ
1. Size of tumor: 0.3 cm (pTis).
2. Nuclear grade: low.
3. Necrosis: absent.
4. Architectural pattern: solid/cribriform.
5. Surgical margins:
   (a) Superior margin: 7 mm.
   (b) Inferior margin: 6 mm.
   (c) Medial margin: 1 mm from ductal carcinoma in situ (slide 1).
   (d) Lateral margin: 45 mm.
   (e) Deep margin: <1 mm from ductal carcinoma in situ (slide 1).
6. Microcalcification: present, tumor/non-tumor.
7. Pathologic stage (AJCC 2010): pTisNx.

	Result	Intensity	Positive %
Estrogen receptor	Intermediate (6/8)	2	1/3–2/3
Progesterone receptor	Negative (0/8)	0	0
C-erbB2	Positive (3+)		
Ki-67	Positive in 25% of tumor cells		

40.2.2 Treatments After Recurrence
See Figs. 268, 269 and 270.

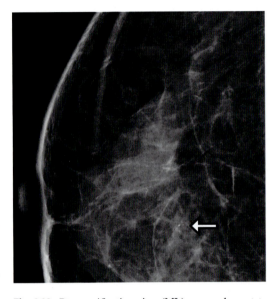

Fig. 268 Rt magnification view (ML): grouped punctate microcalcifications (arrow), showing interval increase in number

Operation
Dec. 2017 Right nipple-areolar complex sparing mastectomy with immediate implant reconstruction, sentinel lymph node biopsy (Fig. 271).

Pathology Report

Microinvasive Ductal Carcinoma
1. Size of invasive component: <0.1 cm (pT1mi).
2. Size of intraductal component: 0.6 cm.

Local Recurrence

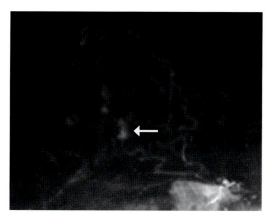

Fig. 269 MRI: irregular enhancing mass at the corresponding area of the microcalcifications on mammography

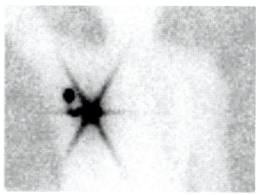

Fig. 270 Lymphoscintigraphy shows visualized sentinel lymph nodes in the right axilla

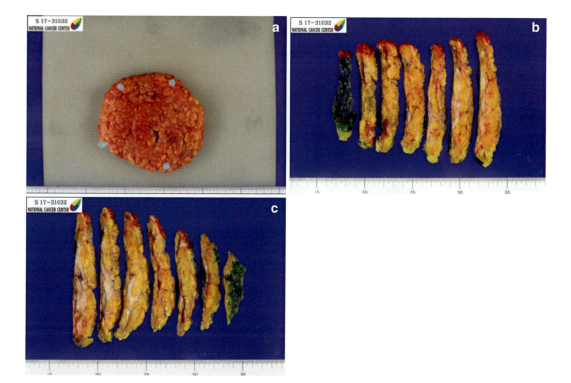

Fig. 271 (**a**) Gross pathology of mastectomy specimen. (**b, c**) The margins get marked and sliced with different colors on each direction

3. Histologic grade: 2/3 (tubule formation: 3/3, nuclear pleomorphism: 2/3, mitotic count: 1/3, 6/10HPF).
4. Intraductal component: present, intratumoral/extratumoral (99%) (nuclear grade: low, necrosis: present, architectural pattern: cribriform/solid/comedo, extensive intraductal component: present).
5. Skin: no involvement of tumor.
6. Surgical margins:
   (a) Deep margin: 2 mm.
   (b) Superficial margin: 2 mm.
7. Lymph nodes: no metastasis in one axillary lymph node (pN0(sn)) (sentinel LN: 0/1).
8. Arteriovenous invasion: absent.
9. Lymphovascular invasion: absent.
10. Tumor border: infiltrative.
11. Microcalcification: present, tumoral/non-tumoral.
12. Pathologic stage (AJCC 2010): pT1miN0(sn).

	Result	Intensity	Positive %
Estrogen receptor	Strong (8/8)	3	>2/3
Progesterone receptor	Negative (0/8)	0	0
C-erbB2	Equivocal (2+)		
Ki-67	Positive in 22% of tumor cells		

Adjuvant Therapy

Anastrozole 1 mg/day for 3.3 years, then tamoxifen 20 mg/day.

41 Case 41

41.1 Patient History and Progress

Female/62 years old, post-menopause.
Screen detected mass lesion on left breast subareolar and retraction of left nipple.
No family history.
No comorbidities.

41.2 Courses of Treatment

Left breast IDC → Operation → Adjuvant therapy → **Right breast recurrence (DCIS).**

41.2.1 Primary Treatment

See Figs. 272, 273 and 274.

Operation

Jul. 2012 Left total mastectomy, sentinel lymph node biopsy (Fig. 275).

Pathology Report

Invasive Ductal Carcinoma
1. Size of invasive tumor: 1.2 cm (pT1c).
2. Size of ductal carcinoma in situ: 3.5 cm.
3. Histologic grade: 2 (tubule formation: 2/3, nuclear pleomorphism: 3/3, mitotic count: 1/3, 3/10HPF).

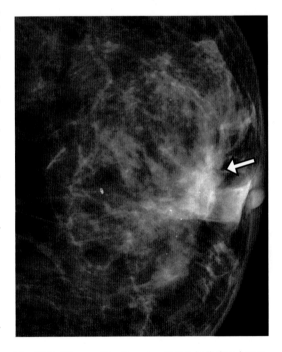

Fig. 272 Lt. magnification view (ML): indistinct irregular hyperdense mass with associated fine pleomorphic microcalcifications in left subareolar area

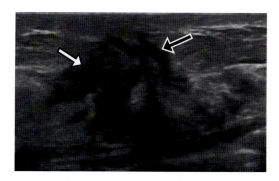

Fig. 273 US: irregular hypoechoic mass (white arrow) with associated ductal dilatations (black arrow) in left subareolar area

4. Intraductal component: present, intratumoral and extratumoral (80%) (nuclear grade: high, necrosis: present, architectural pattern: papillary and cribriform, extensive intraductal component: present).
5. Skin: no involvement of tumor.
6. Nipple: involvement of lactiferous duct by ductal carcinoma in situ.
7. Surgical margins:
   (c) Deep margin: 2 mm.
   (d) Superficial margin: 12 mm.
8. Lymph nodes: no metastasis in 4 axillary lymph nodes (pN0) (sentinel LN: 0/1, axillary LN: 0/3).
9. Vascular invasion: absent.
10. Lymphatic invasion: absent.
11. Tumor border: infiltrative.
12. Microcalcification: present, tumoral.
13. Pathologic stage (AJCC 2010): pT1cN0.

	Result	Intensity	Positive %
Estrogen receptor	Strong (7/7)	3	>2/3
Progesterone receptor	Intermediate (5/7)	3	10%-1/3
C-erbB2	Negative (0)		
Ki-67	Positive in 35% of tumor cells		

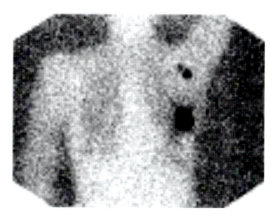

Fig. 274 Lymphoscintigraphy shows visualized sentinel lymph nodes in the left axilla

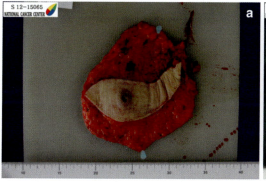
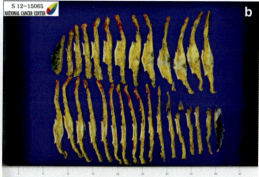

Fig. 275 (**a**) Gross pathology of mastectomy specimen. (**b**) The margins get marked and sliced with different colors on each direction

Adjuvant Therapy

Adjuvant chemotherapy #6 cycles of fluorouracil and doxorubicin and cyclophosphamide.

Tamoxifen 20 mg/day for 2.3 years.

41.2.2 Treatments After Recurrence

See Figs. 276, 277 and 278.

Operation

Apr. 2016 Right nipple-areolar complex sparing mastectomy, sentinel lymph node biopsy (Fig. 279).

Pathology Report

1. Ductal Carcinoma In Situ, residual involving sclerosing adenosis.
   (a) Size of tumor: 3.5 cm.
   (b) Nuclear grade: low.
   (c) Necrosis: present.
   (d) Architectural pattern: papillary/cribriform/comedo.
   (e) Skin and nipple: no involvement of tumor.
   (f) Surgical margins:
      - Deep margin: 3 mm.
      - Superficial margin: 6 mm.
   (g) Lymph nodes: no metastasis in two axillary lymph nodes (pN0(sn)) (sentinel LN: 0/1, axillary LN: 0/1).
   (h) Microcalcification: present, tumoral/non-tumoral.
2. Sclerosing adenosis with microcalcification.

	Result	Intensity	Positive %
Estrogen receptor	Negative (2/8)	1	<1%
Progesterone receptor	Negative (2/8)	1	<1%
C-erbB2	Equivocal (2+) (SISH negative)		
Ki-67	Positive in 20% of tumor cells		

Adjuvant Therapy

Anastrozole 1 mg/day.

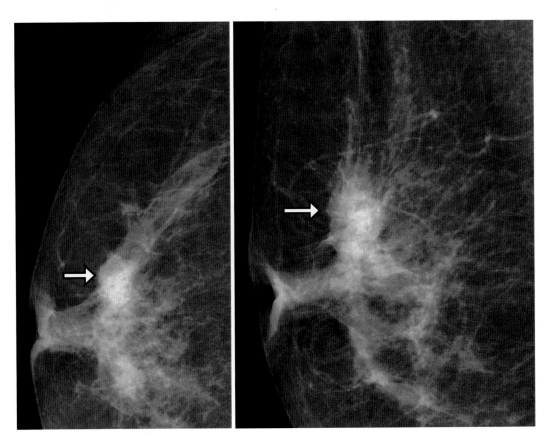

Fig. 276 MG: obscured hyperdense mass in right upper outer quadrant

Local Recurrence

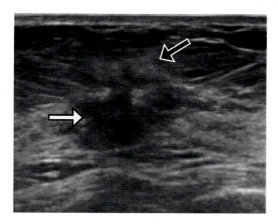

Fig. 277 OPD US: irregular hypoechoic mass (white arrow) with echogenic halo (black arrow)

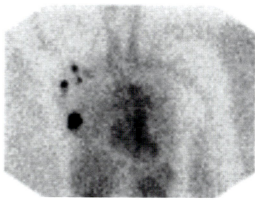

Fig. 278 Lymphoscintigraphy shows visualized sentinel lymph nodes in the right axilla

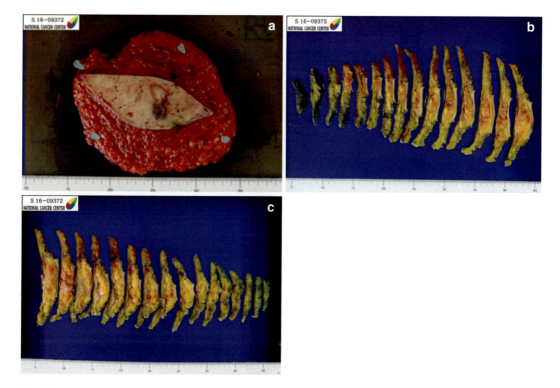

Fig. 279 (a) Gross pathology of mastectomy specimen. (b, c) The margins get marked and sliced with different colors on each direction

42 Case 42

42.1 Patient History and Progress

Female/52 years old, pre-menopause.
　Screen detected mass lesion on right breast 10 o'clock direction.
　Outside result of biopsy: Invasive ductal carcinoma.
　Family history of breast cancer, younger sister at her 44 years old.
　s/p Left breast Nipple sparing mastectomy (invasive lobular carcinoma).
　BRCA 1 and 2 mutation: Not detected.

42.2 Courses of Treatment

Left breast ILC → Operation → Adjuvant therapy → **Right breast recurrence** (IDC).

42.2.1 Primary Treatment
See Fig. 280.

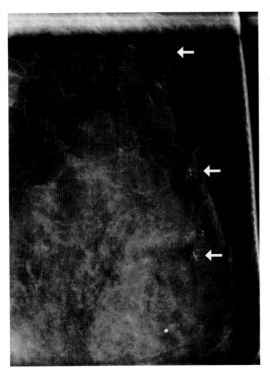

Fig. 280 Lt magnification view (ML): multifocal grouped fine pleomorphic microcalcifications in left upper breast

Operation
Aug. 2017 Left nipple-areolar complex sparing mastectomy with transverse rectus abdominis muscles flap reconstruction (outside).

Pathology Report

Invasive Lobular Carcinoma
1. Size of invasive tumor: 0.2 cm (pT1a).
2. Pathologic stage: pT1aNx.

	Result	Intensity	Positive %
Estrogen receptor	Positive		
Progesterone receptor	Negative		
C-erbB2	Negative (1+)		
Ki-67	Positive in 5% of tumor cells		

Adjuvant therapy.
Tamoxifen 20 mg/day for 0.7 year.

42.2.2 Treatments After Recurrence
See Figs. 281, 282 and 283.

Operation
Apr. 2018 Right breast conserving surgery, sentinel lymph node biopsy (Fig. 284).

Pathology Report

Invasive Ductal Carcinoma
1. Size of tumor: 0.8 cm (pT1b).
2. Histologic grade: 1/3 (tubule formation: 1/3, nuclear pleomorphism: 2/3, mitotic count: 1/3, 5/10HPF)/

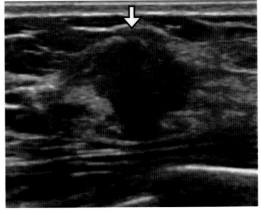

Fig. 281 o/s US: irregular heterogeneous echoic mass

Local Recurrence

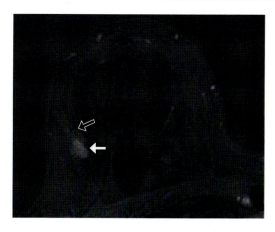

Fig. 282 MRI: irregular heterogeneous enhancing mass (white arrow) with associated non-mass enhancement (black arrow)

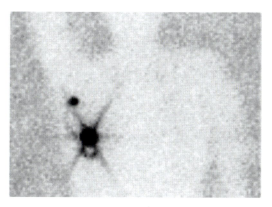

Fig. 283 Lymphoscintigraphy shows visualized sentinel lymph nodes in the right axilla

3. Intraductal component: absent.
4. Skin: no involvement of tumor.
5. Surgical margins:
   (a) Superior margin: 15 mm.
   (b) Inferior margin: 15 mm.
   (c) Medial margin: 10 mm.
   (d) Lateral margin: 20 mm.
   (e) Deep margin: 2 mm.
   (f) Superficial margin: 2 mm.
6. Lymph nodes: no metastasis in one axillary lymph node (pN0(sn)) (sentinel LN: 0/1).
7. Arteriovenous invasion: absent.
8. Lymphovascular invasion: absent.
9. Tumor border: infiltrative.
10. Microcalcification: present, tumoral.
11. Pathological TN category (AJCC 2017): pT1bN0(sn).

	Result	Intensity	Positive %
Estrogen receptor	Intermediate (5/8)	1	1/3–2/3
Progesterone receptor	Weak (4/8)	2	1–10%
C-erbB2	Equivocal (2+) (SISH negative)		
Ki-67	Positive in 2% of tumor cells		

Adjuvant Therapy

Postoperative radiation therapy.
Letrozole 2.5 mg/day with leuprolide.

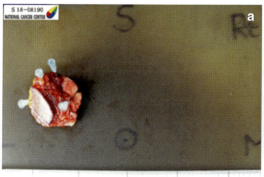
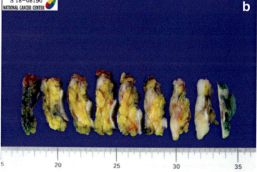

Fig. 284 (**a**) Gross pathology of lumpectomy specimen. (**b**) The margins get marked and sliced with different colors on each direction

43 Case 43

43.1 Patient History and Progress

Female/64 years old, post-menopause.

Screen detected mass lesion on right breast 12 o'clock direction.

Outside result of biopsy: Invasive ductal carcinoma.

Family history of breast cancer, older sister.

Diabetes mellitus, fatty liver, dyslipidemia.

BRCA 1 and 2 mutation: Not detected, ATM VUS (variant of uncertain).

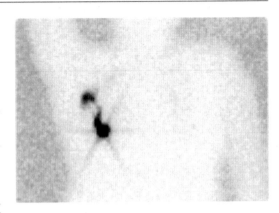

Fig. 286 Lymphoscintigraphy shows visualized sentinel lymph nodes in the right axilla

43.2 Courses of Treatment

Right breast ILC→ Operation → Adjuvant therapy → Left breast recurrence (microinvasive ductal carcinoma).

43.2.1 Primary Treatment
See Figs. 285 and 286.

Operation
May 2014 Right breast conserving surgery, sentinel lymph node biopsy (Fig. 287).

Pathology Report
Invasive Lobular Carcinoma
1. Size of tumor: 1.5 cm (pT1c).
2. Histologic grade: 2/3 (tubule formation: 3/3, nuclear pleomorphism: 2/3, mitotic count: 1/3, 2/10HPF).
3. In situ component: present, extratumoral (40%).
4. Skin: no involvement of tumor.
5. Surgical margins:
    (a) Superior margin: 8 mm.
    (b) Inferior margin: 27 mm.
    (c) Medial margin: positive for lobular carcinoma in situ (Fro 6) (see note).
    (d) Lateral margin: 15 mm.
    (e) Deep margin: 2 mm.
    (f) Superficial margin: 9 mm.
6. Lymph nodes: no metastasis in three axillary lymph nodes (pN0(sn)) (sentinel LN: 0/3).
7. Arteriovenous invasion: absent.
8. Lymphovascular invasion: absent.
9. Tumor border: infiltrative.
10. Microcalcification: absent.
11. Pathologic stage (AJCC 2010): pT1cN0(sn).

Note: 1. Lobular carcinoma in situ is present only in the permanent section of Fro 6.

	Result	Intensity	Positive %
Estrogen receptor	Strong (8/8)	3	>2/3
Progesterone receptor	Strong (8/8)	3	>2/3
C-erbB2	Negative (0)		
Ki-67	Positive in 11% of tumor cells		

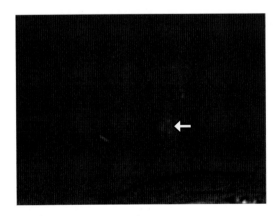

Fig. 285 MRI: irregular heterogeneous enhancing mass in right breast

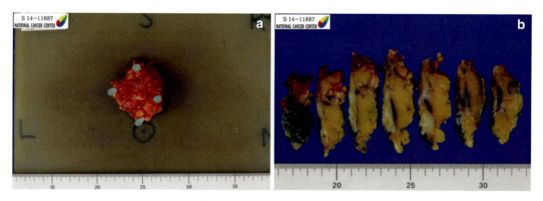

Fig. 287 (**a**) Gross pathology of lumpectomy specimen. (**b**) The margins get marked and sliced with different colors on each direction

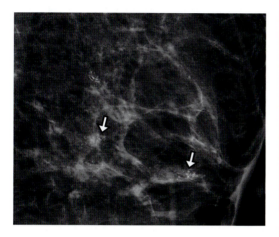

Fig. 288 Lt. magnification view (ML): segmental fine linear microcalcifications in left breast

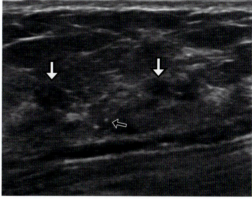

Fig. 289 US: multifocal indistinct hypoechoic masses (white arrows) with microcalcifications (black arrow)

Adjuvant Therapy
Postoperative radiation therapy.
 Anastrozole 1 mg/day for 5 years.

43.2.2 Treatments After Recurrence
See Figs. 288, 289, 290 and 291.

Operation
Jun. 2021 Left breast conserving surgery, sentinel lymph node biopsy (Fig. 292).

Pathology Report
Microinvasive Ductal Carcinoma
1. Size of invasive component: <0.1 cm (pT1mi).
2. Size of intraductal component: 4.0 cm.
3. Histologic grade: not applicable.
4. Intraductal component: present, intratumoral/extratumoral (99%) (nuclear grade: high, necrosis: present, architectural pattern: micropapillary/cribriform/solid/comedo, extensive intraductal component: present).
5. Skin: no involvement of tumor.
6. Surgical margins:
    (a) Superior margin: 5 mm.
    (b) Inferior margin: (see note).
    (c) Medial margin: (see note).
    (d) Lateral margin: 5 mm.
    (e) Deep margin: 2 mm.
    (f) Superficial margin: 2 mm.

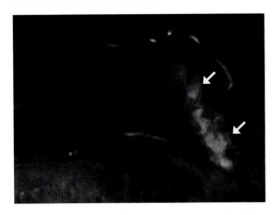

Fig. 290 MRI: segmental heterogeneous non-mass enhancement at the corresponding area of the microcalcifications on mammography

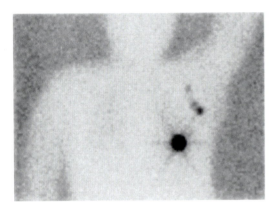

Fig. 291 Lymphoscintigraphy shows visualized sentinel lymph nodes in the left axilla

7. Lymph nodes: no metastasis in one axillary lymph node (pN0(sn)) (sentinel LN: 0/1).
8. Arteriovenous invasion: absent.
9. Lymphovascular invasion: absent.
10. Tumor border: infiltrative.
11. Microcalcification: present, tumoral/non-tumoral.
12. Pathological TN category (AJCC 2017): pT1miN0(sn).

Note: 1. The inferior margin of the lumpectomy specimen (slide 3) is close to ductal carcinoma in situ (<1 mm), but this margin submitted for frozen diagnosis (Fro 3) is free of tumor.

2. The medial margin of the lumpectomy specimen (slide 10) is close to ductal carcinoma in situ (2 mm), but this margin submitted for frozen diagnosis (Fro 4) is free of tumor.

	Result	Intensity	Positive %
Estrogen receptor	Negative (0/8)	0	0
Progesterone receptor	Negative (0/8)	0	0
C-erbB2	Positive (3+)		
Ki-67	Positive in 20% of tumor cells		

Adjuvant Therapy

Postoperative radiation therapy.

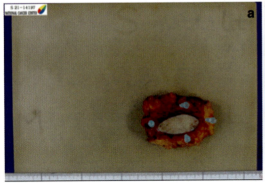
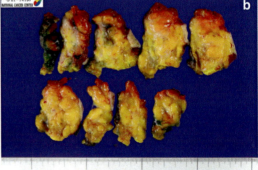

Fig. 292 (**a**) Gross pathology of lumpectomy specimen. (**b**) The margins get marked and sliced with different colors on each direction

44 Case 44

44.1 Patient History and Progress

Female/54 years old, post-menopause.
  Screen detected mass lesion on left breast 2 o'clock direction.
  Outside result of biopsy: Ductal carcinoma.
  No family history.
  No comorbidities.

44.2 Courses of Treatment

Left breast microinvasive ductal carcinoma → Operation → Adjuvant therapy → **Right breast recurrence (IDC).**

44.2.1 Primary Treatment
See Figs. 293, 294, 295 and 296.

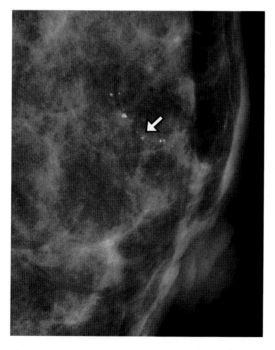

Fig. 293 Lt magnification view (ML): linear fine pleomorphic microcalcifications in left upper breast

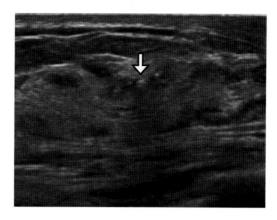

Fig. 294 US: microcalcifications at the corresponding area of the microcalcifications on mammography

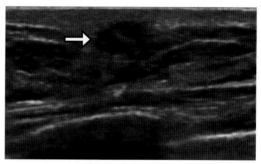

Fig. 295 US: microlobulated hypoechoic mass at 6 o'clock direction of left breast

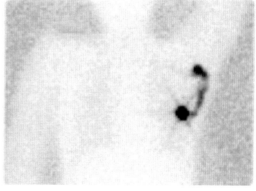

Fig. 296 Lymphoscintigraphy shows visualized sentinel lymph nodes in the left axilla

Operation

First Operation (Feb. 2014) Left breast conserving surgery, sentinel lymph node biopsy (Fig. 297).

Pathology Report

Microinvasive Ductal Carcinoma

1. Size of invasive component: <0.1 cm (pT1mic).
2. Size of intraductal component: 1.2 cm.
3. Histologic grade: 2/3 (tubule formation: 3/3, nuclear pleomorphism: 2/3, mitotic count: 1/3, 3/10HPF).
4. Intraductal component: present, extratumoral (99%) (nuclear grade: low, necrosis: absent, architectural pattern: solid, extensive intraductal component: present).
5. Surgical margins:
   (a) Superior margin: 7 mm.
   (b) Inferior margin: 17 mm.
   (c) Medial margin: positive for ductal carcinoma in situ (Fro 4) (see note).
   (d) Lateral margin: <2 mm from ductal carcinoma in situ (slide 6).
   (e) Deep margin: 4 mm.
   (f) Superficial margin: <1 mm from ductal carcinoma in situ (slide 1).
6. Lymph nodes: no metastasis in one axillary lymph nodes (pN0(sn)) (sentinel LN: 0/1).
7. Venous invasion: absent.
8. Lymphovascular invasion: absent.
9. Tumor border: infiltrative.
10. Microcalcification: present, non-tumoral.
11. Pathologic stage (AJCC 2010): pT1micN0(sn).

Note: 1. Ductal carcinoma in situ is present only in the permanent section of Fro 4.

	Result	Intensity	Positive %
Estrogen receptor	Weak (3/8)	1	1–10%
Progesterone receptor	Negative (0/8)	0	0
C-erbB2	Equivocal (2+)		
Ki-67	Positive in 17% of tumor cells		

Operation

Second Operation (Mar. 2014) Left breast wide excision.

Pathology Report

1. No residual tumor with foreign body reaction.
   (a) Post-lumpectomy status.
2. Atypical ductal hyperplasia, focal (see note).

Note: Atypical ductal hyperplasia is present only in the permanent section of Fro 1.

Adjuvant Therapy

Postoperative radiation therapy.
Tamoxifen 20 mg/day for 5 years.

44.2.2 Treatments After Recurrence

See Figs. 298, 299, 300 and 301.

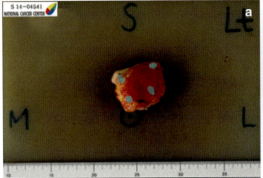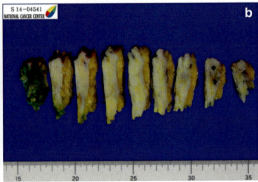

Fig. 297 (**a**) Gross pathology of lumpectomy specimen. (**b**) The margins get marked and sliced with different colors on each direction

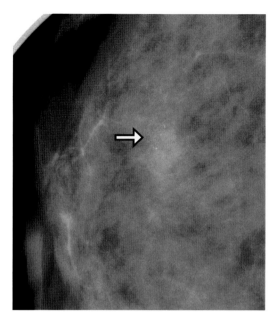

Fig. 298 Rt magnification view (CC): indistinct hyperdense mass with fine pleomorphic microcalcifications

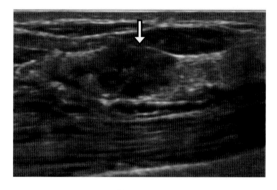

Fig. 299 US: irregular heterogeneous hypoechoic mass with microcalcifications

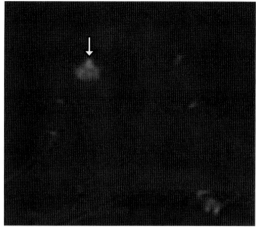

Fig. 300 MRI: irregular heterogeneous enhancing mass

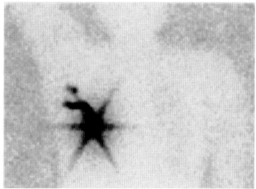

Fig. 301 Lymphoscintigraphy shows visualized sentinel lymph nodes in the right axilla

Operation
Jun. 2020 Right breast conserving surgery, sentinel lymph node biopsy (Fig. 302).

Pathology Report
Invasive Ductal Carcinoma
1. Size of tumor: 1.1 cm (pT1c).
2. Histologic grade: 3/3 (tubule formation: 3/3, nuclear pleomorphism: 2/3, mitotic count: 3/3, 22/10HPF).
3. Intraductal component: present, intratumoral (5%) (nuclear grade: low, necrosis: present, architectural pattern: micropapillary/cribriform/comedo, extensive intraductal component: absent).
4. Skin: no involvement of tumor.
5. Surgical margins:
    (a) Superior margin: 15 mm.
    (b) Inferior margin: (see note).
    (c) Medial margin: 5 mm.
    (d) Lateral margin: 30 mm.
    (e) Deep margin: 5 mm.
    (f) Superficial margin: <1 mm from invasive ductal carcinoma (slides 2 and 3).
6. Lymph nodes: no metastasis in two axillary lymph nodes (pN0(i+)(sn)) (sentinel LN: 0/2).
7. Arteriovenous invasion: absent.

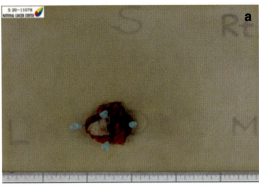
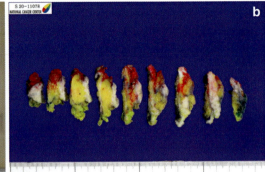

Fig. 302 (**a**) Gross pathology of lumpectomy specimen. (**b**) The margins get marked and sliced with different colors on each direction

8. Lymphovascular invasion: present, intratumoral.
9. Tumor border: infiltrative.
10. Microcalcification: present, tumoral/non-tumoral.
11. Pathological TN category (AJCC 2017): pT1cN0(i+)(sn).

Note: 1. The inferior margin of the lumpectomy specimen (slide 3) is close to invasive ductal carcinoma (3 mm), but this margin submitted for frozen diagnosis (Fro 3) is free of tumor.

2. A few isolated tumor cells are present only in the permanent section of Fro 6 for immunohistochemical staining (pN0(i+)).

	Result	Intensity	Positive %
Estrogen receptor	Strong (8/8)	3	>2/3
Progesterone receptor	Negative (2/8)	1	<1%
C-erbB2	Equivocal (2+) (SISH equivocal)		
Ki-67	Positive in 28% of tumor cells		

Adjuvant Therapy
Postoperative radiation therapy.
Anastrozole 1 mg/day.

45 Case 45

45.1 Patient History and Progress

Female/57 years old, post-menopause.
Screen detected mass lesion on right breast 12 o'clock direction.
Outside result of biopsy: Lobular carcinoma in situ.
Family history of breast cancer, older sister.
Panic disorder.
BRCA 1 and 2 mutation: Not detected.

45.2 Courses of Treatment

Right breast LCIS→ Operation → **Right breast recurrence (DCIS)**.

45.2.1 Primary Treatment
See Fig. 303.

Operation
Jul. 2017 Right breast conserving surgery, left breast mass excision (Figs. 304 and 305).

Pathology Report
<Right>

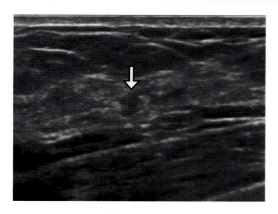

Fig. 303 US: irregular not parallel hypoechoic mass at the 1 o'clock direction of right breast

1. Lobular Carcinoma In Situ
   (a) Size of tumor: up to 0.4 cm, multifocal (pTis).
   (b) Surgical margins:
      - Superior margin: 5 mm.
      - Inferior margin: 5 mm.
      - Medial margin: 5 mm.
      - Lateral margin: (see note).
      - Deep margin: 5 mm.
      - Superficial margin: 5 mm.
   (c) Microcalcification: present, non-tumoral.
   (d) Pathologic stage (AJCC 2010): pTisNx.
2. Atypical ductal hyperplasia.

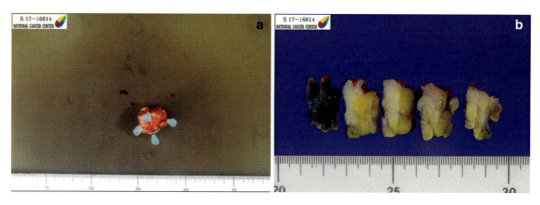

Fig. 304 (a) Gross pathology of right lumpectomy specimen. (b) The margins get marked and sliced with different colors on each direction

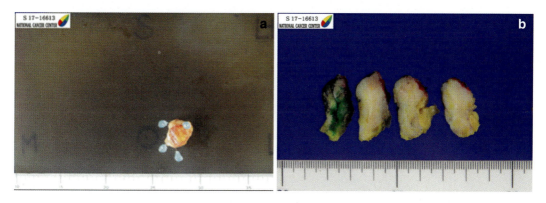

Fig. 305 (a) Gross pathology of left breast excision specimen. (b) The margins get marked and sliced with different colors on each direction

Note: 1. The lateral margin of the lumpectomy specimen (slide 5) is close to lobular carcinoma in situ (<1 mm), but this margin submitted for frozen diagnosis (Fro 5) is free of tumor.

	Result	Intensity	Positive %
Estrogen receptor	Strong (8/8)	3	>2/3
Progesterone receptor	Strong (8/8)	3	>2/3
C-erbB2	Negative (0)		
Ki-67	Positive in 1% of tumor cells		

<Left>
1. Atypical ductal hyperplasia involving intraductal papilloma
2. Fibroadenoma.

45.2.2 Treatments After Recurrence
See Fig. 306.

Operation
Feb. 2020 Right nipple-areolar complex sparing mastectomy (Fig. 307).

Pathology Report

Ductal Carcinoma In Situ
1. Post-lumpectomy status.
2. Size of tumor: 0.3 cm (pTis).
3. Nuclear grade: low.
4. Necrosis: absent.
5. Architectural pattern: cribriform/solid.
6. Skin: no involvement of tumor.
7. Surgical margins:
    (a) Deep margin: 2 mm.
    (b) Superficial margin: 2 mm.
8. Microcalcification: present, tumoral/non-tumoral.
9. Pathological TN category (AJCC 2017): pTis.

	Result	Intensity	Positive %
Estrogen receptor	Strong (8/8)	3	>2/3
Progesterone receptor	Strong (8/8)	3	>2/3
C-erbB2	Negative (1+)		
Ki-67	Positive in 2% of tumor cells		

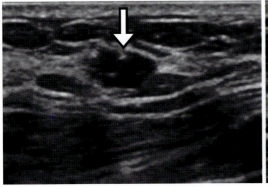 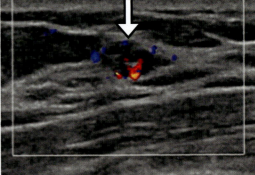

Fig. 306 US: irregular hypoechoic mass with increased vascularity

Local Recurrence

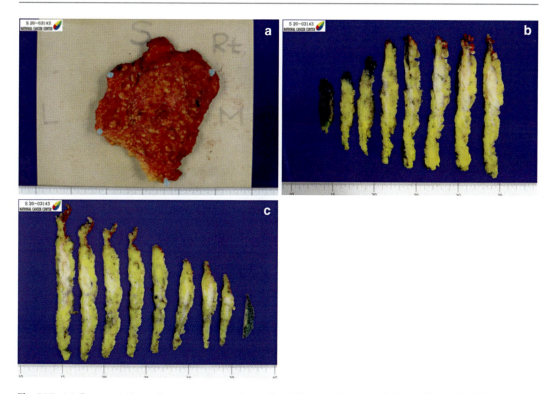

Fig. 307 (**a**) Gross pathology of mastectomy specimen. (**b, c**) The margins get marked and sliced with different colors on each direction

46 Case 46

46.1 Patient History and Progress

Female/69 years old, post-menopause.

Screen detected mass lesion on upper outer portion of right breast.

No family history.

No comorbidities.

46.2 Courses of Treatment

Right breast papillary carcinoma in situ → Operation → Adjuvant therapy → **Right breast recurrence (IDC).**

46.2.1 Primary Treatment

Operation
May 2007 Right breast conserving surgery (Fig. 308).

Pathology Report

Papillary Carcinoma In Situ in background of multiple papilloma (see note)
1. Size of intraductal carcinoma: 0.5 cm (pTis).
2. Nuclear grade: low.
3. Necrosis: absent.
4. Architectural pattern: papillary.
5. Skin: no involvement of tumor.

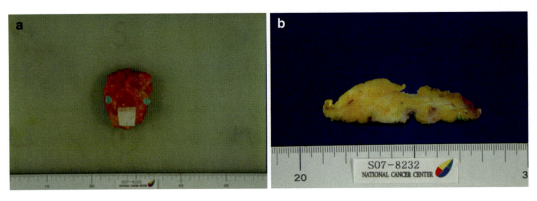

Fig. 308 (a) Gross pathology of lumpectomy specimen. (b) The margins get marked and sliced with different colors on each direction

6. Surgical margins:
   (a) Superior margin: 18 mm.
   (b) Inferior margin: positive for intraductal papilloma.
   (c) Medial margin: 15 mm.
   (d) Lateral margin: 20 mm.
   (e) Deep margin: 2 mm.
7. Microcalcification: present, tumoral/non-tumoral.
8. Pathologic staging: pTis.

Note: The in situ component is mainly present in the needle biopsy specimen.

Adjuvant Therapy
Tamoxifen 20 mg/day for 3.6 years.

46.2.2 Treatments After Recurrence
See Figs. 309, 310, 311 and 312.

Operation
Mar. 2021 Right breast conserving surgery, sentinel lymph node biopsy (Fig. 313).

Pathology Report
Invasive Ductal Carcinoma
1. Size of tumor: 0.8 cm (pT1b).
2. Histologic grade: 2/3 (tubule formation: 3/3, nuclear pleomorphism: 2/3, mitotic count: 1/3, 6/10HPF).
3. Intraductal component: present, intratumoral/extratumoral (30%) (nuclear grade: low, necrosis: absent, architectural pattern: papillary/cribriform, extensive intraductal component: present).
4. Skin: no involvement of tumor.
5. Surgical margins:
   (a) Nipple margin: (see note 1).
   (b) Superior margin: 5 mm.
   (c) Inferior margin: (see note 2).
   (d) Medial margin: (see note 3).
   (e) Lateral margin: 20 mm.
   (f) Deep margin: 2 mm.
   (g) Superficial margin: 2 mm.
6. Lymph nodes: no metastasis in one axillary lymph node (pN0(sn)) (sentinel LN: 0/1).

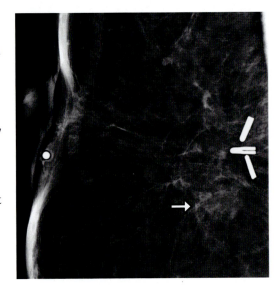

Fig. 309 Rt magnification view (CC): irregular isodense mass with indistinct margin in the center portion of right breast

Local Recurrence

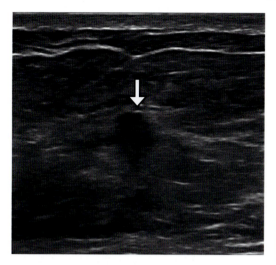

Fig. 310 US: not parallel spiculated hypoechoic mass

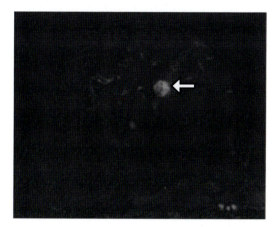

Fig. 311 MRI: round heterogeneous enhancing mass

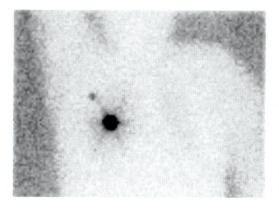

Fig. 312 Lymphoscintigraphy shows visualized sentinel lymph nodes in the right axilla

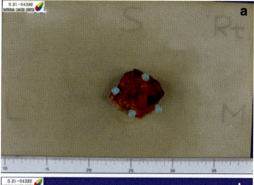

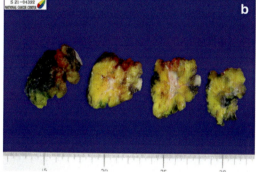

Fig. 313 (a) Gross pathology of lumpectomy specimen. (b) The margins get marked and sliced with different colors on each direction

7. Arteriovenous invasion: absent.
8. Lymphovascular invasion: present, intratumoral.
9. Tumor border: infiltrative.
10. Microcalcification: present, tumoral/non-tumoral.
11. Pathological TN category (AJCC 2017): pT1bN0(sn).

Note: 1. Atypical ductal hyperplasia is present only in the permanent section of Fro 1.

2. The inferior margin of the lumpectomy specimen (slide 8) is close to ductal carcinoma in situ (2 mm), but this margin submitted for frozen diagnosis (Fro 3) is free of tumor.

3. The medial margin of the lumpectomy specimen (slide 6) is close to ductal carcinoma in situ (2 mm), but this margin submitted for frozen diagnosis (Fro 4) is free of tumor.

	Result	Intensity	Positive %
Estrogen receptor	Strong (8/8)	3	>2/3
Progesterone receptor	Strong (8/8)	3	>2/3
C-erbB2	Negative (1+)		
Ki-67	Positive in 10% of tumor cells		

Adjuvant Therapy
Postoperative radiation therapy.
　Anastrozole 1 mg/day.

47　Case 47

47.1　Patient History and Progress

Female/72 years old, post-menopause.
　Screen detected mass lesion on right breast 1 o'clock direction.
　No family history.
　Diabetes mellitus.
　BRCA 1 and 2 mutation: Not detected, ATM VUS (variant of uncertain).
　POLE VUS (variant of uncertain).

47.2　Courses of Treatment

Right breast Infiltrating ductal carcinoma→ Operation → Adjuvant therapy → Left breast recurrence (IDC).

47.2.1　Primary Treatment
See Figs. 314 and 315.

Operation
Aug. 2003 Right breast conserving surgery, axillary lymph node dissection.

Pathology Report
Infiltrating ductal carcinoma.
1. Size of tumor: 2 cm (pT1c).
2. Histologic grade: 2/3 (tubule formation: 2/3, nuclear pleomorphism: 2/3, mitotic count: 2/3).
3. Ductal carcinoma in situ: present, intratumoral (5%) (nuclear grade: low, necrosis: absent, architectural pattern: solid, extensive intraductal component: absent).
4. Skin: no involvement of tumor.
5. Surgical margins: clear:
    (a) Superior margin: 30 mm.
    (b) Inferior margin: 35 mm.
    (c) Medial margin: 35 mm.
    (d) Lateral margin: 25 mm.
    (e) Deep margin: 10 mm.
6. Lymph nodes:
    (a) Metastasis in 2 out of 22 axillary lymph nodes (pN1a) (sentinel LN: 1/2, axillary LN: 1/20).
    (b) Perinodal extension: absent.
    (c) Size of metastatic carcinoma: 6 mm.

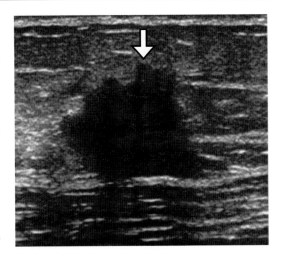

Fig. 314 US: irregular hypoechoic mass with microlobulated margin at the 1 o'clock direction of right breast

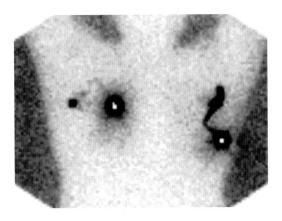

Fig. 315 Lymphoscintigraphy shows visualized sentinel lymph nodes in both axilla

7. Vascular invasion: absent.
8. Lymphatic invasion: absent.
9. Tumor border: infiltrative.
10. Microcalcification: absent.
11. Pathologic staging: pT1cN1a.

	Result	Intensity	Positive %
Estrogen receptor	Intermediate (5/7)	2	1/3–2/3
Progesterone receptor	Weak (2/7)	1	<10%
C-erbB2	Equivocal (2+)		
Ki-67	Positive in 2% of tumor cells		

Adjuvant Therapy

Adjuvant chemotherapy #6 cycles of fluorouracil and doxorubicin and cyclophosphamide.

Postoperative radiation therapy.

Tamoxifen 20 mg/day 1.6 years, anastrozole 1 mg/day for 1 year, tamoxifen 20 mg/day for 2.3 years.

47.2.2 Treatments After Recurrence

See Figs. 316, 317 and 318.

Operation

Mar. 2021 Right breast conserving surgery, sentinel lymph node biopsy (Fig. 319).

Pathology Report

Invasive Ductal Carcinoma

1. Size of tumor: 1.1 cm (pT1c).
2. Histologic grade: 2/3 (tubule formation: 2/3, nuclear pleomorphism: 2/3, mitotic count: 2/3, 11/10HPF).
3. Intraductal component: present, intratumoral/extratumoral (20%) (nuclear grade: low, necrosis: absent, architectural pattern: cribriform, extensive intraductal component: absent).
4. Skin: no involvement of tumor.
5. Surgical margins:
    (a) Superior margin: 10 mm.
    (b) Inferior margin: 10 mm.

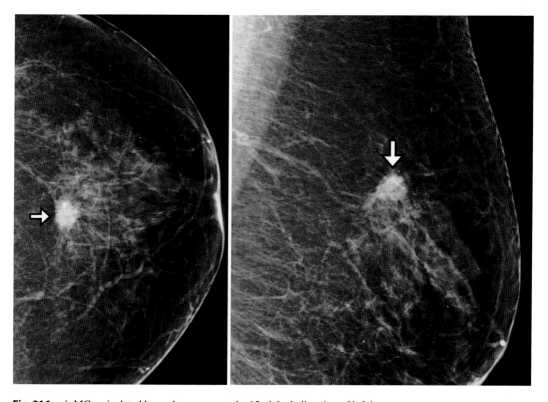

Fig. 316 o/s MG: spiculated hyperdense mass at the 12 o'clock direction of left breast

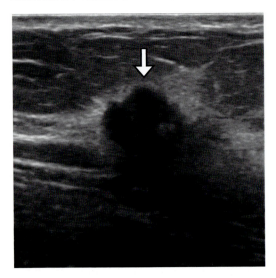

Fig. 317 US: microlobulated round hypoechoic mass

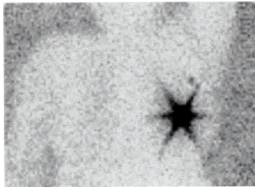

Fig. 318 Lymphoscintigraphy shows visualized sentinel lymph nodes in the left axilla

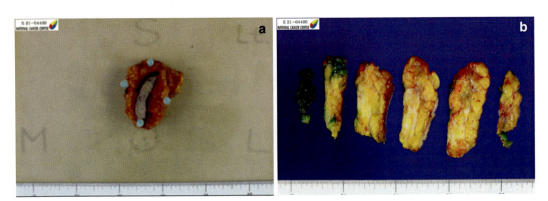

Fig. 319 (a) Gross pathology of lumpectomy specimen. (b) The margins get marked and sliced with different colors on each direction

    (c) Medial margin: 10 mm.
    (d) Lateral margin: 10 mm.
    (e) Deep margin: 2 mm.
    (f) Superficial margin: 2 mm.
6. Lymph nodes: no metastasis in one axillary lymph node (pN0(sn)) (sentinel LN: 0/1).
7. Arteriovenous invasion: absent.
8. Lymphovascular invasion: absent.
9. Tumor border: infiltrative.
10. Microcalcification: present, tumoral/non-tumoral.
11. Pathological TN category (AJCC 2017): pT1cN0(sn).

	Result	Intensity	Positive %
Estrogen receptor	Weak (4/8)	2	1–10%
Progesterone receptor	Weak (4/8)	2	1–10%
C-erbB2	Negative (0)		

Adjuvant Therapy
Postoperative radiation therapy.
    Anastrozole 1 mg/day.

48 Case 48

48.1 Patient History and Progress

Female/42 years old, pre-menopause.
Screen detected mass lesion on left breast 9 o'clock direction.
Outside result of biopsy: Mucinous carcinoma.
No family history.
No comorbdities.

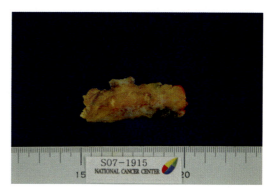

Fig. 322 Gross pathology of lumpectomy specimen

48.2 Courses of Treatment

Left breast Mucinous carcinoma → Operation → Adjuvant therapy → **Left breast recurrence (mucinous carcinoma).**

48.2.1 Primary Treatment
See Figs. 320 and 321.

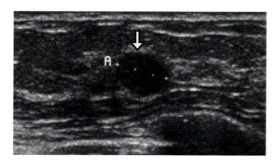

Fig. 320 o/s US: oval hypoechoic mass with microlobulated margin in left breast

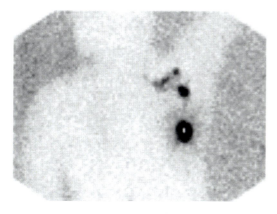

Fig. 321 Lymphoscintigraphy shows visualized sentinel lymph nodes in the left axilla

Operation
Jan. 2007 Left breast conserving surgery, sentinel lymph node biopsy (Fig. 322).

Pathology Report

Mucinous Carcinoma
1. Size of invasive carcinoma: 0.6 cm (pT1b).
2. Size of intraductal carcinoma: 1.5 cm.
3. Histologic grade: 2/3 (tubule formation: 2/3, nuclear pleomorphism: 2/3, mitotic count: 2/3).
4. Ductal carcinoma in situ: present, intratumoral/extratumoral (50%) (nuclear grade: low, necrosis: absent, architectural pattern: cribriform, extensive intraductal component: present).
5. Skin: no involvement of tumor.
6. Surgical margins:
    (a) Superior margin: 8 mm.
    (b) Inferior margin: 15 mm.
    (c) Medial margin: 1 mm from mucinous carcinoma (slide 9) and.
    (d) Positive for atypical ductal hyperplasia (Fro 5) (see note).
    (e) Lateral margin: 10 mm.
    (f) Deep margin: 1 mm.
7. Lymph nodes: no metastasis in 1 axillary lymph nodes (pN0(sn)) (sentinel LN: 0/1).
8. Vascular invasion: absent.
9. Lymphatic invasion: present, intratumoral.
10. Tumor border: pushing.
11. Microcalcification: present, tumoral/non-tumoral.
12. Pathologic staging: pT1bN0(sn).

Note: Atypical ductal hyperplasia is focally present only in the permanent section of Fro 5.

	Result	Intensity	Positive %
Estrogen receptor	Strong (6/7)	3	1/3–2/3
Progesterone receptor	Intermediate (5/7)	2	1/3–2/3
C-erbB2	Negative (1+)		
Ki-67	Positive in 10% of tumor cells		

Adjuvant Therapy
Postoperative radiation therapy.
Tamoxifen 20 mg/day for 5 years.

48.2.2 Treatments After Recurrence
See Figs. 323, 324 and 325.

Operation
Jul. 2015 Left nipple-areolar complex sparing mastectomy with immediate implant reconstruction, sentinel lymph node biopsy (Figs. 326 and 327).

Pathology Report

Mucinous Carcinoma
1. Post-lumpectomy status.
2. Size of tumor: 1.1 cm (rpT1c).
3. Histologic grade: 2/3 (tubule formation: 3/3, nuclear pleomorphism: 2/3, mitotic count: 1/3, 1/10HPF).

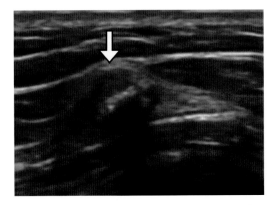

Fig. 323 US: microlobulated irregular isoechoic mass with calcifications at the 10 o'clock direction of left breast

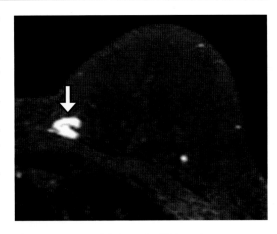

Fig. 324 T2WI MRI: irregular T2 hyperintense mass at the 10 o'clock direction of left breast

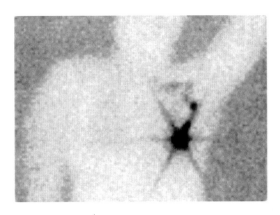

Fig. 325 Lymphoscintigraphy shows visualized sentinel lymph nodes in the left axilla

4. Intraductal component: absent.
5. Skin: no involvement of tumor.
6. Surgical margins:
   (a) Deep margin: <1 mm from mucinous carcinoma (slide 1).
   (b) Superficial margin: 14 mm.
7. Lymph nodes: no metastasis in one axillary lymph node (pN0(sn)) (sentinel LN: 0/1, axillary LN: 0/0).
8. Arteriovenous invasion: absent.
9. Lymphovascular invasion: absent.
10. Tumor border: pushing.
11. Microcalcification: absent.
12. Pathologic stage (AJCC 2010): rpT1cN0(sn).

Local Recurrence

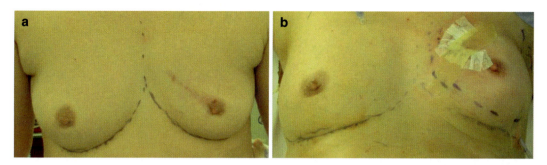

Fig. 326 (**a**) Preoperative and (**b**) immediate postoperative appearance

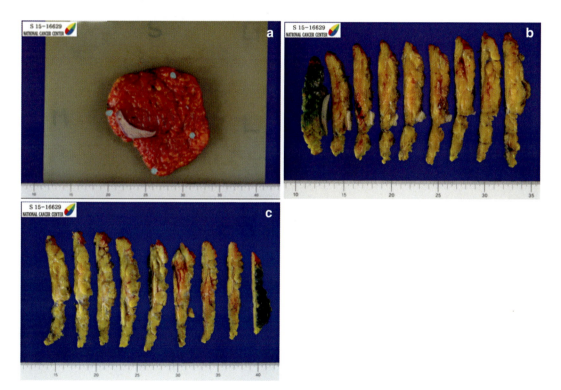

Fig. 327 (**a**) Gross pathology of mastectomy specimen. (**b**, **c**) The margins get marked and sliced with different colors on each direction

	Result	Intensity	Positive %
Estrogen receptor	Strong (7/8)	2	>2/3
Progesterone receptor	Weak (4/8)	2	1–10%
C-erbB2	Negative (0)		
Ki-67	Positive in 6% of tumor cells		

Adjuvant Therapy
Tamoxifen 10 mg/day for 2.2 years.

49 Case 49

49.1 Patient History and Progress

Female/63 years old, post-menopause.
  Self-detected mass lesion on right breast 2 o'clock direction.
  No family history.
  No comorbidities.
  BRCA 1 and 2 mutation: No examination.

49.2 Courses of Treatment

Right breast IDC→ Operation → Adjuvant therapy → **Left breast recurrence (IDC)**.

49.2.1 Primary Treatment
See Figs. 328 and 329.

Operation
Apr. 2004 Right breast conserving surgery, sentinel lymph node biopsy.

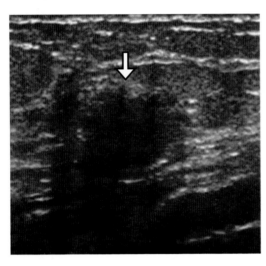

Fig. 328 US: irregular hypoechoic mass with indistinct margin at the 2 o'clock direction of right breast

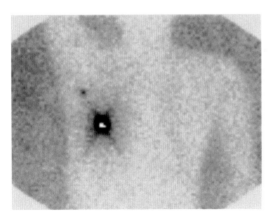

Fig. 329 Lymphoscintigraphy shows visualized sentinel lymph nodes in the right axilla

Pathology Report
Invasive Ductal Carcinoma
1. Size of tumor: 1.5 cm (pT1c).
2. Histologic grade: 2/3 (tubule formation: 2/3, nuclear pleomorphism: 2/3, mitotic count: 2/3).
3. Ductal carcinoma in situ: present, intratumoral/extratumoral (30%) (nuclear grade: low, necrosis: present, architectural pattern: cribriform and comedo, extensive intraductal component: present).
4. Skin: no involvement of tumor.
5. Surgical margins:
   (a) Superior margin: 15 mm.
   (b) Inferior margin: 25 mm.
   (c) Medial margin: 20 mm.
   (d) Lateral margin: 20 mm.
   (e) Deep margin: 5 mm.
6. Lymph nodes: no metastasis in 1 axillary lymph nodes (pN0(sn)) (sentinel LN: 0/1).
7. Vascular invasion: absent.
8. Lymphatic invasion: absent.
9. Tumor border: infiltrative.
10. Microcalcification: present, tumoral/non-tumoral.
11. Pathologic staging: pT1cN0(sn).

	Result	Intensity	Positive %
Estrogen receptor	Strong (6/7)	3	1/3–2/3
Progesterone receptor	Intermediate (4/7)	2	10%-1/3
C-erbB2	Equivocal (2+)		
Ki-67	Positive in 5% of tumor cells		

Adjuvant Therapy
Postoperative radiation therapy.

49.2.2 Treatments After Recurrence
See Figs. 330, 331 and 332.

Operation
Jun. 2018 Left breast conserving surgery, sentinel lymph node biopsy (Fig. 333).

Local Recurrence

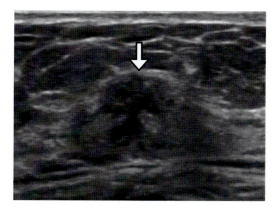

Fig. 330 US: irregular heterogeneous hypoechoic mass at the 10 o'clock direction of left breast

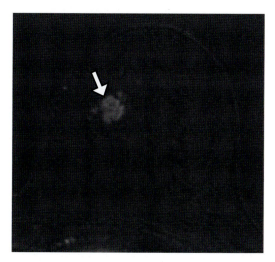

Fig. 331 MRI: irregular heterogeneous enhancing mass

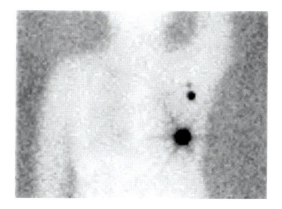

Fig. 332 Lymphoscintigraphy shows visualized sentinel lymph nodes in the left axilla

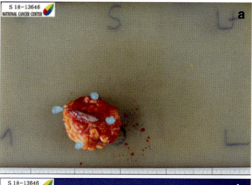

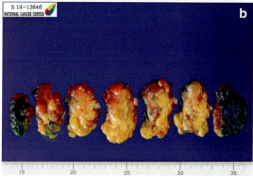

Fig. 333 (**a**) Gross pathology of lumpectomy specimen. (**b**) The margins get marked and sliced with different colors on each direction

Pathology Report

Invasive Ductal Carcinoma

1. Size of tumor: 1.6 cm (pT1c).
2. Histologic grade: 2/3 (tubule formation: 3/3, nuclear pleomorphism: 2/3, mitotic count: 1/3, 4/10HPF).
3. Intraductal component: present, intratumoral (5%) (nuclear grade: low, necrosis: present, architectural pattern: solid, extensive intraductal component: absent).
4. Skin: no involvement of tumor.
5. Surgical margins:
   (a) Superior margin: 19 mm.
   (b) Inferior margin: 11 mm.
   (c) Medial margin: 15 mm.
   (d) Lateral margin: 15 mm.
   (e) Deep margin: 4 mm.
   (f) Superficial margin: 15 mm.
6. Lymph nodes: no metastasis in 2 axillary lymph nodes (pN0(sn)) (sentinel LN: 0/2).
7. Arteriovenous invasion: absent.

8. Lymphovascular invasion: absent.
9. Tumor border: infiltrative.
10. Microcalcification: present, tumoral/non-tumoral.
11. 11) Pathological TN category (AJCC 2017): pT1cN0(sn).

	Result	Intensity	Positive %
Estrogen receptor	Strong (8/8)	3	>2/3
Progesterone receptor	Strong (8/8)	3	>2/3
C-erbB2	Negative (0)		
Ki-67	Positive in 12% of tumor cells		

Adjuvant Therapy

Postoperative radiation therapy.
Anastrozole 1 mg/day.

50 Case 50

50.1 Patient History and Progress

Female/72 years old, post-menopause.

Screen detected mass lesion on right breast 12 o'clock and 8 o'clock direction, left breast 12 o'clock direction.

No family history.

Hypertension, hepatitis B virus carrier, claustrophobia.

50.2 Courses of Treatment

Right breast IDC → Operation → Adjuvant therapy → **Right breast recurrence (IDC).**

50.2.1 Primary Treatment

See Figs. 334, 335 and 336.

Operation

Feb. 2017 Right nipple-areolar complex sparing mastectomy, sentinel lymph node biopsy, left nipple-areolar complex sparing mastectomy (Figs. 337 and 338).

Pathology Report

<Right>
1. Invasive Ductal Carcinoma
   (a) Size of tumor: 1.8 cm (pT1c).
   (b) Histologic grade: 2/3 (tubule formation: 2/3, nuclear pleomorphism: 2/3, mitotic count: 2/3, 10/10HPF).
   (c) Intraductal component: present, intratumoral/extratumoral (30%) (nuclear grade: low, necrosis: absent, architectural pattern: solid, extensive intraductal component: present).
   (d) Surgical margins:
      • Deep margin: 3 mm.
      • Superficial margin: 10 mm.
   (e) Lymph nodes: no metastasis in one axillary lymph node (pN0(sn)) (sentinel LN: 0/1).
   (f) Arteriovenous invasion: absent.
   (g) Lymphovascular invasion: absent.
   (h) Tumor border: infiltrative.
   (i) Microcalcification: present, non-tumoral.
   (j) Pathologic stage (AJCC 2010): pT1cN0(sn).
2. Intraductal Papilloma with usual ductal hyperplasia.

	Result	Intensity	Positive %
Estrogen receptor	Strong (8/8)	3	>2/3
Progesterone receptor	Strong (8/8)	3	>2/3
C-erbB2	Negative (0)		
Ki-67	Positive in 23.8% of tumor cells		

<Left>
Intraductal papilloma with usual ductal hyperplasia.

Adjuvant Therapy

Letrozole 2.5 mg/day for 2.8 years.

50.2.2 Treatments After Recurrence

See Figs. 339 and 340.

Operation

Jan. 2019 Right breast wide excision, sentinel lymph node biopsy (Fig. 341).

Local Recurrence

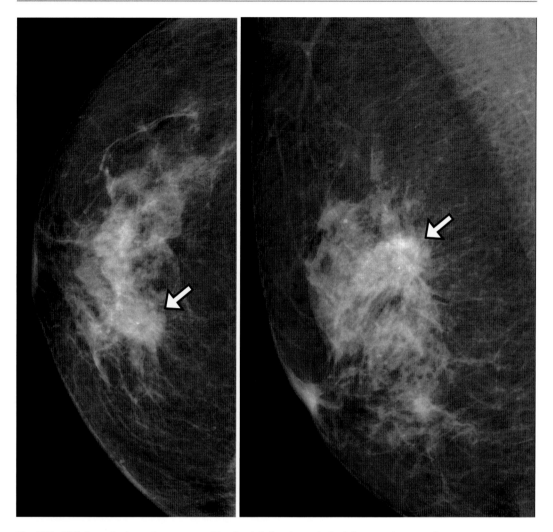

Fig. 334 MG: irregular hyperdense mass with microlobulated margin in right upper inner quadrant

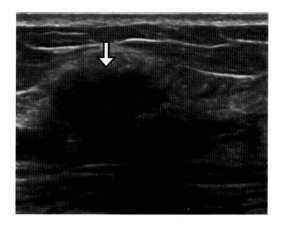

Fig. 335 US: irregular hypoechoic mass with microlobulated margin

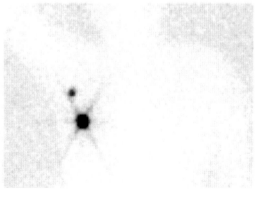

Fig. 336 Lymphoscintigraphy shows visualized sentinel lymph nodes in the right axilla

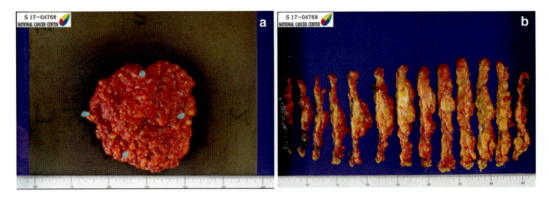

Fig. 337 (**a**) Gross pathology of right mastectomy specimen. (**b**) The margins get marked and sliced with different colors on each direction

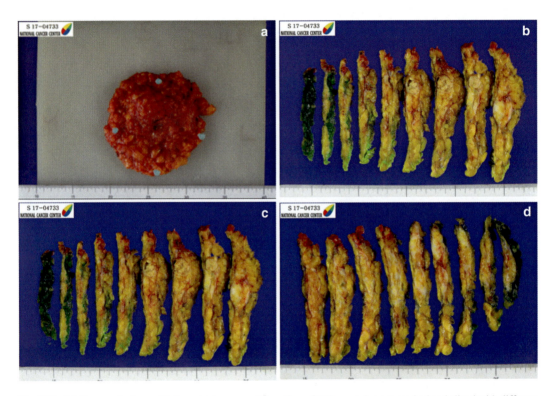

Fig. 338 (**a**) Gross pathology of left mastectomy specimen. (**b, c, d**) The margins get marked and sliced with different colors on each direction

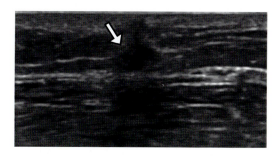

Fig. 339 US: not parallel irregular hypoechoic mass with extension to the overlying skin layer

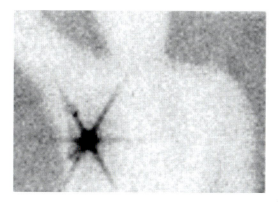

Fig. 340 Lymphoscintigraphy shows visualized sentinel lymph nodes in the right axilla

Pathology Report

Invasive Ductal Carcinoma, clinically recurrent

1. Post-nipple-sparing mastectomy status.
2. Size of tumor: 1.1 cm (rpT1c).
3. Histologic grade: 2/3 (tubule formation: 3/3, nuclear pleomorphism: 2/3, mitotic count: 1/3, 6/10HPF).
4. Intraductal component: absent.
5. Skin: dermal involvement of tumor.
6. Nipple: no involvement of tumor.
7. Surgical margins:
    (a) Superior margin: 10 mm.
    (b) Inferior margin: 10 mm.
    (c) Medial margin: 10 mm.
    (d) Lateral margin: 80 mm.
    (e) Deep margin: 2 mm.
    (f) Superficial margin: 2 mm.
8. Lymph nodes: no metastasis in one axillary lymph node (rpN0(sn)) (sentinel LN: 0/1).
9. Arteriovenous invasion: absent.
10. Lymphovascular invasion: present, intratumoral.
11. Tumor border: infiltrative.

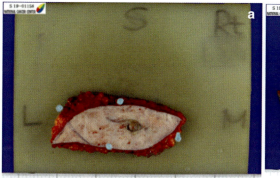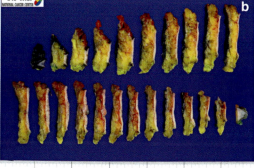

Fig. 341 (**a**) Gross pathology of breast wide excision specimen. (**b**) The margins get marked and sliced with different colors on each direction

12. Microcalcification: present, tumoral/non-tumoral.
13. Pathological TN category (AJCC 2017): rpT1cN0(sn).

	Result	Intensity	Positive %
Estrogen receptor	Strong (8/8)	3	>2/3
Progesterone receptor	Strong (8/8)	3	>2/3

	Result	Intensity	Positive %
C-erbB2	Equivocal (2+) (SISH negative)		
Ki-67	Positive in 31% of tumor cells		

Adjuvant Therapy

Exemestane 25 mg/day.

Metastatic Breast Cancer

Youngmi Kwon, Yunju Kim, Bo Hwa Choi,
Eun-Gyeong Lee, Ji Young You, and Eun Sook Lee

1 Case 1

1.1 Patient History and Progress

Female/49 years old, post-menopause.
   No family history.

Y. Kwon
Department of Radiology, Center for Breast Cancer,
National Cancer Center, Goyang, Gyeonggi,
Republic of Korea
e-mail: ymk@ncc.re.kr

Y. Kim
Department of Pathology, National Cancer Center,
Goyang, Gyeonggi, Republic of Korea
e-mail: radkyj@ncc.re.kr

B. H. Choi
Division of Diagnostic Radiology, Center for Breast Cancer,
National Cancer Center, Goyang, Republic of Korea
e-mail: iawy82@ncc.re.kr

E.-G. Lee
Division of Surgery, Center for Breast Cancer,
National Cancer Center, Goyang, Republic of Korea
e-mail: bnf333@ncc.re.kr

J. Y. You
Division of Breast and Endocrine, Department of
General Surgery, Korea University Medical Center,
Seoul, Republic of Korea
e-mail: joliejean@korea.ac.kr

E. S. Lee (✉)
Center for Breast Cancer, National Cancer Center,
Goyang, Kyonggi-do, Republic of Korea
e-mail: eslee@ncc.re.kr

1.2 Courses of Treatment

Left breast cancer → Operation + Adjuvant therapy → **Chest wall recurrence** → Palliative therapy → **Pleural fissure recurrence** → Palliative therapy.

1.2.1 Primary Treatment

Operation

Mar. 2007 Left modified radical mastectomy.

   Pathology: Invasive ductal carcinoma, stage pT1N0, Size of tumor: 1.5 * 1.0 cm, Lymph node: 0/21.

	Result	Intensity	Positive %
Estrogen receptor	Strong (8/8)	3	>2/3
Progesterone receptor	Strong (8/8)	3	>2/3
C-erbB2	Equivocal (2+)		
Ki-67	Positive in 11% of tumor cells		

Adjuvant Therapy

Adjuvant Chemotherapy #5 cycles (Fluorouracil & Epirubicin & Cyclophosphamide).

   Concurrent Trastuzumab therapy #9 cycles.

   Zoladex for 2 years + Tamoxifen 20 mg/day for 5 years.

© The Author(s), under exclusive license to Springer Nature Singapore Pte Ltd. 2023
E. S. Lee (ed.), *A Practical Guide to Breast Cancer Treatment*,
https://doi.org/10.1007/978-981-19-9044-1_10

1.2.2 Treatments After Recurrence

Chest Wall Recurrence
See Fig. 1.
Feb. 2014 Left chest well excisional biopsy.
Pathology: Invasive ductal carcinoma, clinically recurrent.

	Result	Intensity	Positive %
Estrogen receptor	Strong (8/8)	3	>2/3
Progesterone receptor	Strong (7/8)	3	1/3–2/3
C-erbB2	Equivocal (2+)		
Ki-67	Positive in 21% of tumor cells		
SISH	Negative		

Operation
Apr. 2014 Left chest wall wide excision and bilateral salpingo-oophorectomy.
Pathology: Invasive ductal carcinoma, clinically recurrent, size of tumor: 1.0 cm, residual.

Adjuvant Therapy
Post-operative radiation therapy to chest wall+ Letrozole 2.5 mg/day for 5 years.

Pleural Fissure Recurrence
Mar. 2022 PET-CT: R/O pleural/fissural seedings in left hemithorax.
See Figs. 2 and 3.

Palliative Therapy
Letrozole 2.5 mg/day re-start.

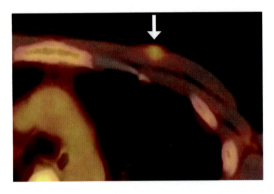

Fig. 1 PET-CT (Feb. 2014): A hypermetabolic lesion at the left chest wall

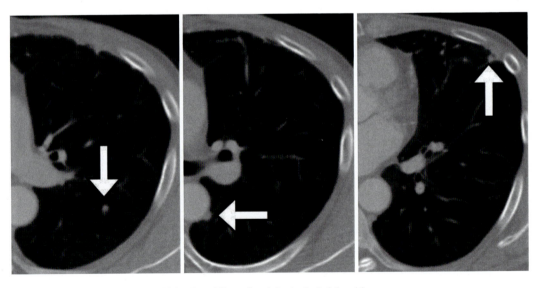

Fig. 2 Chest CT (Mar. 2022): Multiple pleural/fissural nodules in the left hemithorax

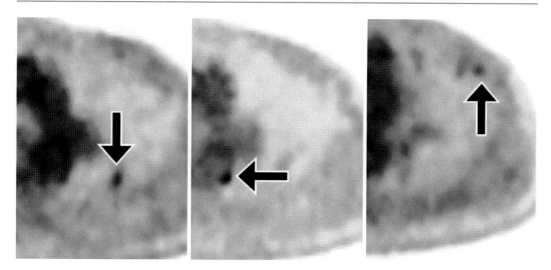

Fig. 3 PET-CT (Mar. 2022): Multiple pleural/fissural nodules with hypermetabolism in the left hemithorax

2 Case 2

2.1 Patient History and Progress

Female/55 years old, post-menopause.
Family history of breast cancer, mother.
BRCA 1 & 2 mutation: No examination.

2.2 Courses of Treatment

Right breast cancer → Operation + Adjuvant therapy → **Lung metastasis** → Palliative therapy → **Progression on rib and lung** → Palliative therapy → **Progression on liver** → Palliative therapy.

2.2.1 Primary Treatment

Radiologic Finding
See Fig. 4.

Operation
Aug. 2012 Right breast conserving surgery, axillary lymph node dissection.
Pathology: Invasive ductal carcinoma, stage pT2(m)N1a.
Size of tumor: 3.5 cm, 1.5 cm, and 0.5 cm, Lymph node: 3/16, size of metastatic carcinoma: 8 mm.

	Result	Intensity	Positive %
Estrogen receptor	Strong (6/7)	2	>2/3
Progesterone receptor	Negative (0/7)	0	0
C-erbB2	Negative (0)		
Ki-67	Positive in 15% of tumor cells		

Adjuvant Therapy
Post-operative radiation therapy + Tamoxifen 20 mg/day for 2.5 years.
Letrozole 2.5 mg/day for 1 year: stop due to skin rash → Change to Tamoxifen 20 mg/day for 1.5 years.

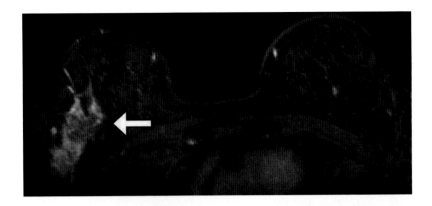

Fig. 4 Breast MRI (Jul. 2012): An irregular enhancing mass in the right breast

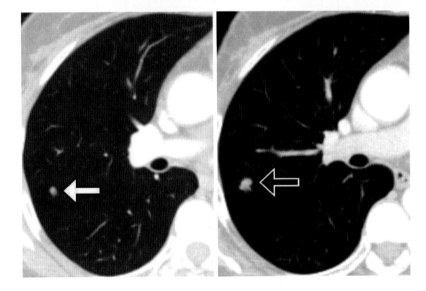

Fig. 5 Chest CT (Jun. 2016, Apr. 2019): A new lung nodule (white arrow) was getting enlarged (black arrow) in the right lung. Wedge resection = Metastatic ductal carcinoma from breast

2.2.2 Treatments After Recurrence

Lung Metastasis

Letrozole 2.5 mg/day for 3 years → Progressive disease on right 8th rib, lung.

Sep. 2017 CT chest r/o lung metastasis.
See Figs. 5 and 6.

Operation

Apr. 2019 Right upper lobe lung wedge resection.

Pathology: Metastatic ductal carcinoma from breast.

Size of tumor: 0.9 × 0.7 × 0.5 cm.

Radiation Therapy

Radiation therapy to Right 8th rib.

Progression on Liver

Fulvestrant 250 mg 1/month + Palbociclib 100 mg/day: Progressive disease on liver → Exemestane 25 mg/day + Everolimus 5 mg/day → Palliative chemotherapy (weekly Paclitaxel #6 cycles): Progressive disease on liver → Doxorubicin & Cyclophosphamide.

See Fig. 7.

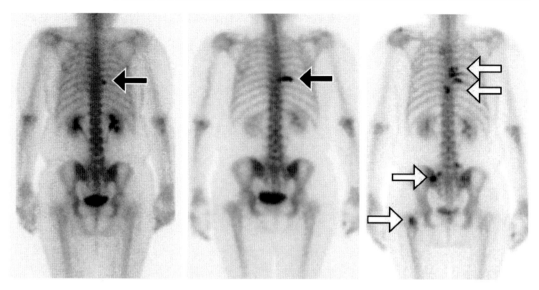

Fig. 6 Bone scan (Aug. 2017, Jan. 2019, Mar. 2022): An increased uptake in the right 8th rib (black arrow) was getting enlarged. Multiple developing increased uptakes in the right ribs, thoracic vertebrae, sternum, left iliac bone, and left femur (white arrows)

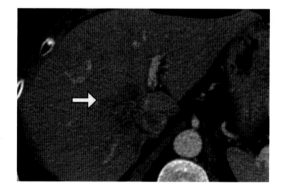

Fig. 7 Abdomen CT (Mar. 2022): Multiple developing low attenuation lesions in the liver (partly shown)

3 Case 3

3.1 Patient History and Progress

Female/62 years old, post-menopause.
  No family history.
  Diabetes mellitus, rheumatoid arthritis.

3.2 Courses of Treatment

Left breast cancer → Neoadjuvant Chemotherapy → Operation → Adjuvant therapy → **Bone, lung, and brain metastasis**.

3.2.1 Primary Treatment
See Fig. 8.

Neoadjuvant Chemotherapy
Neoadjuvant Chemotherapy #8 cycles (Adriamycin + Cyclophosphamide #4 → Docetaxel #4).

Operation
Mar. 2018 Left modified radical mastectomy.
  Pathology: Invasive ductal carcinoma, stage ypT2N1.
  Size of tumor: 2.7 * 2.4 cm, lymph node: 2/5, size of metastatic carcinoma: 4 mm.

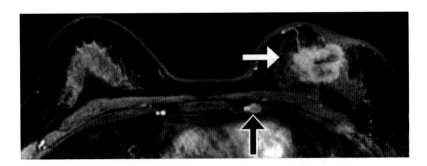

Fig. 8 Breast MRI (Sep. 2017): Irregular enhancing mass in the left breast (white arrow). Enlarged LN at the left internal mammary chain (black arrow). Left total mastectomy = IDC

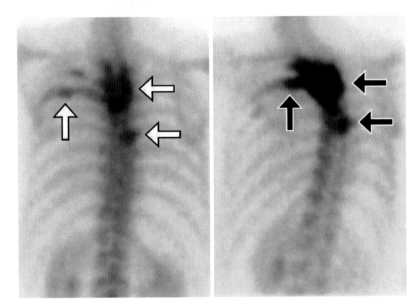

Fig. 9 Bone scan (Apr. 2020, Aug. 2020): Multiple uptakes in the thoracic vertebrae and left ribs (white arrows) were getting increased in intensity (black arrows)

	Result	Intensity	Positive %
Estrogen receptor	Negative (0/8)	0	0
Progesterone receptor	Negative (0/8)	0	0
C-erbB2	Negative (1+)		
Ki-67	Positive in 26% of tumor cells		

Adjuvant Therapy

Post-operative radiation therapy +adjuvant chemotherapy (Xeloda).

3.2.2 Treatments After Recurrence

Bone metastasis → Lung metastasis → Brain metastasis → Progression.

Palliative Therapy

Apr. 2020 Bone scan: multiple bone metastasis in right T2-5, T7 and left 4th–5th ribs.

→ Nab-paclitaxel/atezolizumab #7 cycles: Progressive disease on pleural nodule.

→ Xeloda #7 cycles: Progressive disease on brain → Whole brain radiation therapy.

→ Gemcitabine #2 cycles: Progressive disease on pleural effusion.

→ Eribulin #2 cycles: Progressive disease on pleural effusion.

→ Vinorelbine/carboplatin #3 cycles: clinically progressive disease.

See Figs. 9, 10, 11, and 12.

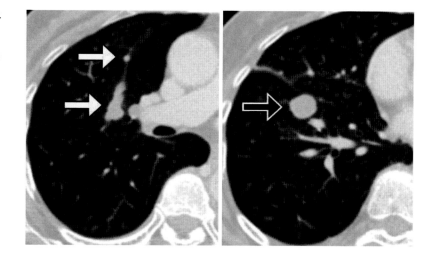

Fig. 10 Chest CT (Apr. 2020): Multiple fissural nodules (white arrows) and lung nodules (black arrow, partly shown) in the right lung

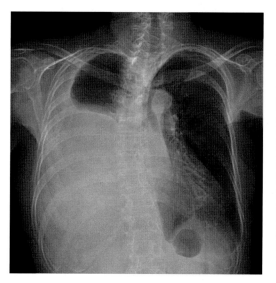

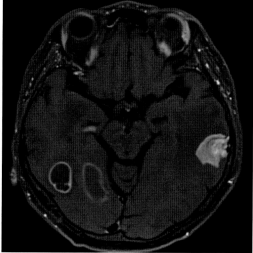

Fig. 11 Chest X-ray (Sep. 2021): Large amount of pleural effusion in the right hemithorax. Pleural fluid cytology = Positive for malignant cells

Fig. 12 Brain MRI (Apr. 2021): Multiple necrotic enhancing lesions in the brain (partly shown)

4 Case 4

4.1 Patient History and Progress

Female/48 years old, pre-menopause.
No family history.
BRCA 1 mutation: detected.
s/p Appendectomy, s/p myomectomy.

4.2 Courses of Treatment

Right breast cancer → Operation → Adjuvant therapy → **Left breast and pleural effusion recurrence**.

4.2.1 Primary Treatment

Operation
Oct. 2008 Right breast conserving surgery, axillary lymph node dissection.
Pathology: Invasive ductal carcinoma, stage T1(m)N1 (2/25).
Size of tumor: 1.7 * 1.5 * 1 cm and 0.5 * 0.4 cm, lymph node: 2/25, size of metastatic carcinoma: 19 mm.

	Result	Intensity	Positive %
Estrogen receptor	Positive	N.A.	N.A.
Progesterone receptor	Positive	N.A.	N.A.
C-erbB2	Negative (1+)		
Ki-67	Positive in 63.51% of tumor cells		

Adjuvant Therapy
Adjuvant chemotherapy #6 cycles → Postoperative radiation therapy + Tamoxifen 20 mg/day for 5 years.

4.2.2 Treatments After Recurrence
Left breast and pleural effusion recurrence.
See Fig. 13.
May 2021 breast, left, needle biopsy:
Invasive ductal carcinoma, histologic grade 2.

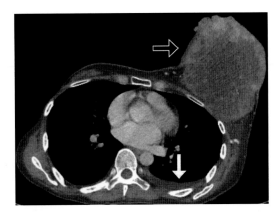

Fig. 13 Chest CT (May 2021): Huge mass in the left breast (black arrow, CNB = IDC) and left pleural effusion (white arrow)

	Result	Intensity	Positive %
Estrogen receptor	Negative (0/8)	0	0
Progesterone receptor	Negative (0/8)	0	0
C-erbB2	Negative (0)		
Ki-67	Positive in 74% of tumor cells		

Clinical stage: cT4N3M1 (pleural effusion).

Palliative Chemotherapy
Palliative chemotherapy #12 cycles (paclitaxel #12 & Cisplatin #9): controlled disease.

Palliative Operation
Feb. 2022 Left total mastectomy, sentinel lymph node biopsy (palliative operation).
Pathology: No residual tumor with foamy histiocytic collection.

1. Post-chemotherapy status
2. Lymph nodes: no metastasis in one axillary lymph node (pN0(sn))
   (sentinel LN: 0/1)

Palliative radiation therapy.
Post-operative radiation therapy.
See Fig. 14.

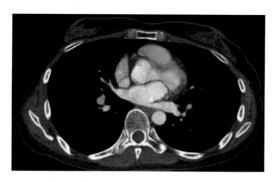

Fig. 14 Post-NAC chest CT (Jan. 2022): Disappearance of the previous left breast mass and left pleural effusion. Left MRM = No residual tumor

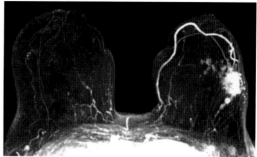

Fig. 15 Breast MRI (Jun. 2015): Multiple malignant enhancing masses in the left breast. US-CNB = IDC

5 Case 5

5.1 Patient History and Progress

Female/70 years old, post-menopause.
 No family history.
 Hypertension.

5.2 Courses of Treatment

Left breast cancer → Neoadjuvant chemotherapy → Operation → Adjuvant therapy → **Lung and liver metastasis**.

5.2.1 Primary Treatment

Jun. 2015 breast, left, needle biopsy:
 Invasive ductal carcinoma, histologic grade 2 with apocrine differentiation.

	Result	Intensity	Positive %
Estrogen receptor	Negative (0/8)	0	0
Progesterone receptor	Negative (0/8)	0	0
C-erbB2	Positive (3+)		
Ki-67	Positive in 24% of tumor cells		

See Figs. 15 and 16.

Neoadjuvant Chemotherapy

Neoadjuvant chemotherapy #8 cycles (Adriamycin + Cyclophosphamide #4 → Docetaxel #4).

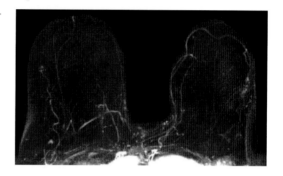

Fig. 16 Post-NAC breast MRI (Dec. 2015): Decreased number and size of the previous masses in the left breast. Left BCS = IDC

Operation

Dec. 2015 Left breast conserving surgery, sentinel lymph node biopsy.
 Pathology: Invasive ductal carcinoma, stage ypT1cN1mi (sn).
 Size of tumor: 1.5 cm, lymph node: 1/3, size of metastatic carcinoma: 1.8 mm.

	Result	Intensity	Positive %
Estrogen receptor	Intermediate (5/8)	2	10%–1/3
Progesterone receptor	Negative (0/8)	0	0
C-erbB2	Negative (1+)		
Ki-67	Positive in 2% of tumor cells		

Adjuvant Therapy

Post-operative radiation therapy + Letrozole 2.5 mg/day for 4.9 years.

5.2.2 Treatments After Recurrence

Lung and Liver Metastasis
Nov. 2020 CT chest: metastasis to lung, liver.
Liver biopsy: Metastatic ductal cancer.

	Result	Intensity	Positive %
Estrogen receptor	Negative (0/8)	0	0
Progesterone receptor	Negative (0/8)	0	0
C-erbB2	Positive (3+)		
Ki-67	N.A.		

Palliative Therapy (Enrolled in Clinical Trial)
→ Clinical trial enrolled (ZW25 + Docetaxel #6 cycles → ZW25 ~).
See Figs. 17, 18, and 19.

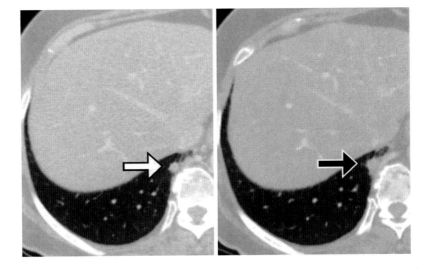

Fig. 17 Chest CT (Feb. 2020, Nov. 2020): A new lung nodule (white arrow) was getting enlarged (black arrow) in the right lung

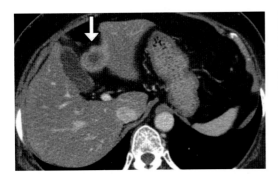

Fig. 18 Abdomen CT (Dec. 2020): Multiple low attenuation lesions with peripheral rim enhancement in the liver (partly shown). US-CNB = Metastatic ductal carcinoma

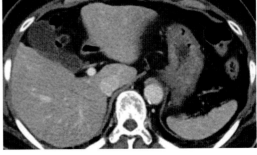

Fig. 19 Abdomen CT (Feb. 2022): Disappearance of the previous metastatic masses in the liver

6 Case 6

6.1 Patient History and Progress

Female/47 years old, pre-menopause.
No family history.

6.2 Courses of Treatment

Right breast cancer → Neoadjuvant chemotherapy → Operation → Adjuvant therapy → **Ipsilateral breast and chest wall recurrence** → Palliative therapy → **Progression on the skin and contralateral axillary lymph nodes**.

6.2.1 Primary Treatment
Aug. 2017 breast, left, needle biopsy:
Invasive ductal carcinoma, histologic grade 2.

	Result	Intensity	Positive %
Estrogen receptor	Negative (0/8)	0	0
Progesterone receptor	Negative (0/8)	0	0
C-erbB2	Positive (3+)		
Ki-67	Positive in 35% of tumor cells		

Clinical stage: cT3N1M0.
See Figs. 20 and 21.

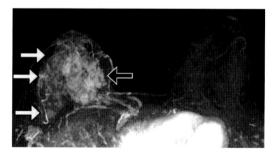

Fig. 20 Breast MRI (Sep. 2017): Conglomerated enhancing masses (black arrow) and non-mass enhancement (white arrows) in the right breast. US-CNB = IDC

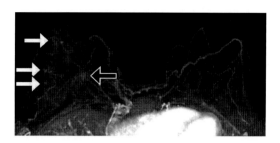

Fig. 21 Post-NAC breast MRI (Jan. 2018): Decreased size of the enhancing masses (black arrow) and non-mass enhancement (white arrows) in the right breast. Right BCS = IDC

Neoadjuvant Chemotherapy
Neoadjuvant chemotherapy #6 cycles (Docetaxel & Carboplatin & Trastuzumab & Pertuzumab).

Operation
Jan. 2018 Right breast conserving surgery, sentinel lymph node biopsy.
Pathology: Invasive ductal carcinoma, stage ypT1aN1mi (sn).
Size of tumor: 0.2 cm, lymph node: 1/1, size of metastatic carcinoma: 2 mm.

	Result	Intensity	Positive %
Estrogen receptor	Negative (0/8)	0	0
Progesterone receptor	Negative (0/8)	0	0
C-erbB2	Positive (3+)		
Ki-67	Positive in 21% of tumor cells		

Adjuvant Therapy
Post-operative radiation therapy + Trastuzumab for 1 year.

6.2.2 Treatments After Recurrence
Ipsilateral breast and chest wall recurrence → Progression on the skin and contralateral axillary lymph nodes.
See Fig. 22.

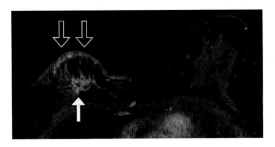

Fig. 22 Breast MRI (May 2020): Multifocal parenchymal non-mass enhancement (white arrow) and skin enhancement (black arrows) in the right breast (partly shown). US-CNB = IDC, Skin shave biopsy = IDC

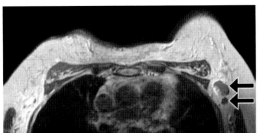

Fig. 23 Breast MRI (May 2021): Multiple enlarged lymph nodes in the left axilla. US-CNB = Metastatic ductal carcinoma

May 2020 Right chest wall skin and breast biopsy.

Pathology: Invasive ductal carcinoma, recurrent.

	Result	Intensity	Positive %
Estrogen receptor	Negative (0/8)	0	0
Progesterone receptor	Negative (0/8)	0	0
C-erbB2	Positive (3+)		
Ki-67	Positive in 40% of tumor cells		

Palliative Therapy

Clinical trial enrolled (ZW25 #20 cycles + Docetaxel #6 cycles): Progressive disease on skin, axillary lymph node.

→ Docetaxel & Trastuzumab & Pertuzumab #6: Progressive disease.

→ Trastuzumab emtansine ~

See Fig. 23.

7 Case 7

7.1 Patient History and Progress

Female/48 years old, pre-menopause.
No family history.

7.2 Courses of Treatment

Left breast cancer → Operation → Adjuvant therapy → **Ipsilateral breast and chest wall recurrence** → Chemotherapy → **Progression on the skin and contralateral axillary lymph nodes**.

7.2.1 Primary Treatment
See Fig. 24.

Operation
Jan. 2019 Left breast conserving surgery, sentinel lymph node biopsy.

Pathology: Invasive ductal carcinoma, stage pT1bN0(sn).

Size of tumor: 0.7 * 0.5 * 0.5 cm, lymph node: 0/2.

	Result	Intensity	Positive %
Estrogen receptor	Negative (2/8)	1	<1%
Progesterone receptor	Negative (2/8)	1	<1%
C-erbB2	Positive (3+)		

	Result	Intensity	Positive %
Ki-67	Positive in 43% of tumor cells		

Adjuvant Therapy

Adjuvant chemotherapy #6 cycles (Cyclophosphamide & Methotrexate & Fluorouracil).

Post-operative radiation therapy.

7.2.2 Treatments After Recurrence

Abdominal Lymph Nodes Metastasis

Mar. 2021 CT abdomen & pelvis: r/o Enlarged lymph node in Rt. external iliac chain and paraaortic area; cannot exclude pathologic lymph node, such as metastasis or lymphoproliferative disorder.

→ Closed follow-up.

See Fig. 25.

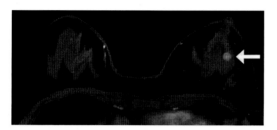

Fig. 24 Breast MRI (Jan. 2019): A round enhancing mass in the left breast. Left BCS = Microinvasive ductal carcinoma

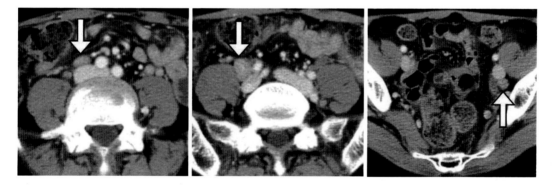

Fig. 25 Abdominopelvic CT (Mar. 2021): Multiple enlarged lymph nodes at the paraaortic and both iliac chains

8 Case 8

8.1 Patient History and Progress

Female/55 years old, post-menopause.
No family history.

8.2 Courses of Treatment

Left breast cancer → Operation → Adjuvant therapy → **Ipsilateral axillary lymph nodes recurrence**.

8.2.1 Primary Treatment
See Fig. 26.

Operation
Mar. 2016 Left breast conserving surgery, sentinel lymph node biopsy.
Pathology: Invasive ductal carcinoma, stage pT2N0(sn).
Size of tumor: 2.5 cm, lymph node: 0/1.

	Result	Intensity	Positive %
Estrogen receptor	Strong (8/8)	3	>2/3
Progesterone receptor	Strong (7/8)	3	1/3–2/3
C-erbB2	Negative (0)		
Ki-67	Positive in 61% of tumor cells		

Oncotype Dx RS Score: 18.

Adjuvant Therapy
Post-operative radiation therapy + Tamoxifen 20 mg/day for 4.8 years.

8.2.2 Treatments After Recurrence

Ipsilateral Axillary Lymph Nodes Recurrence
See Fig. 27.
Mar. 2021 Left axillary lymph node biopsy.
Pathology: Metastatic ductal carcinoma.

	Result	Intensity	Positive %
Estrogen receptor	Strong (8/8)	3	>2/3
Progesterone receptor	Strong (7/8)	3	1/3–2/3
C-erbB2	Negative (0)		
Ki-67	Positive in 29% of tumor cells		

Neoadjuvant Chemotherapy
Neoadjuvant chemotherapy #8 cycles (Adriamycin & Cyclophosphamide #4 → Docetaxel #4).

Operation
Sep. 2021 Left axillary lymph node dissection.
Pathology: No metastasis in twelve axillary lymph nodes.

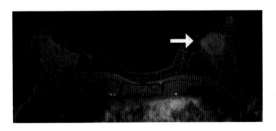

Fig. 26 Breast MRI (Mar. 2016): An irregular enhancing mass in the left breast. Left BCS = IDC

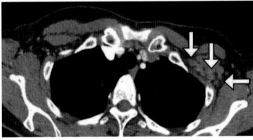

Fig. 27 Chest CT (Feb. 2021): Multiple enlarged lymph nodes in the left axilla. US-CNB = Metastatic ductal carcinoma

Radiation Therapy

Post-operative radiation therapy (axillary and subclavian area) + Letrozole 2.5 mg/day~.

9 Case 9

9.1 Patient History and Progress

Female/57 years old, post-menopause.
No family history.
S/p Myomectomy & bilateral salpingo-oophorectomy.

9.2 Courses of Treatment

Right breast cancer → Operation → Adjuvant therapy → **Ipsilateral axillary lymph nodes recurrence**.

9.2.1 Primary Treatment
See Fig. 28.

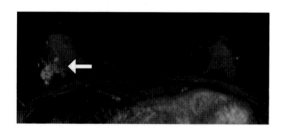

Fig. 28 Breast MRI (Jul. 2019): Mixed enhancing masses and non-mass enhancement in the right breast. Right BCS = IDC

Operation

Jul. 2019 Right breast conserving surgery, sentinel lymph node biopsy.
Pathology: Invasive ductal carcinoma, stage pT1c(2)N0(sn).
Size of tumor: 1.1 cm and 0.5 cm, lymph node: 0/1.

	Result	Intensity	Positive %
Estrogen receptor	Strong (7/8)	2	>2/3
Progesterone receptor	Negative (2/8)	1	<1%
C-erbB2	Negative (0)		
Ki-67	Positive in 23% of tumor cells		

Adjuvant Therapy

Post-operative radiation therapy + Letrozole 2.5 mg/day for 1 year.

9.2.2 Treatments After Recurrence

Ipsilateral Axillary Lymph Nodes Recurrence
See Figs. 29 and 30.
Aug. 2021 Left axillary lymph node biopsy.
Pathology: Metastatic ductal carcinoma.

	Result	Intensity	Positive %
Estrogen receptor	Negative (2/8)	1	<1%
Progesterone receptor	Negative (0/8)	0	0
C-erbB2	Negative (0)		
Ki-67	Positive in 18% of tumor cells		

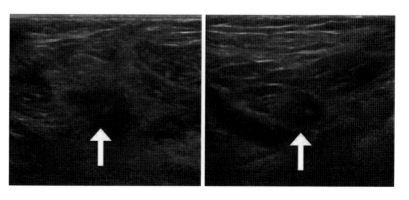

Fig. 29 Breast US (Aug. 2021): Multiple enlarged lymph nodes in the right axilla. US-CNB = Metastatic ductal carcinoma

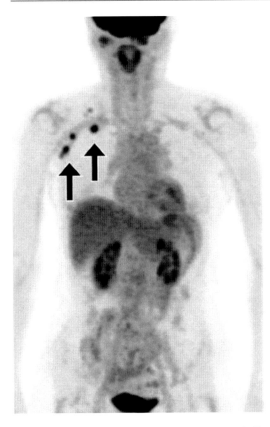

Fig. 30 PET-CT (Sep. 2021): Multiple hypermetabolic lymph nodes in the right axilla

Neoadjuvant Chemotherapy
Neoadjuvant chemotherapy #8 cycles (Adriamycin & Cyclophosphamide #4 → Docetaxel #4).

Operation
Mar. 2022 Left axillary lymph node dissection.
Pathology: No metastasis in seven axillary lymph nodes (right axillary lymph nodes: 0/7).

Radiotherapy
Post-operative radiation therapy (axillary and subclavian area).

10 Case 10

10.1 Patient History and Progress

Female/53 years old, post-menopause.

No family history.
S/p cholecystectomy, s/p knee giant cell tumor excision, s/p interstitial mammoplasty.
S/p otitis media operation.

10.2 Courses of Treatment

Left breast cancer → Operation → Adjuvant therapy → **Ipsilateral breast and lung recurrence** → Palliative therapy → **Progression on lung, left breast.**

10.2.1 Primary Treatment
See Figs. 31, 32, and 33.

Operation
Dec. 2020 Left breast conserving surgery, sentinel lymph node biopsy.
Pathology: Invasive ductal carcinoma, stage pT2N0(sn).
Size of tumor: 2.1 cm, lymph node: 0/1.

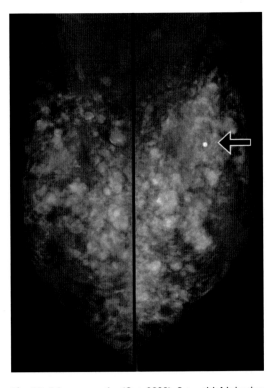

Fig. 31 Mammography (Oct. 2020): Interstitial injection mammoplasty of both breasts. Palpable lump in left breast

Metastatic Breast Cancer

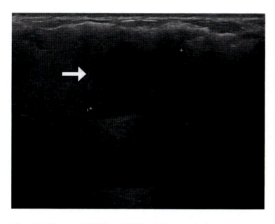

Fig. 32 Breast US (Oct. 2020): A hypoechoic mass at the palpable area of the left breast. US-VAB = IDC

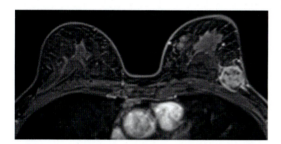

Fig. 33 Breast MRI (Oct. 2020): An oval enhancing mass in the left breast. Left BCS = IDC

	Result	Intensity	Positive %
Estrogen receptor	Negative (0/8)	0	0
Progesterone receptor	Negative (0/8)	0	0
C-erbB2	Negative (1+)		
Ki-67	Positive in 68% of tumor cells		

Adjuvant Therapy
Adjuvant chemotherapy #4 cycles (Docetaxel & cyclophosphamide).

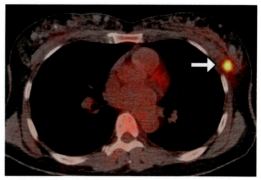

Fig. 34 PET-CT (Mar. 2021): Hypermetabolic nodular lesion at the op bed of the left breast. Excision = IDC

10.2.2 Treatments After Recurrence
Mar. 2021 PET-CT

1. R/O malignancy vs post-op change in left breast upper outer periphery (2h′)
   rec) follow-up or further evaluation.
2. A few solid nodules in BLL; lung metastasis cannot be excluded.

See Fig. 34.

Operation
Apr. 2021 Left wide excision.
Pathology: Invasive ductal carcinoma, stage rpT1b.
Size of tumor: 1.0 cm.

	Result	Intensity	Positive %
Estrogen receptor	Negative (0/8)	0	0
Progesterone receptor	Negative (0/8)	0	0
C-erbB2	Negative (1+)		
Ki-67	Positive in 77% of tumor cells		

→ Chemotherapy #6 cycles (albumin-bound paclitaxel & atezolizumab): Progressive disease on lung, breast.

See Fig. 35.
Oct. 2021 Left breast biopsy.
Pathology: Invasive ductal carcinoma.

	Result	Intensity	Positive %
Estrogen receptor	Negative (2/8)	1	<1%
Progesterone receptor	Negative (0/8)	0	0
C-erbB2	Equivocal (2+)		
Ki-67	Positive in 52% of tumor cells		
SISH	Negative		

Palliative Chemotherapy and Radiation
Chemotherapy #5 cycles (Doxorubicin & Cisplatin).

Radiation therapy to lung~
See Fig. 36.

11 Case 11

11.1 Patient History and Progress

Female/65 years old, post-menopause.
Family history of colon cancer, mother.
BRCA 1 & 2 mutation: Not detected.

11.2 Courses of Treatment

Both breasts cancer → Operation → Adjuvant therapy → **Right axillary lymph node metastasis.**

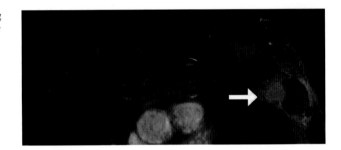

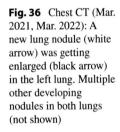

Fig. 35 Breast MRI (Oct. 2021): Enhancing masses at the op bed of the left breast (partly shown). US-CNB = IDC

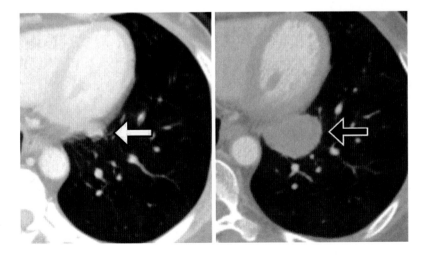

Fig. 36 Chest CT (Mar. 2021, Mar. 2022): A new lung nodule (white arrow) was getting enlarged (black arrow) in the left lung. Multiple other developing nodules in both lungs (not shown)

11.2.1 Primary Treatment
See Fig. 37.

Operation

Jun. 2018 Both nipple-areolar complex sparing mastectomy with immediate implant reconstruction, sentinel lymph node biopsy.

Pathology:

Right> Invasive ductal carcinoma, stage pT1c(2)N0(sn).

Size of tumor: 1.8 cm and 1.7 cm, lymph node: 0/3.

	Result	Intensity	Positive %
Estrogen receptor	Strong (8/8)	3	>2/3
Progesterone receptor	Weak (3/8)	2	<1%
C-erbB2	Equivocal (2+)		
Ki-67	Positive in 22% of tumor cells		
SISH	Equivocal		

HER2/CEP17 gene ratio: 1.93.

Left> Invasive ductal carcinoma, stage pT2N0(sn).

Size of tumor: 2.1 cm, lymph node: 0/2.

	Result	Intensity	Positive %
Estrogen receptor	Strong (8/8)	3	>2/3
Progesterone receptor	Weak (4/8)	2	1–10%
C-erbB2	Equivocal (2+)		
Ki-67	Positive in 34% of tumor cells		
SISH	Tumor heterogeneity		

HER2/CEP17 gene ratio: 2.03.

Adjuvant Therapy

Adjuvant chemotherapy #2 cycles (Docetaxel & cyclophosphamide) → Trastuzumab for 1 year + Letrozole 2.5 mg/day for 2.1 years.

11.2.2 Treatments After Recurrence

Right Axillary Lymph Nodes Recurrence
See Fig. 38.

Nov. 2021 Right axillary lymph node biopsy.
Pathology: Metastatic ductal carcinoma.

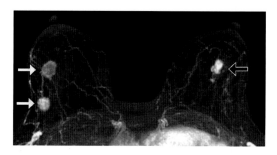

Fig. 37 Breast MRI (May 2018): Malignant masses in the right breast (white arrows) and left breast (black arrow). Both NSM = Both IDC

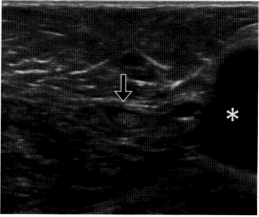

Fig. 38 Breast US (Oct. 2021, Mar. 2022): A new irregular lymph node (white arrow) at the right axillary tail. US-CNB = Metastatic ductal carcinoma. Grossly normalized lymph node (black arrow) after chemotherapy. Right ALND = No metastasis in four axillary lymph nodes. Note the breast implant (*) for reconstruction

	Result	Intensity	Positive %
Estrogen receptor	Strong (8/8)	3	>2/3
Progesterone receptor	Negative (0/8)	0	0
C-erbB2	Equivocal (2+)		
Ki-67	Positive in 25% of tumor cells		
SISH	Positive		

Neoadjuvant Chemotherapy
Chemotherapy #5 cycles (Docetaxel & Carboplatin & Trastuzumab & Pertuzumab).

Operation
Mar. 2022 Right axillary lymph node dissection.
Pathology: No metastasis in four axillary lymph nodes.

Adjuvant Therapy
Trastuzumab & Pertuzumab + Post-operative radiation therapy (axillary and subclavian area).

12 Case 12

12.1 Patient History and Progress

Female/78 years old, post-menopause.
No family history.
Hypertension, diabetes mellitus.

12.2 Courses of Treatment

Left breast cancer → Operation → Adjuvant therapy → **Ipsilateral axillary lymph node recurrence** → **Contralateral breast cancer**.

12.2.1 Primary Treatment
See Fig. 39.

Operation
Apr. 2014 Left total mastectomy, sentinel lymph node biopsy.

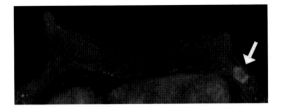

Fig. 39 Breast MRI (Apr. 2014): An irregular enhancing mass in the left breast. Left simple mastectomy = IDC

Pathology: Invasive ductal carcinoma, stage pT2N0(sn).
Size of tumor: 2.0 cm, lymph node: 0/4.

	Result	Intensity	Positive %
Estrogen receptor	Strong (8/8)	3	>2/3
Progesterone receptor	Intermediate (6/8)	2	1/3–2/3
C-erbB2	Equivocal (2+)		
Ki-67	Positive in 26% of tumor cells		
SISH	Negative		

Adjuvant Therapy
Anastrozole 1 mg/day for 4.3 years.

12.2.2 Treatments After Recurrence

Ipsilateral Axillary Lymph Node Recurrence
See Fig. 40.
Aug. 2018 Left axillary lymph node biopsy.
Pathology: Metastatic ductal carcinoma.

	Result	Intensity	Positive %
Estrogen receptor	Strong (7/8)	3	1/3–2/3
Progesterone receptor	Weak (4/8)	3	<1%
C-erbB2	Negative (0)		
Ki-67	Positive in 31% of tumor cells		

Neoadjuvant Chemotherapy
Chemotherapy #8 cycles (Adriamycin + Cyclophosphamide #4 → weekly paclitaxel #4).

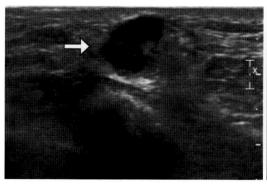 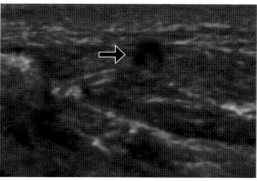

Fig. 40 Breast US (Aug. 2018, Apr. 2019): An enlarged lymph node (white arrow) in the left axilla. US-CNB = Metastatic ductal carcinoma. Normalized size of the biopsy proven metastatic lymph node (black arrow) after chemotherapy. Left ALND = No metastasis in five axillary lymph nodes

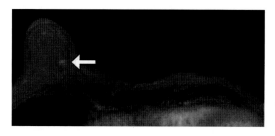

Fig. 41 Breast MRI (Jul. 2021): A new enhancing mass in the right breast

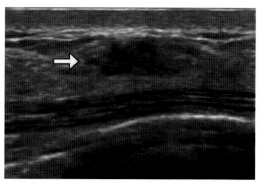

Fig. 42 MRI-directed right breast US (Aug. 2021): An irregular hypoechoic mass at the corresponding area of the MRI abnormality. US-CNB = Ductal carcinoma, Right MRM = DCIS

Operation
Apr. 2019 Left axillary lymph node dissection.
Pathology: No metastasis in five axillary lymph nodes.

Adjuvant Therapy
Post-operative radiation therapy (axillary and subclavian area) + Exemestane 25 mg/day~

Contralateral Breast Cancer
See Figs. 41 and 42.
Aug. 2021 Right breast biopsy.
Pathology: Ductal carcinoma.

Operation
Oct. 2021 Right total mastectomy, sentinel lymph node biopsy.
Pathology: Ductal carcinoma in situ, stage pTisN0(sn).
Size of tumor: 1.6 cm, lymph node: 0/4.

	Result	Intensity	Positive %
Estrogen receptor	Strong (0/8)	0	0
Progesterone receptor	Weak (0/8)	0	0
C-erbB2	Equivocal (2+)		
Ki-67	Positive in 12% of tumor cells		

→ Exemestane 25 mg/day~

Adjuvant Therapy
Exemestane 25 mg/day~

13 Case 13

13.1 Patient History and Progress

Female/39 years old, post-menopause.

Family history of ovarian cancer, paternal aunt.

BRCA 1 mutation: VUS (variant of uncertain).

S/p bilateral salpingo-oophorectomy.

13.2 Courses of Treatment

Right breast cancer → Operation → Adjuvant therapy → **Ipsilateral axillary lymph node recurrence**.

13.2.1 Primary Treatment
See Fig. 43.

Operation

Sep. 2017 Right nipple-areolar complex sparing mastectomy with immediate implant reconstruction, sentinel lymph node biopsy.

Pathology: Invasive ductal carcinoma, stage pT1bN0(sn).

Size of tumor: 0.7 cm, lymph node: 0/2.

	Result	Intensity	Positive %
Estrogen receptor	Intermediate (6/8)	1	>2/3
Progesterone receptor	Strong (8/8)	3	>2/3
C-erbB2	Negative (0)		
Ki-67	Positive in 18% of tumor cells		

Adjuvant Therapy

Tamoxifen 20 mg/day for 3.3 years.

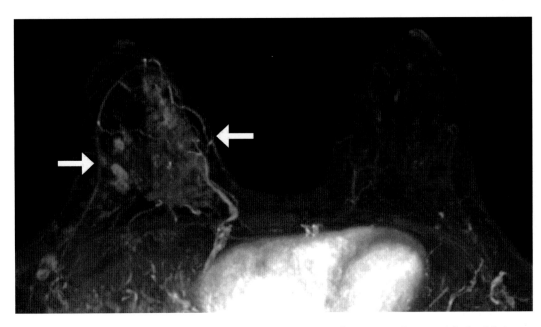

Fig. 43 Breast MRI (Sep. 2017): Multiple irregular enhancing masses and non-mass enhancement in the right breast. Right NSM = IDC

13.2.2 Treatments After Recurrence

See Fig. 44.

Feb. 2021 Right axillary tail biopsy.
Pathology: Metastatic ductal carcinoma.

	Result	Intensity	Positive %
Estrogen receptor	Strong (8/8)	3	>2/3
Progesterone receptor	Strong (8/8)	3	>2/3
C-erbB2	Negative (1+)		
Ki-67	Positive in 44% of tumor cells		

See Figs. 45 and 46.

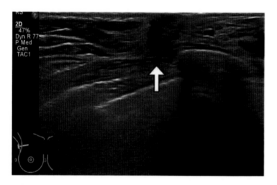

Fig. 44 Breast US (Feb. 2021): An irregular hypoechoic mass with non-parallel orientation at the right axillary tail. US-CNB = Metastatic ductal carcinoma

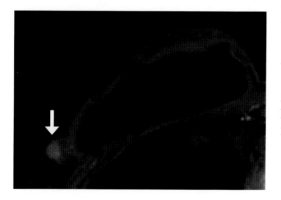

Fig. 45 Breast MRI (Mar. 2021): An enhancing mass at the right axillary tail

Fig. 46 Post-NAC breast MRI (Oct. 2021): No residual enhancing lesion after NAC

Neoadjuvant Chemotherapy

Neoadjuvant chemotherapy #8 cycles (Adriamycin + Cyclophosphamide #4 → Docetaxel #4).

Operation

Oct. 2021 Right axillary tail wide excision and bilateral salpingo-oophorectomy.

Pathology: DUCTAL CARCINOMA IN SITU, stage yrpTis, size of tumor: 0.2 cm.

	Result	Intensity	Positive %
Estrogen receptor	Strong (8/8)	3	>2/3
Progesterone receptor	Strong (8/8)	3	>2/3
C-erbB2	Negative (0)		
Ki-67	Positive in 2% of tumor cells		

Adjuvant Therapy

Post-operative radiation therapy + Letrozole 2.5 mg/day.

14 Case 14

14.1 Patient History and Progress

Female/55 years old, post-menopause.
No family history.
Hepatitis B carrier.

14.2 Courses of Treatment

Right breast cancer → Operation → Adjuvant therapy → **Ipsilateral axillary lymph node recurrence**.

14.2.1 Primary Treatment
See Fig. 47.

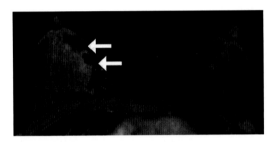

Fig. 47 Breast MRI (Jun. 2014): Segmental non-mass enhancement in the right breast. Right NSM = DCIS

Operation
Jun. 2014 Right nipple-areolar complex sparing mastectomy with immediate implant reconstruction, sentinel lymph node biopsy.
Pathology: DUCTAL CARCINOMA IN SITU, stage pTisN0(sn).
Size of tumor: 6.5 cm, lymph node: 0/1.

	Result	Intensity	Positive %
Estrogen receptor	Intermediate (6/8)	2	1/3–2/3
Progesterone receptor	Strong (7/8)	2	>2/3
C-erbB2	Negative (0)		
Ki-67	Positive in 35% of tumor cells		

Adjuvant Therapy
Tamoxifen 20 mg/day for 0.75 year.

14.2.2 Treatments After Recurrence
See Fig. 48.
Oct. 2017 Right axillary lymph node biopsy.
Pathology: Metastatic ductal carcinoma.

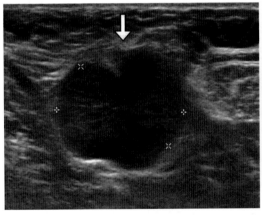
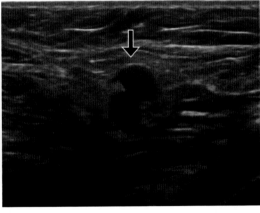

Fig. 48 Breast US (Oct. 2017, May 2018): An enlarged lymph node (white arrow) in the right axilla. US-CNB = Metastatic ductal carcinoma. Decreased size of the biopsy proven metastatic lymph node (black arrow) after chemotherapy. Right ALND = Metastatic ductal carcinoma in one out of nine lymph nodes

	Result	Intensity	Positive %
Estrogen receptor	Strong (8/8)	3	>2/3
Progesterone receptor	Strong (8/8)	3	>2/3
C-erbB2	Negative (0)		
Ki-67	Positive in 27% of tumor cells		

Neoadjuvant Chemotherapy
Neoadjuvant chemotherapy #8 cycles (Adriamycin & Cyclophosphamide #4 → Docetaxel #4).

Operation
May 2018 Right axillary lymph node dissection and bilateral salpingo-oophorectomy.
Pathology: Metastatic ductal carcinoma in 1 out of 9 lymph nodes, size of metastasis: 9 mm.

	Result	Intensity	Positive %
Estrogen receptor	Strong (7/8)	2	>2/3
Progesterone receptor	Negative (2/8)	1	<1%
C-erbB2	Negative (0)		
Ki-67	Positive in 2% of tumor cells		

Adjuvant Therapy
Post-operative radiation therapy + Tamoxifen 20 mg/day~

15 Case 15

15.1 Patient History and Progress

Female/74 years old, post-menopause.
No family history.
Hypertension.

15.2 Courses of Treatment

Right breast cancer → Operation → Adjuvant therapy → **Ipsilateral axillary lymph node recurrence**.

15.2.1 Primary Treatment
See Fig. 49.

Operation
Oct. 2015 Right total mastectomy, sentinel lymph node biopsy.
Pathology: Invasive ductal carcinoma, stage pT2N0(sn).
Size of tumor: 2.5 cm, lymph node: 0/3.

	Result	Intensity	Positive %
Estrogen receptor	Strong (8/8)	3	>2/3
Progesterone receptor	Strong (8/8)	3	>2/3
C-erbB2	Negative (1+)		
Ki-67	Positive in 31% of tumor cells		

Adjuvant Therapy
Tamoxifen 20 mg/day for 5.2 years.

15.2.2 Treatments After Recurrence
See Figs. 50 and 51.

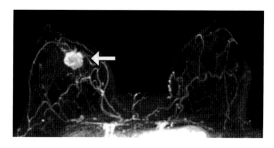

Fig. 49 Breast MRI (Sep. 2015): An irregular enhancing mass in the right breast. Right simple mastectomy = IDC

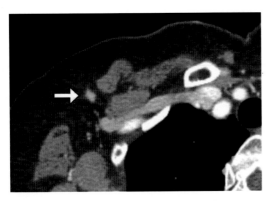

Fig. 50 Chest CT (Jun. 2020): A small irregular lymph node in the right axilla

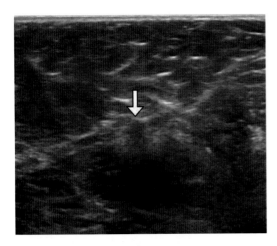

Fig. 51 MRI-directed US (Jul. 2020): A small irregular lymph node at the corresponding area of the CT abnormality. US-CNB = Metastatic ductal carcinoma

Jul. 2020 Right axillary lymph node biopsy.
Pathology: Metastatic ductal carcinoma.

	Result	Intensity	Positive %
Estrogen receptor	Strong (8/8)	3	>2/3
Progesterone receptor	Strong (8/8)	3	>2/3
C-erbB2	Negative (0)		

Operation
Dec. 2020 Right axillary lymph node sampling.
   Pathology: Metastatic ductal carcinoma in 1 out of 7 lymph nodes, size of metastasis: 11 mm.

Adjuvant Therapy
Letrozole 2.5 mg/day~

16   Case 16

16.1   Patient History and Progress

Female/46 years old, post-menopause.
   No family history.
   S/p myomectomy & bilateral salpingo-oophorectomy.

16.2   Courses of Treatment

Left breast cancer → Operation → Adjuvant therapy → **Ipsilateral axillary lymph node recurrence**.

16.2.1   Primary Treatment
See Fig. 52.

Operation
Jul. 2013 Left skin sparing mastectomy with immediate implant reconstruction, sentinel lymph node biopsy.

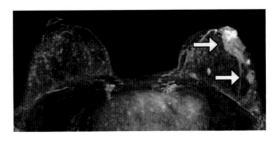

Fig. 52 Breast MRI (Jul. 2013): Two irregular enhancing masses in the left breast. Left SSM = IDC

Pathology: Invasive ductal carcinoma, stage pT2N1a(sn).

Size of tumor: 2.5 cm and 1.0 cm, lymph node: 1/2, size of metastatic carcinoma: 2.1 mm.

	Result	Intensity	Positive %
Estrogen receptor	Strong (8/8)	3	>2/3
Progesterone receptor	Strong (7/8)	3	1/3–2/3
C-erbB2	Equivocal (2+)		
Ki-67	Positive in 49% of tumor cells		
SISH	Negative		

Oncotype Dx RS scores: 29.

Adjuvant Chemotherapy
Adjuvant chemotherapy (Adriamycin + Cyclophosphamide #2 → weekly Paclitaxel #12).

16.2.2 Treatments After Recurrence
See Fig. 53.

Aug. 2015 Soft tissue, left axilla biopsy.
Pathology: Metastatic carcinoma.

	Result	Intensity	Positive %
Estrogen receptor	Strong (7/8)	2	>2/3
Progesterone receptor	Strong (8/8)	3	>2/3
C-erbB2	Negative (1+)		
Ki-67	Positive in 46% of tumor cells		

Neoadjuvant Endocrine Therapy
Tamoxifen 20 mg/day + zoladex.

Operation
Bilateral salpingo-oophorectomy → Progressive disease (Lt. axillary lymph node).

Adjuvant Therapy
Letrozole 2.5 mg/day.
See Fig. 54.

Operation
Aug. 2021 Left axillary lymph node dissection.
Pathology: Metastatic ductal carcinoma in 4 out of 6 lymph nodes, size of metastasis: 25 mm.

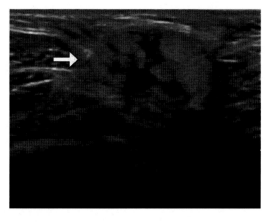

Fig. 53 US for evaluation of a palpable mass in the left axilla (Aug. 2015): An oval mass with heterogeneous echogenicity in the left axilla. US-CNB = Metastatic carcinoma

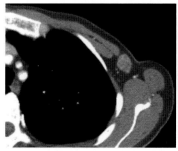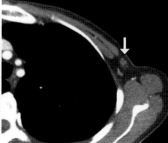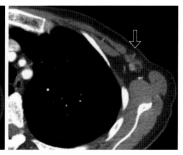

Fig. 54 Chest CT (Aug. 2015, Dec. 2015, Jun. 2021): The biopsy proven metastatic carcinoma in the left axilla had decreased (white arrow) then increased again (black arrow) during palliative therapy. Left ALND = Metastatic ductal carcinoma in four out of six lymph nodes

	Result	Intensity	Positive %
Estrogen receptor	Strong (8/8)	3	>2/3
Progesterone receptor	Negative (0/8)	0	0
C-erbB2	Equivocal (2+)		
Ki-67	Positive in 31% of tumor cells		
SISH	Positive		

Adjuvant Therapy

Post-operative radiation therapy + Letrozole 2.5 mg/day~

17 Case 17

17.1 Patient History and Progress

Female/69 years old, post-menopause.
Family history of breast cancer, daughter.
BRCA 1 mutation: VUS (variant of uncertain).

17.2 Courses of Treatment

Right breast cancer → Operation → Adjuvant therapy → **Ipsilateral axillary lymph node recurrence**.

17.2.1 Primary Treatment
See Fig. 55.

Operation
Oct. 2017 Right breast conserving surgery, axillary lymph node dissection (Level I).
Pathology: Invasive ductal carcinoma, stage pT1c(2)N2.
Size of tumor: 1.8 cm and 1.0 cm, lymph node: 4/8, size of metastasis: 25 mm.

	Result	Intensity	Positive %
Estrogen receptor	Strong (7/8)	3	1/3–2/3
Progesterone receptor	Strong (7/8)	2	>2/3
C-erbB2	Negative (0)		
Ki-67	Positive in 15% of tumor cells		

Adjuvant Therapy
Adjuvant chemotherapy #8 cycles (Adriamycin + Cyclophosphamide #4 → Docetaxel #4).
Post-operative radiation therapy + Letrozole 2.5 mg/day for 3 years.

17.2.2 Treatments After Recurrence
See Fig. 56.
May 2021 Right axillary lymph node biopsy.
Pathology: Metastatic ductal carcinoma.

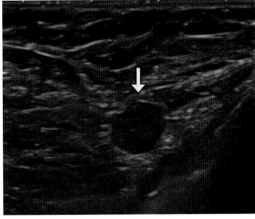

Fig. 56 Breast US (Apr. 2021): A new round lymph node without fatty hilum in the right axilla. US-CNB = Metastatic ductal carcinoma

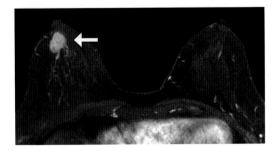

Fig. 55 Breast MRI (Oct. 2017): An irregular enhancing mass in the right breast. Right BCS = IDC

	Result	Intensity	Positive %
Estrogen receptor	Intermediate (6/8)	1	>2/3
Progesterone receptor	Negative (0/8)	0	0
C-erbB2	Negative (0)		
Ki-67	Positive in <1% of tumor cells		

Operation
Jun. 2021 Right axillary lymph node dissection.
Pathology: No metastasis in four axillary lymph nodes.

Adjuvant Therapy
Exemestane 25 mg/day~

18 Case 18

18.1 Patient History and Progress

Female/64 years old, post-menopause.
No family history.
Hypertension, diabetes mellitus.

18.2 Courses of Treatment

Left breast cancer → Operation → **Ipsilateral chest wall recurrence** → Neoadjuvant chemotherapy → operation → targeted therapy → **Ipsilateral lymph node recurrence**.

18.2.1 Primary Treatment
See Fig. 57.

Operation
Dec. 2015 Left breast conserving surgery, sentinel lymph node biopsy.
Pathology: Invasive ductal carcinoma, stage pT1a(Pagets′)N0(sn).

Size of tumor: 0.5 cm, lymph node: 0/1.

	Result	Intensity	Positive %
Estrogen receptor	Negative (0/8)	0	0
Progesterone receptor	Negative (0/8)	0	0
C-erbB2	Positive (3+)		
Ki-67	Positive in 23% of tumor cells		

18.2.2 Treatments After Recurrence
See Figs. 58 and 59.
Nov. 2018 Muscle, left breast biopsy.
Pathology: Invasive ductal carcinoma, clinically recurrent.

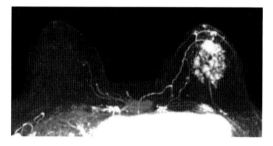

Fig. 57 Breast MRI (Nov. 2015): Mixed masses and non-mass enhancement in the left breast. Left BCS = IDC

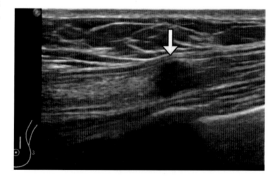

Fig. 58 Breast US (Nov. 2018): An irregular hypoechoic mass in the left pectoralis muscle. US-CNB = IDC

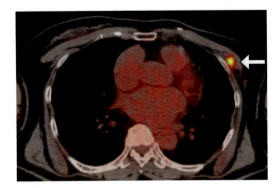

Fig. 59 PET-CT (Dec. 2018): A hypermetabolic mass in the left pectoralis muscle

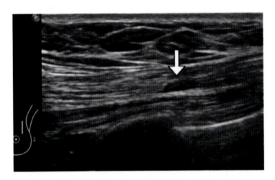

Fig. 60 Post-chemotherapy breast US (Mar. 2019): Decreased size of the IDC in the left pectoralis muscle. Left simple mastectomy = IDC

	Result	Intensity	Positive %
Estrogen receptor	Strong (8/8)	3	>2/3
Progesterone receptor	Intermediate (5/8)	3	1–10%
C-erbB2	Positive (3+)		
Ki-67	Positive in 39% of tumor cells		

Neoadjuvant Chemotherapy
Chemotherapy #3 cycle (Docetaxel & Trastuzumab + Pertuzumab).
   See Fig. 60.

Operation
2019-03-29 Left total mastectomy, axillary lymph node sampling.
   Pathology: Invasive ductal carcinoma, stage yp T1aN1.

Size of tumor: 0.3 cm, lymph node: 3/10, size of metastatic carcinoma: 3 mm.

	Result	Intensity	Positive %
Estrogen receptor	Strong (8/8)	3	>2/3
Progesterone receptor	Negative (2/8)	1	<1%
C-erbB2	Equivocal (2+)		
Ki-67	Positive in 34% of tumor cells		

Adjuvant Therapy
Trastuzumab + Pertuzumab.
   See Fig. 61.
   Nov. 2020 Left axillary lymph node biopsy.
   Pathology: Metastatic ductal carcinoma.

	Result	Intensity	Positive %
Estrogen receptor	Strong (7/8)	3	1/3–2/3
Progesterone receptor	Negative (0/8)	0	0
C-erbB2	Equivocal (2+)		
Ki-67	Positive in 25% of tumor cells		
SISH	Positive		

Operation
Jan. 2020 Left axillary lymph node dissection.
   Pathology: Metastatic ductal carcinoma in three out of eight axillary lymph nodes.

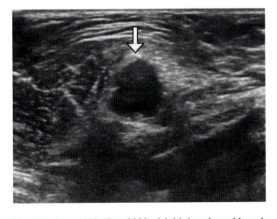

Fig. 61 Breast US (Oct. 2020): Multiple enlarged lymph nodes in the left axilla (partly shown). US-CNB = Metastatic ductal carcinoma

Size of metastatic carcinoma: 20 mm.

	Result	Intensity	Positive %
Estrogen receptor	Strong (8/8)	3	>2/3
Progesterone receptor	Negative (2/8)	1	<1%
C-erbB2	Positive (3+)		
Ki-67	Positive in 30% of tumor cells		

Adjuvant Therapy

Post-operative radiation therapy + Letrozole 2.5 mg/day~

19 Case 19

19.1 Patient History and Progress

Female/45 years old, post-menopause.
No family history.
S/p bilateral salpingo-oophorectomy.

19.2 Courses of Treatment

Right breast cancer → Operation → Adjuvant therapy → **Ipsilateral axillary lymph node recurrence** → Operation → Endocrine therapy → **Progressive disease**.

19.2.1 Primary Treatment
See Fig. 62.

Operation
Mar. 2017 Right nipple-areolar complex sparing mastectomy with immediate implant reconstruction, sentinel lymph node biopsy.

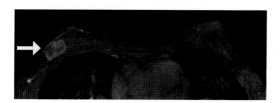

Fig. 62 Breast MRI (Mar. 2017): A heterogeneously enhancing mass in the right breast

Pathology: Invasive ductal carcinoma, stage pT2N1a(sn).
Size of tumor: 2.3 cm, lymph node: 3/5, size of metastatic carcinoma: 7 mm.

	Result	Intensity	Positive %
Estrogen receptor	Strong (7/8)	3	1/3–2/3
Progesterone receptor	Strong (7/8)	3	1/3–2/3
C-erbB2	Negative (0)		
Ki-67	Positive in 26% of tumor cells		

Adjuvant Therapy

Adjuvant chemotherapy #8 cycles (Adriamycin & Cyclophosphamide #4 → Docetaxel #4).

Post-operative radiation therapy + Tamoxifen 20 mg/day for 3.8 years.

19.2.2 Treatments After Recurrence
See Fig. 63.
May 2021 Right axillary lymph node biopsy.
Pathology: Metastatic ductal carcinoma.

	Result	Intensity	Positive %
Estrogen receptor	Strong (8/8)	3	>2/3
Progesterone receptor	Weak (4/8)	2	1–10%
C-erbB2	Negative (0)		
Ki-67	Positive in 6% of tumor cells		

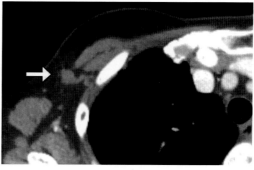

Fig. 63 Chest CT (May 2021): An irregular lymph node in the right axilla

Operation

Jun. 2021 Right axillary lymph node dissection and bilateral salpingo-oophorectomy.

Pathology: Metastatic ductal carcinoma in two out of two axillary lymph nodes.

Size of metastatic carcinoma: 11 mm.

	Result	Intensity	Positive %
Estrogen receptor	Strong (8/8)	3	>2/3
Progesterone receptor	Intermediate (5/8)	2	10%–1/3
C-erbB2	Negative (1+)		
Ki-67	Positive in 7% of tumor cells		

Adjuvant Therapy

Letrozole 2.5 mg/day for 0.75 year → Progressive disease.

See Figs. 64 and 65.

Mar. 2022 Right axillary lymph node biopsy.
Pathology: Metastatic ductal carcinoma.

	Result	Intensity	Positive %
Estrogen receptor	Weak (3/8)	1	1–10%
Progesterone receptor	Negative (0/8)	0	0
C-erbB2	Negative (1+)		
Ki-67	Positive in 11% of tumor cells		

Palliative Chemotherapy

Chemotherapy (Capecitabine~).

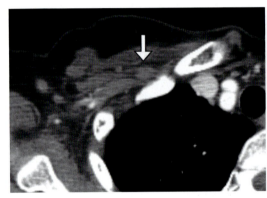
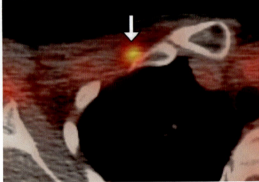

Fig. 64 Chest CT and PET-CT (Mar. 2022): An enlarged lymph node with hypermetabolism at level III of the right axilla

Fig. 65 MRI-directed US (Mar. 2022): An enlarged lymph node at level III of the right axilla

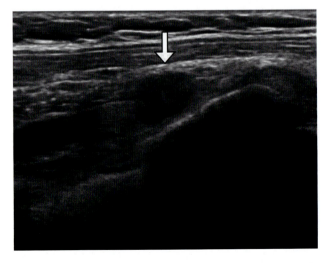

20 Case 20

20.1 Patient History and Progress

Female/61 years old, post-menopause.
Family history of breast cancer, maternal cousin.
BRCA 1 & 2 mutation: Not detected.

20.2 Courses of Treatment

Left breast cancer → Operation → Adjuvant therapy → Ipsilateral axillary lymph node recurrence.

20.2.1 Primary Treatment

Operation
Sep. 1998 Left breast conserving surgery, axillary lymph node dissection.
Pathology: Invasive ductal carcinoma, stage pT1aN0.
Size of tumor: N.A, lymph node: 0/16.

	Result	Intensity	Positive %
Estrogen receptor	Positive	N.A	N.A
Progesterone receptor	Positive	N.A	N.A
C-erbB2	N.A		
Ki-67	N.A		

Adjuvant Therapy
Adjuvant chemotherapy #3 cycles (Cyclophosphamide & Methotrexate & Fluorouracil).
Post-operative radiation therapy +Tamoxifen 20 mg/day for 0.5 year.

20.2.2 Treatments After Recurrence
See Fig. 66.
Sep. 2015 Left infraclavicular lymph node biopsy.
Pathology: Metastatic ductal carcinoma.
Left breast biopsy.
Pathology: Invasive ductal carcinoma, clinically recurrent.

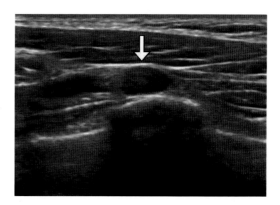

Fig. 66 Breast US (Nov. 2014): A mildly enlarged lymph node at level II of the left axilla

	Result	Intensity	Positive %
Estrogen receptor	Strong (8/8)	3	>2/3
Progesterone receptor	Intermediate (6/8)	2	1/3–2/3
C-erbB2	Negative (0)		
Ki-67	Positive in 32% of tumor cells		

Neoadjuvant Chemotherapy
Neoadjuvant chemotherapy #6 cycles (Adriamycin & Cyclophosphamide #4 → Docetaxel #2).
See Fig. 67.

Operation
Feb. 2016 Left total mastectomy, axillary lymph node sampling.
Pathology: Invasive ductal carcinoma, stage ypT1c(m)N1a.
Size of tumor: up to 1.6 cm, lymph node: 1/2, size of metastatic carcinoma: 7 mm.

	Result	Intensity	Positive %
Estrogen receptor	Strong (8/8)	3	>2/3
Progesterone receptor	Weak (3/8)	1	1–10%
C-erbB2	Negative (0)		
Ki-67	Positive in 12% of tumor cells		

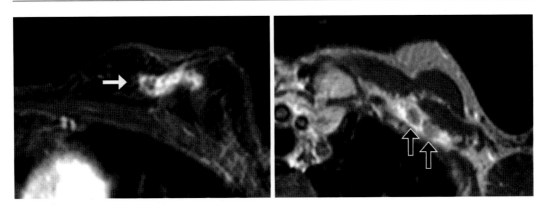

Fig. 67 Breast MRI (Oct. 2015): An irregular enhancing mass in the left breast (white arrow, IDC). Two mildly enlarged lymph nodes at level II and III of the left axilla (black arrows, metastatic ductal carcinoma)

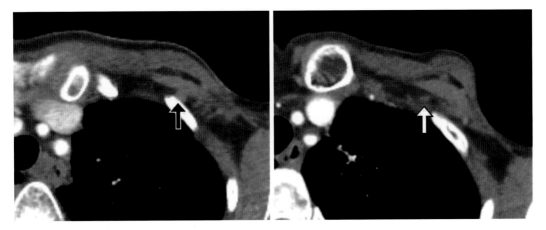

Fig. 68 Chest CT (Sep. 2016, Dec. 2021): A mildly enlarged lymph node (black arrow) had become smaller (white arrow) at level II of the left axilla

Adjuvant Therapy
Post-operative radiation therapy (axilla) +Letrozole 2.5 mg/day~
See Fig. 68.

21 Case 21

21.1 Patient History and Progress

Female/61 years old, post-menopause.
No family history.

21.2 Courses of Treatment

Left breast cancer → Operation → Adjuvant therapy → **Neck node recurrence** → **Lymph nodes, bone metastasis** → **Skull, brain metastasis**.

21.2.1 Primary Treatment

Operation
Apr. 2002 Left breast conserving surgery, sentinel lymph node biopsy.

Pathology: Microinvasive infiltrating duct carcinoma, stage T1miN0(sn).

Size of tumor: N.A, lymph node: 0/2.

	Result	Intensity	Positive %
Estrogen receptor	Positive	Intermediate	60%
Progesterone receptor	Positive	Weak	20%
C-erbB2	Negative (1+)		
Ki-67	N.A		

Adjuvant Therapy
Post-operative radiation therapy +Tamoxifen 20 mg/day for 5 years.

21.2.2 Treatments After Recurrence
See Fig. 69.

Dec. 2015 Left neck lymph node aspiration (level 4).

Pathology: Metastatic ductal carcinoma.

Palliative Therapy
Letrozole 2.5 mg/day → Progressive disease on, lymph node, bone.

Chemotherapy #24 cycles (Paclitaxel) → Progressive disease on brain, skull.

Whole brain radiation therapy.

Fulvestrant + abemaciclib~

See Figs. 70, 71, and 72.

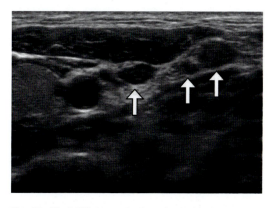

Fig. 69 Neck US for evaluation of palpable lumps (Dec. 2015): Multiple suspicious lymph nodes at the left lower neck

Fig. 70 PET-CT (Apr. 2019): Multifocal hypermetabolic lesions in the liver (white arrow), spleen (black arrow), and bones

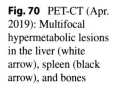
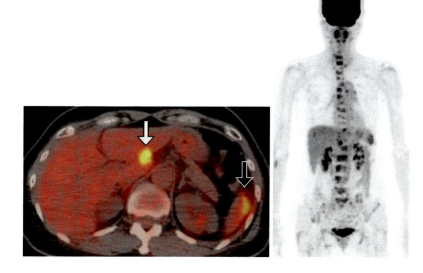

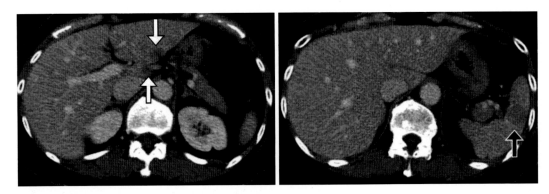

Fig. 71 Abdominopelvic CT (May 2019): Multiple low attenuation lesions in the liver (white arrow, partly shown) and spleen (black arrow)

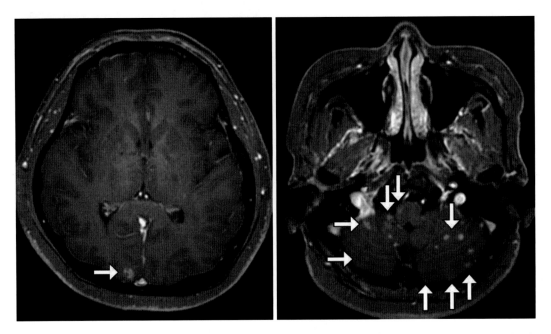

Fig. 72 Brain MRI (Sep. 2020): Multiple enhancing lesions in both cerebellums, brainstem, and both cerebral hemispheres (partly shown)

22 Case 22

22.1 Patient History and Progress

Female/69 years old, post-menopause.
  No family history.
  Hepatitis B carrier.

22.2 Courses of Treatment

Left breast cancer → Operation → Adjuvant therapy → **Right axillary lymph node recurrence → Right breast recurrence → Chest wall → Bone → Pleural effusion metastasis**.

22.2.1 Primary Treatment
See Fig. 73.

Metastatic Breast Cancer

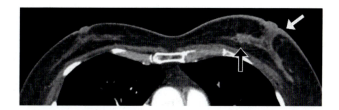

Fig. 73 Chest CT (Oct. 2007): Irregular enhancing lesion (black arrow) and skin thickening (white arrow) of the left breast

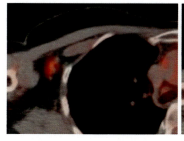
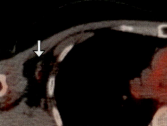
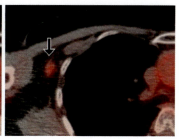

Fig. 74 PET-CT (Apr. 2010, Oct. 2011, Apr. 2014): An enlarged lymph node with hypermetabolism in the right axilla. Size and metabolism of the biopsy proved meta- static lymph nodes had decreased (white arrow) and then increased again (black arrow)

Neoadjuvant Chemotherapy
Neoadjuvant chemotherapy #6 cycles (Fluorouracil + Doxorubicin + cyclophosphamide #3 → Doxorubicin + Docetaxel #3).

Operation
Mar. 2008 Left total mastectomy, axillary lymph node dissection.

Pathology: Invasive apocrine carcinoma, stage ypT1bN2a.

Size of tumor: 1.0 cm, lymph node: 6/6, size of metastatic carcinoma: 10 mm.

	Result	Intensity	Positive %
Estrogen receptor	Negative (0/7)	0	0
Progesterone receptor	Negative (0/7)	0	0
C-erbB2	Negative (1+)		
Ki-67	Positive in 5% of tumor cells		

Adjuvant Therapy
Post-operative radiation therapy.

22.2.2 Treatments After Recurrence

Right Axillary Lymph Node Recurrence
See Fig. 74.

Apr. 2010 Right axillary lymph node biopsy.
Pathology: Metastatic apocrine carcinoma.

	Result	Intensity	Positive %
Estrogen receptor	Negative (0/7)	0	0
Progesterone receptor	Negative (0/7)	0	0
C-erbB2	Negative (1+)		
Ki-67	N.A		

Neoadjuvant Chemotherapy
Chemotherapy #15 cycles (Capecitabine).

Operation
Apr. 2014 Right axillary lymph node dissection.

Pathology: Metastatic ductal carcinoma in eight out of eight axillary lymph nodes, size of metastatic carcinoma: 18 mm.

	Result	Intensity	Positive %
Estrogen receptor	Negative (0/8)	0	0
Progesterone receptor	Negative (0/8)	0	0
C-erbB2	Negative (1+)		
Ki-67	Positive in 6% of tumor cells		

Adjuvant Therapy

Post-operative radiation therapy (axilla).

Right Breast Recurrence

See Fig. 75.
 Feb. 2016 Right breast biopsy.
 Pathology: Invasive ductal carcinoma.

	Result	Intensity	Positive %
Estrogen receptor	Negative (0/8)	0	0
Progesterone receptor	Negative (0/8)	0	0
C-erbB2	Negative (1+)		
Ki-67	Positive in 42% of tumor cells		

Neoadjuvant Chemotherapy

Chemotherapy #8 cycles (paclitaxel + Cisplatin).
 Radiation therapy (breast).
 Chemotherapy #12 cycles (Cyclophosphamide + Methotrexate).
 See Fig. 76.

Operation

Jan. 2017 Right total mastectomy.

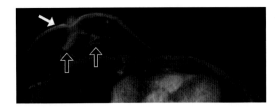

Fig. 75 Breast MRI for evaluation of inflammatory change of the right breast (Feb. 2016): Diffuse non-mass enhancement (black arrows) and skin thickening (white arrow) of the right breast

Fig. 76 Post-chemotherapy breast MRI (Jan. 2017): Decreased enhancing lesions in the parenchyma and skin of the right breast

Pathology: Invasive ductal carcinoma, stage ypT2(m).
 Size of tumor: up to 2.8 cm, multifocal.

	Result	Intensity	Positive %
Estrogen receptor	Negative (0/8)	0	0
Progesterone receptor	Negative (0/8)	0	0
C-erbB2	Negative (1+)		
Ki-67	Positive in 1% of tumor cells		

Chest Wall → Bone → Pleural Effusion Metastasis

Jan. 2018 Right chest wall skin biopsy.
 Pathology: Metastatic ductal carcinoma.

	Result	Intensity	Positive %
Estrogen receptor	Negative (0/8)	0	0
Progesterone receptor	Negative (0/8)	0	0
C-erbB2	Negative (1+)		
Ki-67	Positive in 3% of tumor cells		

Palliative Therapy

Chemotherapy #10 cycles (Harven): Progressive disease.
 Chemotherapy #31 cycles (Capecitabine): Progressive disease on bone.
 Chemotherapy #11 cycles (Gemcitabine): Progressive disease on bone.
 Chemotherapy (Vinorelbine tartrate +Cisplatin)~
 See Figs. 77 and 78.

Metastatic Breast Cancer

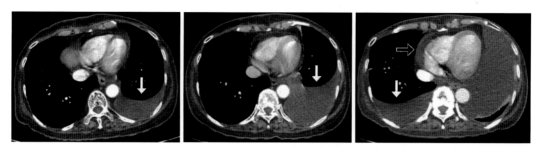

Fig. 77 Chest CT (Jul. 2020, Sep. 2020, Apr. 2022): The amount of pleural effusion was getting increased (white arrow). Cytology of pleural fluid = Positive for malignant cells. Newly developed pericardial effusion (black arrow)

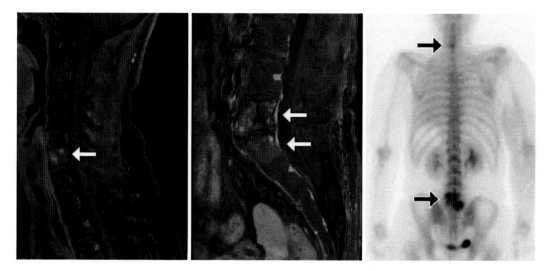

Fig. 78 Spine MRI and bone scan (Aug. 2020): Multiple bone marrow replacing lesions (white arrows) with increased uptake (black arrows) in the vertebrae

23 Case 23

23.1 Patient History and Progress

Female/39 years old, pre-menopause.
 No family history.
 BRCA 1 & 2 VUS (variant of uncertain).

23.2 Courses of Treatment

Left breast cancer → Neoadjuvant chemotherapy → Operation → Adjuvant therapy → **Pericardial effusion, Metastatic lymph nodes** → **Bone, brain metastasis**.

23.2.1 Primary Treatment
See Fig. 79.

Neoadjuvant Chemotherapy
Neoadjuvant chemotherapy #8 cycles (Adriamycin + Cyclophosphamide #4 → Docetaxel #4).

	Result	Intensity	Positive %
Estrogen receptor	Negative (0/7)	0	0
Progesterone receptor	Negative (0/7)	0	0
C-erbB2	Negative (0)		
Ki-67	Positive in 40% of tumor cells		

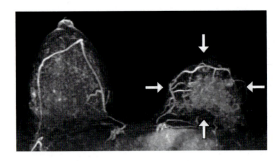

Fig. 79 Breast MRI (Jul. 2012): Conglomerated enhancing masses involving the entire left breast

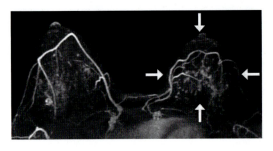

Fig. 80 Post-NAC breast MRI (Jan. 2013): Decreased tumor burden in the left breast

Clinical stage: cT3N1M0.
See Fig. 80.

Operation

Jan. 2013 Left total mastectomy, sentinel lymph node biopsy.

Pathology: Invasive ductal carcinoma, stage ypT1c(m)N0(sn).

Size of tumor: up to 1.5 cm, multifocal, lymph node: 0/4.

	Result	Intensity	Positive %
Estrogen receptor	Weak (3/8)	1	1–10%
Progesterone receptor	Negative (0/8)	0	0
C-erbB2	Negative (0)		
Ki-67	Positive in 21% of tumor cells		

Adjuvant Therapy

Post-operative radiation therapy + Tamoxifen 20 mg/day for 5 years.

23.2.2 Treatments After Recurrence

See Fig. 81.

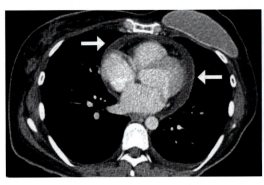
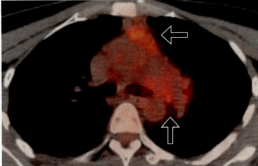

Fig. 81 Chest CT and PET-CT (Apr. 2019): Pericardial effusion (white arrows) and enlarged hypermetabolic mediastinal lymph nodes (black arrows)

Apr. 2019 Chest CT: pericardial effusion, metastatic lymph nodes.

Palliative Therapy

Clinical trial enrolled (Paclitaxel + ipatasertib/placebo #18 cycles): Progressive disease on bone.

Chemotherapy #5 cycles (Capecitabine): Progressive disease on bone.

Chemotherapy #12 cycles (Gemcitabine & Cisplatin): Progressive disease on leptomeningeal, brain.

Intrathecal chemotherapy (Methotrexate).

Chemotherapy (Vinorelbine tartrate & Cisplatin)~

See Figs. 82, 83, 84, and 85.

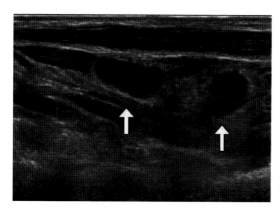
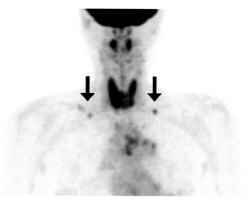

Fig. 82 Neck US and PET-CT (Apr. 2019): Multiple small lymph nodes with irregular margins (white arrows) and mild hypermetabolism (black arrows) at the lower neck

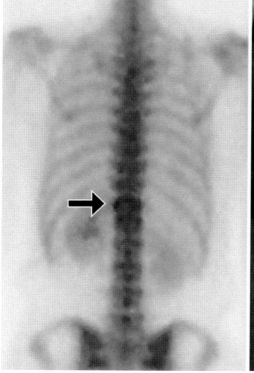
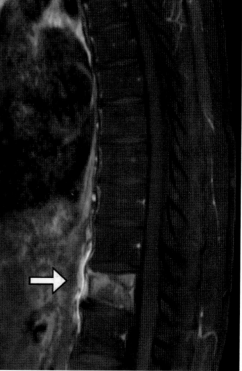

Fig. 83 Bone scan (Oct. 2019) and spine MRI (Dec. 2019): Increased uptake (black arrow) and bone marrow replacing lesion with mild pathologic fracture (white arrow) in the T2 vertebra

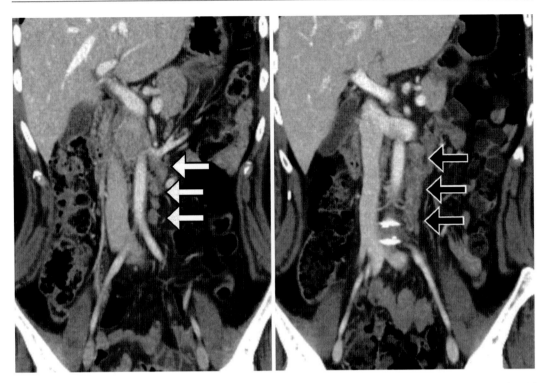

Fig. 84 Abdominopelvic CT (Mar. 2020, Nov. 2020): Multiple lymph nodes (white arrows) were getting enlarged (black arrows) in the abdominopelvic cavity (partly shown)

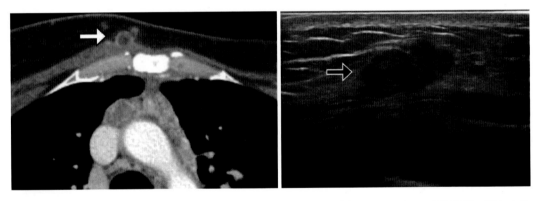

Fig. 85 Chest CT (Sep. 2020) and US (Oct. 2020): A palpable mass at the right parasternal area. US-CNB = Metastatic ductal carcinoma

24 Case 24

24.1 Patient History and Progress

Female/64 years old, post-menopause.
No family history.

24.2 Courses of Treatment

Right breast cancer → Operation → Adjuvant therapy → **Lung metastasis**.

24.2.1 Primary Treatment
See Fig. 86.

Operation
Nov. 2005 Right breast conserving surgery, axillary lymph node dissection.
Pathology: Invasive duct carcinoma, stage T1cN1a.
Size of tumor: 1.9 cm, lymph node: 1/8, size of metastatic carcinoma: 8 mm.

	Result	Intensity	Positive %
Estrogen receptor	Strong (7/7)	3	>2/3
Progesterone receptor	Strong (7/7)	3	>2/3
C-erbB2	Negative (1+)		
Ki-67	Positive in 30% of tumor cells		

Adjuvant Therapy
Adjuvant chemotherapy #8 cycles (Adriamycin + Cyclophosphamide #4 → Docetaxel #4).
Post-operative radiation therapy + Tamoxifen 20 mg/day → Letrozole 2.5 mg/day.

24.2.2 Treatments After Recurrence
See Fig. 87.

Operation
Jan. 2019 Left lower lung wedge resection.
Pathology: Metastatic carcinoma, size of tumor: 0.9 * 0.7 * 0.3 cm.

	Result	Intensity	Positive %
Estrogen receptor	Strong (8/8)	3	>2/3
Progesterone receptor	Intermediate (6/8)	2	1/3–2/3
C-erbB2	Negative (1+)		
Ki-67	Positive in 7% of tumor cells		

Palliative Therapy
Palbociclib #25 cycles + Letrozole 2.5 mg/day~

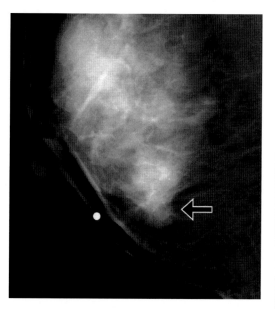

Fig. 86 Right mammography (Oct. 2005): A palpable mass at the lower breast

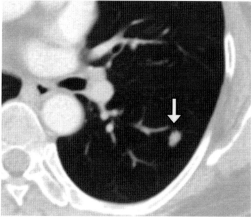

Fig. 87 Chest CT (Dec. 2018): A nodule in the LUL lung

25 Case 25

25.1 Patient History and Progress

Female/46 years old, post-menopause.
Family history of breast cancer, mother.
BRCA 1 & 2 mutation: Not detected.
Hyperthyroidism, s/p bilateral salpingo-oophorectomy.

25.2 Courses of Treatment

Left breast cancer → Operation → Adjuvant therapy → **Ipsilateral breast skin metastasis**.
See Fig. 88.

25.2.1 Primary Treatment

Operation
Apr. 2017 Left nipple-areolar complex sparing mastectomy with immediate implant reconstruction, sentinel lymph node biopsy.
Pathology: Invasive ductal carcinoma, stage T1cN0(sn).
Size of tumor: 1.1 cm, lymph node: 0/1.

	Result	Intensity	Positive %
Estrogen receptor	Strong (8/8)	3	>2/3
Progesterone receptor	Strong (8/8)	3	>2/3
C-erbB2	Negative (0)		
Ki-67	Positive in 7% of tumor cells		

Adjuvant Therapy
Tamoxifen 20 mg/day for 0.75 year.

25.2.2 Treatments After Recurrence

See Figs. 89 and 90.
Jun. 2021 Left breast skin biopsy.
Pathology: Invasive ductal carcinoma, clinically recurrent.

	Result	Intensity	Positive %
Estrogen receptor	Strong (8/8)	3	>2/3
Progesterone receptor	Intermediate (5/8)	2	10%–1/3
C-erbB2	Negative (1+)		
Ki-67	Positive in 40% of tumor cells		

See Fig. 91.

Operation
Jul. 2021 Left breast wide excision, axillary lymph node sampling and bilateral salpingo-oophorectomy.
Pathology: Invasive ductal carcinoma, stage rT1cN0.
Size of tumor: 1.5 cm, lymph node: 0/4.

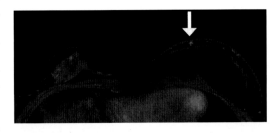

Fig. 89 Breast MRI (Jun. 2020): A tiny enhancing focus (white arrow) in the reconstructed left breast

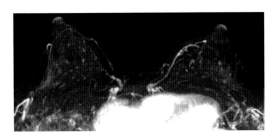

Fig. 88 Breast MRI after multiple vacuum-assisted excisional biopsy in the left breast (Mar. 2017): Mild BPE without definite abnormality of both breasts

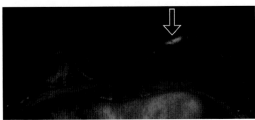

Fig. 90 Breast MRI (Jun. 2020): Increased size of the enhancing skin lesion (black arrow) in the reconstructed left breast

	Result	Intensity	Positive %
Estrogen receptor	Strong (8/8)	3	>2/3
Progesterone receptor	Strong (8/8)	3	>2/3
C-erbB2	Equivocal (2+)		
Ki-67	Positive in 42% of tumor cells		
SISH	Negative		

Oncotype Dx RS scores: 39.

Adjuvant Therapy
→ Adjuvant chemotherapy #4 (Docetaxel & Cyclophosphamide)
→ Letrozole 2.5 mg/day ~

26 Case 26

26.1 Patient History and Progress

Female/54 years old, post-menopause.
No family history.
S/p cholecystectomy, s/p total gastrectomy (gastric cancer), s/p bilateral salpingo-oophorectomy.

26.2 Courses of Treatment

Right breast cancer → Operation → Adjuvant therapy → **Stomach and bone metastasis**.

26.2.1 Primary Treatment
See Fig. 92.

Operation
Jan. 2014 Both total mastectomy, axillary lymph node dissection.
Pathology:
Right> Invasive lobular carcinoma, stage pT3N3a.
Size of tumor: 7 cm, lymph node: 15/17, size of metastatic carcinoma: 13 mm.

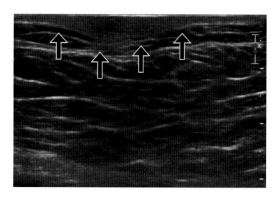

Fig. 91 MRI-directed left US (Jul. 2021): Focal skin thickening at the corresponding area of the MRI abnormality

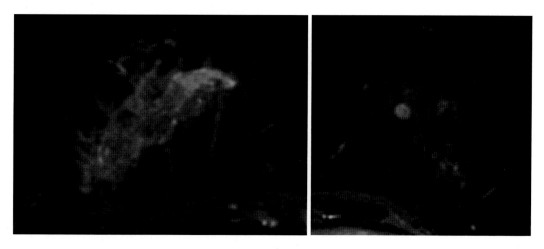

Fig. 92 Breast MRI (Jan. 2020): Segmental heterogeneous non-mass enhancement in the right whole breast and oval heterogeneous enhancing lesion at the 8 o'clock direction of left breast

	Result	Intensity	Positive %
Estrogen receptor	Strong (7/8)	2	>2/3
Progesterone receptor	Strong (8/8)	3	>2/3
C-erbB2	Negative (1+)		
Ki-67	Positive in 29% of tumor cells		

Left> Invasive lobular carcinoma, stage pT1c(m)N1mi.

Size of tumor: up to 1.5 cm, multiple, lymph node: 2/7, size of metastatic carcinoma: 1.5 mm.

	Result	Intensity	Positive %
Estrogen receptor	Strong (7/8)	2	>2/3
Progesterone receptor	Strong (7/8)	3	1/3–2/3
C-erbB2	Negative (0)		
Ki-67	Positive in 17% of tumor cells		

Adjuvant Therapy
Adjuvant chemotherapy #8 cycles (Adriamycin & Cyclophosphamide #4 → Docetaxel #4).

Post-operative radiation therapy +Tamoxifen 20 mg/day for 5 years.

26.2.2 Treatments After Recurrence
See Figs. 93 and 94.

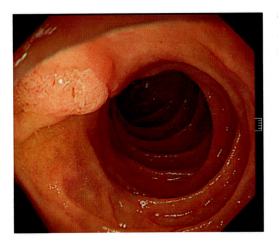

Fig. 93 Esophagogastroduodenoscopy (May 2018): Diffuse infiltrative mass in the stomach

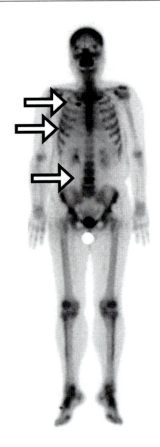

Fig. 94 Bone scan (Jun. 2018): Multifocal increased uptake in the 6th thoracic spinal body and right ribs, suggesting bony metastases

May 2018 Metastasis on stomach, bone.

Stomach biopsy Pathology: Metastatic ductal carcinoma.

	Result	Intensity	Positive %
Estrogen receptor	Intermediate (6/8)	2	1/3–2/3
Progesterone receptor	Strong (7/8)	3	1/3–2/3
C-erbB2	Negative (0)		
Ki-67	Positive in 8% of tumor cells		

Palliative Therapy
Bilateral salpingo-oophorectomy.
  Letrozole 2.5 mg/day + Palbociclib~
Total gastrectomy.

27 Case 27

27.1 Patient History and Progress

Female/74 years old, post-menopause.
No family history.
Hypertension, diabetes mellitus, s/p cholecystectomy (GB stone).

27.2 Courses of Treatment

Left breast cancer → Operation → Adjuvant therapy → **Right shoulder soft tissue metastasis**.

27.2.1 Primary Treatment
See Fig. 95.

Operation
Mar. 2008 Left breast conserving surgery, axillary lymph node dissection.
Pathology: Invasive duct carcinoma, stage T2N1a.
Size of tumor: 3 cm, lymph node: 3/7, size of metastatic carcinoma: 15 mm.

	Result	Intensity	Positive %
Estrogen receptor	Strong (6/7)	3	1/3–2/3
Progesterone receptor	Weak (2/7)	1	<10%
C-erbB2	Equivocal (2+)		
Ki-67	Positive in 15% of tumor cells		
FISH	Negative		

Adjuvant Therapy
Adjuvant chemotherapy #8 cycles (Adriamycin & Cyclophosphamide #4 → Docetaxel #4).
Post-operative radiation therapy + Letrozole 2.5 mg/day for 1 year → Tamoxifen 20 mg/day for 1 year.
Jun. 2021 Right shoulder soft tissue biopsy.
Pathology: Metastatic ductal carcinoma.

	Result	Intensity	Positive %
Estrogen receptor	Strong (8/8)	3	>2/3
Progesterone receptor	Weak (3/8)	1	1–10%
C-erbB2	Negative (1+)		
Ki-67	Positive in 6% of tumor cells		

Palliative Therapy
Clinical trial enrolled (SAR439859/placebo + Letrozole/placebo+ Palbociclib)~

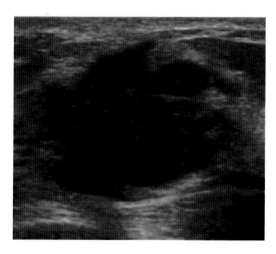

Fig. 95 Breast US (Feb. 2008): Irregular hypoechoic mass at the 9 o'clock direction of left breast

28 Case 28

28.1 Patient History and Progress

Female/51 years old, post-menopause.
No family history.
BRCA 1 & 2 mutation: Not detected, ATM VUS (variant of uncertain).

28.2 Courses of Treatment

Right breast cancer → Operation → Adjuvant therapy → **Right shoulder soft tissue metastasis**.

28.2.1 Primary Treatment
See Fig. 96.

Operation
Feb. 2015 Right breast conserving surgery, sentinel lymph node biopsy.

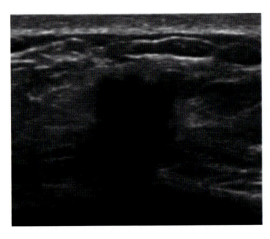

Fig. 96 Breast US (Feb. 2015): Irregular hypoechoic mass with spiculated margin at the 4 o'clock direction of right breast

Pathology: Invasive duct carcinoma, stage T1cN0(sn).
Size of tumor: 1.8 cm, lymph node: 0/1.

	Result	Intensity	Positive %
Estrogen receptor	Strong (7/8)	2	>2/3
Progesterone receptor	Strong (7/8)	2	>2/3
C-erbB2	Negative (1+)		
Ki-67	Positive in 7% of tumor cells		

Adjuvant Therapy
Post-operative radiation therapy + Tamoxifen 20 mg/day.

28.2.2 Treatments After Recurrence
See Fig. 97.

Left Axillary Lymph Node Metastasis
Dec. 2019 Left axillary lymph node biopsy.
Pathology: Metastatic ductal carcinoma.

	Result	Intensity	Positive %
Estrogen receptor	Strong (7/8)	2	>2/3
Progesterone receptor	Weak (3/8)	2	<1%
C-erbB2	Negative (1+)		
Ki-67	Positive in 6% of tumor cells		

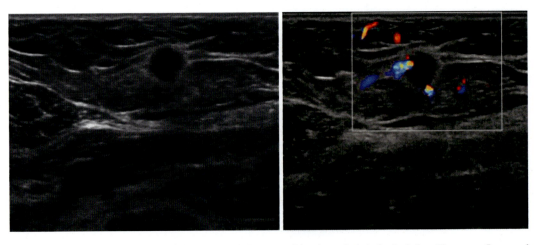

Fig. 97 Breast US (Nov. 2019): Spiculated hypoechoic mass with echogenic halo in the left axillary area. Increased vascularity is seen on color Doppler US

Neoadjuvant Chemotherapy
Neoadjuvant chemotherapy #4 cycles (Adriamycin & Cyclophosphamide).

Operation
Apr. 2020 Left axillary lymph node sampling and bilateral salpingo-oophorectomy.
　Pathology: Metastatic ductal carcinoma in one out of three axillary lymph nodes.
　Size of metastatic carcinoma: 6 mm.

	Result	Intensity	Positive %
Estrogen receptor	Intermediate (5/8)	2	10–1/3
Progesterone receptor	Negative (0/8)	0	0
C-erbB2	Negative (1+)		
Ki-67	Positive in 1% of tumor cells		

Adjuvant Therapy
Post-operative radiation therapy (axilla).

Liver Metastasis
May 2020 Liver MRI: r/o liver metastasis.
　See Fig. 98.

Palliative Therapy
Letrozole 2.5 mg/day + Palbociclib~

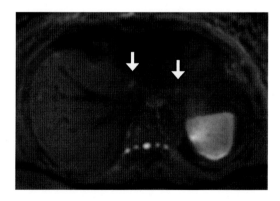

Fig. 98 Liver MRI (Oct. 2020): Two tiny lesions in the segment 2 of liver, showing hyperintensity on diffusion-weighted image

29　Case 29

29.1　Patient History and Progress

Female/41 years old, pre-menopause.
　No family history.

29.2　Courses of Treatment

Right breast cancer → Neoadjuvant chemotherapy → Operation → Adjuvant therapy → **Lung metastasis**.

29.2.1　Primary Treatment
See Fig. 99.

Neoadjuvant Chemotherapy
Neoadjuvant chemotherapy #4 cycles (Adriamycin + Cyclophosphamide) + zoladex.

	Result	Intensity	Positive %
Estrogen receptor	Strong (6/7)	3	1/3–2/3
Progesterone receptor	Strong (6/7)	3	1/3–2/3
C-erbB2	Negative (1+)		
Ki-67	N.A		

Clinical stage: cT3N1M0.

Operation
Oct. 2007 Right total mastectomy, axillary lymph node dissection.
　Pathology: Invasive ductal carcinoma, stage ypT2N0.
　Size of tumor: 2.5 cm, lymph node: 0/6.

	Result	Intensity	Positive %
Estrogen receptor	Strong (6/7)	3	1/3–2/3
Progesterone receptor	Weak (2/7)	1	<10%
C-erbB2	Negative (1+)		
Ki-67	Positive in 5% of tumor cells		

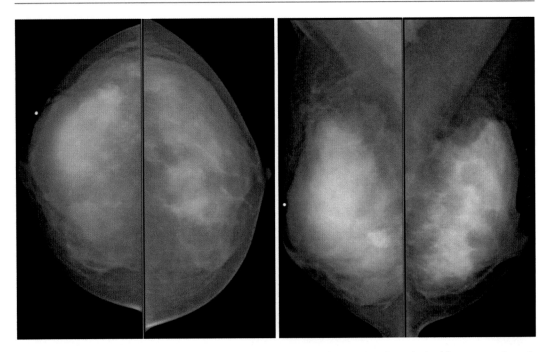

Fig. 99 Mammography (Jul. 2007): obscured irregular isodense mass (marked by BB marker) with punctate microcalcifications in the right upper outer quadrant

Adjuvant Therapy

Chemotherapy #4 cycles (Paclitaxel).

Post-operative radiation therapy +Tamoxifen 20 mg/day for 5 years +zoladex.

29.2.2 Treatments After Recurrence

See Fig. 100.

Aug. 2021 Right bronchus excision.

Pathology: Metastatic ductal carcinoma.

	Result	Intensity	Positive %
Estrogen receptor	Strong (8/8)	3	>2/3
Progesterone receptor	Strong (8/8)	3	>2/3
C-erbB2	Negative (0)		
Ki-67	Positive in 15% of tumor cells		

Aug. 2021 Chest CT:

LN enlargement, right interlobar and right lower paratracheal, metastasis.

Bronchovascular bundle thickening in RUL and centrilobular nodules in RLL, lymphangitic metastasis.

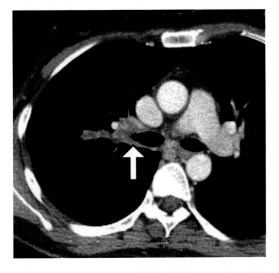

Fig. 100 Chest CT (Aug. 2021): Diffuse peribronchial infiltrates and bronchial wall thickening of right main bronchus

Palliative Therapy

Letrozole 2.5 mg/day + (ribociclib #1→ palbociclib~) + zoladex~

30 Case 30

30.1 Patient History and Progress

Female/50 years old, pre-menopause.
No family history.
Hepatitis B virus carrier, s/p myomectomy.

30.2 Courses of Treatment

Right breast cancer → Operation → Adjuvant therapy → **Bone metastasis**.
See Fig. 101.

30.2.1 Operation
Apr. 2017 Right nipple-areolar complex sparing mastectomy with immediate implant reconstruction, sentinel lymph node biopsy.
Pathology: Invasive duct carcinoma, stage T1c(2)N0(sn).
Size of tumor: 1.3 cm and 0.6 cm, lymph node: 0/2.

	Result	Intensity	Positive %
Estrogen receptor	Strong (7/8)	3	1/3–2/3
Progesterone receptor	Strong (7/8)	3	1/3–2/3
C-erbB2	Negative (0)		
Ki-67	Positive in 5% of tumor cells		

Adjuvant Therapy
Tamoxifen 20 mg/day.

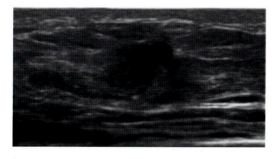

Fig. 101 Breast US (Mar. 2017): 1 cm indistinct irregular hypoechoic mass at the 9 o'clock direction of right breast

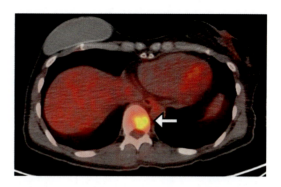

Fig. 102 PET-CT (Feb. 2021): Hypermetabolic bone lesion in 10th thoracic vertebral body, suggesting bony metastasis

30.2.2 Treatments After Recurrence
See Fig. 102.
Feb. 2021 PET-CT: bone metastasis at T10.

Palliative Therapy
Letrozole 2.5 mg/day + ribociclib ~

31 Case 31

31.1 Patient History and Progress

Female/54 years old, post-menopause.
No family history.
BRCA 1: positive for deleterious mutation.
S/p bilateral salpingo-oophorectomy.

31.2 Courses of Treatment

Right breast cancer → Operation → Adjuvant therapy → **Lung metastasis**.

31.2.1 Primary Treatment
See Fig. 103.

Operation
Mar. 2014 Right breast conserving surgery, sentinel lymph node biopsy.
Pathology: Invasive ductal carcinoma, stage pT2N0 (sn).
Size of tumor: 2.3 cm, lymph node: 0/1.

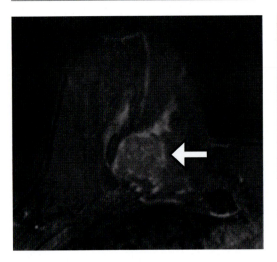

Fig. 103 Breast MRI (Mar. 2014): An irregular enhancing mass with associated non-mass enhancement at the 5–6 o'clock direction of right breast

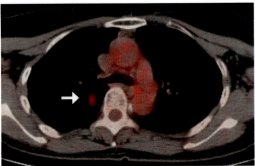

Fig. 104 PET-CT (May 2020): Focal hypermetabolic nodule in right upper lobe

	Result	Intensity	Positive %
Estrogen receptor	Negative (0/8)	0	0
Progesterone receptor	Negative (0/8)	0	0
C-erbB2	Negative (0)		
Ki-67	Positive in 85% of tumor cells		

Adjuvant Therapy

Adjuvant chemotherapy #6 cycles (Fluorouracil & Doxorubicin & Cyclophosphamide).

Post-operative radiation therapy to right breast.

Olaparib & placebo (clinical trial 0040, for 1 year).

Operation

Nov. 2014 Bilateral salpingo-oophorectomy (due to BRCA 1, positive for deleterious mutation).

31.2.2 Treatments After Recurrence

See Fig. 104.

Jun. 2020 Chest CT: R/O metastasis, nodule in right lung upper lobe.

Palliative Therapy

Paclitaxel & Atezolizumab & Ipatasertib & placebo (Jun. 2020 ~ Nov. 2021).

Atezolizumab (Nov. 2021) ~

32 Case 32

32.1 Patient History and Progress

Female/49 years old, peri-menopause.
No family history.

32.2 Courses of Treatment

Left breast cancer → Operation → Adjuvant therapy → **Lung metastasis**.

32.2.1 Primary Treatment

See Fig. 105.

Operation

Jan. 2007 Left breast conserving surgery, sentinel lymph node biopsy.

Pathology: Invasive ductal carcinoma, stage pT2N0 (sn).

Size of tumor: 3.2 cm, lymph node: 0/5.

	Result	Intensity	Positive %
Estrogen receptor	Intermediate (4/7)	2	10%–1/3
Progesterone receptor	Strong (6/7)	3	1/3–2/3–
C-erbB2	Positive (3+)		
Ki-67	Positive in 20% of tumor cells		

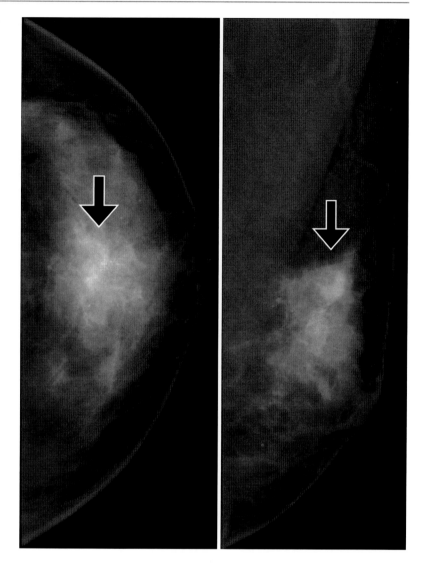

Fig. 105 Mammography (Jan. 2007): Indistinct irregular hyperdense mass with fine pleomorphic microcalcifications at the 12 o'clock direction of left breast on left CC and MLO views

Adjuvant Therapy

Adjuvant chemotherapy # 6 cycles (Fluorouracil & Doxorubicin & Cyclophosphamide).

Post-operative radiation therapy to left breast + Zoladex for 2 years + Tamoxifen 20 mg/day for 5 years.

32.2.2 Treatments After Recurrence

See Fig. 106.

Jul. 2015 Right lung, middle lobe, percutaneous biopsy.

Pathology: Metastatic ductal carcinoma.

	Result	Intensity	Positive %
Estrogen receptor	Strong (7/8)	3	1/3–2/3
Progesterone receptor	Strong (8/8)	3	>2/3
C-erbB2	Positive (3+)		
Ki-67	Positive in 14% of tumor cells		

Palliative Therapy

Palliative therapy # 37 cycles (Paclitaxel & Trastuzumab).

Palliative therapy # 38 cycles (Trastuzumab) ~

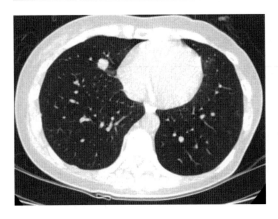

Fig. 106 Chest CT (Jul. 2015): A round nodule in right middle lobe, suggesting pulmonary metastasis

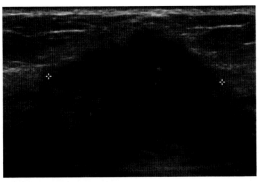

Fig. 107 Breast US (Jun. 2007): Irregular hypoechoic mass with microcalcifications at the 9 o'clock direction of right breast

33 Case 33

33.1 Patient History and Progress

Female/52 years old, peri-menopause.
No family history.

33.2 Courses of Treatment

Right breast cancer → Operation → Adjuvant therapy → **Bone metastasis**.

33.2.1 Primary Treatment
See Fig. 107.

Operation
Jul. 2007 Right modified radical mastectomy at another hospital.
Pathology: Invasive ductal carcinoma, stage pT2N3a.
Size of tumor: 2.7 × 1.4 cm, lymph node: 13/38.

	Result	Intensity	Positive %
Estrogen receptor	Strong (8/8)	3	>2/3
Progesterone receptor	Intermediate (5/8)	2	10%–1/3
C-erbB2	Equivocal (2+)		
Ki-67	Positive in 7% of tumor cells		
SISH	Positive		

Adjuvant Therapy
Adjuvant chemotherapy #8 cycles (Doxorubicin & cyclophosphamide #4 → Docetaxel #4).
Post-operative radiation therapy to right breast +Tamoxifen 20 mg/day for 5 years.

33.2.2 Treatments After Recurrence
See Fig. 108.
Mar. 2018 PET-CT: R/O multiple bone metastasis in T8, T9, L2, L4, L5, sacrum, both pelvic bones, right proximal femur.

Palliative Therapy
Palliative chemotherapy #15 cycles (Pertuzumab & Trastuzumab & docetaxel).
Concurrent Bretra +zoladex (Sep. 2018 ~ Mar. 2019): Progressive disease.
Palliative chemotherapy #38 cycles (T-DM1).
May 2021 Chest CT: T8, spinal canal invasion.

Palliative Therapy
Radiation therapy to L-spine & T-spine & sacrum.
Palliative Capecitabine & lapatinib (Jul. 2021) ~

Metastatic Breast Cancer

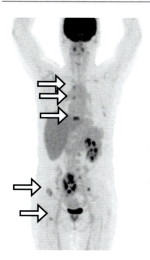
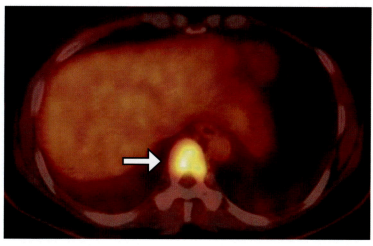

Fig. 108 PET-CT (Mar. 2018): Multifocal increased uptake in thoracic and lumbar spines, sacrum, both pelvic bones and right proximal femur, suggesting multiple bony metastases and hypermetabolic bone lesion in 9th thoracic vertebral body, suggesting bony metastasis

34 Case 34

34.1 Patient History and Progress

Female/42 years old, peri-menopause.
No family history.

34.2 Courses of Treatment

Left breast cancer → Operation → Adjuvant therapy → **Right pleural, liver, right adrenal gland, bone metastasis → Brain metastasis**.

34.2.1 Primary Treatment
See Fig. 109.

Operation
Feb. 2014 Left breast conserving surgery, sentinel lymph node biopsy.
Pathology: Invasive ductal carcinoma, stage pT2N1a (sn), size of tumor: 2.5 cm, lymph node: 1/4 (2.5 mm).

	Result	Intensity	Positive %
Estrogen receptor	Negative (0/8)	0	0
Progesterone receptor	Negative (0/8)	0	0
C-erbB2	Equivocal (2+)		
Ki-67	Positive in 46% of tumor cells		
SISH	Positive		

Adjuvant Therapy
Adjuvant chemotherapy #8 cycles (Doxorubicin & cyclophosphamide #4 → Docetaxel & trastuzumab #4).
Post-operative radiation therapy to left breast.
Concurrent Trastuzumab #13.

34.2.2 Treatments After Recurrence
See Fig. 110.
Feb. 2021 Chest CT: Metastasis to right pleural, liver, right adrenal gland, bone.

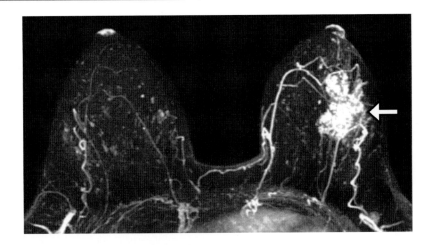

Fig. 109 Breast MRI (Feb. 2014): Irregular heterogeneous enhancing mass at the 12–3 o'clock direction of left breast

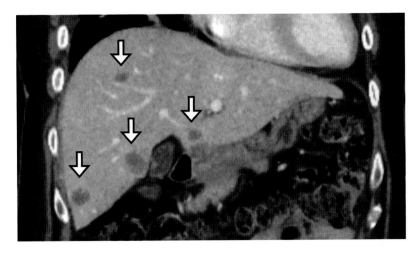

Fig. 110 Liver CT (Mar. 2021): Hypoattenuating masses in the liver, suggesting metastases

Palliative Therapy

Palliative therapy: Zanidatamab + Docetaxel (Mar. 2021 ~ Aug. 2021) →Zanidatamab mono (Sep. 2021 ~ Nov. 2021).

Dec. 2021 Brain MRI> r/o tiny metastasis to brain.

Palliative Therapy

Radiation therapy to brain.

Palliative therapy #6 (Pertuzumab & trastuzumab & Docetaxel) ~

35 Case 35

35.1 Patient History and Progress

Female/51 years old, pre-menopause.

No family history.

S/p hysterectomy & Left salpingo-oophorectomy (benign), s/p total hip replacement arthroplasty.

35.2 Courses of Treatment

Right breast cancer → Operation → Adjuvant therapy → **Bone metastasis**.

35.2.1 Primary Treatment

See Fig. 111.

Operation

Dec. 2013 Right breast conserving surgery, axillary lymph node dissection.

Fig. 111 Breast MRI (Dec. 2013): Segmental heterogeneous non-mass enhancement at the 9–10 o'clock direction of right breast

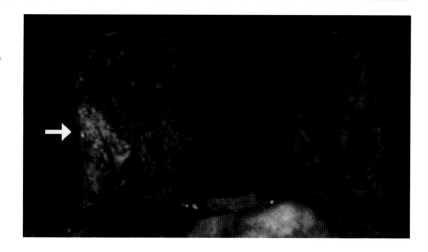

Pathology: Invasive ductal carcinoma, stage pT1bN1a.

Size of tumor: 0.8 cm, 0.5 × 0.3 cm, lymph node: 1/6 (8 mm).

	Result	Intensity	Positive %
Estrogen receptor	Strong (8/8)	3	>2/3
Progesterone receptor	Negative (0/8)	0	0
C-erbB2	Negative (1+)		
Ki-67	Positive in 16% of tumor cells		

Oncotype Dx test: 23 (Recurrence Score).

Adjuvant Therapy
Post-operative radiation therapy to right breast zoladex for 2 years +Tamoxifen 20 mg/day for 5 years.

35.2.2 Treatments After Recurrence
See Figs. 112 and 113.

Sep. 2017 PET-CT: R/o metastasis to C2 vertebra.

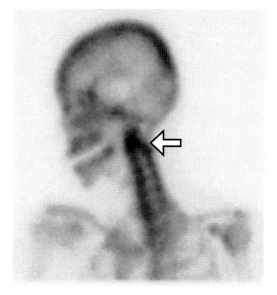

Fig. 112 Bone scan (Sep. 2017): Increased uptake in the upper C-spine

Palliative Therapy
Bilateral salpingo-oophorectomy.

Radiation therapy to C-spine + Letrozole & Palbociclib & zometa (2017-11-03~).

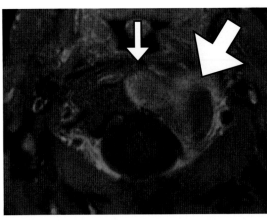
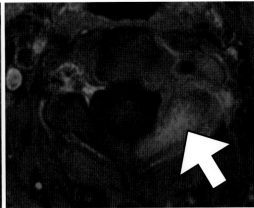

Fig. 113 C-spine MRI (Sep. 2017): Infiltrative enhancing lesion in the C2 vertebra vertebral body and left lateral arc, suggesting bony metastasis

36 Case 36

36.1 Patient History and Progress

Female/55 years old, post-menopause.
No family history.
S/p bilateral salpingo-oophorectomy, diabetes mellitus.

36.2 Courses of Treatment

Right breast cancer → Operation → Adjuvant therapy → **Lung metastasis**.

36.2.1 Primary Treatment
See Fig. 114.

Operation
Sep. 2008 Right breast conserving surgery, axillary lymph node dissection.
Pathology: Invasive ductal carcinoma, stage pT2N1a.
Size of tumor 2.3 cm, lymph node: 1/15 (5 mm).

	Result	Intensity	Positive %
Estrogen receptor	Strong (7/7)	3	>2/3
Progesterone receptor	Intermediate (5/7)	2	1/3–2/3

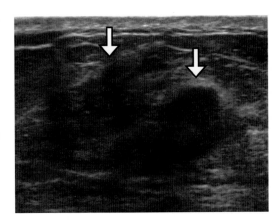

Fig. 114 Breast US (Sep. 2008): Indistinct heterogeneous echoic mass at the 12 o'clock direction of right breast

	Result	Intensity	Positive %
C-erbB2	Equivocal (2+)		
Ki-67	Positive in 10% of tumor cells		
SISH	Negative		

Adjuvant Therapy
Adjuvant chemotherapy #8 cycles (Doxorubicin & cyclophosphamide #4 → Docetaxel #4).
Post-operation radiation to right breast + Tamoxifen 20 mg/day for 5 years.

36.2.2 Treatments After Recurrence
See Fig. 115.

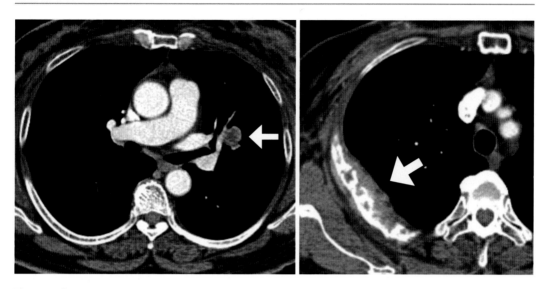

Fig. 115 CT chest (Jul. 2017): Hypodense nodule in left upper lobe, suggesting metastasis and bone metastasis, right 4th rib

Jul. 2017 PET-CT: R/O metastasis to left lung lobe and right 3rd rib & 4th rib.

Aug. 2017 Left lung, upper lobe, percutaneous biopsy: Metastatic ductal carcinoma.

	Result	Intensity	Positive %
Estrogen receptor	Strong (8/8)	3	>2/3
Progesterone receptor	Intermediate (6/8)	2	1/3–2/3
C-erbB2	Negative (0)		
Ki-67	Positive in 22% of tumor cells		

Palliative Therapy

Clinical trial: Capecitabine #19: Progressive disease.

Nov. 2018 Bilateral salpingo-oophorectomy.

Palliative therapy: Letrozole +Palbociclib (Dec. 2018) ~

37 Case 37

37.1 Patient History and Progress

Female/59 years old, post-menopause.
No family history.

Hypertension, s/p right vertebral artery, transient ischemic attack.

37.2 Courses of Treatment

Right breast cancer → Operation → Adjuvant therapy → **Lung metastasis**.

37.2.1 Primary Treatment
See Fig. 116.

Operation

May 2013 Right breast conserving surgery, axillary lymph node dissection.

Pathology: Invasive ductal carcinoma, stage pT2N1a.

Size of tumor: 2.0 cm, lymph node: 3/30 (15 mm).

	Result	Intensity	Positive %
Estrogen receptor	Intermediate (6/8)	2	1/3–2/3
Progesterone receptor	Intermediate (6/8)	2	1/3–2/3
C-erbB2	Positive (3+)		
Ki-67	Positive in 27% of tumor cells		

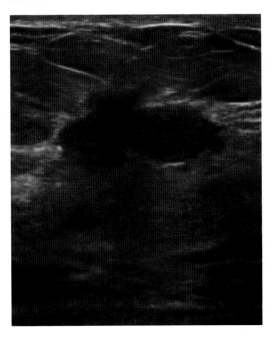

Fig. 116 Breast US (May 2013): Irregular hypoechoic mass with angular margin at the 11 o'clock direction of right breast

Adjuvant Therapy
Adjuvant chemotherapy #8 cycles (Doxorubicin & cyclophosphamide #4 → Docetaxel & trastuzumab #4).

Post-operative radiation therapy to right breast.

Concurrent Trastuzumab # 4 + Tamoxifen 20 mg/day for 85 days.

37.2.2 Treatments After Recurrence
See Figs. 117 and 118.

Feb. 2014 PET>R/O metastasis to lung, lymph node, and right pleural effusion.

Palliative Therapy
Palliative therapy: Letrozole & trastuzumab (Feb. 2014) ~

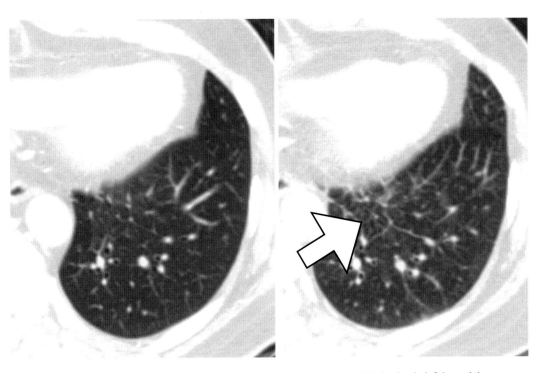

Fig. 117 Chest CT (Aug. 2013, Feb. 2014): Newly developed interlobular septal thickening in left lower lobe, suggesting lymphangitic metastasis

Metastatic Breast Cancer

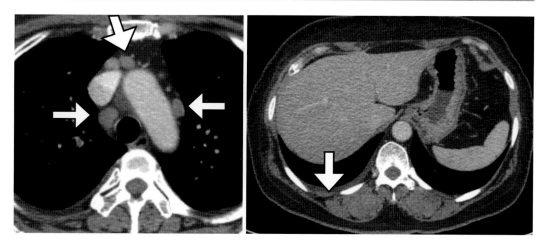

Fig. 118 Chest CT (Feb. 2014): Enlarged mediastinal LNs, suggesting metastases and right malignant pleural effusion

38 Case 38

38.1 Patient History and Progress

Female/70 years old, post-menopause.
No family history.

38.2 Courses of Treatment

Both breasts cancer → Operation → Adjuvant therapy → **Liver metastasis**.

38.2.1 Primary Treatment
See Figs. 119 and 120.

Operation
Dec. 2008 Bilateral breast conserving surgery, axillary lymph node dissection.
Pathology:
Right breast> Invasive ductal carcinoma, stage pT2N2a, size of tumor: 4.5 cm, lymph node: 6/9 (12 mm).

	Result	Intensity	Positive %
Estrogen receptor	Weak(2/7)	1	<10%
Progesterone receptor	Negative (0/7)	0	0

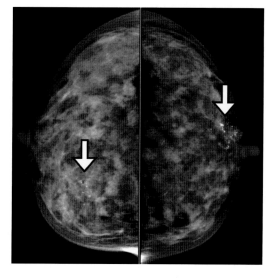

Fig. 119 Mammography (Dec. 2008): Grouped fine pleomorphic microcalcifications in right inner breast and the subareolar area of left breast

	Result	Intensity	Positive %
C-erbB2	Positive (3+)		
Ki-67	Positive in 15% of tumor cells		

Left breast> Ductal carcinoma in situ, stage pTisN0, size of tumor: 2.0 cm, lymph node: 0/7.

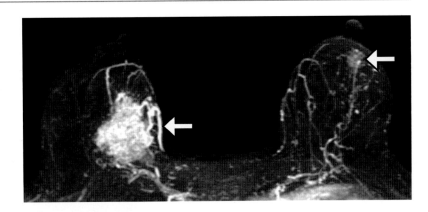

Fig. 120 Breast MRI (Dec. 2008): Irregular heterogeneous enhancing mass at the 1–3 o'clock direction of right breast and irregular homogeneous enhancing mass in the subareolar area of left breast

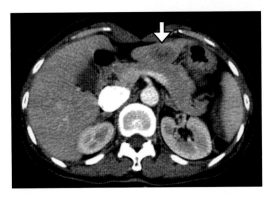

Fig. 121 Liver CT (Sep. 2011): Hypoattenuating mass in the lateral segment of liver, suggesting metastasis

	Result	Intensity	Positive %
Estrogen receptor	Negative (0/7)	0	0
Progesterone receptor	Negative (0/7)	0	0
C-erbB2	Positive(3+)		
Ki-67	Positive in 5% of tumor cells		

Adjuvant Therapy

Adjuvant chemotherapy #8 cycles (Doxorubicin & cyclophosphamide #4 → Docetaxel #4).

Post-operative radiation therapy to right breast & supraclavicular lymph node + Letrozole for 5 years, concurrent Trastuzumab #18.

38.2.2 Treatments After Recurrence

See Fig. 121.

Aug. 2011 PET> R/O metastasis to liver.

Palliative Therapy

Palliative therapy (clinical trial): Trastuzumab & Paclitaxel (Sep. 2011~ Mar. 2012).

Trastuzumab mono (Mar. 2012~ Oct. 2019): Partial response (end of treatment).

39 Case 39

39.1 Patient History and Progress

Female/51 years old, peri-menopause.
No family history.
BRCA 1 & 2 mutation: Not detected.
Hepatitis B virus carrier, hypertension.

39.2 Courses of Treatment

Right breast cancer → Neoadjuvant chemotherapy → Operation → Adjuvant therapy → **Left breast and lung metastasis**.

39.2.1 Primary Treatment

See Fig. 122.

Jul. 2007 Outside slide review > Right infiltrating duct carcinoma.

Neoadjuvant Chemotherapy

Neoadjuvant chemotherapy #4 cycles (Doxorubicin & cyclophosphamide #4).

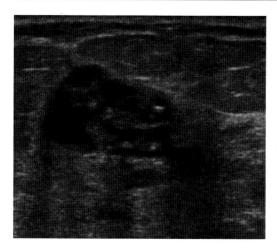

Fig. 122 Breast US (Jul. 2007): Microlobulated hypoechoic mass with microcalcifications at the 12 o'clock direction of right breast

Operation
Oct. 2007 Right breast conserving surgery, sentinel lymph node biopsy.

Pathology: Invasive ductal carcinoma, stage ypT1cN0 (sn).

Size of tumor: 1.5 × 1.0 cm, lymph node 0/1.

	Result	Intensity	Positive %
Estrogen receptor	Negative(0/7)	0	0
Progesterone receptor	Negative(0/7)	0	0
C-erbB2	Equivocal (2+)		
Ki-67	Positive in 10% of tumor cells		
SISH	Negative		

Adjuvant Therapy
Post-operative radiation to right breast.

39.2.2 Treatments After Recurrence
See Fig. 123.

Feb. 2021 Left 12 o'clock biopsy: Invasive ductal carcinoma.

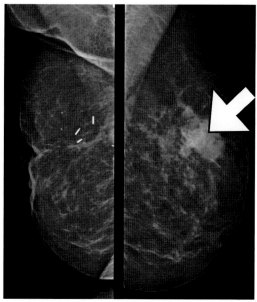

Fig. 123 Mammography (Feb. 2021): Irregular hyperdense mass in the upper portion of left breast

Left axillary lymph node biopsy: Metastatic ductal carcinoma.

	Result	Intensity	Positive %
Estrogen receptor	Negative (0/8)	0	0
Progesterone receptor	Negative(0/8)	0	0
C-erbB2	Positive (3+)		
Ki-67	Positive in 43% of tumor cells		

See Fig. 124.

Mar. 2021 PET-CT> R/O metastasis to lung, left supraclavicular lymph node & lower neck.

Palliative Therapy
Palliative therapy (clinical trial): Zanidatamab + Docetaxel (Apr. 2021~ Sep. 2021).

Zanidatamab mono (Sep. 2021) ~

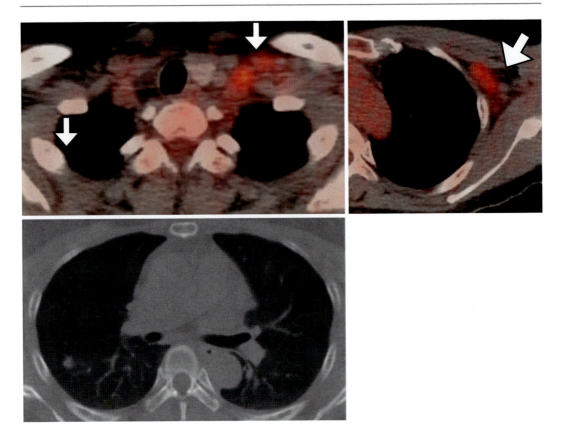

Fig. 124 PET-CT (Mar. 2021): Hypermetabolic activity in the left supraclavicular lymph nodes, and left axillary lymph nodes and nodule in right upper lobe, suggesting pulmonary metastasis

40 Case 40

40.1 Patient History and Progress

Female/54 years old, post-menopause.
  No family history.
  S/p bilateral salpingo-oophorectomy.

40.2 Courses of Treatment

Right breast cancer → Neoadjuvant chemotherapy → Operation → Adjuvant therapy → **Lung metastasis**.

40.2.1 Primary Treatment
See Fig. 125.

Oct. 2014 Outside slide review> Right invasive ductal carcinoma.

Right axillary lymph node, metastatic ductal carcinoma.

	Result	Intensity	Positive %
Estrogen receptor	Strong (8/8)	3	>2/3
Progesterone receptor	Strong (8/8)	3	>2/3
C-erbB2	Negative (0)		
Ki-67	Positive in 76% of tumor cells		

Neoadjuvant Chemotherapy
Neoadjuvant chemotherapy #8 cycles (Doxorubicin & cyclophosphamide #4 → Docetaxel #4).

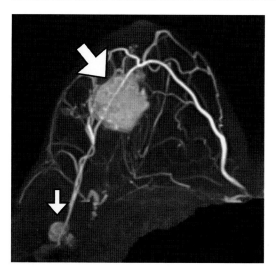

Fig. 125 Breast MRI (Oct. 2014): Irregular homogeneous enhancing mass in right upper outer quadrant. Enlarged lymph nodes in right axillary area, suggesting metastasis

Operation
Apr. 2015 Right breast conserving surgery, axillary lymph node dissection.

Pathology: Invasive ductal carcinoma, stage ypT1cN1mi.

Size of tumor: 1.4 cm, lymph node 2/9 (2 mm).

Adjuvant Therapy
Post-operative radiation to right breast + Tamoxifen 20 mg/day for 2 years.

40.2.2 Treatments After Recurrence
See Fig. 126.

Jun. 2017 PET-CT> R/O metastasis in right lung lobe.

Palliative Therapy
Clinical trial: Capecitabine # 30 cycles: Progressive disease.

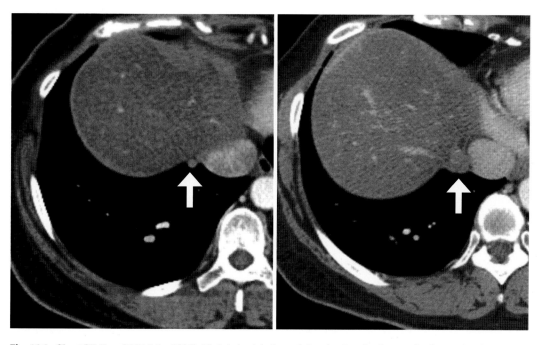

Fig. 126 Chest CT (Jun. 2017, May 2019): Nodule in right lower lobe, abutting diaphragmatic pleura, showing interval increase in size

Jun. 2019 Bilateral salpingo-oophorectomy.
Palliative therapy: Letrozole + Palbociclib (Jul. 2019) ~

41 Case 41

41.1 Patient History and Progress

Female/52 years old, peri-menopause.
  No family history.
  S/p Tuberculosis.

41.2 Courses of Treatment

Left breast cancer → Operation → Adjuvant therapy → Lung, liver, and bone metastasis.

41.2.1 Primary Treatment
See Fig. 127.

Operation
Nov. 2015 Left breast conserving surgery.

Pathology: Invasive ductal carcinoma, stage pT2N2a.
Size of tumor: 2.4 cm, lymph node: 5/12 (11 mm).

	Result	Intensity	Positive %
Estrogen receptor	Strong (7/8)	3	1/3–2/3
Progesterone receptor	weak (4/8)	2	1–10%
C-erbB2	Positive (+3)		
Ki-67	Positive in 19% of tumor cells		

Adjuvant Therapy
Adjuvant chemotherapy # 8 cycles (Doxorubicin & cyclophosphamide #4 → Docetaxel & Trastuzumab #4).
Post-operative radiation to left breast + Tamoxifen 20 mg/day for 2.5 years.
Concurrent Trastuzumab # 14.

41.2.2 Treatments After Recurrence
See Figs. 128 and 129.
Oct. 2018 PET-CT> R/O multiple metastasis in both lungs, bone, and liver.

Palliative Therapy
Palliative therapy # 23 cycles (Docetaxel & Trastuzumab & Pertuzumab).
Feb. 2020 Brain MRI> Metastasis in brain.

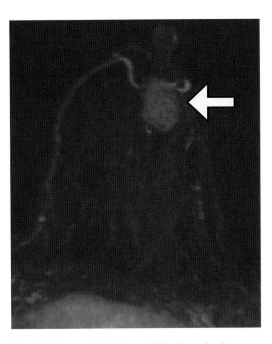

Fig. 127 Breast MRI (Oct. 2015): Irregular homogeneous enhancing mass at the 1 o'clock direction of left breast

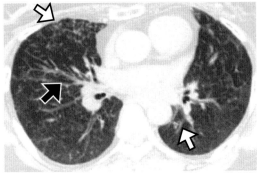

Fig. 128 Chest CT (Sep. 2018): Interlobular septal line thickening and bronchovascular bundle thickening (black arrow), tiny nodules (white arrows) in bilateral lungs, suggesting hematolymphangitic metastasis

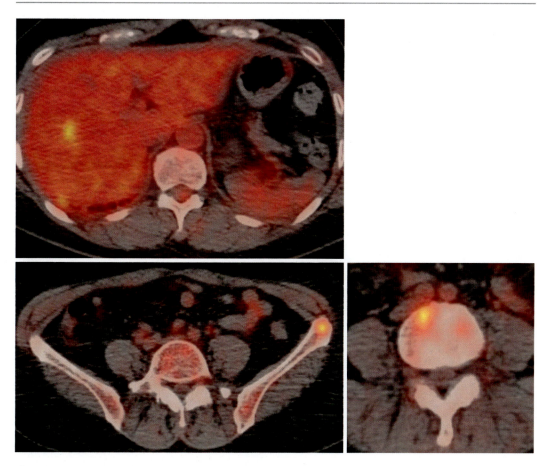

Fig. 129 PET-CT (Oct. 2018): Hypermetabolic activity in the liver, suggesting hepatic metastasis and hypermetabolic activity in the left ilium and 4th lumbar vertebral body, suggesting body metastases

Palliative Therapy
Radiation to whole brain.

Palliative therapy # 11 cycles (Lapatinib & Capecitabine): Progressive disease.

Palliative therapy # 4 cycles (Trastuzumab emtansine).

42 Case 42

42.1 Patient History and Progress

Female/57 years old, post-menopause.
No family history.
Arrhythmia (taking on medicine).

42.2 Courses of Treatment

Left breast cancer → Operation → Adjuvant therapy → **Lung metastasis**.

42.2.1 Primary Treatment
See Fig. 130.

Operation
Jun. 2008 Left breast conserving surgery, sentinel lymph node biopsy.

Pathology: Invasive ductal carcinoma, stage pT1aN0 (sn).

Size of tumor: 0.6 cm, 0.5 × 0.3 cm, lymph node: 0/2.

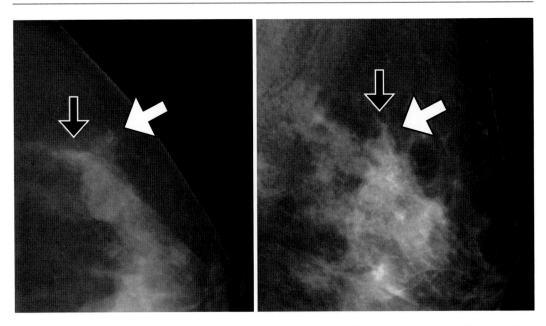

Fig. 130 Mammography (May 2008): Irregular isodense mass (white arrow) and regional microcalcifications (black arrow) in left upper outer quadrant

	Result	Intensity	Positive %
Estrogen receptor	Strong (6/7)	3	1/3–2/3
Progesterone receptor	Strong (7/7)	3	>2/3
C-erbB2	Equivocal (2+)		
Ki-67	Positive in 5% of tumor cells		
FISH	Negative		

Adjuvant Therapy

Adjuvant chemotherapy #6 cycles (Fluorouracil-5 & Doxorubicin & Cyclophosphamide).

Post-operation radiation to left breast + Tamoxifen 20 mg/day for 5 years.

42.2.2 Treatments After Recurrence

See Fig. 131.

Mar. 2021 Pleural fluid, cytology: Metastatic carcinoma.

Palliative Therapy

Palliative therapy: Letrozole & Ribociclib (Jan. 2021 ~ Mar. 2021).

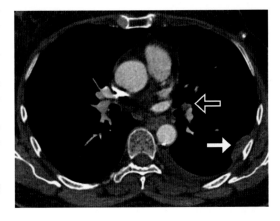

Fig. 131 Chest CT (Jan. 2021): Hypoattenuating pleural nodule (white arrow) in left lower lobe and enlargement of left interlobar lymph node (black arrow), suggesting pleural and lymph node metastasis

Palliative therapy: Letrozole & Palbociclib (Mar. 2021 ~ Dec. 2021).

Palliative therapy: Capecitabine # 3 (Feb. 2022 ~ Mar. 2022): Progressive disease.

Palliative therapy: Paclitaxel & Cisplatin (Apr. 2022) ~

43 Case 43

43.1 Patient History and Progress

Female/54 years old, post-menopause.
Family history of breast cancer, sister.
BRCA 1 & 2 mutation: Not detected.
S/p bilateral salpingo-oophorectomy.

	Result	Intensity	Positive %
Estrogen receptor	Strong (7/7)	3	>2/3
Progesterone receptor	Strong (7/7)	3	>2/3
C-erbB2	Negative (1+)		
Ki-67	Positive in 8% of tumor cells		

43.2 Courses of Treatment

Right breast cancer → Operation → Adjuvant therapy → **Brain metastasis**.

43.2.1 Primary Treatment
See Fig. 132.

Operation
Jun. 2012 Right breast conserving surgery, sentinel lymph node biopsy.
Pathology: Invasive ductal carcinoma, stage pT1cN0 (sn).
Size of tumor: 1.5 cm, lymph node: 0/2.

Adjuvant Therapy
Post-operation radiation to right breast + Tamoxifen 20 mg/day for 3 years.
Concurrent Zoladex for 1 year.

43.2.2 Treatments After Recurrence
See Fig. 133.
Jun. 2015 Brain MRI> R/O metastasis in leptomeningeal.
Jun. 2015 Cerebrospinal fluid cytology: Atypical cells.

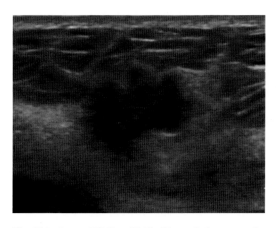

Fig. 132 Breast US (Jun. 2012): Hypoechoic mass at the 10 o'clock direction of right breast

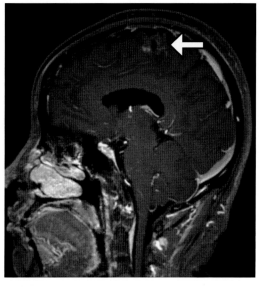

Fig. 133 Brain MRI (Jun. 2015): Small acute hemorrhagic lesion with dense leptomeningeal enhancement in left superior frontal gyrus, suggesting leptomeningeal metastasis with focal cortical hemorrhage

Palliative Therapy

Jul. 2015 Bilateral salpingo-oophorectomy.
  Palliative therapy: Letrozole (Jul. 2015) ~

44 Case 44

44.1 Patient History and Progress

Female/49 years old, post-menopause.
  No family history.
  S/p bilateral salpingo-oophorectomy.

44.2 Courses of Treatment

Right breast cancer with bone metastasis →
Palliative therapy.
  See Fig. 134.
  See Fig. 135.

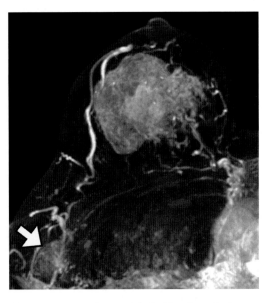

Fig. 134 Breast MRI (Jan. 2018): Huge irregular heterogeneous enhancing mass in right breast. Enlarged lymph nodes (white arrow) in the right axillary area, suggesting metastases

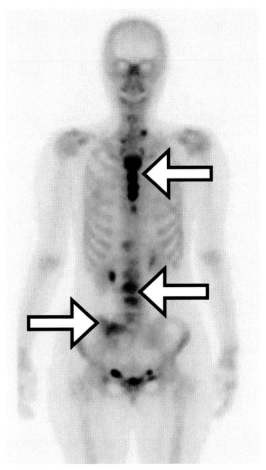

Fig. 135 Bone scan (May 2018): Multifocal increased uptake in sternum, lumbar vertebral bodies, and right pelvic bone, suggesting bony metastases

Right invasive ductal carcinoma, stage IV (metastasis in bone).

	Result	Intensity	Positive %
Estrogen receptor	Strong (8/8)	3	>2/3
Progesterone receptor	Negative (0/8)	0	0
C-erbB2	Negative (1+)		
Ki-67	Positive in 57% of tumor cells		

44.2.1 Palliative Therapy

Feb. 2018 Bilateral salpingo-oophorectomy.

Palliative therapy: Letrozole & Palbociclib # 16: Progressive disease.

Jul. 2019 Palliative operation: Right nipple-sparing mastectomy, axillary lymph node dissection.

Pathology: Invasive ductal carcinoma, stage ypT1cN1a.

Size of tumor: 2.0 cm, lymph node: 3/7 (2 mm).

	Result	Intensity	Positive %
Estrogen receptor	Strong (7/8)	3	1/3–2/3
Progesterone receptor	Negative(0/8)	0	0
C-erbB2	Equivocal (2+)		
Ki-67	Positive in 66% of tumor cells		
SISH	Negative		

Palliative therapy: Capecitabine (Sep. 2019 ~ Dec. 2019): Progressive disease.

See Fig. 136.

Jan. 2020 Liver biopsy: Metastatic ductal carcinoma.

	Result	Intensity	Positive %
Estrogen receptor	Strong (8/8)	3	>2/3
Progesterone receptor	Weak (4/8)	2	1–10%
C-erbB2	Negative (1+)		
Ki-67	Positive in 2% of tumor cells		

Palliative therapy: DS-8201aU 303 # 8: Progressive disease (liver).

Concurrent proton therapy: radiation to liver.

Palliative therapy: Albumin-bound Paclitaxel # 8: Progressive disease.

Palliative therapy: Fluorouracil-5 & Doxorubicin & cyclophosphamide # 5.

Palliative therapy: Eribulin.

Dec. 2021 Death.

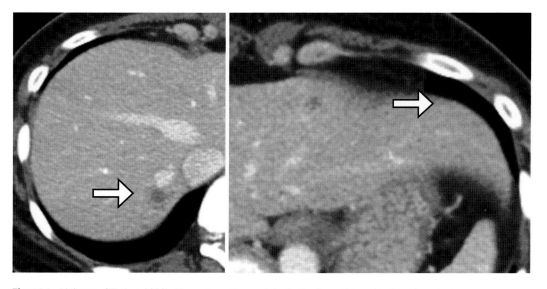

Fig. 136 Abdomen CT (Jan. 2020): Hypoattenuating nodules in the liver, suggesting hepatic metastases

45 Case 45

45.1 Patient History and Progress

Female/49 years old, pre-menopause.
No family history.

45.2 Courses of Treatment

Left breast cancer with lung and bone metastasis → Palliative therapy.
See Figs. 137, 138, and 139.
Left invasive ductal carcinoma, stage IV (metastasis in lung, bone).

	Result	Intensity	Positive %
Estrogen receptor	Strong (8/8)	3	>2/3
Progesterone receptor	Negative (2/8)	1	<1%
C-erbB2	Equivocal (2+)		
Ki-67	Positive		

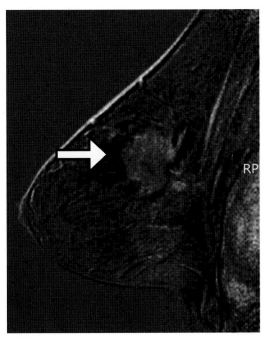

Fig. 137 Breast MRI (Jun. 2013): Irregular heterogeneous enhancing mass at the 12 o'clock direction of left breast

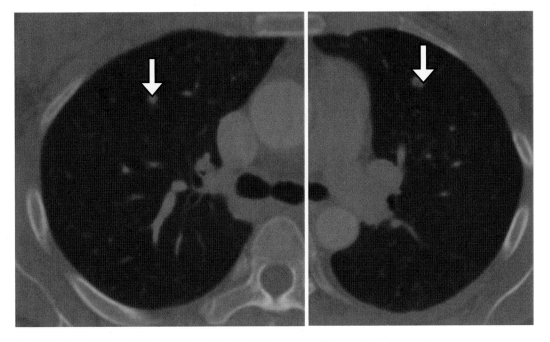

Fig. 138 Chest CT (Jun. 2013): Multiple nodules in both lungs, suggesting pulmonary metastases

Metastatic Breast Cancer

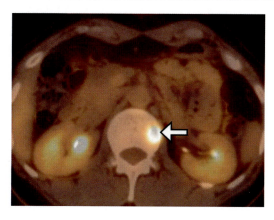

Fig. 139 PET-CT (Jun. 2013): Hypermetabolic activity in the 1st lumbar vertebral body, suggesting bony metastasis

Palliative therapy: Paclitaxel & Trastuzumab # 24.

Dec. 2014 Left breast conserving surgery, sentinel lymph node biopsy.

Pathology: Invasive ductal carcinoma, stage ypT2N0 (sn).

Size of tumor: 2.3 cm, lymph node: 0/2.

	Result	Intensity	Positive %
Estrogen receptor	Weak (4/8)	2	1–10%
Progesterone receptor	Negative (0/8)	0	0
C-erbB2	Negative (0)		
Ki-67	Positive in 8% of tumor cells		

Palliative therapy: fluorouracil & Doxorubicin & cyclophosphamide # 6.

Post-op radiation to left breast & subclavicular lymph node + Tamoxifen 20 mg/day (Apr. 2015 ~ Jul. 2018).

Jul. 2018 Chest CT> increased nodule in lung, hepatic metastasis.

Palliative therapy: Trastuzumab emtansine # 5 cycles: Progressive disease.

Palliative therapy: Lapatinib & Capecitabine # 39 cycles: Progressive disease.

Palliative therapy: Gemcitabine & Cisplatin (Feb. 2021) ~

46 Case 46

46.1 Patient History and Progress

Female/61 years old, post-menopause.
  No family history.
  s/p appendectomy, hypertension.

46.2 Courses of Treatment

Right breast cancer with bone metastasis → Palliative therapy.
See Figs. 140 and 141.

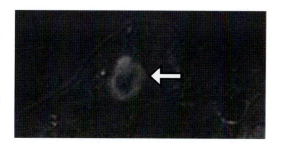

Fig. 140 Breast MRI (Jan. 2019): Irregular rim enhancing mass at the 7 o'clock direction of right breast

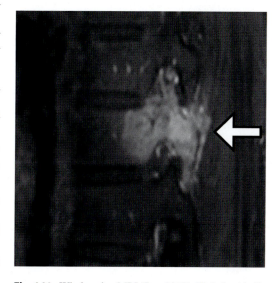

Fig. 141 Whole spine MRI (Jan. 2019): Ill-defined infiltrative bony enhancing lesion in the vertebral body and post arc of the 10th thoracic vertebra, suggesting bony metastasis

Right invasive ductal carcinoma, Stage IV (R/O metastasis in bone, T-spine 10).

	Result	Intensity	Positive %
Estrogen receptor	Strong (8/8)	3	>2/3
Progesterone receptor	Strong (8/8)	3	>2/3
C-erbB2	Equivocal (2+)		
Ki-67	Positive in 43% of tumor cells		
SISH	Negative		

Palliative therapy: Letrozole & Palbociclib # 29.

Dec. 2021 Right breast conserving surgery, sentinel lymph node biopsy.

Pathology: Invasive ductal carcinoma, stage ypT1bN0 (sn).

Size of tumor: 0.9 cm, lymph node: 0/2.

	Result	Intensity	Positive %
Estrogen receptor	Negative (0/8)	0	0
Progesterone receptor	Negative (0/8)	0	0
C-erbB2	Positive (3+)		
Ki-67	Positive in 34% of tumor cells		

Palliative chemotherapy #4 cycles (Doxorubicin & Cyclophosphamide).

Post-op radiation to right breast & T-spine 10.

47 Case 47

47.1 Patient History and Progress

Female/46 years old, pre-menopause.
No family history.

47.2 Courses of Treatment

Right breast cancer → Neoadjuvant chemotherapy → Operation → Adjuvant therapy → **Ipsilateral breast recurrence** → **Lung metastasis**.

47.2.1 Primary Treatment

See Fig. 142.

Feb. 2012 Outside slide review> Left invasive ductal carcinoma.

	Result	Intensity	Positive %
Estrogen receptor	Negative (0/8)	0	0
Progesterone receptor	Negative 0/8)	0	0
C-erbB2	Positive (3+)		
Ki-67	Positive in 5% of tumor cells		

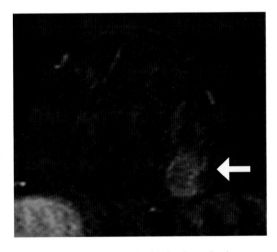

Fig. 142 Breast MRI (Feb. 2013): Irregular heterogeneous enhancing mass in the left upper outer quadrant

Neoadjuvant Chemotherapy
Neoadjuvant chemotherapy #8 cycles (Doxorubicin + cyclophosphamide #4 → Docetaxel + Trastuzumab #4).

Operation
Aug. 2013 Left breast conserving surgery, sentinel lymph node biopsy.
Pathology: Ductal carcinoma in situ (residual), stage yp TisN0 (sn).
Size of tumor: up to 0.5 cm, lymph node: 0/3.

	Result	Intensity	Positive %
Estrogen receptor	Negative (0/8)	0	0
Progesterone receptor	Negative 0/8	0	0
C-erbB2	Positive (3+)		
Ki-67	Positive in 19% of tumor cells		

Adjuvant Therapy
Post-operative radiation to left breast & subclavicular lymph node.
Concurrent Trastuzumab # 18.

47.2.2 Treatments After Recurrence

Ipsilateral Breast Recurrence
See Fig. 143.
Apr. 2016 Left breast biopsy> Invasive ductal carcinoma.

	Result	Intensity	Positive %
Estrogen receptor	Negative (0/8)	0	0
Progesterone receptor	Negative 0/8	0	0
C-erbB2	Positive (3+)		
Ki-67	Positive in 84% of tumor cells		

Adjuvant Chemotherapy
Adjuvant chemotherapy #8 cycles (Paclitaxel & Trastuzumab # 8).

Operation
Nov. 2016 Left simple mastectomy with implant reconstruction.
Pathology: Invasive ductal carcinoma, stage rpT2.
Size of tumor : 2.5 cm.

Adjuvant Therapy
Adjuvant therapy: Paclitaxel & Trastuzumab # 32 cycles.

Lung Metastasis
See Fig. 144.
Mar. 2018 Chest CT> metastasis in lung.
Palliative therapy: Trastuzumab emtansine # 11: Progressive disease.
Palliative therapy: Lapatinib & Capecitabine # 16: Progressive disease.

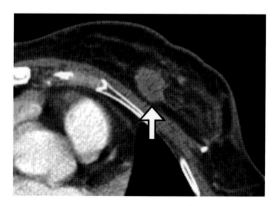

Fig. 143 Chest CT (Apr. 2016): Newly developed irregular enhancing mass in left breast, suggesting recurrent tumor

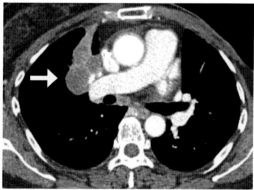

Fig. 144 Chest CT (Aug. 2020): Mildly enhancing hypoattenuating mass in right upper lobe, suggesting pulmonary metastasis

Concurrent radiation to internal mammary lymph node.

Clinical trial: Herzuma & Vinorelbine tartrate #4: Progressive disease.

Palliative therapy: Gemcitabine & Cisplatin #5: Progressive disease.

Clinical trial: PF-06804103 #1: withdraw due to side effects.

Palliative therapy: Irinotecan & Cisplatin # 6: Partial response.

Rest for 3 months.

Palliative therapy: Trastuzumab & Eribulin #2.

Radiation to lung.

Palliative therapy: Abraxane #2: Progressive disease.

Palliative therapy: Mitomycin #2: Progressive disease.

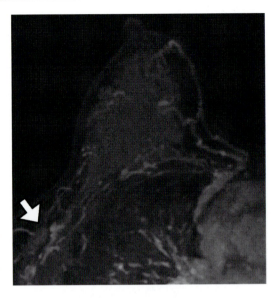

Fig. 145 Breast MRI (May 2014): Huge irregular heterogeneous enhancing mass in right breast

48 Case 48

48.1 Patient History and Progress

Female/45 years old, post-menopause.
No family history.
BRCA 1 & 2 mutation: Not detected.
S/p bilateral salpingo-oophorectomy.

48.2 Courses of Treatment

Right breast cancer with mediastinum and bone metastasis → Palliative therapy.

See Fig. 145.

Enlarged lymph nodes (white arrow) in the right axillary area, suggesting metastases.

See Figs. 146 and 147.

Right invasive ductal carcinoma, stage IV (R/O metastasis in bone).

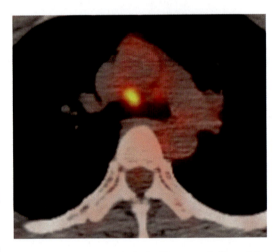

Fig. 146 PET-CT (May 2014): Hypermetabolic activity in the mediastinal lymph node, suggesting metastasis

Metastatic Breast Cancer

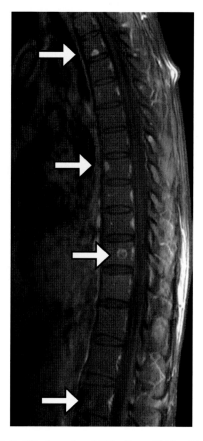

Fig. 147 Whole spine MRI (Jun. 2014): Multiple enhancing lesions in thoracic and lumbar vertebrae, suggesting bony metastases

	Result	Intensity	Positive %
Estrogen receptor	Strong (8/8)	3	>2/3
Progesterone receptor	Intermediate (5/8)	2	10%–1/3
C-erbB2	Negative (0)		
Ki-67	Positive in 54% of tumor cells		

Neoadjuvant chemotherapy #8 cycles (Doxorubicin + Cyclophosphamide #4 → Docetaxel #4).

Dec. 2014 Right breast conserving surgery.

Pathology: Invasive ductal carcinoma, stage ypT2N2a.

Size of tumor: 3.0 × 1.5 cm, lymph node: 4/4 (10 mm).

	Result	Intensity	Positive %
Estrogen receptor	Intermediate (6/8)	2	1/3–2/3
Progesterone receptor	Negative (0/8)	0	0
C-erbB2	Negative (0)		
Ki-67	Positive in 1% of tumor cells		

Post-operative radiation to right breast & internal mammary lymph node + Tamoxifen 20 mg/day & zoladex.

Mar. 2015 Bilateral salpingo-oophorectomy. Tamoxifen 20 mg/day only.

Mar. 2016 PET-CT> metastasis in multiple bone.

Palliative therapy: Letrozole (Mar. 2016 ~ Nov. 2017: Progressive disease).

Palliative therapy: Exemestane & Everolimus.

Oct. 2018 Chest CT> metastasis in liver.

Palliative therapy: Paclitaxel & Cisplatin #21: Progressive disease.

Palliative therapy: Fulvestrant & Abemaciclib (Feb. 2020)~

49 Case 49

49.1 Patient History and Progress

Female/55 years old, post-menopause.

No family history.

S/p bilateral salpingo-oophorectomy, s/p Left pelvis cementoplasty.

49.2 Courses of Treatment

Right breast cancer with bone metastasis → Palliative therapy.

See Figs. 148 and 149.

Right invasive ductal carcinoma, stage IV (metastasis in bone).

	Result	Intensity	Positive %
Estrogen receptor	Strong (8/8)	3	>2/3
Progesterone receptor	Strong(8/8)	3	>2/3
C-erbB2	Negative (1+)		
Ki-67	Positive in 75% of tumor cells		

Clinical trial: Tamoxifen 20 mg/day & Goserelin 3.6 mg (Dec. 2014 ~ Jan. 2017): Progressive disease.

Jan. 2017 Palliative right breast conserving surgery & bilateral salpingo-oophorectomy.

Pathology: Invasive ductal carcinoma, stage yp T1p.

Size of tumor: 1.4 cm.

	Result	Intensity	Positive %
Estrogen receptor	Strong (8/8)	3	>2/3
Progesterone receptor	Weak (4/8)	3	<1%
C-erbB2	Negative (1+)		
Ki-67	Positive in 30% of tumor cells		

Palliative therapy: Letrozole & Palbociclib (Jan. 2017) ~

Post-operative radiation to pelvic bone.

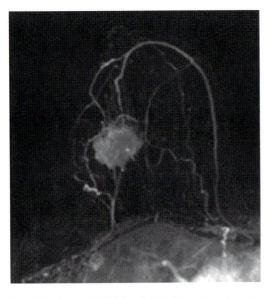

Fig. 148 Breast MRI (Nov. 2014): Irregular enhancing mass at the 11 o'clock direction of right breast

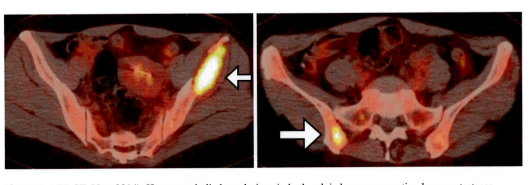

Fig. 149 PET-CT (Nov. 2014): Hypermetabolic bone lesions in both pelvic bones, suggesting bony metastases

50 Case 50

50.1 Patient History and Progress

Female/47 years old, post-menopause.
No family history.
S/p bilateral salpingo-oophorectomy, diabetes mellitus.

50.2 Courses of Treatment

Left breast cancer with lung metastasis → Palliative therapy.
See Figs. 150 and 151.
Left invasive ductal carcinoma, stage IV (metastasis in ovary, s/p bilateral salpingo-oophorectomy).

	Result	Intensity	Positive %
Estrogen receptor	Negative (0/8)	0	0
Progesterone receptor	Weak (3/8)	1	1–10%
C-erbB2	Negative (1+)		
Ki-67	Positive in 52% of tumor cells		

Palliative therapy: Letrozole & Palbociclib #11.
Jan. 2021 Left breast conserving surgery.
Pathology: Invasive ductal carcinoma, stage ypT2N1a.
Size of tumor: 2.5 cm, lymph node: 1/7 (6 mm).

	Result	Intensity	Positive %
Estrogen receptor	Negative (02/8)	1	<1%
Progesterone receptor	Negative (2/8)	1	<1%
C-erbB2	Negative (0)		
Ki-67	Positive in 59% of tumor cells		

Palliative chemotherapy # 4 cycles (Docetaxel & cyclophosphamide #4).
Post-operative radiation to left breast & subclavicular lymph node + Tamoxifen 20 mg/day (May 2021)~

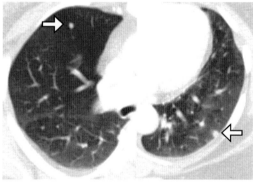

Fig. 151 Chest CT (Feb. 2020): Several nodules, both lungs, suggesting pulmonary metastases

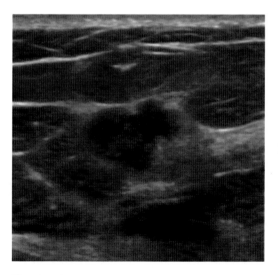

Fig. 150 Breast US (Nov. 2019): Irregular hypoechoic mass with echogenic halo at the 11 o'clock direction of left breast

Treatment Roadmap and Summaries

Eun Sook Lee

See Fig. 1.

- Breast cancer treatment is highly affected by the patient's status of illness, overall health, and socioeconomic condition, but it is also influenced by the insurance policy of the society to which the patient belongs and the political and economic situation of the country.
- South Korea receives a relatively high-level, guideline-compliant treatment because the entire population is under the national health insurance system, but there is a slight gap in

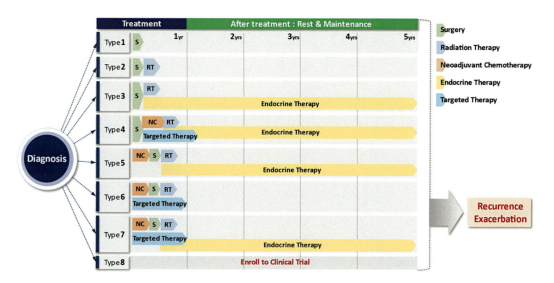

Fig. 1 Treatment types after breast cancer diagnosis

E. S. Lee (✉)
Center for Breast Cancer, National Cancer Center, Goyang, Kyonggi-do, Republic of Korea
e-mail: eslee@ncc.re.kr

- the immediate adoption of newly developed therapeutics such as immune checkpoint inhibitors, antibody-drug conjugate, and many other agents.
- For primary breast cancers, most patients are treated well according to the guidelines, but there is still a shortage in patients with metastatic cancer.
- Fortunately, we are actively involved in many global clinical trials and patients who have metastasis and are heavily treated are benefiting from many new treatments, but globally, the health disparity is clearly an ongoing problem.